CATHOLIC
IN HEALTH CARE

CATHOLIC WITNESS IN HEALTH CARE

PRACTICING MEDICINE IN TRUTH AND LOVE

Edited by John M. Travaline & Louise A. Mitchell

Foreword by Ashley K. Fernandes

THE CATHOLIC UNIVERSITY OF AMERICA PRESS
Washington, D.C.

Copyright © 2017
Catholic Medical Association

All rights reserved
The paper used in this publication meets the minimum requirements of American
National Standards for Information Science—Permanence of Paper for Printed Library
Materials, ANSI Z39.48-1984.

∞

Library of Congress Cataloging-in-Publication Data
Names: Travaline, John M., 1963– editor. |
Mitchell, Louise A. (Louise Annette), editor.
Title: Catholic witness in health care : practicing medicine in truth and love /
edited by John M. Travaline and Louise A. Mitchell ; foreword by Ashley K. Fernandes.
Description: Washington, D.C. : The Catholic University of America Press, [2017] |
Includes bibliographical references and index.
Identifiers: LCCN 2017014471 | ISBN 9780813229836 (pbk. : alk. paper)
Subjects: | MESH: Religion and Medicine | Catholicism | Delivery of Health Care |
Religion and Psychology | Theology
Classification: LCC BL65.M4 | NLM BL 65.M4 | DDC 615.8/52—dc23
LC record available at https://lccn.loc.gov/2017014471

Nihil Obstat:
Doctor Susan M. Timoney, STD
Censor Deputatus
Imprimatur:
Most Reverend Barry C. Knestout
Auxiliary Bishop of Washington
July 5, 2016
The *nihil obstat* and *imprimatur* are official declarations that a book
or pamphlet is free of doctrinal or moral error. There is no implication that those
who have granted the *nihil obstat* and the *imprimatur* agree with the content,
opinions, or statements expressed therein.

To my wife, Cathy, and our
children, John and his wife, Regina,
Catherine, Megan, and Emily

With gratitude for making this,
and all of my work, possible
JMT

To my mother, Mary Ann Finkelstein

Always supportive and always loved
LAM

To our colleagues, students,
and patients who witness to us
JMT and LAM

CONTENTS

List of Tables and Figure ix

Foreword by Ashley K. Fernandes xi

Preface xv

Acknowledgments xvii

PART I. ELEMENTS OF CATHOLIC CARE

1. Foundations of Authentic Medical Care 3
   J. Brian Benestad

2. A Catholic Anthropology and Medical Ethics 31
   Peter J. Colosi

3. Pastoral Care of the Sick and Dying 70
   Reverend Philip G. Bochanski

PART II. WITNESS IN PRACTICE: THE CLINICAL CONTEXT

4. Reproductive Health and the Practice of Gynecology 105
   Kathleen M. Raviele

5. Fertility Care Services 170
   Richard J. Fehring

6. Catholic Witness in Pediatrics 209
   Christopher O'Hara

7. Caring for Older Adults 261
   Sister Mary Diana Dreger and James S. Powers

8. Catholic Perspectives on Caring for the Critically Ill 288
   Stephen E. Hannan, Peter A. Rosario, Dennis M. Manning,
   E. Wesley Ely, and Deacon John M. Travaline

9. Challenges for Catholic Surgeons 316
   Leonard P. Rybak and Christopher Perro

10. A Spiritual Perspective in Rehabilitation Medicine 346
    José A. Santos

11. Catholic Psychologists and the Spiritual Dimension 367
    Wanda Skowronska

12. The Catholic Pharmacist 393
    Reverend Patrick Flanagan and Robert A. Mangione

PART III. TOWARD A SHIFTING CULTURE

13. Apprenticed to Christ: The Formation of
    Catholic Medical Students 415
    Medical Student

14. Ethics in Clinical Research 439
    Deacon William V. Williams

15. A Model of Catholic Care—"The Casa" 477
    Domenico Francesco Crupi, Francesco Giuliani,
    Jere D. Palazzolo, and Gianluigi Mazzoccoli

Contributors 503
Index 505

TABLES AND FIGURE

Table 5-1. Unintended Pregnancy Rates 183

Table 5-2. Classic and Recent NFP Efficacy Studies 184

Table 8-1. Fourteen-Day Series 305

Table 12-1. Pharmacy Schools of Institutions of Higher Learning
That Are Catholic or in the Catholic Tradition 395

Table 15-1. View of Hospital Mission 494

Table 15-2. View of the Dominant Hospital Value 495

Table 15-3. Reasons for Choosing to Work at the Casa 495

Figure 15-1. Three-Pillar Model for Casa USA 497

Ashley K. Fernandes, MD, PhD

FOREWORD

We live in a time of extreme moral pluralism. It is not simply a time in which men and women merely disagree civilly about whether a person ought to be able to do X, Y, or Z; rather, it is an age in which physicians, philosophers, and the secular culture call the very words "person" and "ought" into question. It is a time in which there seems to be no shared philosophical anthropology—no answer to that seminal question asked in both East and West since the dawn of man but posed most beautifully by the Psalmist—"*What is man*, O Lord, that thou art mindful of him?"

In fact, many of us practicing medicine or engaged in teaching medicine today are taught that the only "goods" that matter are the patient's biomedical or physiological good—and her *own* conception of the good. Dr. Edmund Pellegrino's two other "goods" the physician ought to strive for—human flourishing, and a person's spiritual good—are relegated to sociological curiosity, or worse, are ridiculed entirely.

There are data to confirm these observations, but contemporary anecdotes are even more powerful: A physician who performs abortions jokes on hidden camera that she "wants a Lamborghini" from her compensation for the sale of fetal tissue. California's governor in 2015, on signing a bill legalizing physician-assisted suicide, notes that people would find the "right" to this option a "comfort." An obstetrics and gynecology physician, after failing a Catholic medical student for following her conscience and religious convictions, received this *supportive* comment on her blog as a warning to other "like-minded" students: "Do not confuse religion with ethics. They are completely separate. One need not have religion in order to be an ethical person, and your religion should not be a factor in the decisions you make in your job. If religion comes into play at all, it is the health-care recipient whose religion matters, not yours . . . your religion drives only your choices for your own personal health care, not for the people you are serving."

There is a triple threat to medical ethics—a materialist or nihilistic anthropology, moral relativism, and apathy—that can make the future of truly Catholic medicine seem dark. But it was Ralph Waldo Emerson who once said, "When it is dark enough, you can see the stars." Thus, into the growing darkness we have been gifted with Dr. John Travaline and Louise Mitchell's remarkably compiled and edited *Catholic Witness in Health Care: Practicing Medicine in Truth and Love*. Travaline and Mitchell have put together the first-ever Catholic medical ethics textbook written by physicians, bioethicists, and theologians that is at once accessible to the learned lay person and also a tremendous resource for those who practice medicine, students of the health sciences, and philosophers and clergy who require a scholarly, practical guide to authentic Catholic medicine and ethics.

Their title is telling. To be a "Catholic witness" is to relate, in light of the Church's teaching, what both *experience and reason* in medicine have shown us. It is unhappily the case that much Catholic bioethics nowadays is heterodox; that is, it is not faithful to the Church's Magisterium. Further, it often happens that Catholic bioethics gets hijacked by nonpractitioners and turned into an intellectual exercise—puzzles over praxis. But "practicing medicine" is, of course, at the heart of what it means to be a *Catholic* health-care professional.

We come into contact with and experience our patients' real wounds—physical, mental, and, often, spiritual. To fulfill our vocation to heal the whole person, we must do more than be a technician who fiddles with a complex machine that happens to be a human. We must also do more than preach, and certainly more than "preach to the choir." Rather, the title reminds us that truth and love are two sides of the same coin, for each tempers the other; no man, relying on only one of the two, can live a godly life, because Christ Himself was the perfect embodiment of both. Medicine, a generated art, was hewn out by the reason of man and permeated with the medical professional's love for his patient as a child of God.

Travaline and Mitchell have provided a summary for each chapter in this volume. These summaries provide a scholarly, authoritative, and definitive voice, which unifies the polyphony of the "Church's scientific choir." Dr. Travaline has written and edited in a way that reflects his own decades of practice in medicine, academic and scholarly life, education, and theology (as a deacon in the Roman Catholic Church) and, of course, in a way that reflects his role as a family man who understands the importance of a proper understanding of bioethics in the life and health of the everyday family in the twenty-first century.

The majority of the authors of this book are clinicians—physicians, a nurse, a psychologist, and a pharmacist—of whom one may boast outstanding accomplishments both in the sciences and in medical ethics. Philosophers and theologians also contribute—with powerful effect—showing that medicine does not stand alone but may be richly complemented by reason *and* faith. The introductory chapters provide solid principles and anthropologic background for any study of Catholic medical ethics. Subsequent chapters cover topics in pediatrics, obstetrics and gynecology (including fertility awareness), pediatrics, geriatrics, and pharmacy. Travaline and Mitchell have made a tremendous contribution through their authors' addressing oft-ignored topics in medical ethics—Catholic or otherwise—and have included Catholic guidance in critical care, surgery, rehabilitation, and mental health. Chapters on medical student formation and clinical research ethics, as well as a model for putting Catholic health care into practice, round out this unique book.

For two decades I have hoped for a written tool that would demonstrate the harmony of faith and science in the practice of medicine. Travaline and Mitchell, along with their authors, have delivered a gift to the Church, and something that is necessary to help educate our next generation of Catholic health-care professionals.

In these times, courage is required for a person to practice the kind of truly Catholic love that medicine often demands. This volume, it is my hope, will give the reader that courage and will spur action that will be the volume's ultimate legacy. For Catholic love does not blink in the face of disease, disability, or discrimination. We, as Catholics in health care, must always *act*—and in acting, even in the midst of the storm, we hold firmly to a mast of truth and reason, while reaching in love with our other hand to the most vulnerable of our society; indeed, we must have the courage to risk everything for this person in front of us.

For those committed to Christ and his Church, reading this substantial, groundbreaking volume is only a beginning for coming to understand the human drama and mystery that is medicine. The knowledge and perspective gained herein must be infused with the grace that comes from steadfast prayer and animated in clinical practice with a truly distinctive Catholic love. This Catholic love of the human person does not fail, nor does it run from a fight; it is a star in the darkness; it is, as St. Thomas Aquinas taught us centuries ago, a love that "takes up where knowledge leaves off."

PREFACE

Endeavoring to educate physicians about Catholic doctrine pertaining to the practice of medicine, the first Catholic Physicians Guild was founded in Boston in 1912. In 1927, a guild formed in Brooklyn, and soon other gatherings of Catholic physicians, accompanied by priests serving as spiritual directors, formed guilds in many cities. In 1932, the National Federation of Catholic Physicians Guilds formed to unite the seven guilds that existed at the time. Over the next several years, the organization grew, helping physicians to mature in faith and providing spiritual counsel and moral guidance for them. By 1961 there were one hundred guilds, and in 1963 the federation was the sixth largest medical organization in the country. By 1967, it had ten thousand physician members. Following the promulgation of *Humanae Vitae*, however, the federation was severely fractured as controversy over contraception intensified. Membership declined to a low of three hundred physicians in only two guilds. Despite its relatively small numbers, the federation continued to meet annually, and it remained faithful to the Magisterium. In 1997, it changed its name to the Catholic Medical Association (CMA); and over time, a re-structuring of the organization fostered revival of local guilds. These guilds brought a renewed focus on the Catholic physician who sought to be rooted more deeply in the vocation to practice medicine in accord with authentic teachings of the Church and to witness to the sanctity of life, the inalienable rights of the person, and common good of society in which all may flourish. Today there are again one hundred guilds. It was within this milieu that *Catholic Witness in Health Care* was conceived.

Early in its gestation, as we were surveying much of the literature in Catholic medical ethics, we discovered an important unmet need in this genre. Specifically, we recognized there was no guide for practicing medical personnel that was written in large part *by* practicing medical professionals. It is easy to find many books written by ethicists and moral theologians and some by physicians trained in these disciplines; but there is very little to virtually nothing penned by practicing physicians to the extent that is offered in this book. Most of the comparative books dealing with Catholic health care and biomedical ethics do so from a moral theology perspective, not from the perspective of practicing clinicians or ministers in the field. *Catholic Witness in Health Care* was written, therefore, to help bridge this gap. Specifically, it was written to address practical clinical matters that practitioners encounter, and it posits authentic Catholic responses to those practical clinical matters.

Catholic Witness achieves its purpose within a three-part structure. Introductory chapters in the first part discuss foundational elements of Catholic care; they touch upon Scripture, moral philosophy, theology, anthropology, and pastoral care. In the second part, Catholic clinicians illuminate the practice of authentic Catholic medical care in various medical disciplines. Part 3 offers unique perspectives concerning medical education, research, and practice, conceived as elements that, within a shifting culture, are ordered toward an authentically Catholic medical ethos. It is highly recommended that readers begin with part 1, to set the foundations for authentically Catholic medical care. Readers then may select chapters to suit their interest, using them as reference, as explanations for particular practices, or as interesting perspectives on how to mesh one's life in faith with a particular discipline of medicine. At the beginning of each chapter, a summary provides a guide to the chapter's particular content.

In *Catholic Witness* we present an expression of authentic Catholic health care from the perspective of practicing clinicians. The title for this presentation was chosen to denote a compilation of medical content, information, experiences, and reflections, all at the service of witness—testimony to authentic practice of medicine by those with personal knowledge acquired through experience in the health-care field. We hope it will attract individuals to see a robust rendering of what living one's Catholic faith in the health-care world might look like.

There is a long history of physicians who have sought enrichment in their faith and spiritual life while being at the same time engaged in the noble profession of medicine. We are encountering a renewed fervor among physicians and others in health care who are seeking to practice medicine in accord with authentic Catholic values. More and more we hear from Catholic physicians searching to better understand their faith and have it be a part of medical practice. *Catholic Witness* is our contribution to this search.

On the Solemnity of Saints Peter and Paul
June 29, 2016
Philadelphia, Pennsylvania

ACKNOWLEDGMENTS

There are innumerable people to be acknowledged for their assistance in the production of this book, from its conception to its delivery into the hands of its reader. We can call to mind only a few. Dr. Kathy Raviele is credited with inspiring the idea for this book when she was serving as president of the Catholic Medical Association; she suggested that the Association take to the next level a previously published book on medical ethics written by a prominent Catholic physician. The encouragement and prayerful support of the project (once it was under way) from John Brehany, then executive director of the CMA, and subsequently his successor, Mario Dickerson, have been greatly appreciated. The members of the CMA Executive Board over the years of the writing of this book are equally appreciated. Current President of the CMA, Dr. Les Ruppersberger, along with current members of the board of directors—Drs. Marie-Alberte Boursiquot, Bill Mueller, John Schirger, Michael Parker, Peter Morrow, Paul Braaton, David Hilger, Tom McGovern, Michelle Stanford, and Craig Treptow—are to be acknowledged for their support, especially during the past few months when they helped us get this project finally across the goal line. We are grateful also for the prayerful support of the Most Reverend James Conley, our episcopal advisor, and the national chaplain for the CMA, Rev. Fr. Matthew Gutowski.

From the outset, it was intended that this book would be written largely by Catholic physicians who were in the clinics, in the hospitals, practicing their respective areas of medicine, witnessing to the Catholic faith, and trying to be true to their identity as Catholics who were also physicians. To these physicians, as well as to the nonphysician authors of this book—who in their respective ways also contributed so much to the book, helping to situate it in an authentically Catholic framework—we are most grateful.

We are also indebted to Janice Steinhagen, whose professional contribution to this work was to bring, out of the variety of writing styles of the authors, a more unified voice to the book. We are thankful to the anonymous reviewers of the book, who conveyed insightful comments and needed encouragement to us. We are most grateful to the staff at the Catholic University of America Press, especially John Martino. We also are grateful for the work of Rev. Msgr. Charles Antonicelli, judicial vicar for the Archdiocese of Washington, D.C. We offer our thanks to Dr. Susan M. Timoney, censor deputatus, and to the Most Rev. Barry C. Knestout, and, for granting ecclesiastical approval and permission for this publication, we thank His Eminence Donald Cardinal Wuerl.

Finally, without the unwavering support of Cathy Travaline, John's wife, and their children, the necessary effort devoted to this project would not have been possible. And to Mary Ann Finkelstein, Louise's mother, who has been supportive always of her "folly" of quitting the lucrative computer programming industry in mid-life to pursue the mystery of God in advanced studies in moral theology and bioethics. To all of those named, and unnamed, who contributed to this project, we are most sincerely thankful.

PART I

ELEMENTS OF CATHOLIC CARE

J. Brian Benestad

1. FOUNDATIONS OF AUTHENTIC MEDICAL CARE

The first part of this book aims to provide day-to-day health-care practitioners with some background necessary for a reasonable understanding of patient care in the context of practitioners' living out their faith in the activities of their medical professions. In this first chapter of this section, Professor Benestad explores the scriptural, theological, and philosophical foundations of Christian medical care. Scripture shows the dignity of the human person, the goodness of health, and the nobility of the healing professions; it reveals the meaning of suffering, the charity of Christ's healing of others, and his suffering and sacrifice for our redemption. Theology emphasizes the dignity of the human person, the necessity of virtue in both health-care professional and patient, and the meaning of suffering as a sharing in Christ's suffering and redemptive mission, and as a means to growth in virtue. Philosophy provides the ends and purposes of medicine—to preserve and restore health—and emphasizes the professionalism of the physician, who must be knowledgeable in his or her area of competence and must also take into account the nonphysical dimension of the patient—the soul. *An ethic of love* and the parable of the Good Samaritan draw all of this together into the Catholic view of the medical profession.—*Editors*

Introduction

The foundations of a Catholic approach to good medical care are, of course, found in Scripture, Church teaching, and reason. These three sources present a Catholic understanding of good medical care by clarifying the doctor-patient relationship and by specifying the duties of both the physician and the patient. Physicians need both knowledge and virtue, especially the charity of the Good Samaritan, to do their job well; patients also need virtues—notably, fortitude and patience to bear their sufferings and the virtue of faith to believe that putting up with them will bring about their own closer union with Christ.

In order that we may approach our subject systematically, this chapter is divided into three parts: scriptural foundations, Church teaching, and reason, a necessary complement to Church teaching. My treatment of these subjects will be not exhaustive but sufficient to bring out considerations essential for clarifying a Catholic understanding of good medical care. In the first part we will look at the Old Testament books of Genesis, Sirach, Job, and Isaiah and then the New Testament texts that deal with healings. In the second part, we will explore three subjects of Church teaching that are indispensable for thinking about the doctor-patient relationship: the dignity of the human person, virtue, and suffering. Finally, we will point out some of the things that reason, inspired by the Catholic faith, has to say about the following topics: the four principles of medical ethics popularized by the Kennedy Institute of Ethics at Georgetown University; the restoration of health as the goal of medicine; the duty of doctors to teach patients how to stay well or to recover their health; and the understanding of medicine as a profession. I reflect on the Kennedy Institute's four principles, not to provide a way into Catholic bioethics, but to indicate how these principles, if used incautiously, can lead Catholics astray.

Scriptural Foundations

Old Testament

The Book of Genesis

The Bible's fundamental teaching on the dignity of the human person is found first of all in Genesis 1:26: "Then God said, 'Let us make man in our image, after our likeness.'"[1] We find this concept again in the story of the covenant with Noah: "Whoever sheds the blood of man, by man shall his blood be shed; for God made man in his own image" (Gn 9:6). These passages express the truth that all human beings are endowed with great dignity and have an obligation to live in accordance with that dignity by avoiding sin, striving for holiness, and, even, preserving their health as far as possible. This teaching of Genesis stands in contrast to the prevailing secular view that the primary way to promote dignity is to respect the autonomy of the individual. Such a view presumes the acceptance of moral relativism.

The Book of Sirach

The dignity of human beings should also guide our understanding of the good of health, the evil of sickness, the duties of the sick, and the high calling of the physician to heal and comfort. The Book of Sirach addresses these matters. "There is no wealth better than health of body, and there is no gladness better than joy of heart" (Sir 30:16). The wise author, a man of practical wisdom, urges his readers to avoid giving in to sorrow, "for sorrow has destroyed many, and there is no profit in it" (Sir 30:23); and he goes on to name other unhealthy vices: "Jealousy and anger shorten life, and anxiety brings on old age too soon" (Sir 30:24). "Many have died of gluttony, but he

---

1. *The Holy Bible*, Revised Standard Version, Second Catholic Edition. All quotations from Sacred Scripture are from this edition of the Bible.

who is careful to avoid it prolongs his life" (Sir 37:31). The serene person, however, has a good appetite, enjoys his food, and profits from it (Sir 30:15–25). One can infer from Sirach that all the capital sins (pride, avarice, gluttony, lust, sloth, envy, anger) adversely affect a person's health and, of course, undermine one's relationship with God. Furthermore, Sirach implies that good physicians will try to understand everything that might affect their patients' health, including vices. This means that physicians need not only a scientific education but also a thorough understanding of human nature. In other words, physicians must be able to discern, in a particular patient, whether a problem in the soul (psyche) is the principal cause of an illness.

The beginning of chapter 38 in Sirach (vv. 1–15) specifically addresses physician and patient. The biblical author tells us that God made medicines available on the earth and created the physician, who acquires considerable skills. Even so, healing itself "comes from the Most High" (Sir 38:2). More precisely, God makes use of the physician to heal and take away pain. Sirach tells the patient, "My son, when you are sick, do not be negligent, but pray to the Lord and he will heal you" (Sir 38:9). The biblical author further exhorts the sick to "cleanse [their] heart from all sin," to offer sacrifices to God, and never lose hope in the help the physician can give (Sir 38:10–12). To physicians, Sirach gives hope for success in their medical practice and urges them to pray for a good outcome in their work. "There is a time when success lies in the hands of physicians, for they too will pray to the Lord that he should grant them success in diagnosis and in healing for the preservation of life" (Sir 38:13). It is good to desire health, to pray for help in overcoming sickness, and to do whatever is reasonable to preserve or recover health, including renouncing sins that impair health.

The question naturally arises whether the wisdom contained in Sirach is fully appreciated and put into practice by many Christian physicians and patients. How many bioethicists and students of bioethics emphasize the duty to stay healthy (as distinguished from the enthusiasm for fitness), the need for prayer by both physician and patient, and the adverse effect of vices on people's health? In how many bioethics anthologies would you find selections from the Book of Sirach or the Book of Job?

The Book of Job

In the Book of Job we encounter another aspect of health care, the problem of suffering. A rich, esteemed, and upright man suddenly loses his goods, his children, and finally his good health. At first he is patient, rebuffing his wife's exhortation to curse God and die: "Shall we receive good at the hand of God, and shall we not receive evil?" (Jb: 2:10). But after three of his friends visit and tell him that he must have sinned if he is undergoing suffering, Job curses the day of his birth. These friends give voice to the common belief that God rewards good deeds and punishes bad deeds in this life. Despite Job's protestations of innocence, his friends do not question their belief that a person afflicted with suffering must have committed serious sins. Job responds by questioning God's justice in causing or allowing him to suffer so much despite his innocence. In fact, Job finally issues a challenge to God:

Oh that I had one to hear me! (Here is my signature! Let the Almighty answer me!) Oh, that I had the indictment written by my adversary! Surely I would carry it on my shoulder; I would bind it on me as a crown; I would give him an account of all my steps; like a prince I would approach him. (Jb 31:35–37)

The reference to a princely approach to God indicates that Job considers himself justified in accusing God of unfairness. His bold challenge to God comes after a lengthy description of his own upright behavior in which he explains how he has kept God's commandments and acted justly and lovingly.

God responds to Job over the course of four chapters (Jb 38–41). He gives no explanation of why the innocent suffer, but he also does not address Job as a sinner, for which Job feels gratitude and reassurance. God does explain to Job that he is simply a creature immersed in a mysterious creation governed by God's unfathomable wisdom. Job says in response:

I know that you can do all things, and that no purpose of yours can be thwarted.... Therefore, I have uttered what I did not understand, things too wonderful for me, which I did not know.... I had heard of you by the hearing of the ear, but now my eye sees you; therefore I despise myself, and repent in dust and ashes. (Jb 42:2, 3, 5–6)

Job is so humbled by his encounter with God that he does not ask why the innocent undergo pain and suffering, nor does he even ask to be liberated from his hardships. Job now sees that the reason for his suffering is beyond his ken and entrusts himself to God's providence.

God, in turn, addresses Job's three friends; he denounces them for defaming God and implies that their treatment of Job as a sinner was wrong and offensive. God tells them to go to Job, make an offering for themselves and ask Job to pray for them so that they will not incur divine punishment. The Lord accepts Job's prayer for his friends and then restores his goods, children, and health. Job receives twice as many goods as he previously possessed, has more children and grandchildren, and lives to a ripe old age.

The Book of Job does not provide a full answer to the problem of suffering, but it does provide some important insights. Job is innocent yet suffers grievously, so no one should think one's own sufferings or those of others are necessarily punishment for sins. Job's repentance and restoration show that trust in the love and wisdom of God in the midst of pain will eventually bear fruit. In addition, God's rebuke to Job's friends implicitly shows that we should offer loving support to our suffering friends. In his encyclical *Spe Salvi, On Christian Hope*, Pope Benedict XVI describes the dimensions of loving support beautifully and concretely:

Indeed, to accept the other who suffers, means that I take up his suffering in such a way that it becomes mine also. Because it has now become a shared suffering, though, in which another person is present, this suffering is penetrated by the light of love. The Latin word *con-solatio*, "consolation," expresses this beautifully. It suggests *being with* the other in his solitude, so that it ceases to be solitude.[2]

---

2. Pope Benedict XVI, *Spe Salvi, On Christian Hope*, Encyclical Letter, November 30, 2007, no. 38.

Job's three friends failed to "be with" Job in his suffering; rather, they stood apart from Job, left him lonely, and judged him guilty of sin because of his suffering. Finally, while Job's faith in God persisted throughout his ordeal, it deepened and matured with the realization that no one may question God's fairness or justice.

One might naturally ask whether God would look with favor on the right kind of plea for deliverance from affliction. The psalms give perhaps the clearest answer to that question. Psalm 13 provides an example of how the faithful should pray in the midst of affliction.

> How long, O Lord? Will you forget me forever?
> How long will you hide your face from me?
> How long must I bear pain in my soul
> and have sorrow in my heart all the day?
> How long shall my enemy be exalted over me?
> Consider and answer me, O Lord my God;
> lighten my eyes, lest I sleep the sleep of death;
> lest my enemy say, "I have prevailed over him";
> lest my foes rejoice because I am shaken.
> But I have trusted in your merciful love;
> my heart shall rejoice in your salvation.
> I will sing to the Lord,
> because he has dealt bountifully with me.

Though the psalmist teaches God's faithful to give voice to their pain and to cry out for deliverance, they must not blame God for their situation. Instead, they should approach him in thanksgiving for the gifts he has already given, trusting in the steadfastness of his merciful love, no matter what happens.

Reading the Book of Job should, at the very least, challenge health-care professionals to find ways to support their patients in their suffering, especially when they are very much alone. Patients can learn to tolerate their pain without grumbling against God and to be grateful for the growth in dignity and faith that comes from bearing suffering with patient endurance. As Psalm 13 teaches, they may also cry out for deliverance from their suffering, if they maintain their trust in God's merciful love and a heart full of thanksgiving for the many benefits received from God during their lifetime.

The Book of the Prophet Isaiah

In Isaiah we read the story of Hezekiah, king of Judah, who falls sick; at the point of death, he prays to the Lord, reminding him that he has served him long and faithfully. The Lord hears his prayer and grants him fifteen more years of life. After he is healed, Hezekiah describes how he benefitted from his sickness: "Behold, it was for my welfare that I had great bitterness, but you have held back my life from the pit of destruction, for you have cast all my sins behind my back" (Is 38:17). Hezekiah clearly associates his healing with the forgiveness of his sins.

Chapter 53 of Isaiah contains the extraordinary account of the Lord's Suffering Servant, who voluntarily suffers on behalf of others:

> Surely, he has borne our griefs
> and carried our sorrows;
> yet we esteemed him stricken,
> struck down by God and afflicted.
> But he was wounded for our transgressions,
> he was bruised for our iniquities;
> upon him was the chastisement that made us whole,
> and with his stripes we are healed.
> All we like sheep have gone astray;
> we have turned everyone to his own way
> and the Lord has laid on him
> the iniquity of us all. (Is 53:4–6)

The *Catechism of the Catholic Church* (no. 1502) explains that the prophet Isaiah "intuits that suffering can also have a redemptive meaning for the sins of others." A note in the Revised Standard Version of the Bible further explains Isaiah's prophecy: "By the Servant's vicarious suffering, he restores all people to God."[3] This prophecy is ultimately fulfilled in the life, death, and resurrection of Jesus Christ, whose suffering brings forgiveness and healing to all people. The New Testament, to which we now turn, makes plain that all people are invited to unite their sufferings with those of Jesus.

New Testament

We read in the New Testament that Jesus spent much of his ministry curing the sick. For example, Matthew tells us: "And Jesus went about all the cities and villages teaching in their synagogues and preaching the gospel of the kingdom, and healing every disease and every infirmity."[4] In Mark, too, we find that Jesus sympathizes with all the sick whom he encounters: "Whatever villages or towns or countryside he entered, they laid the sick in the marketplaces and begged him that they might touch only the tassel on his cloak, and as many as touched it were healed" (Mk 6:56). Luke reports that Jesus healed Simon's mother-in-law, then ministered to the crowds: "At sunset, all who had people sick with various diseases brought them to him. He laid his hands on each of them and cured them" (Lk 4:40). John makes the point that Jesus did not hesitate to heal on the Sabbath, narrating the story of his healing of the man who had been crippled for thirty-eight years (Jn 5:1–8). John also relates how Jesus raised his friend Lazarus from the dead (Jn 11:1–44). In sum, Jesus shows great compassion for the sick throughout his ministry.

The Gospel of Matthew hearkens back to the Suffering Servant of Isaiah: "'He took our infirmities and bore our diseases'" (Mt 8:17). The *Catechism* comments, "By his passion and death on the cross Christ has given a new meaning to suffering: it can henceforth configure us to him and unite us with his redemptive Passion."[5] This, of

---

3. This explanatory note is found in *The New Oxford Annotated Bible with the Apocrypha* (Revised Standard Version), eds. Herbert G. May and Bruce M. Metzger (New York: Oxford University Press, 1973), 888.

4. Mt 9:35; see also Mt 4:24 and Mt 14:35–36.

5. *Catechism of the Catholic Church*, 2nd edition, trans. United States Conference of Catholic Bishops (Washington, D.C.: USCCB, 1997), no. 1505.

course, means that all patients and health-care professionals can attempt to model their lives on the life of Christ, thus contributing to the healing and salvation of the world. In difficult moments, when patients and their caregivers feel they have nothing more to give, this teaching can provide much hope and comfort.

Jesus so identified with the sick that he even tells his disciples, "I was sick and you visited me" (Mt 25:36). We understand this to mean that caring for the sick is caring for Christ himself. This profound reality should inspire caregivers to serve their patients with the greatest care and compassion they can muster.

While Jesus healed many sick and infirm people, the *Catechism* notes that he did not heal them all. "His healings were signs of the coming kingdom of God. They announced a more radical healing: the victory over sin and death through his Passover. On the cross Christ took upon himself the whole weight of evil and took away the 'sin of the world.'"[6] We might infer from this that healing all the sick might have obscured Christ's deeper message: the conquest of sin and death is more important than liberation from sickness and suffering.

Even so, healing was a prominent part of Christ's ministry, as well as that of his apostles and disciples. "So they went out and preached that men should repent. And they cast out many demons, and anointed with oil many that were sick and healed them" (Mk 6:12–13). Part of the mission Jesus entrusted to his apostles, along with proclaiming the coming of God's kingdom, was to "heal the sick, raise the dead, cleanse lepers, cast out demons" (Mt 10:7–8). The Church today continues the work of healing the sick, not usually by dramatic miracles, but through personal care, especially by care in Catholic hospitals. She also ministers to the sick through intercessory prayer and the sacraments, especially the Eucharist and the Anointing of the Sick, through which the sick encounter Christ, "the physician of souls and bodies."[7] Like Christ, the Church attends to both the souls and the bodies of the faithful. In administering the Anointing of the Sick, the Church prays not only for the spiritual well-being of the sick person but also for a restoration of health "if it would be conducive to his salvation."[8]

Church Teaching

In order to shed more light on the principles that should guide the clinical encounter between the patient and the physician, let us examine three elements of Church teaching: the dignity of the human person, the meaning of virtue, and the mystery and benefit of suffering.

The Dignity of the Human Person

Rev. Albert Moraczewski writes, "Upon this truth, namely, the *inherent* dignity and sacredness of human life, rests [sic] the principles of medical ethics and morals."[9]

---

6. Ibid., quoting Jn 1:29.
7. Ibid.
8. Ibid., no. 1512.
9. Albert S. Moraczewski, OP, "The Human Person and the Church's Teaching Authority," in *Catholic*

Moraczewski speaks of inherent dignity because it is intrinsic to all human beings, whether society recognizes it or not. Out of respect for their own human dignity and that of their patients, health-care professionals try to restore health and relieve suffering. They rely on principles of medical ethics and on their personal virtue to guide them in the service of the human person.

All persons, by virtue of their humanity, possess inherent and permanent dignity. Moreover, people realize their human dignity fully by the way they live; in other words, human dignity is also a kind of excellence that one acquires. Dr. Leon Kass explains the distinction between the two kinds of dignity as basic human dignity— the dignity of human being—and full human dignity—the dignity of being human. Society's acceptance of the reality of basic dignity, which can never be lost or diminished, is crucial if people are to be protected from being made candidates for euthanasia or physician-assisted suicide because, for example, they have no control of their bladder. That kind of deficit should never be considered a loss of "personal" dignity. It is a suffering just like the loss of a limb, eyesight, or hearing. Physical and mental deficits do not cause a loss of personal dignity, but are a normal part of human aging. Did Jesus suffer a loss of personal dignity because he was nailed to a cross? Kass, a non-Christian, described the crucified Jesus as "the epitome of dignity" because he accepted his suffering "as *sacrificial* and as *redemptive*."[10] Kass mentions, as an example of full human dignity, the greater dignity of using freedom well, which is to be contrasted with the basic dignity of having freedom.

Those who reject the distinction between the two kinds of dignity do so in most cases, I suspect, for the best of reasons. They are fearful that as a result of the distinction the basic dignity of some people will be compromised, opening the door to such evils as physician-assisted suicide and poor treatment of the poor and marginalized. This is not the place to answer that argument in any detail. Suffice it to say that Catholics must make the case that nothing we do or suffer will ever undermine our basic dignity. It remains permanent because Scripture teaches that we are created in the image of God, redeemed by Jesus Christ, and destined for eternal life.

The Second Vatican Council affirms the existence of flourishing dignity when discussing every Christian's obligation to obey his or her conscience: "Man has a law in his heart inscribed by God, to obey which is his very dignity, and according to which he will be judged."[11] The text implies that people diminish their dignity by not obeying their conscience; we see this reflected in the common phrase "to act beneath one's dignity." People continually realize their dignity by seeking the truth, obeying conscience, resisting sin, practicing virtue, and repenting when they succumb to

---

Health Care Ethics: A Manual for Practitioners, 2nd ed., ed. Edward J. Furton, Peter J. Cataldo, and Albert S. Moraczewski, OP (Philadelphia: The National Catholic Bioethics Center, 2009), 4.

10. Leon Kass, "Defending Human Dignity," in *Human Dignity and Bioethics: Essays Commissioned by the President's Council on Bioethics* (Washington, D.C.: President's Council on Bioethics, 2008), 318, emphasis in original.

11. Vatican Council II, *Gaudium et Spes, Pastoral Constitution on the Church in the Modern World*, December 7, 1965, no. 16.

temptation. In other words, dignity is not merely a permanent possession, unaffected by the way people live. A life of sin continually diminishes dignity; a lifetime of seeking perfection continually enhances it. Still another illuminating passage from *Gaudium et Spes* confirms the latter point: "it devolves on humanity to establish a political, social, and economic order which will, to an even better extent, serve man and help individuals as well as groups to affirm and perfect the dignity proper to them."[12]

The *Catechism of the Catholic Church*, in the beginning of Part 3, "Life in Christ" (no. 1700), also provides evidence that dignity must be realized in the way people live. "The dignity of the human person is rooted in his creation in the image and likeness to God (*article 1*); it is fulfilled in his vocation to divine beatitude (*article 2*). It is essential to a human being freely to direct himself to this fulfillment (*article 3*)." Another revealing passage from the CCC (no. 1706) reads: "Living a moral life bears witness to the dignity of the human person." Finally, let us note that there is a close connection between dignity and perfective action, as the CCC shows by including discussion of the image of God, happiness, freedom, the morality of acts and of passions, of conscience and sin, all under the chapter titled "The Dignity of the Human Person." In *Rerum Novarum*, his encyclical on capital and labor, Pope Leo XIII made the same point, using language characteristic of St. Thomas Aquinas: "True dignity and excellence in men resides in moral living, that is, in virtue."[13] St. Leo the Great's famous Christmas sermon memorably echoes this sentiment: "Christian, recognize your dignity and, now that you share in God's own nature, do not return to your former base condition by sinning."[14] It is significant that this exhortation opens the section on morality in the new *Catechism of the Catholic Church*. Christians are urged to realize their human dignity by avoiding sin and living in accordance with the divine nature which Christ's salvation has purchased for them. We even see this understanding of human dignity in the secular world. Visitors to Arlington National Cemetery are greeted by a sign that reads, "Conduct yourselves with dignity and respect at all times." This statement is a tacit acknowledgment of the way in which good behavior enhances dignity.

The latter part of this chapter will attempt to reveal what realized dignity looks like in a health-care setting: health-care professionals doing their best and patients struggling to get well and bearing their pains with grace. Let us turn now to a Catholic explanation of virtue, the practice of which is necessary for both doctors and patients in order to insure a good clinical encounter.

Virtue

The word "virtue" is largely absent from public discourse today. People more readily speak of values, rights, good character, moral or ethical conduct, fairness, and integrity. Even in Catholic circles, virtue is no longer as familiar as it should be. In my own

---

12. Vatican Council II, *Gaudium et Spes*, no. 9: "ad dignitatem sibi propriam affirmandum et excolendam."

13. Pope Leo XIII, *Rerum Novarum, On Capital and Labor*, Encyclical Letter, May 15, 1891, no. 37.

14. St. Leo the Great, *Sermo 21 in nat. Dom.*, 3, quoted in *Catechism of the Catholic Church*, no. 1691.

experience, asking a freshman theology class at a Catholic university to name a virtue usually elicits dead silence. If encouraged to take a guess, students might say "cleanliness," no doubt thinking of the proverb "cleanliness is next to godliness." Or they might name "patience," again referring to a familiar maxim: "patience is a virtue." In all my years of teaching, no one has ever responded with the names of the cardinal and theological virtues: prudence, justice, temperance, fortitude; and faith, hope, and charity. This is not to say that many students, and other Americans, for that matter, do not practice these virtues in their everyday lives. It more likely indicates that they simply are unable to describe their thoughts, desires, words, and deeds in terms of virtue.

Nevertheless, publications such as Alasdair MacIntyre's *After Virtue* have given rise to "virtue talk" and "virtue theory" in academic circles. The greater emphasis on social justice has gradually increased interest in the older concepts of the common good and virtue. And the revival of core curricula in universities has, in many instances, led to the rediscovery of older books in which virtue is a common theme.

The best-known book on virtue is Aristotle's *Nicomachean Ethics*. Familiarity with this book is an excellent preparation for coming to the Catholic understanding of virtue. The ancient Greek philosopher defines moral virtue in this way: "Virtue, then, is a settled disposition determining choice [or literally, a choosing habit], lying in a mean relative to us, this being determined by a rational principle, as the prudent person would determine it."[15] Aristotle saw virtue not just as knowledge of principles but as a habit that inclines a person to act in a certain way, guided by prudence. For example, when doctors are on duty in the hospital, they must not work under the influence of alcohol. Prudence would tell physicians that the virtue of temperance or moderation should incline them to remain sober. If a doctor understood good behavior but had the habit of intemperance, that habit might prompt excessive drinking if an opportunity presented itself. The story of my third child's birth illustrates this point: the attending obstetrician appeared to be under the influence. He came in to examine my wife and told her that she had hours to wait. After he left the room, an experienced nurse on duty immediately told my wife that she would deliver in five or ten minutes. She was right, and the doctor was late for the delivery, despite a rush call by the nurses.

Because virtue is a habit, it requires a certain training, preferably beginning at an early age, to fully develop. Virtuous habits are the foundation of whatever character formation takes place later, such as that developed during medical training. With good role models, young medical students can acquire or reinforce those settled dispositions that will enable them to do their duty. But this will not always be possible if, for example, a medical student has a settled disposition to love gain more than the patient. This kind of physician can be induced by self-interest to neglect the good of his patient. Drs. Edmund Pellegrino and David Thomasma write: "If managed care

---

15. Aristotle, *Nicomachean Ethics*, trans. Martin Ostwald (New York: The Library of Liberal Arts, 1962), bk. 2, chap. 6 [1106b36–1107a3].

calls us to be indifferent to the needs of patients or makes us instruments of economics or profit, we must resist."[16] Without virtuous habits, some physicians will be incapable of resisting, even if they have taken a course on medical ethics in medical school. Mere knowledge of ethical principles does not necessarily incline a person to follow them if they conflict with self-interest.

By contrast, Kantian ethics regards early training in virtuous habits by parents and educators as an infringement on human dignity. The Kantian approach to ethics would not approve a medical school's efforts to inculcate students with virtuous dispositions, even indirectly. What most offends the modern mind about Aristotle's concept of virtue is his assertion that the young need to be educated in virtue before they are able to work on becoming virtuous themselves. Modern man's radical investment in autonomy precludes all but self-education in such a personal endeavor. For Aristotle and Plato, human beings are social or political animals who need the help of the community to acquire virtue. In denying the social nature of human beings, much modern thought gravitates toward moral self-education by autonomous individuals. This explains in part why the principle of autonomy has become the ultimate trump card in medical ethics.

Christian theologians such as Ambrose, Augustine, and Aquinas define virtue in these terms: order in the soul, well-ordered reason, proper control of the passions by reason, good use of free choice, living according to nature and in accordance with reason, compliance with God's will or the divine law, love of God and neighbor, and friendship of man for God.

St. Augustine describes virtue as "the perfect love of God." He refines this definition by adding that virtue is fourfold:

Temperance is love giving itself wholeheartedly to that which is loved; fortitude is love enduring all things willingly for the sake of that which is loved; justice is love serving alone that which is loved, and thus ruling rightly; and prudence is love choosing wisely between that which helps it and that which hinders it.[17]

This love of God is an attitude and activity that engages a person's whole mind, heart, and soul. Augustine goes so far as to say, "When the divine majesty has begun to reveal itself in the measure proper to man while an inhabitant of earth, then such ardent charity is engendered and such a flame of divine love bursts forth that all vices are burned away and man is purged and sanctified."[18] The fervor of charity consumes vices such as envy, gluttony, drunkenness, avarice, and anger. In other words, a passionate love of God gives a person motivation to overcome sinful habits, always, of course, with the necessary help of God's grace.

In various works Augustine explains how people necessarily do what they love. In

---

16. Edmund D. Pellegrino and David C. Thomasma, *The Christian Virtues in Medical Practice* (Washington, D.C.: Georgetown University Press, 1996), 145.

17. St. Augustine, *The Catholic and Manichean Ways of Life* (*De Moribus Ecclesiae Catholicae et de Moribus Manichaeorum*), trans. Donald A. Gallagher, FOTC, vol. 56 (Washington, D.C.: The Catholic University of America Press, 1966), ch. 15, no. 5.

18. Ibid., ch. 30, no. 64.

his justly famous *Confessions*, he writes: "My love is my weight, wherever I go my love is what brings me there."[19] Augustine explains his own conflicting drives: on the one hand, his pride, lust, desire for acclaim, and wish to avoid blame; and on the other hand, his love of wisdom and of God, which eventually drove out his love for vices.

Augustine's teaching on love can illuminate the Catholic understanding of medical care. Physicians who love serving the good of their patients and stay current in their field are not swayed in their medical judgment by pharmaceutical or insurance companies, they respect confidentiality, and they avoid harming their patients by what Dr. Greg Burke calls "negligence due to sloth (laziness), pride (lack of appropriate consultation), or lack of temperance (impairment due to the use of illicit drugs or alcohol)."[20] In other words, the love of serving God through the care of their patients (or simply the love of patients by the nonbelieving doctor) can motivate physicians to cultivate the virtues of prudence, justice, temperance, and fortitude.

Thomas Aquinas says that everything taught in the Gospel pertains to virtue;[21] he says further that virtue makes both people and their work good. He quotes a definition originating with Peter Lombard: "Virtue is a good quality of the mind, by which we live rightly, of which no one can make bad use, which God works in us without us."[22] Aquinas writes that this definition "expresses perfectly the whole nature of virtue," because it includes all the causes of virtue. The formal cause of virtue is a good quality, or more simply, a "good habit." Since Aquinas is defining virtue in general terms, without reference to function, he does not specify an object of virtue or "matter about which it is concerned." He discusses only the ultimate subject of virtue or "the matter in which" virtue is found: that is, the mind or reason. Virtue is not found in human appetites unless they follow the commands of reason. Aquinas's words "by which we live rightly" indicate that the end of virtue is a good operation. His words "of which no one can make bad use" refer to virtue consisting of habits that continually incline a person to the good. The efficient cause of virtue is God, as is expressed by the phrase "which God works in us without us." Both the theological virtues (faith, hope, and charity) and cardinal virtues (prudence, justice, temperance, and fortitude) can be infused by God "without acts on our part, but not without our consent."[23] In other words, free will must cooperate with divine grace.

Possession of the cardinal, or principal, virtues not only gives the ability to be good "but also causes the performing of a good action," says Aquinas. These virtues bring about "rectitude of appetite,"[24] which is the perfection of virtue. Intellectual virtue, by contrast, simply enables a person to perform a good action; the intellectually virtuous person may choose to use or not use the virtues, except for prudence. The

19. St. Augustine, *Confessions*, trans. F. J. Sheed (Indianapolis: Hackett Publishing Company, 1993), bk. XIII, ch. 9.

20. Greg F. Burke, "The Conscience of the Physician," *Ethics and Medics* 29, no. 1 (January 2004), 3.

21. St. Thomas Aquinas, *Summa theologiae* [ST], II-II, q. 117, a. 1. Quotes are from *Summa Theologica* (New York: Benziger Brothers, 1947).

22. Ibid., I-II, q. 55, a. 4.

23. Ibid., q. 55, a. 4, ad 6.

24. Ibid., q. 61, a. 1.

theological virtues are similar to the cardinal virtues, since they also cause "the performing of a good action." Like Augustine, Aquinas stresses the involvement of heart and mind in the practice of virtue. He explains: "If a passion follows a judgment of reason as commanded by reason, the passion helps in the carrying out of the command of reason."[25] In other words, at its pinnacle, virtue prompts the enthusiastic performance of good deeds.

While Aquinas seems to follow Aristotle's treatment of virtue very closely, he teaches that Christians are held to a higher standard of virtue than what Aristotle prescribes. Simply stated, charity should direct the practice of all the virtues, as it does in the moral theology of Augustine. In their book *The Christian Virtues in Medical Practice*, Drs. Pellegrino and Thomasma explain how "the theological virtues reshape both the natural virtues and the philosophical principles on which clinical ethical decisions are made."[26] Like Kass, they hold that medicine, as defined by the healing relationship between physician and patient, first requires the practice of certain virtues by all physicians, Christian or not. In an earlier edition of the book, they explain further:

If these ends of medicine are to be attained, certain character traits are required of the physician, like compassion, fidelity to trust, honesty, intellectual humility, benevolence, and courage. These are, to use Aristotle's term, the "excellences" or virtues that enable the physician to do the work of medicine well. Among these virtues, prudence plays a special role because of the nature of medicine as an activity. Medicine, or more properly healing, is a practical enterprise requiring a fusion of ethical competence and moral judgment.[27]

If physicians are Christian, they are called not only to practice the virtues intrinsic to the art of medicine but also to allow the practice of faith, hope, and charity to inform and support all the natural virtues. Pellegrino and Thomasma are acutely aware of how difficult it is to be a model physician day in and day out. Today, they say, doctors

talk of rationing the care we give, especially to the most vulnerable among us—the poor, the elderly, the chronically handicapped, the infants, the mentally ill, and the retarded. *We shrink from the sacrifice—of our time, emotions, energies, and money—that the care of the sick so much requires.*[28]

The natural virtues can falter under the pressures that physicians face, but the Christian virtues, especially charity, close the gap between knowing the right thing to do and having the motivation to do it in difficult circumstances. Marie Nolan adds, "Charity and patience are needed to care for some patients who by their defiance or hostility may evoke anger in the caregiver."[29]

25. Ibid., q. 59, a. 3, ad 3.

26. Pellegrino and Thomasma, *The Christian Virtues in Medical Practice*, 25.

27. Edmund Pellegrino and David Thomasma, *The Virtues in Medical Practice* (Washington, D.C.: Georgetown University Press, 1993), 86.

28. Pellegrino and Thomasma, *The Christian Virtues in Medical Practice*, 86, emphasis added.

29. Marie T. Nolan, RN, "The Professional-Patient Relationship," in Furton, Cataldo, and Moraczewski, *Catholic Health Care Ethics*, 252.

Patients themselves need various virtues to bear their suffering, and it is that subject to which we now turn.

Suffering

Salvifici Doloris, On the Christian Meaning of Suffering, the apostolic letter by Pope John Paul II (now St. John Paul) on suffering, is a comprehensive presentation of the proper Christian attitude toward one's own suffering and that of others. I cannot do justice to the apostolic letter in this chapter, but I will try to present enough of it to guide both physician and patient, especially the latter. The introduction takes note of the fact that "suffering seems to be, and is, almost *inseparable from man's earthly existence*."[30] Otherwise stated, everyone gets a chance to suffer. It is, however, a mystery why some suffer much more than others. People react well or badly to their few or many sufferings. St. Paul tell us that he came to rejoice in his sufferings when he understood their salvific meaning: "In my flesh I complete what is lacking in Christ's afflictions for the sake of his body, that is, the Church" (Col 1:24). To have St. Paul's attitude requires, of course, an informed, strong faith.

The Quest for an Answer to the Question of the Meaning of Suffering

The Book of Job in the Old Testament shows that God expects human beings to ask searching questions about the way things are in the world. As we saw, the Book of Job tells the story of a man who undeservedly suffers the death of his children and the loss of his property, his livestock, and his health. His three friends make things worse by telling him that he is justly suffering because of his serious sins. Since Job knows that he is innocent of their charges, the unjust remarks by his friends increase his moral suffering. For Job's friends, "suffering can have meaning only as a punishment for sin."[31]

Many Old Testament writings do, in fact, show suffering to be punishment inflicted on human beings because of their sins. While this is true in many cases, the Book of Job shows that not all suffering is deserved. God even rebukes Job's friends for unjustly accusing him and testifies to Job's innocence. "His suffering is the suffering of someone who is innocent; it must be accepted as a mystery, which the individual is unable to penetrate completely by his own intelligence."[32] The Book of Job, while not providing a complete answer to the problem of suffering, can convince the innocent that their sufferings are not punishment for their sins. This knowledge can spare them the additional suffering of self-flagellation for sins that they did not commit. God's Word about suffering in the Book of Job, then, is a clear statement that there can be "suffering without guilt." This can be a very consoling truth for human

---

30. Pope John Paul II, *Salvifici Doloris, On the Christian Meaning of Suffering*, Apostolic Letter, February 11, 1984, no. 3, emphasis in original.

31. Ibid., no. 10.

32. Ibid., no. 11.

beings who find themselves in painful situations. Another lesson is that Job's suffering has the nature of a test. "And if the Lord consents to test Job with suffering, He does it *to demonstrate the latter's righteousness.*"[33]

Sharers in the Suffering of Christ

After turning to the New Testament, John Paul II reflects on sharing in the suffering of Christ, presenting his main point in two short sentences. "Christ *has* also *raised human suffering to the level of the Redemption.* Thus each man, in his suffering, can also become a sharer in the redemptive suffering of Christ."[34] Just as the Church participates in the salvific work of Christ, so human beings through their suffering can unite themselves to Christ's redemptive suffering. So, "*human suffering itself has been redeemed.*"[35] In faith, Christians now know that none of their suffering is ever in vain, because it allows them "to share in the work of the Redemption." Bearing suffering thus enables people to help their fellow human beings attain salvation.

Faith in Christ's resurrection and the certainty of their own resurrection gives suffering Christians the courage to persevere in the midst of all kinds and degrees of suffering. They know in faith that their suffering benefits not only others but themselves as well. John Paul comments on the latter point, "Thus to share in the sufferings of Christ is, at the same time, to suffer for the kingdom of God. In the eyes of the just God, before his judgment, those who share in the suffering of Christ become worthy of this kingdom."[36] The Acts of the Apostles summarizes some of the teaching of Paul and Barnabas on the personal benefits of suffering in these words: "through many tribulations we must enter the kingdom of God."[37] The Apostle Peter adds an additional insight in speaking about the possibility of joy in suffering: " 'But rejoice insofar as you share Christ's suffering, that you may also rejoice and be glad when his glory is revealed.' "[38] In quoting Peter, John Paul II does not mean to imply that suffering is not always a trial. It always is, but joy is still possible in the midst of the trial. The lives of the saints bear witness to these truths in striking ways.

Another way to speak of the joy in the midst of trials is to say that "Christ's resurrection has revealed … the *glory* [of the future age] *that is hidden in the very suffering of Christ* …," which glory, when present in human suffering, expresses "man's spiritual greatness."[39] That glory is present not only in the martyrs for the faith but also in many others "who, at times even without belief in Christ, suffer and give their lives for the truth and for a just cause. In the sufferings of all these people the great dignity of man is strikingly confirmed."[40] This way of speaking of dignity, as we saw, means that it is not only a given but also a quality that is enhanced by the way one

---

33. Ibid., emphasis in original.
34. Ibid., no. 19, emphasis in original.
35. Ibid., emphasis in original.
36. Ibid., no. 21.
37. Acts 14:22, quoted in John Paul II, *Salvifici Doloris*, no. 21.
38. 1 Pt 4:23, quoted in John Paul II, *Salvifici Doloris*, no. 22.
39. John Paul II, *Salvifici Doloris*, no. 22, emphasis in original.
40. Ibid.

lives. In other words, human beings ennoble themselves when they live and die for justice and truth, thereby revealing the great dignity to which all can aspire in their life and death.

The Good Samaritan Attends to Every Kind of Suffering

Pope John Paul II revealingly titles the chapter before his conclusion "The Good Samaritan." The parable of the Good Samaritan in Luke 10:25–37 teaches us to attend to the suffering of our neighbors when *by chance* we have the opportunity to do so. "*Everyone who stops beside the suffering of another person*, whatever form it may take, is a Good Samaritan."[41]

Because he puts his whole heart into helping his neighbor, the Good Samaritan, John Paul II is able to say, is the kind of person who is capable of making a gift of himself to another, which is the only way persons are able to find themselves (to use the language of *Gaudium et Spes*, no. 24). Otherwise stated, people need to provide relief to others in order to practice solidarity, to fulfill Christ's commandment to love one another—in short, to perfect their dignity as human persons.

As his first example of institutionalized Good Samaritan work, John Paul II mentions the profession of doctor, nurse, and related health-care personnel. He implies that the ethic intrinsic to medicine can be described, at least partially, as that of the Good Samaritan. The work of doctor and nurse is then both a profession and a vocation. I recently came across a wonderful example of the profession of medicine in Good Samaritan mode. In the pages of the *National Catholic Bioethics Quarterly*, Dr. Greg Burke wrote about the obligation of physicians vis-à-vis patients who check out of a hospital against medical advice (AMA). When one of his patients prematurely left the hospital while being treated for a gastrointestinal hemorrhage, Dr. Burke called him on the phone and expressed concern for his well-being. The patient returned for regular treatment following Dr. Burke's Good Samaritan initiative. The doctor's care prompted the patient to take better care of himself. Dr. Burke drew this conclusion: "[The doctor's] devotion to the good of those entrusted to his care should not be compromised by an AMA discharge. The relationship does not end at the hospital door."[42]

After mentioning the Good Samaritan work of other unspecified institutions, Pope John Paul II says that the Gospel parable is really a kind of universal ethic. People of all religions and all points of view find the story of the Good Samaritan to be compelling. "In view of all this, we can say that the parable of the Good Samaritan of the Gospel has become *one of the essential elements of moral culture and universally human civilization*."[43] In other words, all over the world non-Christian individuals and institutions have acted like the Good Samaritan and thus have indirectly given their assent to the teaching of the famous Lucan parable.

John Paul II discerns Good Samaritan work being carried out in three ways: by organizations (both religious and nonreligious), by individuals toward strangers, and

41. Ibid., no. 28, emphasis in original.
42. Greg F. Burke, "Medicine," *National Catholic Bioethics Quarterly* 11, no. 1 (Spring 2011): 149.
43. John Paul II, *Salvifici Doloris*, no. 29, emphasis in original.

by family members. Part of the Church's apostolate is to be a Good Samaritan to those in need. Sometimes, single individuals with particular qualities and skills are most suited to relieve suffering in a personal way. Family members may help one another within one family or deliver help to other families in need.

Not surprisingly, St. John Paul II compares the work of the Good Samaritan to that of Christ himself, whose good works "became especially evident in the face of human suffering."[44] The pope further states that Good Samaritan work is necessary for the attainment of salvation. He makes this point by quoting Matthew 25 on the Last Judgment: "'Come, O blessed of my Father, inherit the kingdom prepared for you from the foundation of the world; for I was hungry and you gave me food, I was thirsty and your gave me to drink, I was a stranger and you welcomed me, . . . I was in prison and you came to me.'"[45] In order to attain eternal life everyone must come to the relief of suffering individuals, as the Good Samaritan did.

John Paul II goes so far as to say that "suffering is present in the world in order to release love, in order to give birth to works of love towards neighbor, in order to transform the whole of human civilization into a 'civilization of love.'"[46] Otherwise stated, most people have to be moved by the suffering of others to attain the level of love required for salvation.

John Paul II concludes this chapter with a memorable formulation of Christ's teaching on the meaning of suffering: He "taught man *to do good by his suffering* and *to do good to those who suffer*."[47] By doing these two things, human beings participate in the salvific dimension of Christ's suffering. In other words, whether personally suffering or relieving the suffering of someone else, individuals "'complete' with their own suffering 'what is lacking in Christ's affliction.'"[48]

After this brief review of Church teaching on three of the most important topics pertaining to a Catholic understanding of good medical care, we are now ready to examine some major contributions of reason to the subject.

Reason Alone as a Supplement to Church Teaching

On the Four Principles of Medical Ethics

Hospital ethics committees in non-Catholic hospitals are likely to discuss the relevant issues of such cases in the light of four principles: autonomy, beneficence, non-maleficence, and justice. This four-principles approach has had a strong influence on medical ethics for about forty years. The well-known Kennedy Institute of Ethics at Georgetown University has taught this approach to thousands of health professionals in an intensive bioethics course since the mid-1970s. "This course," say Drs. Edmund Pellegrino and David Thomasma, "has had a strong influence on

---

44. Ibid., no. 30.
45. Mt 25:34–36, quoted in John Paul II, *Salvifici Doloris*, no. 30.
46. John Paul II, *Salvifici Doloris*, no. 30.
47. Ibid., emphasis in original.
48. Ibid., no. 31, quoting Col 1:24.

the teaching and research of health professionals and ethicists who teach in medical schools, colleges, and universities, or consult in clinical settings."[49] It is not within the purview of this chapter to explain in detail what the Kennedy Institute means by these four principles. I will, however, say that their interpretation depends on people's understanding of the good and that Catholics in situations where they are invoked must be very careful not to be led astray, for example, by the principle of autonomy, or to leave out essential considerations. Some examples follow.

Over the years reliance on the four principles has resulted in a primary emphasis on autonomy. Many people initially welcomed this focus as a way of both overcoming problems created by doctors' paternalism and empowering patients to maintain control of their lives during their illness. The following story illustrates a doctor's failure to respect patient autonomy: After being diagnosed with breast cancer, a woman in my neighborhood went to consult with a general surgeon in our area who had a sterling reputation for competence. He recommended a mastectomy and a sentinel node biopsy to find out if the cancer had spread to the lymph nodes. The woman scheduled the surgery, checked into the hospital, and several hours later was informed that the hospital forgot to order the radioactive dye required to do the biopsy. The surgery was canceled, and she decided to head for Sloan Kettering Memorial in New York, the well-known cancer hospital. There she discovered that her local surgeon had not told her that he had practically no experience in doing sentinel node biopsies. Nor had he mentioned that an experienced breast surgeon might possibly be better able than he to obtain sufficiently clear margins by means of a lumpectomy, followed by radiation. Sentinel node biopsies, if not done properly, can create a lifelong problem of swelling in the arm for the patient. If our local surgeon had truly respected the woman's autonomy, he would have told her all she needed to know in order to make an informed decision.

But patients need more than autonomy, especially when by itself it can work against their good health. Some physicians interpret "autonomy" so loosely as to abdicate their own duty to inform, even to persuade, patients to act in their own best interests. Medical students are sometimes taught to just lay out options before their patients and let them choose, without much guidance being offered. Patients with common sense often realize that, without the authoritative guidance of a knowledgeable physician, they do not have enough information to discern their best options. What is needed is an approach that offers a mean between paternalism and imprudent deference to uninformed patient autonomy.

The four-principles approach instructs doctors to respect the dignity and autonomy of their patients, to benefit them as much as possible, to do no harm, and to avoid any kind of injustice. But what constitutes benefit, harm, and justice is often a subject of dispute. For example, whereas Catholic hospitals regard providing abortion and sterilization services as doing harm to patients, many secular hospitals regard the provision of these procedures as beneficial. Dr. Peter Cataldo observes: "Health care is always provided according to a particular vision of what is good for the patient as

---

49. Pellegrino and Thomasma, *The Virtues in Medical Practice*, 188.

a human person;" this disconnect concerning abortion and sterilization, he says, "is a function of two different views of serving the human good of the patient."[50] It is not bad medicine, as some allege, when Catholic hospitals follow Catholic teaching.

The principle of double effect helps Catholic practitioners recognize the doing of harm in the practice of medicine. For example: is it a benefit or harm to remove a cancerous uterus if a woman is pregnant? Is it a benefit or harm to remove a healthy uterus if a woman has a dangerous heart condition that could not tolerate a pregnancy? Application of the principle of double effect answers these questions. Medical personnel may perform an action that has both good and bad effects if four conditions are met. First, the action performed must be good in itself, or at least indifferent; second, only the good effect is intended; third, the good effect must not come about through the bad effect; and fourth, there must be a proportionate reason to tolerate the bad effect. The removal of the cancerous uterus fulfills all four conditions, while the removal of the healthy uterus to prevent a pregnancy violates the third condition.

In their *Ethical and Religious Directives for Catholic Health Care Services*, the U.S. Catholic bishops propose helpful principles for discerning what beneficence should mean in difficult situations. For example, let us take a look at directives 56 and 57.

56. A person has a moral obligation to use ordinary or proportionate means of preserving his or her life. Proportionate means are those that in the judgment of the patient offer a reasonable hope of benefit and do not entail an excessive burden or impose excessive expense on the family or the community.

57. A person may forgo extraordinary or disproportionate means of preserving life. Disproportionate means are those that in the patient's judgment do not offer a reasonable hope of benefit, or entail an excessive burden, or impose excessive expense on the family or the community.[51]

These two directives help patients discern how to fulfill their obligation to preserve their own life through reasonable measures. The proper interpretation of ordinary and extraordinary, proportionate and disproportionate will be examined later in the book. Suffice it to say for now that patients and family members who fully adhere to these directives may legitimately arrive at different conclusions when trying to decide whether the "expected benefits are greater than the anticipated burdens."[52]

These principles can prove helpful in case studies and quandary ethics if they are applied intelligently and if there is agreement on what is good and what is harmful for patients. However, mere knowledge of these principles is insufficient, as they do not cover all the situations faced in medical practice; nor does mere knowledge insure that health-care providers live by these principles. Some scholars, therefore, propose supplementing these principles with virtue ethics, because virtue enables people to observe moral principles. Rev. David Beauregard explains, "The perfection [through

---

50. Peter J. Cataldo, "The Moral Fonts of Action and Decision Making," in Furton, Cataldo, and Moraczewski, *Catholic Health Care Ethics*, 10.

51. United States Conference of Catholic Bishops, *Ethical and Religious Directives for Catholic Health Care Services*, 5th ed. (Washington, D.C.: USCCB, 2009).

52. Editorial summary of Albert S. Moraczewski, OP, and Greg F. Burke, MD, "Assessing Benefits and Burdens," in Furton, Cataldo, and Moraczewski, *Catholic Health Care Ethics*, 202.

the practice of virtue] of the acting agent, who must carry out the laws, rules, and procedures of good medicine, is essential to the good of the patient."[53]

Virtue should also guide an important but neglected aspect of medical care: the way doctors and nurses routinely treat patients during the course of the day.[54] Hospital ethics committees rarely deal with this seemingly mundane subject. But quality care of the patient "can be ensured only by virtuous medical professionals interested in the good of the patient and the enjoyable development and exercise of their talents."[55] Merely proclaiming the four principles in a hospital setting will accomplish little unless they are supplemented and corrected when necessary, and individuals are disposed by virtue to observe them.

Medicine's Principal Goal: To Preserve and Restore Health

It is now time to see what reason by itself has to say on the ends or purposes of medicine and to discern medicine's intrinsic ethic. Dr. Leon Kass writes that the physician is tempted to embrace four false goals for his craft: (1) satisfying patient desires; (2) social adjustment or obedience, or more ambitiously, civic or moral virtue; (3) the alteration of human nature, or of some human natures; and (4) the prolongation of life, or the prevention of death.[56] Examples of gratifying patients include performing vasectomies and providing physician-assisted suicide. Under civic virtue Kass includes such things as the taming of juvenile delinquents and the prevention of crime or war. The third false goal includes eugenic uses of artificial insemination. If the fourth false goal is sought, then medicine will focus on attacking "the diseases that are the leading causes of death rather than the leading causes of ill health." Kass's comment on the last false goal suggests that the real end of medicine is health.[57] The venerable Hippocratic Oath made the same observation a long time ago in saying, "I will apply dietetic measures for the benefit of the sick according to my ability and judgment. I will keep them from harm and injustice."

To clarify his meaning, Kass rejects the view that health is simply a social construct or a mere convention determined by majority consensus at a particular time. He explains:

Health is a natural standard or norm, . . . a state of being that reveals itself in activity as a standard of bodily excellence or fitness, relative to each species and to some extent to individuals, recognizable if not definable, and to some extent attainable. If you prefer a more simple formulation, I would say that health is "the well-working of the organism as a whole," or again, "an activity of the living body in accordance with its specific excellences."[58]

---

53. David Beauregard, OMV, "Virtue in Bioethics," in Furton, Cataldo, and Moraczewski, *Catholic Health Care Ethics*, 28.

54. Hospital administrators send out questionnaires to patients asking them how well they have been treated during a doctor's visit or a hospital stay. However, the virtuous actions of health-care professionals cover more than simply patient satisfaction.

55. Beauregard, "Virtue in Bioethics," 28.

56. Leon R. Kass, *Toward a More Natural Science* (New York: Free Press, 1985), 159–62.

57. Ibid., 162.

58. Ibid., 173.

When understood in this way, the attainment of health depends on good habits of body and soul. A proper diet, moderate drinking, daily exercise, sufficient sleep, not smoking, eating breakfast, keeping one's weight down all contribute to good health.[59] These healthful measures, however, cannot be maintained over the long haul without cultivating virtuous habits, such as temperance, fortitude, love of one's self, and love of family.

Kass makes much of the fact that many diseases are caused or worsened by the patient's way of life.

Some disorders of the body are caused, in part, by primary problems of the soul (psyche); the range goes from the transitory bodily effects of simple nervousness and tension headaches, through the often severe somatic symptoms of depression (e.g., weight loss, insomnia, constipation, impotence), to ulcers and rheumatoid arthritis. . . . Most chronic lung diseases, much cardiovascular disease, most cirrhosis of the liver, many gastrointestinal disorders (from indigestion to ulcers), numerous muscular and skeletal complaints (from low-back pain to flat feet), venereal disease, nutritional deficiencies, obesity and its consequence, and certain kinds of renal and skin infections are in important measure self-induced or self-caused—and contributed to by smoking, overeating, overdrinking, eating the wrong foods, inadequate rest and exercise, and poor hygiene.[60]

If, in fact, people often generate their own health problems, then it makes sense to talk first of a patient's duty to stay healthy before discussing the doctor's duty to help the sick and the healthy. While much public discourse emphasizes the *right* to health care, too little attention is paid to the *responsibility* of preserving health. Certainly, some situations severely limit what people can do for themselves, and living a healthy lifestyle can be hindered by threats from environmental pollution and everyday stresses. Even so, people can take steps to promote their own emotional and physical health, and they can avoid spreading disease or causing injury to others.

Some people will attend to their health in order to look good or feel good. Most people will need incentives, such as the desire to be free from physical limitations or from the mental preoccupations that come with illness. Others may be prompted to stay healthy so as not be a burden on their families or on society. Still others care for their health out of gratitude for the gift of life itself: the joys of learning, the love of family and friends, and the rewards of helping others. A deep sense of gratitude moves Christians and other religious people to nurture their health as a sign of reverence toward God. In short, trying to stay well is a way of loving one's self, loving one's neighbor, and even of being civic-minded.

From a Christian perspective, the highest purpose of health is to help the believer finish the task assigned by God; seen in this light, trying to stay well is a virtue. St. Ignatius, the founder of the Jesuits, at one time in his life abused his health by severe penances. Later, as Superior General of the Jesuits, he wrote to a fellow Jesuit: "If one takes proper care of his body he will have enough strength for works of zeal and

59. Ibid., 177.
60. Ibid., 175, 176.

charity, and for the help and edification of his neighbor. If he does not do so, he will grow weak and feeble, and be of little advantage to the neighbor."[61] Pellegrino and Thomasma address this subject with insight into the principle of autonomy:

Charity-illuminated autonomy would also recognize the obligation to preserve health and nurture the gift of life all around us, not to endanger or abuse it. This is true of the environment as well as for personal life. There is, thus, no absolute freedom to reject treatment that is clearly beneficial unless there is some overriding burden, and persons cannot fail to take preventive measures that are under their control.[62]

Persuading Patients to Cherish Health

Many institutions can work to persuade people to take care of their health. Although civic associations, government agencies, and political leadership may attempt to do this through rhetoric or legislation, the more effective results come from families, churches, and schools. In the United States today, however, these institutions are facing serious challenges to their missions. The breakdown of the family, the abandonment of real moral education in public schools, and the declining influence of institutional religion all pose serious obstacles to any true education in virtue, including the virtue of taking reasonable steps to preserve one's health.

Apart from the efforts of civil institutions, physicians can always play a role in helping their patients stay well. Traditionally, however, medicine has been more preoccupied with curing disease than with teaching ways to maintain health. Pediatrics might be the one exception to this generalization, as pediatricians have always focused on promoting their young patients' growth and development. If the effort to stay well is to become more widespread and lasting, then primary care physicians also must focus on teaching their adult patients to take better care of themselves.

This education of patients must avoid the two extremes of paternalism and exclusive focus on patient autonomy. Sensible patients trust authoritative, not authoritarian, guidance offered by knowledgeable physicians. The doctor should neither lecture patients as though they were children nor withhold information they need to make well thought out decisions about their care. The doctor serves, not merely the patient, but the *good* of the patient. Kass puts it this way:

[The doctor] is a leader and a teacher, one who leads the activities of healing and one who teaches patients and the community about regaining and maintaining healthy functioning. The word "doctor" literally means "teacher," from the Latin verb *docere*, to teach, in this case one who teaches the wisdom and wonders of the body to patient and pupil alike.[63]

This view of the doctor, when properly understood, is perfectly compatible with the principle of autonomy. Drs. Pellegrino and Thomasma explain:

61. St. Ignatius Loyola, *Counsels for Jesuits: Selected Letters and Instructions of Saint Ignatius Loyola*, ed. Joseph Tylenda, SJ (Chicago: Loyola University Press, 1985), 113.

62. Pellegrino and Thomasma, *The Christian Virtues in Medical Practice*, 122.

63. Kass, *Toward a More Natural Science*, 200.

Autonomy must be restored to its original meaning of having to take responsibility for one's choice, rather than making one's choice the standard of right and wrong. We respect autonomy because it is the freedom to do the good and to give oneself, not the freedom to determine what is right and wrong.[64]

In other words, patients need information and support to make responsible decisions for themselves. The principle of autonomy serves patients badly when they invoke it to justify decisions that harm their well-being. When this happens, the conscientious physician will try to persuade patients to do what will contribute to their health or diminish their suffering. Plato said the same thing about the doctor more than two thousand years ago in his *Laws*: "He doesn't give orders until he has in some sense persuaded; when he has on each occasion tamed the sick person with persuasion, he attempts to succeed in leading him back to health."[65]

Doctors will more successfully persuade patients if they genuinely esteem them. Writing in *Catholic Health Care Ethics*, Dr. Kevin Murrell relies on St. Paul to make his point about the importance of esteem. Paul says, "Love one another with mutual affection; anticipate one another in showing honor" (Rm 12:10). The lesson for physicians is that they "must practice humility, especially in their hearts, and habitually think of their brethren (their patients in this case) with esteem."[66] Physicians who esteem their patients will show them respect, avoid saying negative things about them behind their backs, honor confidentiality, and place confidence in them. Dr. Murrell further comments: "In showing our confidence in our patients and colleagues, we encourage them to put all their resources and abilities into the task ahead of them. Where this esteem and confidence are lacking, one usually finds mistrust."[67] When doctors show confidence in their patients, the patients will in turn put confidence in their doctors, taking to heart their instructions for recovering health and staying well.

Serving the good of the patient requires more of doctors than competence in their area of specialty. They must also know what they do not know and be humble enough to consult with other doctors when it may be necessary or possibly helpful, keeping in mind the healthy functioning of the human body as a whole. Rev. Albert Moraczewski and Dr. Greg Burke elaborate on this idea: "It is incumbent on the clinician, therefore, to maintain certification in his specialty, review the relevant literature, and consult colleagues when appropriate, . . . and be willing to change his mind on the basis of new data, and never be 'married' to a diagnosis."[68] This advice implies that a doctor must possess the virtue of humility in order to consult with other doctors and the fortitude to face the toil of keeping up in one's field.

Treating an ailment in one part of the patient's body without paying sufficient

---

64. Pellegrino and Thomasma, *The Christian Virtues in Medical Practice*, 146.

65. Plato, "Athenian Stranger," in Plato, *Laws*, 702b–e, quoted in Kass, *Toward a More Natural Science*, 211.

66. Kevin J. Murrell, MD, "Confidentiality," in Furton, Cataldo, and Moraczewski, *Catholic Health Care Ethics*, 19.

67. Ibid., 20.

68. Albert S. Moraczewski, OP, and Greg F. Burke, MD, "Assessing Benefits and Burdens," in Furton, Cataldo, and Moraczewski, *Catholic Health Care Ethics*, 199–200.

attention to the treatment's effect on the rest of the body is imprudent. Doctors must be curious about the well-working of the whole body and pay close attention to what patients say about their own problems. Consider this case: a specialist decided to change a person's blood pressure medicine for a very good reason: to keep his heart rate from going too low. From past experience, the patient knew that stopping his blood pressure medicine would immediately cause his blood pressure to spike, a fact he explained to the specialist, to no avail. Sure enough, the blood pressure spike occurred and persisted. Meanwhile, however, the specialist had gone on vacation and none of his partners wanted to deal with problem. So the patient contacted his family physician via e-mail, and together, by trial and error, they managed to lower the blood pressure. Although the specialist might have been a very dedicated physician, he should have paid more attention to his patient's observations and to the workings of the body as a whole. A better response would have been, "I am going on vacation, so we need a back-up plan if your blood pressure goes up significantly and remains elevated."

Physicians may be inattentive to the workings of the body as a whole, and they also may not appreciate "the riches and mysteries of the human soul."[69] The lack of this knowledge can lead to misdiagnosis when a real illness is caused by a problem in the soul (psyche). Examples of this kind of problem can be found in illnesses caused or aggravated by anger, sadness, depression, marital and family tensions, and horrible crimes such as murder. Think of the effect of murder on Lady Macbeth as described by Shakespeare. Physicians must recognize when they need the help of a patient's pastor or the hospital chaplain, for lack of hope or of a will to survive can imperil a patient's recovery from illness or surgery. The philosophically naive view, held by many scientists, that the soul is a leftover medieval concept has no bearing on the fact of psychic influences on the body; in fact, the mind and the soul do have an influence on the well-working of the body, for good or for ill.

Serving the patient's good also requires that doctors do their best in the face of obstructive governmental regulations and insurance companies. Even when patients cannot be restored to health, doctors still have a duty to stand by them. Kass explains: "Relief of suffering stands, next to health, as a crucial part of the medical goal, and medicine has always sought to comfort when it cannot heal."[70] Comforting patients involves not only the prescription of medication to relieve pain but also appropriate encouragement. In addition, Christian doctors can pray with and for their patients, especially in difficult circumstances. Pellegrino expands on this point:

The Christian, physician, then, is not ashamed to pray, to ask God to show how to heal in this case, how to use medical knowledge to heal, how to make the patient whole again in body, mind, and spirit. The physician does not fear to pray with the patient, to call upon the patient's spiritual resources, or to ask the chaplain's assistance.[71]

---

69. Kass, *Toward a More Natural Science*, 199.
70. Ibid., 204.
71. Pellegrino and Thomasma, *The Christian Virtues in Medical Practice*, 45.

On the Profession of Medicine

The very nature of medicine requires an extraordinary commitment by the physician to the well-being of patients, whether or not patients bring their problems upon themselves. The doctor must never treat such patients with less care than those clearly not responsible for their condition. Medicine is aptly referred to as a "profession," a term derived from two Latin words, *pro* and *fateor*, which mean "to declare publicly or to confess devotion on behalf of." In becoming a physician, a person joins a profession which dedicates itself to healing the sick, relieving suffering, and helping people to stay well. Kass comments: "A profession, to speak precisely, would be an activity or occupation to which its practitioner publically professes, that is confesses, his devotion. . . . It is a matter not only of the mind and hand but also of the heart, not only of the intellect and skill, but also of character."[72] Kass explains that the term "profession" has been especially applied to the work of medicine, law, and theology, which respectively study human nature, ethics and politics, and God. To live fully the inherent meaning of their professions, the doctor, lawyer, and theologian must acquire knowledge, character, and devotion to the ideals of their respective fields: health for patients, justice for individuals, and truth about God for humanity.

Lawyers have been criticized from time immemorial for neglecting justice in favor of self-interest. No one pays much attention to theologians, and, therefore, few people would know how devoted they are to the highest truth. Medicine probably has a higher popular standing than the other two professions, but today more and more people question the physician's devotion to patients. We should not be surprised that people are unable or unwilling to live up to the ideals of these three professions; all three require a great deal of knowledge, good character, and demanding service. Nevertheless, we should expect theologians, lawyers, and physicians to abide by the ideals of their respective professions.

In a discussion of euthanasia in his book *Life, Liberty and the Defense of Dignity: The Challenge for Bioethics*, Kass sheds more light on the medical profession and the ethic intrinsic to its practice. He argues that, despite widespread belief to the contrary, the legalization of euthanasia and physician-assisted suicide will not promote human dignity and will instead harm the profession of medicine. Putting physicians in the position of killing legally, even with the patient's consent, will have a disastrous impact on the doctor's self-understanding and on patient trust. Kass rightly says that "the medical profession's devotion to heal and refusal to kill—its ethical center—will be permanently destroyed, and with it patient trust and physician self-restraint."[73] Patient trust of doctors is already decreasing, and will certainly be further eroded if physicians subtly (or not so subtly) suggest death to patients as their best option.

If, in fact, there must be an ethic intrinsic to the profession of medicine, physicians must practice virtue, even if scholars are unable to agree either on virtue's mean-

---

72. Kass, *Toward a More Natural Science*, 214, 215.
73. Leon Kass, *Life, Liberty and the Defense of Dignity: The Challenge for Bioethics* (San Francisco: Encounter Books, 2002), 227.

ing or its ultimate foundation. Since such agreement is unlikely in our pluralistic society, some argue that recourse to virtue ethics is not possible or wise. I contend, however, that the correct practice of medicine not only requires that doctors practice virtue but also teaches all people how they should relate to each other. In an address to physicians on the profession of medicine, Pope Paul VI made the same point on the basis of rational observation.

Love your profession! It is for you a great school. It sensitizes you to the suffering of your brothers and sisters, it helps you to understand and respect them, it purifies the most noble impulses of your heart by the devotion and spirit of sacrifice it requires of you. *Further, your activity is still a great lesson for the whole of society: it is still and will be always the example of generous kindness towards brothers and sisters that, more than every word, leads people and carries them along, moves the coldest hearts and offers the life of the community a cause for confidence and moral stability.*[74]

Patients who rightly expect virtuous behavior from physicians and nurses should come to see that the practice of medicine actually teaches them how to behave toward their fellow human beings.

The beautiful words of Paul VI point to still another dimension of the medical profession, its eminent contribution to the common good of society. As David Gallagher writes,

each person contributes to the common good through his professional work, including homemaking. The division of labor means that each, by his particular expertise, contributes something to the common good of society, giving rise to the obligation to exercise one's professional work primarily as a service to the rest of society.[75]

The *Catechism*, echoing the thoughts of Pope John XXIII, defines the common good as "the sum total of social conditions which allow people either as groups or individuals to reach their perfection more fully and more easily."[76] Health and health care are clearly very important elements of the common good, since they allow people to have a life, so to speak. Without health and the care that both restores and preserves health, people would be severely hindered in what they could do for themselves and for others. Physicians and other health-care professionals make an outstanding contribution to the common good, not only by providing care, but also by the virtues they evince in carrying out their work. As Paul VI said, the devotion and sacrifices of the dedicated physician provide "a great lesson for the whole of society" in how to live a fully human life. In other words, the dedicated physician perfects his or her dignity and shows others how to do the same. The more people perfect their dignity, the

---

74. Pope Paul VI, "Allocution à des médecins," quoted in Pellegrino and Thomasma, *The Christian Virtues in Medical Practice*, 138n42, emphasis added. I modified the translation of this papal address, made by Pellegrino and Thomasma, on the basis of the French original that they provided. See Pope Paul VI, "Allocution à des medecins," in *Documents Pontificaux de Paul VI* (St. Maurice, Switzerland: Editions Saint-Augustin, 1970), 701.

75. David M. Gallagher, "The Common Good," in Furton, Cataldo, and Moraczewski, *Catholic Health Care Ethics*, 31.

76. *Catechism of the Catholic Church*, no. 1906.

better for society as a whole, since the common good is ultimately the good of every single individual. The ultimate common good is, of course, the communion of all the saints with the triune God in eternal life.

Medicine is a profession that requires not only scientific competence but also good character. Thus it should be clear why a part of this chapter explains in some detail what character-building virtue looks like.

Conclusion

In this chapter, we have been able to take a good look at the doctor-patient relationship through the lens of Scripture, Church teaching, and reason. The limits imposed by this single chapter did not allow for a discussion of several important subjects (e.g., doctors' allowing sufficient time to see each patient, informed consent, advance directives, etc.). However, these matters can be addressed in the light of Scripture, which provides guidance for clinical encounters that will remain valid until the end of time; in the light of Church teaching on the dignity of the human person, on virtue, and on suffering; and in the light of reason, which discerns, among other things, the responsibilities of both doctor and patient. Medicine is a profession that requires consistent devotion of doctors to their patients; and the ethic intrinsic to the practice of medicine, an ethic of love, provides "a great lesson for the whole of society" (in the words of Pope Paul VI) in how to live a life fully in accord with the dignity of the human person and with the teaching of the parable of the Good Samaritan.[77]

Bibliography

Aristotle. *Nicomachean Ethics*. Translated by Martin Ostwald. New York: Library of Liberal Arts, 1962.

Augustine. *The Catholic and Manichean Ways of Life* (*De Moribus Ecclesiae Catholicae et de Moribus Manichaeorum*). Translated by Donald A. Gallagher. FOTC, vol. 56. Washington, D.C.: The Catholic University of America Press, 1966.

———. *Confessions*. Translated by F. J. Sheed. Indianapolis: Hackett, 1993.

Beauregard, David, OMV. "Virtue in Bioethics." In Furton, Cataldo, and Moraczewski, *Catholic Health Care Ethics*, 27–29.

Benedict XVI, Pope. *Spe Salvi, On Christian Hope*. Encyclical Letter. November 30, 2007.

Burke, Greg F. "The Conscience of the Physician." *Ethics and Medics* 29, no. 1 (January 2004): 2–3.

———. "Medicine." *National Catholic Bioethics Quarterly* 11, no. 1 (Spring 2011): 147–53.

Cataldo, Peter J. "The Moral Fonts of Action and Decision Making." In Furton, Cataldo, and Moraczewski, *Catholic Health Care Ethics*, 9–12.

Catechism of the Catholic Church. 2nd edition. Translated by the United States Conference of Catholic Bishops. Washington, D.C.: USCCB, 1997.

Furton, Edward J., Peter J. Cataldo, and Albert S. Moraczewski, OP, eds. *Catholic Health Care Ethics: A Manual for Practitioners*. 2nd edition. Philadelphia: National Catholic Bioethics Center, 2009.

Gallagher, David M. "The Common Good." In Furton, Cataldo, and Moraczewski, *Catholic Health Care Ethics*, 29–31.

Ignatius Loyola. *Counsels for Jesuits: Selected Letters and Instructions of Saint Ignatius Loyola*. Edited by Joseph Tylenda, SJ. Chicago: Loyola University Press, 1985.

77. Paul VI, "Allocution à des médecins."

John Paul II, Pope. *Salvifici Doloris, On the Christian Meaning of Suffering.* Apostolic Letter. February 11, 1984.

Kass, Leon R. *Toward a More Natural Science.* New York: Free Press, 1985.

——. *Life, Liberty and the Defense of Dignity: The Challenge for Bioethics.* San Francisco: Encounter Books, 2002.

——. "Defending Human Dignity." In *Human Dignity and Bioethics: Essays Commissioned by the President's Council on Bioethics*, 297–331. Washington, D.C.: President's Council on Bioethics, 2008.

Leo XIII, Pope. *Rerum Novarum, On Capital and Labor.* Encyclical Letter. May 15, 1891.

Moraczewski, Albert S., OP. "The Human Person and the Church's Teaching Authority." In Furton, Cataldo, and Moraczewski, *Catholic Health Care Ethics*, 3–8.

Moraczewski, Albert S., OP, and Greg F. Burke, MD. "Assessing Benefits and Burdens." In Furton, Cataldo, and Moraczewski, *Catholic Health Care Ethics*, 199–202.

Murrell, Kevin J., MD. "Confidentiality." In Furton, Cataldo, and Moraczewski, *Catholic Health Care Ethics*, 19–23.

Nolan, Marie T., RN. "The Professional-Patient Relationship." In Furton, Cataldo, and Moraczewski, *Catholic Health Care Ethics*, 251–4.

Pellegrino, Edmund D., and David C. Thomasma. *The Virtues in Medical Practice.* Washington, D.C.: Georgetown University Press, 1993.

——. *The Christian Virtues in Medical Practice.* Washington, D.C.: Georgetown University Press, 1996.

Thomas Aquinas. *Summa theologica.* 3 vols. New York: Benziger Brothers, 1947, 1948.

United States Conference of Catholic Bishops. *Ethical and Religious Directives for Catholic Health Care Services.* 5th edition. Washington, D.C.: USCCB, 2009.

Vatican Council II. *Gaudium et Spes, Pastoral Constitution on the Church in the Modern World.* December 7, 1965.

Peter J. Colosi

2. A CATHOLIC ANTHROPOLOGY AND MEDICAL ETHICS

Any serious attempt to practice medicine in a manner consistent with what is truly good for a patient must be rooted firmly in a proper understanding of the human person. Professor Colosi methodically outlines the key elements of a truly Catholic anthropology and then places it in the context of medical practice. He begins with a real, and very practical, question posed in 2011 to Pope Benedict XVI concerning the personhood of a son in a state of permanent unconsciousness. Weaving this example through his explication of the foundational Catholic teachings on the human person, Colosi sets the stage upon which medical practitioners can act in their daily caring for patients. He does not, however, leave us simply to ponder the foundational propositions. Rather, he makes the connection between this abiding Catholic understanding of the human person and an ethos appropriate for every person privileged to care for another. In the last section of the chapter, Colosi takes up the issue of euthanasia and physician-assisted suicide. Using the example posed at the beginning of his chapter, he leads the reader to gain a clear understanding of the reasons underlying the imperative for a Catholic ethos in medicine.—*Editors*

Introduction: Catholic Anthropology

MARIA TERESA: Your Holiness, has the soul of my son Francesco, who has been in a vegetative coma since Easter Sunday 2009, left his body, seeing that he is no longer conscious, or is it still near him?

POPE BENEDICT XVI: Certainly his soul is still present in his body. The situation, perhaps, is like that of a guitar whose strings have been broken and therefore can no longer play. The instrument of the body is fragile like that, it is vulnerable, and the soul cannot play, so to speak, but remains present. I am also sure that this hidden soul feels your love deep down, even if unable to understand the details, your words, etc. He feels the presence of love.

Your presence, therefore, dear parents, dear mother, next to him for hours and hours every day, is the true act of a love of great value because this presence enters into the depth of that hidden soul. Your act is thus also a witness of faith in God, of faith in man, of faith, let us say, of commitment, to life, of respect for human life, even in the saddest of situations. I encourage you, therefore to carry on, to know that you are giving a great service to humanity with this sign of faith, with this sign of respect for life, with this love for a wounded body and a suffering soul.[1]

This exchange occurred on Good Friday in 2011, when Pope Benedict XVI made history by being the first pope to appear on a television program to answer questions in a Q & A format. His answer to Maria Teresa can serve as a springboard to the discussion of a Catholic anthropology and its relation to medical ethics. Notice that the pope's answer to Maria Teresa is also beautiful and moving. He responds to her not solely with a moral commandment, although that is certainly present, but also with love. His answer, we could say, is imbued with a Catholic ethos.[2]

Before turning directly to anthropology, let us outline briefly the relationship between moral teachings and the Catholic ethos that should be at the foundation of a Catholic approach to biotechnology, medicine, and health care. The main purpose of official Church documents dealing with bioethics, such as *Donum Vitae*[3] and *Dignitas Personae*,[4] is to present a list of the Church's precise indications on the tough moral questions, that is, a list of which specific actions are allowed and which are prohibited.[5] Reading those documents closely, however, one finds woven throughout them profound, if brief, meditations on the meanings of love, person, family, suffering, and many other topics pertaining to the deepest meaning of life. The presence of those meditations, in documents whose main purpose is to outline which specific actions are prohibited and which are allowed, makes understandable a sentence in the conclusion of *Donum Vitae* that at first reading seems surprising in a document full of definitive

1. Vatican Radio, "Pope Benedict XVI Answers Questions on Special Television Broadcast," April 22, 2011, http://en.radiovaticana.va/storico/2011/04/22/pope_benedict_xvi_answers_questions_on_special_television_broadcast/en1-480959.

2. Ethos is the general tenor and spirit of a society, and it forms the way institutions in that society are run. According to Pope John Paul II, one can deduce that ethos in any given society by pondering its structures and institutions. The deduction then leads ultimately back to the hearts and minds of the individual persons in the society. See Pope John Paul II, *Man and Woman He Created Them: A Theology of the Body*, trans. Michael Waldstein (Boston: Pauline Books and Media, 2006), 264–321, esp. 266 (Audiences 34–48, esp. 34:5).

3. Congregation for the Doctrine of the Faith, *Donum Vitae, Instruction on Respect for Human Life in Its Origin and on the Dignity of Procreation*, February 22, 1987, http://www.vatican.va/roman_curia/congregations/cfaith/documents/rc_con_cfaith_doc_19870222_respect-for-human-life_en.html.

4. Congregation for the Doctrine of the Faith, *Dignitas Personae, Instruction on Certain Bioethical Questions*, September 8, 2008, http://www.vatican.va/roman_curia/congregations/cfaith/documents/rc_con_cfaith_do_20081208_dignitas-personae_en.html.

5. The phrases "moral indication" and "precise moral indication" are the technical way the Church refers to the concise answer to specific moral questions. In some cases the answer can be a simple "yes" or "no." For an example, see Congregation for the Doctrine of the Faith, *Responses to Certain Questions of the United States Conference of Catholic Bishops Concerning Artificial Nutrition and Hydration*, August 1, 2007, http://www.vatican.va/roman_curia/congregations/cfaith/documents/rc_con_cfaith_doc_20070801_risposte-usa_en.html. Two unique features of such documents are their precision and concision. This is a gift from the Church to the world, for through these documents we receive clear moral guidance. However, as we will see, there is still an important task to be accomplished in explaining the underlying reasons for the truth and goodness of the precise moral indications. This task must be fulfilled in order that the faithful can more fully live in the truth.

moral conclusions, "The precise indications which are offered in the present Instruction are not meant to halt the effort of reflection but rather to give it renewed impulse."[6]

One might wonder what further reflection could be needed, since the primary purpose of such documents is to present the most recent medical and scientific advances, to analyze them, and carefully to pronounce definitively on the moral licitness or illicitness of each. The reason for renewed reflection is given in the same conclusion:

[T]he Congregation for the Doctrine of the Faith addresses an invitation with confidence and encouragement to theologians, and above all to moralists, that they study more deeply and make ever more accessible to the faithful the contents of the teaching of the Church's Magisterium in the light of a valid anthropology in the matter of sexuality and marriage and in the context of the necessary interdisciplinary approach. Thus they will make it possible to understand ever more clearly the reasons for and the validity of this teaching.[7]

And so, the renewed reflection is *not* needed with respect to the determined precise indications, since they cannot change. Rather, the Church calls for renewed reflection so that the underlying *reasons for* and the deep *goodness of* the truth of the precise indications may be understood and expressed to the faithful; in this way, the faithful are enabled to interiorize the goodness of the truth and thus to live it fully and freely, so that "[a]s a result, love of neighbor will no longer be for them a commandment imposed, so to speak, from without, but a consequence deriving from their faith, a faith which becomes active through love."[8]

In a culture or a medical school that is not colored with the backdrop of a Catholic ethos, precise moral indications can stand out like random, odd, disconnected, individual commands. For this reason, renewed reflection is desperately needed, and the imparting of a Catholic ethos and valid anthropology that reveal the reasonability and goodness of the Church's moral teachings needs to be given prominence in Catholic medical and health-care training. This is so because "[b]ehind every 'no' in the difficult task of discerning between good and evil, there shines a great 'yes' to the recognition of the dignity and inalienable value of every single and unique human being called into existence."[9] The goal, therefore, of this chapter is, within the context of a Catholic ethos, to explore the qualities of human persons that give them dignity and to understand how the inherent dignity of persons is related to medical ethical questions.

Dr. Edmund Pellegrino, in an article outlining the various moral approaches in the patient-doctor relationship, made the following statement about love and morality in that context:

---

6. Congregation for the Doctrine of the Faith, *Donum Vitae*, conclusion.

7. Ibid.

8. Pope Benedict XVI, *Deus Caritas Est, On Christian Love*, Encyclical Letter, December 25, 2005, no. 31, http://www.vatican.va/holy_father/benedict_xvi/encyclicals/documents/hf_ben-xvi_enc_20051225_deus-caritas-est_en.html.

9. Congregation for the Doctrine of the Faith, *Dignitas Personae*, no. 36.

Charity does not ignore ethical principles nor substitute vague moral sentiment for rational ethical decisions. It does, however, ask how each principle applies in the light of the Sermon on the Mount or the example of Jesus' daily healing of the sick. It emphasizes the kind of persons we ought to be rather than the solution to a particular moral puzzle.[10]

Notice that Dr. Pellegrino is careful to point out that precise moral conclusions are not relegated to the sidelines, nor are they violated, when love is given pride of place in medical ethics. The ethical principles are in fact *applied*. And so, when he says that charity in ethics does not focus on the solution to a moral puzzle, this can in no way be interpreted as a rejection of the Church's moral teaching, nor of the work needed to come to those precise moral indications. Instead, his remark should be understood, I think, as a warning not to separate correct moral conclusions from a Catholic ethos. There are many important reasons for avoiding such a separation, and one of them is that the moral truths will not be understood with the depth needed in order for them to be fully lived and obeyed in love.

In other words, love deepens our awareness of the goodness and truth of the precise indications listed in *Donum Vitae* and *Dignitas Personae*. Toward the end of the chapter, we will look at how this applies to two real life situations, one dealing with the beginning of life and the other with end of life. Let us turn first, then, to the main topic of this chapter, Catholic anthropology.

Anthropology

The term "anthropology," as used in the context of moral teaching, means the study of what it is to be a human person. The relation of such an anthropology to medical ethics lies in the fact that human persons have a lofty value, an intrinsic dignity, which makes a connection between the human person and ethics. Put simply, since a person is such a worthy entity, some ways of treating persons are violations of their dignity and thus are morally wrong. *Catholic* anthropology refers to the deepened understanding, which the Catholic faith has provided, of what it is to be a human person.

There is something very interesting about this last point: even though we now see more clearly what it means to be a human person because of the Catholic faith, this new understanding is quite accessible to people who do not share that faith. This is because we are all human persons, and therefore the truths about being a human person "ring true" when we hear them.[11]

---

10. Edmund D. Pellegrino, MD, "The Catholic Physician in an Era of Secular Bioethics," *The Linacre Quarterly* 78, no. 1 (February 2011): 13–28.

11. See Pope John Paul II, *Evangelium Vitae, On the Value and Inviolability of Human Life*, Encyclical Letter, March 25, 1995, no. 2. http://www.vatican.va/holy_father/john_paul_ii/encyclicals/documents/hf_jp-ii_enc_25031995_evangelium-vitae_en.html.

Dignity

There is a marked difference between kicking a rock down the street and kicking a person who is walking toward you on the same street. Few would find anything wrong with randomly kicking the rock, yet most people would agree that performing the same action on a person is clearly wrong. This elementary observation gives rise to a question: what exactly is the difference between a rock and a person such that the former makes no moral claim on me not to kick it, while the latter does? Or put another way, why do people have more worth than rocks? Many thinkers throughout history have asked not only why people have more worth than rocks, but why they have more worth than any other type of entity in the created world.

The question that Maria Teresa posed to Pope Benedict XVI is deeply related to this question. She wanted to know if her son, who is in a severely debilitated state, still has the dignity that we readily recognize in healthy people; and the pope's answer was a resounding "yes."

As stated above, the goal of this chapter is to explore the qualities of human persons that give them dignity, and through that exploration come to an understanding concerning how the inherent dignity of persons is related to medical ethical questions within a Catholic ethos. To assist in this study, we will start with the definitions of three philosophical terms that will be used in our analysis:

- *Ontology* comes from the Greek word for "being" (ontos), and one branch of ontology studies the nature or essence of beings, that is, the *kinds* of beings there are.
- *Axiology* comes from one of the Greek words for "good" (axios), and this refers to the goodness, worth, or value of a being. The relationship between ontology and axiology is that the worth of a being (axiology) depends on what kind of being it is, that is, on its existence and nature (ontology).
- *Ethics* is a branch of philosophy with many dimensions, including virtue and vice, good and bad, happiness and misery, and the study of right and wrong in human action. Ethics is related to ontology and axiology in that moral claims are made by beings of high worth.

For simplicity's sake, take the example above concerning the rock and the person. In that case, the moral claim "thou shalt not kick me" is issued by the person walking toward you by that person's very being and worth. The rock, by contrast, issues no such moral claim, since the kind of being it is does not grant it lofty worth.

Consider the opening sentences of *Dignitas Personae*, the Church's most recent magisterial document on moral questions in the field of bioethics. The opening sentence employs all three of the concepts just defined:

The dignity of a person must be recognized in every human being from conception to natural death. This fundamental principle expresses *a great "yes" to human life* and must be at the center of ethical reflection on biomedical research, which has an ever-greater importance in today's world.[12]

---

12. Congregation for the Doctrine of the Faith, *Dignitas Personae*, no. 1, emphasis in original.

The term "dignity" in the quotation is an *axiological* expression, which indicates the lofty worth of persons. The term "person" is an *ontological* expression referring to a certain kind of being (in this case, *human* persons, and so "human person" and "human being" are both *ontological* expressions). Since the very nature of human persons grants them such high value, the document asserts that this dignity of persons "*must* be recognized"; this is an *ethical* expression, for it draws our attention to our moral obligations to respect human persons.

Catholic Anthropology and Ethics
versus Utilitarianism

In his encyclical letter *Fides et Ratio*, Pope John Paul II wrote of the relationship between moral theology and philosophy:

> In order to fulfill its mission, moral theology must turn to a philosophical ethics which looks to the truth of the good, to an ethics which is neither subjectivist nor utilitarian. Such an ethics implies and presupposes a philosophical anthropology and a metaphysics of the good.[13]

In this passage, the pope refers to ontological, axiological, and ethical realities, invoking their truth in order to refute subjectivist and utilitarian views, which stand at the basis of the culture of death. There is a difference between moral subjectivism, also known as moral relativism, and utilitarianism. The pope warns against both of these in this quotation. What subjectivism/relativism and utilitarianism have in common is the rejection of both traditional Judeo-Christian morality, in particular the absolute moral laws it announces, and the sanctity of human life and intrinsic dignity of persons, which is the foundation of those laws and which those laws protect and safeguard. Where they differ is that subjectivism/relativism is amoral, whereas utilitarianism is a theory of ethics. Ethics attempts to formulate moral norms (characterized by the words *ought* or *should* or *must*), and when ethical writers formulate such norms they provide reasons which back up their claim that they have formulated a moral norm. Utilitarians are no different than other ethicists in this regard. Subjectivists/relativists, on the other hand, reject the very idea of moral norms.

These are the three basic principles that make up utilitarianism:

- *The consequentialist principle*: the rightness, or wrongness, of an action is determined by the goodness or badness of the results that flow from it.[14]
- *The hedonist principle*: the only thing that is good in itself is pleasure, and the only thing bad in itself is pain.[15]
- *The principle of extent*: one must take into account the number of people affected by the action.[16]

---

13. Pope John Paul II, *Fides et Ratio, On the Relationship between Faith and Reason*, Encyclical Letter, September 14, 1998, no. 98, http://www.vatican.va/holy_father/john_paul_ii/encyclicals/documents/hf_jp-ii_enc_15101998_fides-et-ratio_en.html.

14. Anthony Quinton, *Utilitarianism* (London: Duckworth, 1989), 1.

15. Ibid.

16. Jeremy Bentham, "An Introduction to the Principles of Morals and Legislation," in *The English Philosophers from Bacon to Mill*, ed. Edwin A. Burtt (New York: Random House: 1939), 804.

The following simple formulation of ethical utilitarianism emerges: the rightness of an action is determined by its contribution to the happiness (pleasure) of the greatest number of people affected by it.

Utilitarians, therefore, reject the notion that there are exceptionless moral norms. That is, they do not believe in moral claims of the type mentioned above; rather, they think that any act which brings about what they consider "the greater good" is what ought to be done. Utilitarian philosopher Peter Singer has encapsulated this position:

from trite rules against lying and stealing to such noble constructions as justice and human rights . . . , when the debunked principles have been scrutinized, found wanting, and cleared away, we will be left with nothing but the impartial rationality of the principle of equal consideration of interests.[17]

In the Catholic view, however, the dignity of persons gives rise to moral claims that may never be violated, because doing so violates people.[18] And so, even though utilitarianism calls for calculating "the greater good," it can also be termed a form of ethical relativism in the sense that it rejects *absolute* moral norms, which it would *always* be wrong to violate.

Greek Philosophy and the Christian Concept of "Person"

Catholic anthropology expresses an understanding of human persons that is both philosophical and rooted in faith. Joseph Cardinal Ratzinger (later Pope Benedict XVI) wrote:

The concept of "person," as well as the idea that stands behind this concept, is a product of Christian theology. In other words, it grew in the first place out of the interplay between human thought and the data of Christian faith, and so entered intellectual history. The concept of person is . . . one of the contributions to human thought made possible and provided by Christian faith. It did not simply grow out of mere human philosophizing, but out of the interplay between philosophy and the antecedent given of faith, especially Scripture.[19]

The concept of the dignity of persons is rooted in ancient Greek philosophy, from which it sprang in the interplay between that thought and Christian faith. Aristotle (384–322 BC) did not use the phrase "human person" or "person," but he explained man as a rational animal.[20] Aristotle's definition is a classical definitional formulation which has two parts: proximate genus and specific difference.[21] In this way Aris-

17. Peter Singer, *The Expanding Circle* (Oxford: Clarendon Press 1981), 151. For an example of another contemporary thinker who holds this views, see Shelly Kagan, *The Limits of Morality* (Oxford: Clarendon Press, 1989).

18. I have developed at much greater length this distinction between utilitarian and Catholic ethics as it related to questions of human suffering in my article "John Paul II and Christian Personalism vs. Peter Singer and Utilitarianism: Two Radically Opposed Conceptions of the Nature and Meaning of Suffering," *Ethics Education* 15, no. 1 (2009): 20–41.

19. Joseph Cardinal Ratzinger, "Concerning the Notion of Person in Theology," *Communio* 17 (1990): 439.

20. See Aristotle, *Nicomachean Ethics*, I.7 (1098a3–5).

21. See Aristotle, *Topics*, IV.1–4 [120b11–125b14]; Aristotle, *Metaphysics*, VII.12 [1037b8–1038a35].

totle distinguishes man from the animals: the closest genus to man, he says, is animal. This serves to pick out a broad category of beings, namely, animals, within which are all animals, humans included. In the second step of the definition, Aristotle takes note of the one thing that makes human beings different from all the other animals in that larger group: our rational nature. Put differently, human beings form a unique species among the animals because we have a rational nature (our specific difference), while none of the other animals do.

It should be noted here that, while Aristotle is accurate in his analysis, later thinkers in the Christian tradition will choose "person" as the proximate genus and then select "embodied" as the specific difference for human beings. This difference is very important from a medical ethical point of view and is expressed this way in *Donum Vitae*:

By virtue of its substantial union with a spiritual soul, the human body cannot be considered as a mere complex of tissues, organs, and functions, nor can it be evaluated in the same way as the body of animals; rather it is a constitutive part of the person who manifests and expresses himself through it.[22]

This is the basic approach of John Paul II, for example, in the opening of his *Theology of the Body*, where he points out that the Book of Genesis indicates man's *difference from* the animals:

Although man is so strictly tied to the visible world, nevertheless the biblical narrative does not speak of his likeness with the rest of creatures, but only with God ("God created man in his image; in the image of God he created him," Gen 1:27). In the cycle of the seven days of creation, a precise step-by-step progression is evident; man, by contrast, is not created according to a natural succession, but the Creator seems to halt before calling him to existence, as if he entered back into himself to make a decision: "Let us make man in our image, in our likeness" (Gen 1:27).[23]

Here the pope makes the point that man is different *in kind* from the animals, a point that does not fully come across in the Aristotelian definition. Whereas Aristotle correctly points out that "rational nature" distinguishes man from the *animals* as his closest genus, John Paul II emphasizes that man is a *person* and is distinguished in Genesis from the Divine Persons in various ways; for example, by being embodied (although later the Second Person of the Trinity will take on a body also), and by being contingent, that is, by existing as a limited being.

It is important to note that, for John Paul II, even our bodies are different in kind from the animals, and our bodies are integral to the image of God that we are. Our bodies, according to the pope, have a spousal meaning, which the animals lack, namely, the ability to express love. This becomes very clear in the case of sexual relations, where for animals sex is exclusively for reproduction, but for persons sex is for procreation and also to foster, express, deepen, and renew the love between the spouses.

---

22. Congregation for the Doctrine of the Faith, *Donum Vitae* (1987), introduction, no. 3.
23. John Paul II, *Man and Woman He Created Them*, 135 (Audience 2:4).

The human body, with its sex—its masculinity and femininity—seen in the very mystery of creation, is not only a source of fruitfulness and procreation, as in the whole natural order, but contains "from the beginning" the "spousal" attribute, that is, *the power to express love: precisely that love in which the human person becomes a gift* and—through this gift—fulfills the very meaning of his being and existence.[24]

Returning to the Greek roots of the dignity of persons: before Aristotle, Socrates (469–399 BC) taught that it is better to suffer injustice than to commit injustice. By this he meant that the harm done to oneself *by* oneself in committing immoral deeds is a worse harm than that done to oneself when another commits an immoral deed *against* one. This is because a person who commits immoral actions *by means of those very acts* turns himself into a morally bad person. Socrates pointed out, however, that simply undergoing bad treatment does not make one into an evil person. Put simply, if someone robs you, that event does not turn you (the victim) into an evil person; whereas, if you rob someone, that act of theft has an effect on you: it makes you morally bad, it turns you into a dishonest human being. Likewise, the performance of morally good actions has an effect on the one who performs them, making him or her into a person with morally good character traits.

Socrates taught that a person who has become morally bad has an "unhealthy soul" and that one who has become morally good has a "healthy soul." In his view, a person's most important goal is having a healthy soul. He taught that since the soul becomes unhealthy by acting unjustly, it follows that if one were somehow faced with the choice, for example, between being a thief or being the one robbed, one would be much better off choosing to be the one robbed, so as not to ruin the health of one's soul by stealing.[25]

The Second Vatican Council document *Gaudium et Spes* is in perfect agreement with this Socratic insight, holding that the effect of morally bad actions on the agent's

---

24. Ibid., 185–86 (Audience 15:1). Another text in which John Paul II expresses his idea that the Aristotelian approach is correct but incomplete is this one: "Contemporary mentality has become accustomed to think and speak about sexual drives, thereby transferring to the terrain of human reality what is proper to the world of living beings, to the *animalia*. Now, a deepened reflection on the concise text of Genesis 1–2 allows us to show with certainty and conviction that 'from the beginning' a clear and unambiguous boundary is drawn between the world of the animals (*animalia*) and man created in the image and likeness of God.... Thus, *the application to man* of this *category*, a substantially naturalistic one, which is contained in the concept and expression of '*sexual drive*,' *is not entirely appropriate and adequate*. Of course, one can apply this term on the basis of a certain analogy; in fact, man's particularity in comparison with the whole world of living beings (*animalia*) is not such that, understood from the point of view of species, he cannot be qualified in a fundamental way as an *animal* as well, but as an *animal rationale* [rational animal]. For this reason, despite this analogy, the application of the concept of 'sexual drive' to man—given the dual nature in which he exists as male and female—nevertheless greatly limits and in some sense 'diminishes' what the same masculinity-femininity is in the personal dimension of human subjectivity. It limits and 'diminishes' also that for which both, the man and the woman, unite so as to be one flesh (see Gen 2:24). To express this appropriately and adequately, one must also use *an analysis different from the naturalistic one*" (*Man and Woman He Created Them*, 437–38 [Audience 80:3–4], emphasis in original).

In order to understand the "different analysis" referred to in the quotation, this article is very helpful: Karol Wojtyła, "Subjectivity and the Irreducible in the Human Being," in *Person and Community: Selected Essays*, trans. Theresa Sandok, OSM (New York: Peter Lang, 2008), 209–217. This article is available online: http://robertaconnor.blogspot.com/2012/07/karol-wojtyla-person-and-community_29.html.

25. See Socrates's argument about this point with Thrasymachus in book I of *The Republic of Plato*, trans. Allan Bloom (New York: Basic Books, 1991), 3–34.

soul is worse than the suffering inflicted on the person who is harmed. The reason for this is that moral evil is different in kind and worse than the evil of physical or psychological suffering. The passage from *Gaudium et Spes* gives a list of such actions and concludes with this Socratic insight, adding a point about God:

Whatever is opposed to life itself, such as any type of murder, genocide, abortion, euthanasia, or willful self-destruction, whatever violates the integrity of the human person, such as mutilation, torments inflicted on body or mind, attempts to coerce the will itself; whatever insults human dignity, such as subhuman living conditions, arbitrary imprisonment, deportation, slavery, prostitution, the selling of women and children; as well as disgraceful working conditions, where people are treated as mere instruments of gain rather than as free and responsible persons; all these things and others like them are infamies indeed. They poison human society, and they do more harm to those who practice them than to those who suffer from the injury. Moreover, they are a supreme dishonor to the Creator.[26]

We see very clearly the difference between an ethics based on Catholic anthropology and one based on utilitarianism: Since pleasure is the sole good according to utilitarians, and since their idea is to maximize pleasure, they conclude that action based on the criterion of the absolute moral norms of traditional ethics can constitute moral failure, namely, in those cases where it increases suffering or pain. And so, they are willing to violate traditional Judeo-Christian morality if they calculate that doing so will achieve the foundational principles of the utilitarian system. This is the reason for which utilitarian ethics tosses all traditional absolute moral laws out of ethics: it sees no difference between a boulder killing a person and one person killing another person so long as in both cases some "greater good" results.

In some instances, according to traditional Judeo-Christian morality, there will be times when suffering will have to be endured in order to avoid violating the moral law.[27] In these cases, there are two reasons to follow this course: (a) to respect the dignity of the person who would be violated if you broke the moral law, and (b) to avoid becoming an immoral person by violating the moral law. There is a well-known example in which Peter Singer uses his utilitarian method to calculate that to kill a newborn, hemophiliac baby is morally justified on the grounds that, if the newborn is killed, the mother will be able to afford to have another, healthy baby.[28] On the one hand, then, Singer is an ethical relativist in that he rejects moral absolutes, since, for example, he is willing to kill innocents; but on the other, he himself thinks that he is not an ethical relativist, since he is committed to the objective goal of reducing the overall suffering of as many people as possible, at any cost.

As we have seen, the idea, often stated in Church documents, that immoral or harmful actions harm the doer was developed philosophically long before Christian-

---

26. Vatican Council II, *Gaudium et Spes, Pastoral Constitution on the Church in the Modern World*, no. 27.

27. In his apostolic letter *Salvifici Doloris, On the Christian Meaning of Human Suffering*, February 11, 1984, Pope John Paul II expresses a strikingly sensitive awareness to the difficulty of the question of suffering and all possible responses to it. The letter is available at http://www.vatican.va/holy_father/john_paul_ii/apost_letters/documents/hf_jp-ii_apl_11021984_salvifici-doloris_en.html.

28. Peter Singer, *Practical Ethics* (Cambridge: Cambridge University Press, 1993), 186.

ity; it was expressed in Western thought by Socrates, who taught that it is better to suffer injustice than to commit it. This Socratic insight brings to light the fact that there are different dimensions of human dignity, and in particular these two: ontological dignity and moral dignity. Professor Juan Miguel Palacios has expressed this distinction well:

On the one hand, then, the person is partly endowed with dignity by the mere fact of his existence as person, and this fact makes him merit to be treated in a certain manner, which can already be regarded as a form of moral(ly relevant) dignity. But, on the other hand, any person makes himself worthy or unworthy morally in a more proper sense in turning into such or such a person—into a good or into an evil person, as we say in plain English—in virtue of the moral acts which he performs.[29]

And so, with Socrates and Aristotle, we have two basic features of human existence: rationality and morality, which make us ontologically different from, and more worthy than, any beings that do not have these capacities.

In an earlier work, written before he became Pope John Paul II, Karol Wojtyła confirmed this basic Greek insight, observing that it actually reveals that human beings are different in kind from the animals:

In the human person, cognition and desire acquire a spiritual character and therefore assist in the formation of a genuine interior life, which does not happen with the animals. *Inner life means spiritual life. It revolves around truth and goodness.* And it includes a whole multitude of problems, of which two seem central: what is the ultimate cause of everything, and how to be good and possess goodness at its fullness.[30]

---

29. Juan Miguel Palacios, "El problema de la fundación metafísica de los derechos humanos," *Revista de filosofía*, 6, no. 2, (1983): 261; as quoted in Josef Seifert, "The Right to Life and the Fourfold Root of Human Dignity," in *The Nature and Dignity of the Human Person as the Foundation of the Right to Life*, ed. Juan de Djos Vial Correa and Elio Sgreccia (Vatican City: Libreria Editrice Vaticana, 2002), 209n33. Seifert's article is an excellent delineation of four distinct but related sources of human dignity. Seifert's article is available online here: http://www.academiavita.org/_pdf/assemblies/08/the_nature_and_dignity_of_the_human_person. pdf. Leon Kass makes a distinction similar to that of Palacios, between "basic human dignity" and "full human dignity." (See Leon Kass, "Defending Human Dignity," in *Human Dignity and Bioethics: Essays Commissioned by the President's Council on Bioethics* (Washington, D.C.: President's Council on Bioethics, 2008), 297–331.) Kass holds that all human beings have basic human dignity, whereas full human dignity entails an accomplishment, for example, to become morally good. Basic human dignity grounds the right to life of all human beings. Kass develops the distinction further in a helpful way, showing how the two are integrated and mutually dependent on each other. One possible shortcoming of Kass's analysis is that he defines basic human dignity as "low" and full human dignity as "high," at one point saying, "everything high about human life—thinking, judging, loving, willing, acting—depends absolutely on everything low—metabolism, digestion, respiration, circulation, excretion" (325). Although at points in his article Kass detects rationality as co-present in the low, basic human dignity, I would say that the ontological dignity mentioned by Palacios is inalienable and includes much more than the low features mentioned by Kass. A fuller account of the ontological worth of persons should therefore be included in what Kass calls basic human dignity. Expanding on the ideas laid out in the magisterial texts cited in this chapter, which bring out the ontological sources of the dignity of persons, Josef Seifert has delineated quite clearly various sources of the dignity of persons, bringing out the loftiness of the ontological or inalienable sources which should have been included by Kass in what he terms "basic human dignity." See Josef Seifert, "Is the Right to Life or Is Another Right the Most Fundamental Human Right—The 'Urgrundrecht'? Human Dignity, Moral Obligations, Natural Rights and Positive Law," *Journal of East-West Thought* 3, no. 4 (Winter 2013): 11–31, http://www.cpp.edu/~jet/Documents/JET/Jet9/Seifert11-31.pdf.

30. Karol Wojtyła, *Love and Responsibility* (San Francisco: Ignatius Press, 1993), 22–23, emphasis in original.

The term "person" was not used by Aristotle and Socrates, at least not in the sense that we use it today. As Cardinal Ratzinger has shown,[31] and as St. Thomas Aquinas (1225–1274) explained before him, the term "person" developed because of the interplay between human thought and Christian faith. St. Thomas Aquinas says:

> Although this name *person* may not belong to God as regards the origin of the term, nevertheless it excellently belongs to God in its objective meaning. For as famous men were represented in comedies and tragedies, the name *person* was given to signify those who held high dignity. Hence, those who held high rank in the Church came to be called *persons*. Then by some the definition of person is given as *hypostasis distinct by reason of dignity*.[32] And because subsistence in a rational nature is of high dignity,[33] therefore every individual of the rational nature is called a *person*. Now the dignity of the divine nature excels the dignity of every other nature; and thus the name *person* preeminently belongs to God.[34]

Cardinal Ratzinger has explained the history of the term person by pointing out that Tertullian (c. 160–c. 225) defined God as *una substantia—tres personae* (one substance—three persons), and that with this definition, "the word 'person' entered intellectual history for the first time with its full weight."[35]

Drawing on the work of Carl Andresen,[36] Cardinal Ratzinger explains that the Greek word *prosopon* (and also the Latin word *persona*) originally were terms that meant what we now mean by the word "role" as used in theater. In the dramas of ancient times, playwrights introduced roles, or characters, to speak the drama, in contrast to simple narration. These dramatic or dialogical roles gave more life to the drama, in accordance with the developed literary theory of the time.[37] When Christian theologians who were familiar with this literary theory began to delve into the Scriptures, they made a striking discovery:

> In their reading of Scripture, the Christian writers came upon something quite similar. They found that, here too, events progress in dialogue. They found, above all, the peculiar fact that

---

31. Ratzinger, "Concerning the Notion of Person in Theology."

32. Here St. Thomas is referring to Alexander of Hales (c. 1183–1245), who said, "The person is a substance which is distinguished through a property related to dignity." See Alexander of Hales, *Glossa*, 1, 23, 9.

33. Here St. Thomas is recalling the definition of person given by Boethius (480–524), "Person is an individual substance of a rational nature," in Latin, "*Persona est rationalibis naturae individua substantia.*" See Boethius, *Contra Eutychen et Nestroium*, ch. 3. Boethius's definition of person is the foundation out of which Christian reflection on the matter, since his time on, has been based. Note that in his definition Boethius broadens the proximate genus to the category of substance, whereas Aristotle had used animal. We will see as we proceed through to the Christian understanding of person to our present day, that while John Paul II accepts the Boethian definition, he broadens it dramatically to include dimensions of personal being that had not been discussed by Boethius, or by many of the commentators on his definition.

34. St. Thomas Aquinas, *Summa theologiae* I, q. 29, a. 3, ad 2. All quotes are taken from *Summa theologica*, trans. the Fathers of the English Dominican Province (New York: Benzinger Brothers, 1947).

35. Ratzinger, "Concerning the Notion of Person in Theology," 440. For two other helpful and recent tracings of the history of the term person to its current meaning, see also, Josef Seifert, *Essere e Persona* (Milan: Vita e Pensiero, 1989), ch. 9; and Joseph Koterski, SJ, "Boethius and the Theological Origins of the Concept of Person," *American Catholic Philosophical Quarterly* 78, no. 2 (Spring 2004): 203–24.

36. Carl Andresen, "Zur Entstehung und Geschichte des Trinitarischen Personenbegriffs" [On the origin and history of the Trinitarian concept of person], *Zeitschrift für die Neutestamentliche Wissenschaft* 52 (1961): 1–38.

37. See Ratzinger, "Concerning the Notion of Person in Theology," 441.

God speaks in the plural or speaks with himself (e.g., "Let *us* make man in our image and likeness," or God's statement in Genesis 3, "Adam has become like one of *us*," or Psalm 110, "The Lord said to my Lord," which the Greek Fathers take to be a conversation between God and his Son). The Fathers approach this fact, namely, that God is introduced in the plural as speaking with himself, by means of prosopographic exegesis which thereby takes on a new meaning. Justin [Martyr], who wrote in the first half of the second century (d. 165), already says: "The sacred writer introduces different *prosopa*, different roles." However, now the word no longer means "roles," because it takes on a completely new reality in terms of faith in the Word of God. The roles introduced by the sacred writer are realities, they are dialogical realities. The word "*prosopon*" = "role" is thus at the transitional point where it gives birth to the idea of person.[38]

This historical development of the term "person" has profound implications for understanding the dignity of persons. St. Thomas Aquinas, and Boethius before him, focused on rationality as the source of personal dignity. Boethius defined "person" as "an individual substance of a rational nature."

Western philosophy has long pointed to the rational nature of human beings as the basis for their lofty worth, or dignity, which grounds the moral respect owed to all people. This means that any being who possesses rational nature is owed absolute respect. But what is "rational nature"? The exact definition differs somewhat among the philosophers who have defended it, but their explanations share a few key elements.

First, rational nature includes the ability to transcend oneself in such a way as to relate meaningfully to the whole world. We perform acts of self-transcendence through our intellect, will, and affections. These dimensions of the human person are called "faculties" or "capacities," and they allow us to relate to the world outside of us and to other people in meaningful ways. St. Bonaventure (c. 1217–1274), a medieval theologian who understood the faculties of the soul in this way, used them to describe the nature of wisdom:

Wisdom is a light coming down from the Father of Lights within the soul, and by radiating through it made it in the form of God and the house of God. This descending light makes the intellective power beautiful, the affective power delightful, and the operative power strong.[39]

---

38. Ibid.

39. Quoted in John R. White, "St. Bonaventure and the Problem of Doctrinal Development," *The American Philosophical Quarterly* 85, no. 1 (Winter 2011): 191. White gives the original Latin as follows: "*Coll. In Hex.* 2 n. 1V, 336a: 'sapientia est lux descendens a Patre luminum in animam et radians in eam facit animam deiformem et domum Dei. Ista lux descendens facit intellectivam speciosam, affectivam amoenam, operativam robustam.'" This issue of *The American Catholic Philosophical Quarterly*, edited by Timothy B. Noone, is dedicated entirely to the thought of St. Bonaventure. In his introduction, Noone explains that St. Bonaventure is "one of the greatest of medieval philosophers," but that "[p]erhaps no other medieval figure has been so undeservedly neglected," and expresses his "sincere hope that this collection will once more draw Bonaventure into the discussion of our medieval inheritance, whether within the history of medieval philosophy or theology or in contemporary thought and its critical evaluation" ("editor's introduction," 5–6).

It is often said that in their philosophical and theological writings, St. Thomas Aquinas (1225–1275) gives a primacy to knowledge, and St. Bonaventure (1217–1274) gives a primacy to love; of course, both doctors emphasize both dimensions of human experience quite deeply. I will occasionally draw on both of these great medieval thinkers in this chapter, and also on the saint who is the source of the emphasis of love in the work of St. Bonaventure, St. Francis of Assisi. A more contemporary author who follows this Bonaventurian three-part understanding of the faculties of the human soul is Dietrich von Hildebrand (1889–1977). Hildebrand has

These three faculties make us different from all other beings in the world. For example, only fellow humans can, using their intellect, follow a lecture, make judgments about it, and ask questions after it. Only humans participate in the moral life, by freely using the will to choose to perform actions, which then lead to character traits that can be called morally good or evil.[40] Only human beings can be moved and then respond with the deepest of emotions to beauty in works of art and in nature, because of their affective capacity.

The idea, then, is that any being who possesses these rational capacities has the lofty worth we call dignity. It follows from this that persons may not be treated in certain ways that violate that dignity. Put simply: since a rock does not have a free will, an intellect, or affectivity, you may kick it without committing an immoral act; but since a person possesses a rational nature, kicking a person is an immoral act.

It is also wrong to kick animals, in part because they feel pain. Animals have a nature that is higher than that of rocks. Anyone who has ever owned a dog, for example, knows well that dogs that spend a lot of time around persons exhibit forms of intelligence and emotions that are similar, though only analogous, to human ones. However, although animals relate to the world around them in a way that rocks cannot, and although they become humanized in a way through spending time with persons, they do not have the ability to transcend themselves in the way that persons do. This difference is one, but not the only, reason why it is incorrect to refer to animals as persons. This is also one of the reasons why animals do not make absolute moral claims on us to respect their lives, or not to buy and sell them, or not to "put them down." It is morally wrong to buy or sell a human person, to kill a person for food or other uses, or to kill a person through euthanasia. Though animals do deserve respect, it is not intrinsically immoral to treat them in these ways.

Self-Transcendence

Animals cannot engage in conversational dialogue; they do not become morally virtuous or vicious, and they do not perceive, become moved by, or respond to the beauty of a sunset. Any being with these capabilities reveals itself as possessing a rational nature; it is thus of a higher rank than beings that lack these capabilities.

Aristotle once said that the human soul can become all things.[41] He did not mean that each human being is infinite, but rather that, since human beings have a rational nature, they can come to know the very essences of things with their minds.

---

written an insightful essay emphasizing the affective power, showing that while the Greeks rightly pointed to the intellect and the will, they were lacking in their development of affectivity as a source of human transcendence and rationality. See Dietrich von Hildebrand, *The Heart: An Analysis of Human and Divine Affectivity* (South Bend, Ind.: St. Augustine's Press, 2006).

40. Max Scheler held this view too: "[o]nly persons can (originally) be morally good or evil; everything else can be good or evil only *by reference to persons*, no matter how indirect this 'reference' [*Hinsehen*] may be." Max Scheler, *Formalism in Ethics and Non-Formal Ethics of Values*, trans. Manfred S. Frings and Roger L. Funk (Evanston, Ill.: Northwestern University Press, 1973), 85.

41. See Aristotle, *De anima*, III.8. Also quoted in Aquinas, *Summa theologiae* I, q. 54, a. 4, obj. 1.

Human beings are open to the whole world, able to grasp the inner essences and meaning of things. This is possible precisely because of the three faculties of rationality; in other words, the richness of our inner lives enables us to be in profound relation with the whole world. In *Love and Responsibility*, Karol Wojtyła explains this concept:

[T]he person as a subject is distinguished from even the most advanced animals by a specific inner self, an inner life, characteristic only of persons.... *Inner life means spiritual life. It revolves around truth and goodness....* [I]t is just because of his inner being, his interior life, that man is a person, but it is also because of this that he is so much involved in the world of objects, the world 'outside.'...*A person is an objective entity, which as a definite subject has the closest contacts with the whole (external) world and is most intimately involved with it precisely because of its inwardness, its interior life.*[42]

The *Catechism of the Catholic Church* describes the human person in this way.

With his openness to truth and beauty, his sense of moral goodness, his freedom and the voice of his conscience, with his longings for the infinite and for happiness, man questions himself about God's existence.[43]

And the *Compendium of the Social Doctrine of the Church* puts it this way:

Openness to transcendence belongs to the human person: man is open to the infinite and to all created beings. He is open above all to the infinite—God—because with his intellect and will he raises himself above all the created order and above himself, he becomes independent from creatures, is free in relation to created things and tends towards total truth and the absolute good. He is open also to others, to the men and women of the world, because only insofar as he understands himself in reference to a "thou" can he say "I." He comes out of himself, from the self-centered preservation of his own life, to enter into a relationship of dialogue and communion with others. *The human person is open to the fullness of being, to the unlimited horizon of being.* He has in himself the ability to transcend the individual particular objects that he knows, thanks effectively to his openness to unlimited being. In a certain sense, the human soul is—because of its cognitive dimension—all things.[44]

In commenting on the way in which the philosopher Max Scheler (1874–1928) expresses the difference between animals and human beings in this regard, philosopher John Crosby says that human beings

can stop considering things as potential sources of food, or as potential dangers, and begin to wonder *what things are in their own right.* With this we begin wondering what things *essentially* are. We begin wondering what the place of each thing within the whole of being is; for what a thing is in its own right, and essentially, is in part determined by its place within the whole. We now set off on a journey that can never come to an end, for we can never encompass the whole of being, and so we can never be finished with understanding things in their

---

42. Karol Wojtyła, *Love and Responsibility*, 22–23, emphasis in original.

43. *Catechism of the Catholic Church*, 2nd ed., trans. United States Conference of Catholic Bishops (Washington, D.C.: USCCB, 1997), no. 33.

44. Pontifical Council for Justice and Peace, *Compendium of the Social Doctrine of the Church* (Vatican City: Libreria Editrice Vaticana, 2004), no. 130, emphasis in original, http://www.vatican.va/roman_curia/pontifical_councils/justpeace/documents/rc_pc_justpeace_doc_20060526_compendio-dott-soc_en.html.

own right; and we can certainly never be finished with loving them according to the value they have in their own right.[45]

This is no way intended to express anything negative toward animals nor does the Church see them negatively—in fact, the Church finds many points of agreement with the environmentalist movement (though not in some of its most radical forms). Rather, it emphasizes that there is indeed a difference in kind between people and animals, which becomes clear when we consider how each relates to the world. This difference then yields an insight into the lofty worth of human persons, which is known as their dignity and which grounds the inviolability of each person.

Consider Peter Jackson's 2005 remake of the movie *King Kong*, in which Kong was portrayed on two separate occasions as being deeply moved by a beautiful sunset. This is depicted in the movie by giving King Kong the facial expressions that humans have when they see such beauty. In these scenes, the character Ann Darrow says to Kong, "Yes, beauty!" Whoever wrote those scenes clearly accepts the basic premise of Western philosophy that having a rational capability is a source of lofty worth. Such scenes are devised to sway the minds of movie-goers into believing that King Kong has much more worth than an ordinary ape. By giving King Kong a dimension of rational nature (affectively sensing the beauty of a sunset), the film's creators display a deep appreciation for the truth that humans and animals are different in kind, and they reveal that appreciation for beauty gives the being that possesses it a higher worth, one that real-life animals do not possess.

If the rational nature of persons is seen as evidence of a lofty worth, it raises the question whether human beings who lack the ability to exercise that rational nature still have dignity. This question is at the heart of Maria Teresa's question to Pope Benedict about her son. This question also arises with respect to embryos, especially the tiniest of human embryos who have not yet formed a brain. This question leads us into the union of body and soul that constitutes the human person and into questions related to consciousness.

Body/Soul Unity and the Question
of Consciousness

Another source of human personal dignity is our existence as both spiritual and bodily realities. The spiritual soul is not the brain, nor are the intellect, will, and affective powers. These elements of the human person cannot be identified with the brain or with any other material dimension of our body. The brain is something physical: grey matter, blood, synapses, etc. These parts of the brain are all things that can be seen under a microscope; whereas the intellect and the soul *are not physical*. The spiritual soul is real, but it is in no way material.

---

45. John F. Crosby, "The Human Person as *Gottsucher* in the Thought of Max Scheler," in *El Amor a La Verdad: Toda Verdad y en Todas Las Cosas. Ensayos en Honor de Josef Seifert, a Sus 65 Años de Edad/The Love of Truth, Every Truth and in Every Thing, Essays in Honor of Josef Seifert on His 65th Birthday*, ed. Carlos Augusto (Santiago, Chile: Pontificia Universidad Católica de Chile, 2010), 270. Emphasis in original.

This concept may be clarified by a few points about angels. (By the way, even if a reader does not believe in angels, this example is used to convey the *meaning* of the answer.) Angels have an intellect—but they are brainless. Angels have no gray matter, no synapses, no blood, no neurons—and, for that matter, no fingernails. But they most certainly have an intellect, a will, and affective abilities. With these they know, love, and serve God. How can they do those things if they have no brain? They can because the intellect, will, and affective abilities reside in the spiritual soul, not in the brain, and they are all immaterial.

A further question that arises here concerns the exact connection between the intellect and the brain. This is a deep question, and the answer from a Catholic anthropological perspective is this: God created some personal beings (human beings) so that they must have a healthy brain in order for their intellects to fully function. However, other personal beings (angels and demons) are not created that way; they can use their intellects perfectly well even though they are brainless. So the relation between the brain and the intellect is one of *condition* but not one of *causality*. Our brain is not the cause of our intellect; it is simply a condition for its full functioning when we are embodied.

Thus, Pope Benedict's answer to Maria Teresa clarifies the fact that, although her son's brain is so damaged that his intellect cannot function fully, this does not mean either that his intellect is gone or that he is gone. It means only that he cannot fully utilize his intellect, which nonetheless remains a faculty of his spiritual soul, which is still present. Maria Teresa's son is alive and is fully a person, even though he is wounded. When he dies, his soul will be separated from his body, awaiting the resurrection. At the resurrection, he will be restored, in a glorified state, to the bodily/spiritual union that is Francesco.

John Paul II expressed this concept in a 2004 statement:

I feel the duty to reaffirm strongly that the intrinsic value and personal dignity of every human being do not change, no matter what the concrete circumstances of his or her life. A man, even if seriously ill or disabled in the exercise of his highest functions, is and always will be a man, and he will never become a "vegetable" or an "animal." Even our brothers and sisters who find themselves in the clinical condition of a "vegetative state" retain their human dignity in all its fullness.[46]

This is a clear answer to the difficult question of the unity and integrity of body and soul, as addressed from a Catholic anthropological perspective. For this anthropological reason—namely, that the person is fully present, though in a wounded state—the moral teaching of the Church calls for continual loving and medical care (ordinary means), and rejects the killing of these patients by either passive or active euthanasia (which will be defined in a later chapter). Romano Guardini once expressed the reason for this quite concisely, when he said: "The prohibition against taking human

46. He said this in an address, "To the Participants in the International Congress on 'Life-Sustaining Treatments and Vegetative State: Scientific Advances and Ethical Dilemmas,'" given March 20, 2004. http://w2.vatican.va/content/john-paul-ii/en/speeches/2004/march/documents/hf_jp-ii_spe_20040320_congress-fiamc.html.

life expresses in the most acute form the prohibition of treating a man as if he were a thing."[47]

Personal Uniqueness

The rational nature of persons is not the sole source of their dignity. One phrase that appears frequently in the pre-papal and papal writings of both John Paul II and Benedict XVI, as well as in the *Compendium of the Social Doctrine of the Church,* is "the uniqueness and unrepeatability of persons." This phrase reveals another source of the dignity of persons, one deeply related to their rational nature, but not identical to it. In one of his pre-papal writings, John Paul II emphasized this point:

> The person would be an individual whose nature is rational—according to Boethius's full definition *persona est rationalis naturae individua substantia*. Nevertheless, in our perspective it seems clear that neither the concept of the "rational nature" nor that of its individualization seems to express fully the specific completeness expressed by the concept of person. The completeness we are speaking of here seems to be something that is unique in a very special sense rather than concrete. In everyday use we may substitute for a person the straightforward [term] "somebody." It serves as a perfect semantic epitome because of the immediate connotations it brings to mind—and with them the juxtaposition and contrast to "something."[48]

Wojtyła does not reject Boethius's definition of person, since all persons have a rational nature that is a source of human dignity.[49] Yet he asserts that the definition is insufficient, as it is not an *exhaustive* definition of personal being. Boethius's definition is a general statement about all people, and is therefore incapable of expressing the uniqueness of each person, since it expresses only a trait common to all persons.

We all know that to focus exclusively on one trait of another person is to ignore, and possibly even to violate, that person. A very serious case of this is racism, in which a person's race is used as a reason to ignore or mistreat that person. Another case would be treating people with disabilities in disrespectful ways. It is interesting to note, however, that not only neutral facts like skin color, or unfortunate facts like the inability to walk, but also positive facts, if focused on *exclusively*, can cause us to violate others. If we like another person only insofar as they help our team win, but would ignore them if they were not proficient at the sport in question, we overlook the person. In Wojtyła's view, Boethius's definition does not deliberately disrespect people but, if taken as exhaustive, it will unavoidably overlook people. This is so be-

---

47. Romano Guardini, "I diritti del nascituro," *Studi cattolici* (May/June 1974), quoted in Joseph Ratzinger, *Christianity and the Crisis of Cultures*, trans. Brian McNeil (San Francisco: Ignatius Press, 2006), 69.

48. Karol Wojtyła, *The Acting Person*, trans. A. Potocki, ed. A.-T. Tymienicka (Dordrecht: D. Reidel Publishing Company, 1979), 73–74.

49. For example, in *Love and Responsibility*, 22, Wojtyła states, "[Man] is a rational being, which cannot be said of any other entity in the visible world, for in none of them do we find any trace of conceptual thinking. Hence Boethius' famous definition of a person as simply an individual being of a rational nature (*individua substantia rationalis naturae*). This differentiates a person from the whole world of objective entities, this determines the distinctive character of a person."

cause, while rational nature is a very noble trait, it is a trait nonetheless and in itself does not capture the unique person. Furthermore, some people cannot exercise their rational nature. This does not mean that they do not possess it, only that they cannot exercise it fully, which was part of the point of Benedict's answer to Maria Teresa. The other part of his point was that the boy, in all of his uniqueness, is still there.

Another contemporary writer who upholds the dignity inherent in a person's uniqueness is Christoph Cardinal Schönborn. In his book *God's Human Face*, Cardinal Schönborn makes the point that the theological developments of the fourth century "are among the greatest feats in the history of human thought," and he adds that the most prominent feature of their developments was the concept of person.[50]

With this definition of personhood, there is initiated a transition that becomes understandable only against the background of the Christian conception of man: the particular individual, and the unique reality of this singular human being, moves to the center of interest. No longer is the generality of the essence deemed the higher reality, but rather the individual personality.... The uniqueness of the individual no longer is seen so much as a restriction because limited, of a necessarily general essence—a basic tendency of Greek philosophy—but rather as the more important and significant reality.... What triggered and motivated this process was without doubt the awareness, within the context of Judeo-Christian revelation, that each man is unique.[51]

Putting together these passages of John Paul II and Schönborn, one could say that Boethius's definition of person expresses a truth about all persons, namely, that they have a rational nature. However, this definition is still too strongly influenced by the Greek tendency to focus on generalities, and it thereby overlooks the actual heart of personal being.

To further plumb John Paul II's meaning on this matter, we can note a term that appears over and over again in his writings. This term appears in two distinct formulations: "the mystery of *the* person" and "the mystery of *each* person." Wojtyła holds that this mystery of persons ultimately is revealed to us in Christ; and he explains it philosophically in a way that is accessible to believers and non-believers alike. In a February 1968 letter to Henri de Lubac, Karol Wojtyła wrote:

I devote my very rare free moments to a work that is close to my heart and devoted to the metaphysical sense and mystery of the PERSON. It seems to me that the debate today is being played on that level. The evil of our times consists in the first place in a kind of degradation, indeed a pulverization, of the fundamental uniqueness of each human person. This evil is even much more of the metaphysical order than of the moral order. To this disintegration, planned at times by atheistic ideologies, we must oppose, rather than sterile polemics, a kind of "recapitulation" of the inviolable mystery of the person.[52]

50. Christoph Schönborn, *God's Human Face*, trans. Lothar Krauth (San Francisco: Ignatius Press, 1994), 14, see also 14–28.

51. Ibid., 21–22.

52. A section of a personal letter from Wojtyła to Henri de Lubac, quoted in Henri de Lubac, *At the Service of the Church: Henri de Lubac Reflects on the Circumstances that Occasioned His Writings*, trans. Anne Elizabeth Englund (San Francisco: Ignatius Press, 1989), 171–72.

The first of Wojtyła's formulations—the mystery of *the* person—is a general one. It describes the person's status—in religious terms, as the highest point in the created world explained in Genesis; in non-religious terms, as the loftiness of our nature. The intellect, will, and affections of human persons allow them to transcend themselves, to find the truth in knowledge; to seek the good through practice of the virtues; and to rejoice in the beautiful, through the appreciation of such things as a beautiful sunset. This nature *is* a reason why human persons have lofty worth and are deserving of moral respect.

John Paul's second formulation—the mystery of *each* person—refers to *the individual* mystery of every unique person. Thus, another profoundly deep source of the person's lofty worth is his or her uniqueness.[53] One way to understand this is to ask yourself why you love a person whom you love. If asked to come up with a few sentences that explain why you love a particular person, you might answer "it's because of their laugh" or "I love their walk." But it is not the laughter or the walking as such that one loves—it is the *person* who is laughing or walking, who is *expressed in* the laugh or the walk, whom you love. That laughter or walk expresses the uniqueness of the person. While all forms of love (friendship, sibling/sibling, parent/child, spousal) have many essential differences, they share a common thread: they begin with a glimpse of the uniqueness of the other person, which inspires the love, which in turn enables the lover to better appreciate the loved one's uniqueness, *ad infinitum*.

Our rational nature is indeed an intrinsic source of the dignity at the foundation of the moral respect owed to persons. Yet even a rational nature *as such* is not a person, even though there is no person without a rational nature. No one, upon meeting a new friend or falling in love, declares, "Guess what; today I met another functioning intellect!" or, "I met a free will!" No, they say, "Today I met a person. This person was expressed to me through an intellect and will, a laugh and a walk. Yes, all other persons have these things, too, but I met a unique, new person." One knows the real uniqueness of the people that one loves, and one can abstractly understand that the people one does not know are also unique.

This is helpful in building recognition that in the world there are things that we know but that cannot be expressed in words, and the best example of this is the uniqueness of a specific person. While we may know a reality or even love it, some realities cannot be captured in words.

There is a distinct difference between knowing that a human being has a rational

---

53. While Karol Wojtyła/John Paul II never developed a rigorous philosophy of the uniqueness of persons, the numerous references to this idea expressed in his pastoral and theological texts reveal a striking similarity to and deep absorption of this key, perhaps most important idea. I have collected quite a few of such quotes and attempted to show the relation to Max Scheler's work in Peter J. Colosi, "The Uniqueness of Persons in the Life and Thought of Karol Wojtyła/Pope John Paul II, with Emphasis on His Indebtedness to Max Scheler," in *Karol Wojtyła's Philosophical Legacy,* ed. Nancy Mardas Billias, Agnes B. Curry, and George F. McLean, (Washington, D.C.: Council for Research in Values and Philosophy, 2008), 61–99. Following Max Scheler, John F. Crosby has developed this idea of the uniqueness of persons in a deep and original way; he refers to the uniqueness of persons as their "incommunicability." See John F. Crosby, *Personalist Papers* (Washington, D.C.: The Catholic University of America Press, 2004), chs. 1 and 7; and Crosby, *The Selfhood of the Human Person* (Washington, D.C.: The Catholic University of America Press, 1996), ch. 2.

nature and knowing the very person of another. In his analysis of the philosopher Max Scheler's approach to the uniqueness of persons (Scheler calls this uniqueness the "individual value essence" of people),[54] Joshua Miller puts it this way:

In the first place, coming to know the unique person is at the same time a gaining of insight into her *individual value essence*. This essence comes to us as a distinct feeling in the heart; the person impresses herself on our heart in a way that no one else does. It also often comes to us in our imagination; we literally picture the person, especially her face, as a kind of incarnation of this *individual value essence*.[55]

In order to grasp more fully the relation between knowledge of the heart and health-care ethics, it is necessary to consider yet another source of personal dignity: relationality.

Relationality

The Holy Trinity and Person-to-Person Relationships

John Paul II, while fully granting that rationality is a profound source of personal dignity, nonetheless called the Boethian definition to task for failing to grasp the uniqueness of each person. Ratzinger, while also holding the view that rationality is a source of personal dignity, also criticizes the Boethian definition of person as deficient, but his criticism differs from John Paul II's criticism:

54. Max Scheler, who lived from 1874 to 1928, was one of the original phenomenologists in the circle that included, among others, Edmund Husserl, Edith Stein, and Dietrich von Hildebrand. For a helpful introduction to the life, writings, personality, and thought of Scheler, to be recommended is the special issue devoted to him of the *American Catholic Philosophical Quarterly* 79, no. 1 (Winter 2005), ed. John F. Crosby. Pope John Paul II wrote his *Habilitation* thesis about Max Scheler, and Scheler's thought had a deep influence on John Paul II's work. George Weigel has provided insightful and thorough historical evidence of this through a concise retelling of the interesting way in which Wojtyła came to study Scheler, the reasons for which he translated Scheler's Formalism into Polish, and numerous anecdotal stories gleaned from personal interviews with Wojtyła's brightest students, fellow colleagues, and, of course, with the man himself. See George Weigel, *Witness to Hope: The Biography of Pope John Paul II* (New York: Harper Collins, 1999), 124–39. With respect to Wojtyła's *Habilitation* thesis, which could be considered the equivalent of writing a second doctoral dissertation, I know of no English translation of this work, written originally in Polish. The following are the references for the Italian and the German translations: Karol Wojtyła, *Valuazioni sulla Possibilità di Costruire l'Etica Cristiana sulle Basi del Sistema di Max Scheler*, in *Metafisica della Persona, Tutte le Opere Filosofiche e Saggi Integrative*, ed. Giovanni Reale and Tadeusz Styczeń, trans. Sandro Bucciarelli (Milan: Bompiani, 2003), 248–449. Karol Wojtyła, *Über die Möglichkeit eine christliche Ethik in Anlehnung an Max Scheler zu schaffen*, ed. Juliusz Stroynowski, in *Primat des Geistes: Philosophische Schriften* (Stuttgart-Degerloch: Seewald Verlag, 1980), 35–197.

Karol Wojtyła/Pope John Paul II often expresses his indebtedness to Scheler. Consider, for example, this explanation of his sources for *The Acting Person*: "Granted the author's acquaintance with traditional Aristotelian thought, it is however the work of Max Scheler that has been a major influence upon his reflection. In my overall conception of the person envisaged through the mechanisms of his operative systems and their variations, as presented here, may indeed be seen the Schelerian foundation studied in my previous work" (viii).

55. Joshua Miller, "Scheler on the Twofold Source of Personal Uniqueness," *American Catholic Philosophical Quarterly* 79, no. 1 (Winter 2005): 167, emphasis in original.

Boethius's concept of the person, which prevailed in Western philosophy, must be criticized as entirely insufficient. Remaining on the level of the Greek mind, Boethius defined "person" as *naturae rationalis individua substantia*, as the individual substance of a rational nature. One sees that the concept of person stands entirely on the level of substance. This cannot clarify anything about the Trinity or about Christology; it is an affirmation that remains on the level of the Greek mind, which thinks in substantialist terms.[56]

Whereas John Paul II emphasized the *uniqueness* of each person as missing from the Boethian definition, Ratzinger emphasizes the notion of personal *relations* as missing from the Boethian definition. Relation is just as important and integral to being a person as uniqueness;[57] in fact, it is impossible for unique persons to exist without relations to other persons, just as it is impossible for relationships to exist without unique persons.[58] Of course, Robinson Crusoe can be isolated on an island and in that sense not be in immediate relation to other people. But the fact that God has existed for all eternity as three persons means that it is de facto impossible for there ever to be only one person. Also, the three persons of the Trinity are eternally in relation with each other. In fact, Ratzinger cites late patristic writers who, in their efforts to understand the Trinity (one God and three Persons) and the nature of Christ (one Person with two natures, divine and human), held the view that the three Divine Persons *are* their relations.

According to Augustine and late patristic theology, the three persons that exist in God are, in their nature, relations. They are, therefore, not substances that stand next to each other, but they are real existing relations, and nothing besides. I believe this idea of the late patristic period is very important. In God, person means relation. Relation, being related, is not something superadded to the person, but it *is* the person itself. In its nature, the person exists only *as* relation. Put more concretely, the first person does not generate, in the sense that the act of generating a Son is added to the already complete person; but the person *is* the deed of generating, of giving itself, of streaming itself forth. The person is identical with this act of self-donation.[59]

Theologians have debated, and will continue to debate, the question of how exactly the uniqueness of each of the three persons of the Holy Trinity remains when they are explained entirely in terms of relation. How can a relationship come "before" the terms relating to each other? This is a realm of profound mystery. The glossary entry for the word "Trinity" in the *Catechism of the Catholic Church* puts it this way:

Trinity: The mystery of one God in three Persons: Father, Son and Holy Spirit. The revealed truth of the Holy Trinity is at the very root of the Church's living faith as expressed in the Creed. The mystery of the Trinity in itself is inaccessible to the human mind and is the object of faith only because it was revealed by Jesus Christ, the divine Son of the eternal Father.[60]

56. Ratzinger, "Concerning the Notion of Person in Theology," 448.

57. Cardinal Ratzinger states, "The Christian concept of God has as a matter of principle given the same dignity to multiplicity as to unity. While antiquity considered multiplicity the corruption of unity, Christian faith, which is a Trinitarian faith, considers multiplicity as belonging to unity with the same dignity" ("Concerning the Notion of Person in Theology," 453).

58. John Crosby explains that uniqueness, or incommunicability, is precisely what makes the deepest forms of interpersonal relations possible. See Crosby, *The Selfhood of the Human Person*, 54–58.

59. Ratzinger, "Concerning the Notion of Person in Theology," 444.

60. *Catechism of the Catholic Church*, glossary entry for "Trinity," 902.

This chapter is not the place to attempt a solution to the debate concerning the primacy of distinction or relation with respect to the persons of the Holy Trinity, and so, for our purposes, it is enough to see that the three persons are indeed distinct and that their relations are so utterly foundational to their reality that some of the greatest Fathers of the Church have defined the persons by this relationality. The *Catechism* provides this succinct formulation:

The Church uses (I) the term "substance" (rendered also at times by "essence" or "nature") to designate the divine being in its unity; (II) the term "person" or "hypostasis" to designate the Father, Son and Holy Spirit in the real distinction among them; and (III) the term "relation" to designate the fact that their distinction lies in the relation of each to the others.[61]

Since man is made in God's image, and God is a Trinity of Persons, relationship is also a profound dimension of human personal being, without which our dignity cannot be fully conceived. In other words, since we are truly made in the image and likeness of God (Gn 1:26), and since God is Trinitarian, relationship and communion must not be neglected in any discussion of our dignity. And the idea of persons who are, in their very essence, relational beings has profound meaning in the realms of procreation and end-of-life care.

Since the Persons of the Trinity are defined in their very personhood as relations, and since human persons are made in the image and likeness of God, then relation and relationships must be one of the supreme sources of, and reasons for, the dignity of persons. Of course, human persons are not completely defined in terms of relation, as the Divine Persons are; but this difference between human persons and Divine Persons in no way diminishes the importance of relation to human dignity. Ratzinger expresses the point in this way:

[I]n God there are three persons—which implies, according to the interpretation offered by theology, that persons are relations, pure relatedness. Although this is in the first place a statement about the Trinity, it is at the same time the fundamental statement about what is at stake in the concept of person. It opens the concept of person into the human spirit and provides its foundation and origin.[62]

Referring to the history of the concept of personhood, Ratzinger continues:

First, the concept of "person" grew out of reading the Bible, as something needed for its interpretation. It is a product of reading the Bible. Secondly, it grew out of the idea of dialogue; more specifically, it grew as an explanation of the phenomenon of the God who speaks dialogically. The Bible, with its phenomenon of the God who speaks, the God who is *in* dialogue, stimulated the concept of "person." ... [T]he fundamental phenomenon into which we are placed by the Bible is the God who speaks and the human person who is addressed, the phenomenon of the partnership of the human person who is called by God to love in the word. The idea of "person" expresses in its origin the idea of dialogue and the idea of God as the dialogical being. It refers to God as the being who lives in the word and consists of the word as "I" and "you" and "we." In the light of this knowledge of God, the true nature of humanity became clear in a new way.[63]

61. Ibid., no. 252.
62. Ratzinger, "Concerning the Notion of Person in Theology," 447.
63. Ibid., 443.

The "true nature of humanity" he refers to here means that we are intended to live, as does the Holy Trinity, in relation with God and in relation with one another.

In John Paul II's *Theology of the Body*, he comments on the Book of Genesis, expressing the image of God in just these communal terms:

If we ... want to retrieve ... from the account of the Yahwist text the concept of "image of God," we can deduce that *man became the image of God not only through his own humanity, but also through the communion of persons*, which man and woman form from the very beginning. The function of the image is that of mirroring the one who is the model, of reproducing its own prototype. Man becomes an image of God not so much in the moment of solitude as in the moment of communion. He is, in fact, from the "beginning" not only an image in which the solitude of one Person, who rules the world, mirrors itself, but also and essentially the image of an inscrutable divine communion of Persons.[64]

A few years earlier, in the Vatican Council II document *Gaudium et Spes* (the *Pastoral Constitution on the Church in the Modern World*), the Church also expressed this idea.

Indeed, the Lord Jesus, when He prayed to the Father, "that all may be one ... as we are one" (Jn 17:21–22) opened up vistas closed to human reason, for He implied a certain likeness between the union of the divine Persons, and the unity of God's sons in truth and charity. This likeness reveals that man, who is the only creature on earth which God willed for itself, cannot fully find himself except through a sincere gift of himself.[65]

This is of course reminiscent of Christ's words in the gospel: "Whoever seeks to preserve his life will lose it, but whoever loses it will save it" (Lk 17:33).

This understanding gives rise to the notion of self-donation, of making of oneself a gift to others and to God, which in turn becomes a deep source of genuine fulfillment. It also gives rise to the beautiful idea of persons relating to each other face-to-face, as it were, in "I-thou" relationships, and to the notion of "we." Since God is three persons and not only two, we recognize, as Cardinal Ratzinger pointed out, that we are one human family.

This trinitarian "we," the fact that even God exists only as a "we," prepares at the same time the space of the human "we." The Christian's relation to God is not simply ... somewhat one-sidedly, "I and Thou," but, as the liturgy prays for us every day, *"per Christum in Spiritu Sancto ad Patrem"* (through Christ in the Holy Spirit to the Father). Christ, the one, is here the "we" into which Love, namely the Holy Spirit, gathers us and which means simultaneously being bound to each other and being directed toward the common "you" of the one Father.[66]

---

64. John Paul II, *Man and Woman He Created Them*, 163, (Audience 9:3), emphasis in original.
65. Vatican Council II, *Gaudium et Spes*, no. 24.3.
66. Ratzinger, "Concerning the Notion of Person in Theology," 453.

Knowledge of the Heart and the
Relationality of Persons

It is only with the heart that one can see rightly; what is essential is invisible to the eye.

Antoine de Saint-Exupéry[67]

The heart has its reasons which reason does not know.

Blaise Pascal[68]

Benedict XVI once referred to the "impact produced by the response of the heart in the encounter with beauty, which is a true form of knowledge." While emphasizing the indispensability of exact and precise scientific thought, he said that to disdain or reject that impact of the heart as a source of genuine knowledge would be to impoverish our knowledge. He added that it is a pressing need of our time to rediscover this form of knowledge.[69] Strikingly, in this text he was criticizing *theologians* who have disdained this knowledge of the heart, and who, through their exclusive reliance on rational deduction, miss a profound reality. However, his critique could be applied to all the sciences, and especially, in our day, to the empirical sciences, in particular biotechnology and health-care ethics.

What is this knowledge that comes through the heart, and why would science need to be informed by it? To examine this question, consider a young married couple, pregnant for the first time and filled with excitement, anticipation, and trepidation. They ask each other questions: "Who is this new person?" "What will he or she be like? "How will we raise this child?" Now, in contrast, consider the scientists who create and kill many embryos at a time. For example, in April 2010, a widely reported experiment by scientists at Newcastle University in London revealed that human embryos with three genetic parents had been created in a technique designed to avoid defects related to mitochondrial DNA.[70] In this procedure, two zygotic embryos are created through IVF, and both have their pronuclei removed. The nuclear DNA removed from the zygote whose original egg had defective mitochondrial DNA is implanted into the enucleated zygotic embryo conceived by a donor woman whose egg had healthy mitochondria; the pronuclei from that zygote are discarded. The resultant developing embryo has about 98 percent of its DNA from the original couple and the rest from the mitochondria in the donor egg, thus giving the embryo three

---

67. Antoine de Saint-Exupéry, *The Little Prince,* trans. Katherine Woods (London: Piccolo Books, 1974), 70.

68. Blaise Pascal, *Pascal's Pensées*, trans. Martin Turnell (London: Harvill Press, 1962), §277, p. 163.

69. Benedict XVI, "The Feeling of Things, the Contemplation of Beauty," in *The Essential Pope Benedict XVI, His Central Writings and Speeches*, ed. John F. Thornton and Susan B. Varenne (San Francisco: HarperSanFrancisco, 2007), 49: "Being struck and overcome by the beauty of Christ is a more real, more profound knowledge than mere rational deduction. Of course, we must not underrate the importance of theological reflection, of exact and precise theological thought; it remains absolutely necessary. But to move from here to disdain or to reject the impact produced by the response of the heart in the encounter with beauty as a true form of knowledge would impoverish us and dry up our faith and our theology. We must rediscover this form of knowledge; it is a pressing need of our time."

70. Lyndsay Craven et al., "Pronuclear Transfer in Human Embryos to Prevent Transmission of Mitochondrial DNA Disease," *Nature* 465 (2010): 82–85.

genetic parents. This procedure is immoral on numerous levels,[71] but most telling are these words from Professor Douglass Turnbull, the lead researcher:

What we've done is like changing the battery on a laptop. None of the information on the hard drive has been changed. A child would have correctly functioning mitochondria but in every other respect would get all their genetic information from their father and mother. This technique could allow us to prevent the diseases occurring.[72]

None of the 160 embryos created by the Newcastle team was allowed to live, neither the eighty whose defective mitochondrial DNA was replaced nor the eighty who supplied healthy mitochondrial DNA, which means that 160 human beings were killed in this experiment. The attitude expressed here forgets the fundamental truth that human persons are bodily/spiritual unities in their very being, and that all medical moral decisions must be made based on this truth. Each of the tiny humans discarded in that experiment was a distinct human being with a body and a soul, an utterly unique person. *Donum Vitae* expresses the point this way:

Each human person, in his absolutely unique singularity, is constituted not only by his spirit, but by his body as well. Thus, in the body and through the body, one touches the person himself in his concrete reality. To respect the dignity of man consequently amounts to safeguarding this identity of the man "*corpore et anima unus*," as the Second Vatican Council says (*Gaudium et Spes*, no. 14.1). It is on the basis of this anthropological vision that one is to find the fundamental criteria for decision making in the case of procedures which are not strictly therapeutic, as, for example, those aimed at the improvement of the human biological condition.[73]

There is a clear and striking difference between the exuberant response of the young expectant parents and the lack of any such response from Professor Turnbull, even though both grant with equal certainty that the embryos are new human beings. The young couple represent a contemplative wonderment at the presence of a new person, and the researchers represent manipulative disregard for the persons on whom they experiment.

---

71. See the commentary by Fr. Stephen Wang on Mark Henderson's, "Babies with Three Parents May Be Key to Preventing Genetic Disorders," *Times Online* (London), April 15, 2010, http://www.timesonline.co.uk/tol/news/science/genetics/article7097547.ece, in which Wang reveals the immoral dimensions of this research and unmasks the sophistical use of language: Stephen Wang, "The Distortion of Language in Bioethical Debate," *Bridges and Tangents Blog*, March 11, 2011, http://bridgesandtangents.wordpress.com/2011/03/15/the-distortion-of-language-in-bioethical-debate. For another critique of the research from a moral perspective, see David Prentice, "UK Scientists Clone 3-Parent Embryos," *Family Research Council Blog*, April 15, 2010, http://www.frcblog.com/2010/04/uk-scientists-clone-3-parent-embryos. Prentice's post also contains a helpful diagram showing how the procedure is carried out.

72. Quoted in Henderson, "Babies with Three Parents."

73. Congregation for the Doctrine of the Faith, *Donum Vitae* (1987), introduction, no. 3. This passage is a quotation from Pope John Paul II, *Address at the Conclusion of the 35th General Assembly of the World Medical Association*, 29 October 1983: *Acta Apostolicae Sedis* 76 (1984), 393. *Donum Vitae* is available online, http://www.vatican.va/roman_curia/congregations/cfaith/documents/rc_con_cfaith_doc_19870222_respect-for-human-life_en.html. Accessed, December 14, 2012.

Gift or Product? Man's Relation to
Himself in General

Mindful of Benedict XVI's admonition that knowledge of the heart is an urgent need of our time, we could perhaps say that the attitude of the young couple, as contrasted with that of scientists who create, manipulate, and destroy embryos in the laboratory, is captured in these words from Pope John Paul II. He calls us

to *foster*, in ourselves and in others, *a contemplative outlook*. Such an outlook arises from faith in the God of life, who has created every individual as a "wonder" (cf. Ps 139:14). It is the outlook of those who see life in its deeper meaning, who grasp its utter gratuitousness, its beauty and its invitation to freedom and responsibility. It is the outlook of those who do not presume to take possession of reality but instead accept it as a gift, discovering in all things the reflection of the Creator and seeing in every person his living image (cf. Gen 1:27; Ps 8:5).[74]

A person imbued with this attitude sees creation, life, and other persons as gifts to be received and held in awe. The scientists at Newcastle are imbued with an attitude that could be described as the direct opposite of John Paul II's and Ratzinger's. Their stance is described by Ratzinger:

Man becomes a product, and this entails a total alteration of man's relation to his own self. He is no longer a gift of nature or of the Creator God; he is his own product. Man has descended into the very wellsprings of power, to the sources of his own existence. The temptation to construct the "right" man at long last, the temptation to experiment with human beings, the temptation to see them as rubbish to be discarded—all this is no mere fantasy of moralists opposed to "progress."[75]

Ratzinger's quote asks us to consider these questions: Do we conceive of others as gifts or as products? Do we see others as unique mysteries to be wondered at or as possessions to be manipulated? What we answer to those questions determines whether we approach the world and others as humble co-creatures or as self-proclaimed gods. John Paul II ponders the same general question in the other direction, showing that there has also been a fundamental shift in attitude toward the world which affects our view of persons:

In the field of scientific research, a positivistic mentality took hold which not only abandoned the Christian vision of the world, but more especially rejected every appeal to a metaphysical or moral vision. It follows that certain scientists, lacking any ethical point of reference, are in danger of putting at the center of their concerns something other than the human person and the entirety of the person's life. Further still, some of these, sensing the opportunities of technological progress, seem to succumb not only to a market-based logic, but also to the temptation of a quasi-divine power over nature and even over the human being.[76]

In his first encyclical, *Redemptor Hominis*, John Paul II put it more dramatically:

---

74. John Paul II, *Evangelium Vitae*, no. 83.

75. Jürgen Habermas and Joseph Ratzinger, *The Dialectics of Secularization* (San Francisco: Ignatius Press, 2006), 65. This dialog took place just before Ratzinger was elected pope in 2005.

76. John Paul II, *Fides et Ratio*, no. 46.

The man of today . . . lives increasingly in fear. He is afraid that what he produces . . . can radically turn against himself; he is afraid that it can become the means and instrument for an unimaginable self-destruction, compared with which all the cataclysms and catastrophes of history known to us seem to fade away.[77]

At first blush, this seems to refer directly to the possibility of a nuclear holocaust. However, it can certainly also be applied to the field of biotechnology. This fundamental attitude shift—from seeing each person as a unique gift in the universe, to be treasured and cared for, to seeing other people as products and possessions to be manipulated at will—has the potential to turn man against himself on a grand scale. At the other end of the spectrum, maintaining respect for each person in the fields of health care and biotechnology can build a civilization of love.

These reflections need to be tied to our practice in both beginning and end of life issues, as one attitude or its opposite can lead to very different decisions and actions in those fields.

Applications: Euthanasia and Physician-Assisted Suicide

Peter Singer and His Care for His Mother: Personal Uniqueness and Human Relations in Action

A powerful bit of empirical evidence for the truth and goodness of Catholic teaching on euthanasia can be found, surprisingly, in the words of Peter Singer, professor of bioethics at Princeton University's Center for Human Values, and perhaps the most influential contemporary proponent of euthanasia. When his own mother was approaching the end of her life, Singer hired a team of home health-care aides, spending tens of thousands of dollars to care for his mother, even though she clearly fit his definition of a "non-person human."[78] When asked about his actions by a reporter for *The New Yorker*, Singer responded, "I think this has made me see how the issues of someone with these kinds of problems are really very difficult. . . . Perhaps it is more difficult than I thought before, because it is different when it's your mother."[79]

According to Singer's own long-held views, he should have either killed his mother or not spent any money on her, since she fit his standard of a non-person. In fact, however, he spent a great deal of money on her care, money that his writings indicate should have gone only to those deemed persons according to his logic. Many people, including myself, published criticisms of Singer for this;[80] we were in turn taken to

---

77. John Paul II, *Redemptor Hominis, The Redeemer of Man*, Encyclical Letter, March 4, 1979, no. 15.

78. For Singer's view that many classes of humans, including "profoundly and irreparably intellectually disabled human being[s]," such as his mother was, are not persons and may (and sometimes ought to) be killed, see Singer, *Practical Ethics,* 85–87; and Peter Singer, *Unsanctifying Human Life,* ed. Helga Kuse (Oxford: Blackwell Publishers, 2002), 239–40.

79. Singer made this remark in a profile piece about him by Michael Specter titled, "The Dangerous Philosopher," *The New Yorker*, September 6, 1999, 46–55.

80. See Richard John Neuhaus, "A Curious Encounter with a Philosopher from Nowhere," *First Things* 120 (February 2002): 77–82; Peter Berkowitz, "Other People's Mothers, The Utilitarian Horrors of Peter Singer," *New Republic* (January 10, 2000): 27–37, http://www.peterberkowitz.com/otherpeoplesmothers.htm; and

task on the premise that instances of hypocrisy do not refute a theory—which is true, they do not.[81] That is, Singer's failure to follow his own theory does not necessarily prove it false; many people, for all sorts of reasons, do not follow theories, even true ones, but the theories can be true nonetheless.

But this "critique of the critique" misses the point altogether. The point in bringing up Singer's caring actions and his remark "it is different when it's your mother" is not primarily to accuse him of hypocrisy.[82] The point is, his statement reveals that he *saw* something in *reality* (the dignity of his mother), and it was *love* (which is precisely what is different when it is your mother) that made him see it. The *relationship* with his mother opened his eyes to the truth of her dignity. This new awareness then *influenced* his moral decision making in a profoundly meaningful way: it caused him to behave in a manner exactly opposite of that prescribed by his theory. In fact, in the case of his mother he acted according to the principles of Catholic health care: he refused to euthanize her, and instead he cared for her. His statement offers a glimpse into the idea, discussed above, that relationships are so intrinsic to personal being and personal dignity that they form the very foundation of ethical knowledge. If relationships are ignored, then ethics becomes skewed. One of Singer's critics authored an article titled "Other People's Mothers,"[83] which both conveys the moral blindness of those who make ethics anonymous and also captures with concision the underlying meaning of Singer's "hypocrisy." That is, utilitarianism tries to get us into the position of thinking and feeling about our own family members in the exact same way we feel about the people we do not know, in order to make an unbiased calculation. But the truth is that we are supposed to let the intensity of love we feel for our family members "flow over" into and influence our relations with all people. Pope John Paul II put the point this way: "If the family is so important for the civilization of love, it is because of the particular closeness and intensity of the bonds which come to be between persons and generations within the family."[84]

Singer serves as a flash point in the stark contrast between utilitarian and Christian ethics. He has publically criticized Mother Teresa of Calcutta because she described her love for others as love for each of a succession of individuals, rather than as "love for mankind merely as such." "If we were more rational," Singer wrote, "we

---

Peter J. Colosi, "What's Love Got to Do with It: The Ethical Contradictions of Peter Singer," 2005, Catholic Education Resource Center, http://www.catholiceducation.org/articles/euthanasia/eu0034.html.

81. See Richard McDonough, "The Abuse of the Hypocrisy Charge in Politics," *Public Affairs Quarterly* 23, no. 4 (October 2009): 296–98.

82. It should be noted that the charge of hypocrisy applies more strongly to Singer than to other thinkers in light of this assertion, on page 2 of his *Practical Ethics*: "[E]thics is not an ideal system that is noble in theory but no good in practice. The reverse of this is closer to the truth: an ethical judgment that is no good in practice must suffer from a theoretical defect as well, for the whole point of ethical judgments is to guide practice." Singer himself, then, holds the view that hypocrisy—not actually putting into practice one's ethical theory—is reason enough to reject the theory. Nonetheless, he did not reject his theory, which proved useless in his very own practice. Still, hypocrisy is, in fact, not the main point in the discussion of his remark; rather, the connection between love and ethics is.

83. Berkowitz, "Other People's Mothers."

84. Pope John Paul II, *Letter to Families*, February 2, 1994, no. 13, http://www.vatican.va/holy_father/john_paul_ii/letters/1994/documents/hf_jp-ii_let_02021994_families_en.html.

would use our resources to save as many lives as possible, irrespective of whether we do it by reducing the road toll or by saving specific, identifiable lives."[85] In his view, Mother Teresa was irrational because she did not spend her energy calculating auto accident rates against various speed limit options, since in doing so she could have helped more people. Notice that if Mother Teresa had taken Singer's advice, she never would have *met* the people she helped, she never would have had personal relationships with them. This distancing of people from each other, which characterizes the utilitarian approach to suffering and which stands in contrast to the Christian approach, was captured very well by G. K. Chesterton in his biography of St. Francis of Assisi.

He [St. Francis] was a lover of God and he was really and truly a lover of men; possibly a much rarer mystical vocation. A lover of men is very nearly the opposite of a philanthropist; indeed the pedantry of the Greek carries something of a satire on itself. A philanthropist may be said to love anthropoids. But as St. Francis did not love humanity but men, so he did not love Christianity but Christ.[86]

Perhaps Mother Teresa is a saint whom we deeply admire, not primarily because she put bandages on people, but because of the look she gave each person she bandaged. "Mankind" is not something one can love; individual persons can be loved. Chesterton continues:

To him [St. Francis], a man was always a man and did not disappear in a dense crowd any more than in a desert. He honored all men; that is, he not only loved but respected them all. What gave him his extraordinary personal power was this: that from the pope to the beggar, from the sultan of Syria in his pavilion to the ragged robbers crawling out of the wood, there was never a man who looked into those brown burning eyes without being certain that Francis Bernardone was really interested in him; in his own inner individual life from the cradle to the grave; that he himself was being valued and taken seriously, and not merely added to the spoils of some social policy or the names in some clerical document.[87]

This is not to suggest that social policy is irrelevant; one only has to look at the rich tradition of the social doctrine of the Catholic Church to see how much the Church participates in the debates and discussions of those policies. Rather, this idea at the heart of Christian teaching is that each person is precious and unrepeatable, with his or her own inner life, and is therefore inviolable. All individual actions and all policy decisions directed toward suffering must take this fact into account; individual persons must not be ignored. The utilitarian approach, by contrast, attempts to calculate a sort of quantitative "amount" of mass suffering in order then to diminish that total quantity. That approach rejects the idea that each individual's inviolability is a foundational principle of health-care ethics.

After enduring much criticism for not following his theory in the case of his own mother, Singer finally declared that he acted in a morally *wrong* way by taking care of her.

---

85. Singer, *The Expanding Circle*, 157.

86. G. K. Chesterton, *St. Francis of Assisi* (Nashville, Tenn.: Sam Torode Books Arts, 2010), 4.

87. Ibid., 52–53.

Suppose, however, that it were crystal clear that the money could do more good elsewhere. Then I would be doing wrong in spending it on my mother, just as I do wrong when I spend, on myself or my family, money that could do more good if donated to an organization that helps people in much greater need than we are. I freely admit to not doing all that I should; but I could do it, and the fact that I do not do it does not vitiate the claim that it is what I should do.[88]

While this is a profoundly unfortunate statement in its own right, it also has the problem of answering the wrong question. He responds to the question of *whether* he disobeyed his own dictates, which he obviously had done, which he freely admitted, and which we already knew. But he did not address the question of *why* he had done so. He still has not answered that. Perhaps the true answer to that question is this: Singer was able to recognize that persons, with all of their worth, are still present even when their consciousness is diminished or absent and that there is an absolute moral law not to kill them. Put another way, he realized that the person of his mother was before him still, and his love for her opened his eyes to that fact.

Singer has justified his actions by explaining that his siblings wanted to take care of his mother and so he acquiesced to their wishes.[89] Still, even if that were part of his reason, it begs the question of his meaning when he said, "it is different when it's your mother." Singer probably did not mean that he recognized in her case the innate rational capacity for conceptual thought, which she could use to understand syllogisms if she would just wake up. It is also unlikely that he meant that, in the case of one's mother, one has to consider the wishes of family members who will choose the "immoral act" (according to his theory) of caring for her. It is more likely that his love for his mother opened his eyes to *her*, the very person of his mother, who she alone is and who was before him still, in a vulnerable state; this awareness expanded his ethical knowledge and thus caused him to change his behavior in her case. That experience, then, should have prompted Singer to reconsider his premises and rework his theory, both about the nature of human persons and about the existence of absolute moral laws. Unfortunately, he did not ponder the experience philosophically, but instead abandoned it, going so far as to accuse himself in print of acting immorally by caring for his mother—for the sake, presumably, of saving his theory. As a philosopher, he should not have run from the answer imbedded in his response "it is different when it's your mother"; he should instead have reflected on it. Had he done so, he might have concluded that, in addition to rational knowledge that uses the intellect, another type of knowledge exists—knowledge of the heart. This sort of knowledge is often held in suspicion by people with highly developed rational capacities, but it is no less a legitimate and necessary form of knowledge.

88. Peter Singer, "Outsiders: Our Obligations to Those Outside Our Borders," in *The Ethics of Assistance*, ed. Dean Chatterjee (Cambridge: Cambridge University Press, 2004), 29.

89. For example, Fr. Richard John Neuhaus once pointed out to Singer in a debate that "it is a cockeyed ethical theory that is embarrassed by a son's caring for his elderly mother." Singer responded, according to Neuhaus, by explaining that "the extensive care he had provided his mother was not entirely his idea, that there were family pressures and so forth." Neuhaus commented: "The striking thing is that he was more interested in defending his curious theory than in defending his commendable care for his mother" (Neuhaus, "A Curious Encounter with a Philosopher from Nowhere," 79).

Singer, in his remark, seems to express an intuitive insight into the very answer that Benedict XVI gave to Maria Teresa about her debilitated son: "Certainly his soul is still present in his body."[90]

Are Euthanasia and Physician-Assisted Suicide Compassionate?

If we have no peace, it is because we have forgotten we belong to one another.

St. Teresa of Calcutta[91]

Interestingly, on the question of the morality of euthanasia, both the pro-euthanasia movement and the Catholic Church claim to have love and compassion on their side of the argument. One thing is certain: since they advocate exactly the opposite behavior, one of them must be wrong. But which is it? Does it fit with the nature of love and compassion to end the extreme pain of a suffering person by injecting her with enough morphine to kill her? Or, does it fit with the nature of love never to kill another person? Here it behooves us to ask why a person who is in extreme pain or who is unconscious should never be killed, and why such a person still deserves care and medical treatment. The answer is twofold: First, persons unconscious or in extreme pain are still persons, in just the same sense as those who are not. Second, those who kill people in either of these categories are, by doing so, transformed in a way that is detrimental to their own inner lives and to society as a whole. In other words, from a moral point of view there is no difference between killing a sick person and killing a healthy person: they are both persons with dignity and so is the one who kills them. On this latter point *Gaudium et Spes* is perfectly clear; after listing a catalogue of crimes against life, it asserts that all such actions "poison human society, and they *do more harm to those who practice them than to those who suffer from the injury.* Moreover, they are a supreme dishonor to the Creator."[92]

Such actions have an effect on the soul of the agent that is even worse than the violation and death endured by the person killed. Socrates already knew this. Euthanasia is morally wrong because of both the violation of the vulnerable sick person and the moral evil that accrues to the soul and, in fact, to society when euthanasia is administered.

90. Vatican Radio, "Pope Benedict XVI Answers Questions." Professor Singer, it should be noted, is an atheist, and this experience of his seems to me to confirm the following passage of *Evangelium Vitae*, "The Church knows that this *Gospel of Life*, which she has received from her Lord, has a profound and persuasive echo in the heart of every person—believer and non-believer alike—because it marvelously fulfills all the heart's expectations while infinitely surpassing them. Even in the midst of difficulties and uncertainties, every person sincerely open to truth and goodness can, by the light of reason and the hidden action of grace, come to recognize in the natural law written in the heart (Cf. Rom. 2: 14–15) the sacred value of human life from its very beginning until its end, and can affirm the right of every human being to have this primary good respected to the highest degree. Upon this right, every human community and the political community itself are formed" (John Paul II, *Evangelium Vitae*, no. 2).

91. This quotation is from an essay written by Mother Teresa for the Architects of Peace Project. See https://legacy.scu.edu/ethics/architects-of-peace/Teresa/essay.html.

92. Vatican Council II, *Gaudium et Spes*, no. 27, quoted in John Paul II, *Evangelium Vitae*, no. 3; emphasis added.

The premise that love is a mere sentimental force which can push a moral agent equally in favor of or against euthanasia is false. Those in favor of euthanasia typically argue from love and compassion for their view. But, whatever form of "love" the pro-euthanasia movement refers to, it cannot be that movement of the heart about which the Church—in the passages we have reflected on—and Dr. Pellegrino—in the passage quoted in the introduction to this chapter—are speaking. It must be made very clear that a radical and contrary opposition exists between these two claims to love. This opposition remains hidden in superficial presentations of euthanasia.

The place to begin is to note that love has more than one opposite. The most obvious opposite of love is hatred. Many, perhaps most, people who opt to participate in euthanasia do not have feelings of hatred for the person killed. A second opposite of love is use—that is, the reduction of another person to an object; to use another person is to treat them as if their only worth comes from whether or not they satisfy my interests.[93] A third opposite of love is abandonment. Here we find the primary reason why euthanasia is the opposite of loving a person. This is strikingly revealed in the fact that the request to be killed is actually a plea for two basic things: to be loved and to have relief from pain. As soon as a sick person's pain is managed and/or that person feels loved, the person no longer asks to be killed and is grateful that the request was not heeded.[94] Suffering is an unavoidable and overwhelming fact of life. John Paul II has developed the idea that one of the deepest meanings to be found within it is its ability to "unleash love," which, if realized in individual cases, will eventually result in an entire civilization of love.[95] Yet, we can be strongly tempted to think that people who are sick have lost their worth and do not deserve love and care. For this reason the *Catechism of the Catholic Church* insists: "Those whose lives are diminished or weakened deserve special respect."[96] This is not because they are worth more than the healthy, but because it is too easy for the healthy to forget that the ill or weak still have all of their personal dignity. As soon as love comes into the picture, the right attitude toward individuals returns, and that attitude never includes killing a person and always includes caring for a person.

In his first encyclical letter, *Deus Caritas Est*, Pope Benedict XVI said this in the context of his discussion of health-care professionals:

Going beyond exterior appearances, I perceive in others an interior desire for a sign of love, of concern. This I can offer them not only through the organizations intended for such purposes.... Seeing with the eyes of Christ, I can give to others much more than their outward necessities; I can give them the look of love which they crave.[97]

---

93. This is the opposite to love critically analyzed in Karol Wojtyła's work *Love and Responsibility*.

94. For ample evidence of this, see Wesley J. Smith, *Forced Exit: The Slippery Slope from Assisted Suicide to Legalized Murder* (Dallas, Tex.: Spence Publishing, 2003).

95. See John Paul II, *Salvifici Doloris*, nos. 28–30. I develop his idea of suffering unleashing love in Colosi, "John Paul II and Christian Personalism vs. Peter Singer and Utilitarianism." See also Colosi, "John Paul II and Max Scheler on the Meaning of Suffering," *Logos: A Journal of Catholic Thought and Culture* 12, no. 3 (Summer 2009): 17–32.

96. *Catechism of the Catholic Church*, no. 2276.

97. Benedict XVI, *Deus Caritas Est*, no. 18; see also no. 31, on the need for the human look, beyond technical prowess.

Love has a *cognitive dimension* that opens our eyes to the dignity of persons and to the many sources of that dignity.[98] Love also gives us the eyes to see more deeply the goodness of the precise moral indications that, as Dr. Pellegrino notes, are not to be ignored when charity is made paramount.

There is also a broader, cultural reason for the wrongness of euthanasia, namely, that euthanasia necessarily causes killing on a wide scale and thus increases rather than decreases suffering. The link between the legalization of euthanasia and large-scale killing is not correctable through "guidelines," because it follows from an inner and unavoidable logic. Historically, large-scale killing has always followed on the coattails of legalized euthanasia, and the two crimes have a logical connection.[99] Typically, those who argue in favor of euthanasia are keen to promote what they call "guidelines," which are intended to limit the categories of living people who are allowed to be killed legally. This emphasis on "guidelines" is rooted in a certain knowledge of history, for euthanasia advocates will grant that the legalization of euthanasia—for example, in pre-war Germany—can be seen as a causal factor in the building of the concentration camps. They say, however, that humanity can learn from history and that with the proper guidelines such atrocities can be avoided.

But the deeper question is whether there is an intrinsic reason for which legalized euthanasia *necessarily* leads to widespread killings and atrocities. It does, and the reason is this: To kill or abandon one single human person is, in a certain sense, just as horrible as killing or abandoning thousands. Since persons are irreplaceably precious, killing one of them represents a crime of infinite magnitude. Just as in mathematics infinity added to infinity does not make a greater number, so killing many persons is not a "greater" evil in a quantitative sense. It is not the case that immorality kicks in only when a certain death toll is reached.

Dr. Maria Fedoryka put the point this way: "Killing many persons should be understood as a 'greater' evil in the sense that it is repeating many times over an already infinite crime of violating a unique person."[100] So, if the killing of any person is allowable, the sole foundation on which mass killing could be opposed has been removed from the moral analysis. Only a person who understands this can truly bring about what John Paul II calls a "civilization of love."

---

98. Cf. Peter J. Colosi, "Christian Personalism vs. Contemporary Utilitarianism: The Cognitive Dimension of Love and Its Relation to Moral Decision Making," in *El Amor a la Verdad: Toda Verdad y en Todas las Cosas. Ensayos en Honor de Josef Seifert, a sus 65 Años de Edad*, ed. Carlos Augusto (Santiago, Chile: Pontificia Universidad Católica de Chile, 2010), 391–406.

99. Wesley J. Smith provides a detailed historical account of this trajectory as it played out in pre-war Germany, giving ample evidence of the link between the legalization of euthanasia and the move to the concentration camps. Recognizing that it is unlikely that concentration camps will spring up after World War II, Smith considers possible scenarios of how the logic leading from the medicalization of killing to widespread killing might play out in our day. See Wesley J. Smith, *Forced Exit*, 81–106.

100. Maria Fedoryka, Ph.D., email exchange with author in 2004, during the preparation of "Unleashing Love: Why We Care for Those Who Suffer," *Franciscan Way* (Fall 2004): 10–15, http://www.calameo.com/books/0000568542048477sbd68.

Conclusion

The Magisterium also seeks to offer a word of support and encouragement for the perspective on culture which considers science an invaluable service to the integral good of the life and dignity of every human being. The Church therefore views scientific research with hope and desires that many Christians will dedicate themselves to the progress of biomedicine and will bear witness to their faith in this field.[101]

The Catholic Church is in favor of science and has a long history of participation in health care, and she urges her members to continue in these fields with vigor! There are, however, two diametrically opposed approaches that one can take in such participation. The one that dominates our world today is a utilitarian-calculative method of determining rightness or wrongness; it is based on the narrow realm of technological know-how that works on the principle "if we *can* do it, then we *may* or even *must* do it." The utilitarian-calculative method of determining right and wrong means that no act is in itself good or bad and that God and objective moral laws are removed from ethical decision making in biotechnology and health care. When this happens, all that is left is power.

These philosophies are characterized by their positivist—and therefore anti-metaphysical— character, so that ultimately there is no place for God in them. They are based on a self-limitation of the positive reason that is adequate in the technological sphere but entails a mutilation of man if it is generalized. The result is that man no longer accepts any moral authority apart from his own calculations.[102]

This attitude, which Cardinal Ratzinger criticizes, brings about a fundamental shift from thinking of other people as gifts to be received and cherished to thinking of them as products to be dominated or discarded. Stated in the terms we have used in this chapter, the anthropology that is the foundation of utilitarian ethics is a view of the human person that is diametrically opposed to a Catholic anthropology. In a quotation that we looked at above from his dialogue with German atheistic philosopher Jürgen Habermas, Ratzinger described this opposition well, and it is worth quoting again:

Man becomes a product, and this entails a total alteration of man's relation to his own self. He is no longer a gift of nature or of the Creator God; he is his own product. Man has descended into the very wellsprings of power, to the sources of his own existence. The temptation to construct the "right" man at long last, the temptation to experiment with human beings, the temptation to see them as rubbish to be discarded—all this is no mere fantasy of moralists opposed to "progress."[103]

In other words, once this shift has occurred, anything is allowed, and man begins to clone, perform abortions, spawn chimeras, and build atomic bombs. Furthermore, an inner change occurs in the hearts of the people in a society that has accepted this view.

---

101. Congregation for the Doctrine of the Faith, *Dignitas Personae*, no. 3.
102. Ratzinger, *Christianity and the Crisis of Cultures*, 40.
103. Habermas and Ratzinger, *The Dialectics of Secularization*, 65.

If an entirely immanentistic, technocratic worldview is the reigning ethos, then the entire culture will be blind to the anthropological truths about human persons. But, as we've seen in the examples given above, there is a contemplative attitude open to transcendence, which, if present in the ethos of a culture, will open that culture to profound dimensions of reality, including a deep knowledge of the underlying reasons for absolute moral truths. This then will inspire people to strive to live according to those truths because they themselves understand the goodness of those truths for life and society. If medical schools and health-care systems incorporate into themselves a Catholic ethos, this too will result in genuine moral and anthropological *knowledge* as a kind of superabundant fruit of that ethos, which will then enrich the common good.

Let us return to Dr. Pellegrino's words, "Charity does not ignore ethical principles nor substitute vague moral sentiment for rational ethical decisions," and conclude by saying that the many, though not exhaustive, sources of the dignity of persons discussed in this chapter have been deeply thought out by the popes and reflected upon by the Church and Catholic philosophers and theologians, and it is very important that this rich body of knowledge become more well known in the medical field. At the heart of a Catholic worldview is an attitude that engenders openness to seeing these anthropological realities—realities that, quite surprisingly, are occasionally clearly glimpsed by atheists like Singer when genuine love enters the picture. The authors who have explored Christian anthropological truths do not rely on "vague moral sentiment" but have probed the depths of human experience and existence and given deeply reasonable answers to foundational questions surrounding medical and health-care ethics in the philosophical and theological results of their studies. If incorporated into authentic Catholic medical schools, health-care facilities and hospitals, these insights would, I am certain, inspire in the hearts of students and practitioners that which Pope Benedict called for when he said:

Individuals who care for those in need must first be professionally competent: they should be properly trained in what to do and how to do it, and committed to continuing care. Yet, while professional competence is a primary, fundamental requirement, it is not of itself sufficient. We are dealing with human beings, and human beings always need something more than technically proper care. They need humanity. They need heartfelt concern. Those who work for the Church's charitable organizations must be distinguished by the fact that they do not merely meet the needs of the moment, but they dedicate themselves to others with heartfelt concern, enabling them to experience the richness of their humanity. Consequently, in addition to their necessary professional training, these charity workers need a "formation of the heart": they need to be led to that encounter with God in Christ which awakens their love and opens their spirits to others. As a result, love of neighbour will no longer be for them a commandment imposed, so to speak, from without, but a consequence deriving from their faith, a faith which becomes active through love (cf. Gal 5:6).[104]

---

104. Benedict XVI, *Deus Caritas Est*, no. 31.

Bibliography

Andresen, Carl. "Zur Entstehung und Geschichte des Trinitarischen Personenbegriffs" [On the origin and history of the Trinitarian concept of person]. *Zeitschrift für die Neutestamentliche Wissenschaft* 52 (1961): 1–38.

Aristotle. *The Complete Works of Aristotle*. The Revised Oxford Translation. 2 vols. Edited by Jonathan Barnes. Bollingen Series 71. Princeton, N.J.: Princeton University Press, 1995.

Benedict XVI, Pope. *Deus Caritas Est, On Christian Love*. Encyclical Letter. December 25, 2005.

——. "The Feeling of Things, the Contemplation of Beauty." In *The Essential Pope Benedict XVI, His Central Writings and Speeches*, edited by John F. Thornton and Susan B. Varenne, 47–55. San Francisco: HarperSanFrancisco, 2007.

Bentham, Jeremy. "An Introduction to the Principles of Morals and Legislation." In *The English Philosophers from Bacon to Mill*, edited by Edwin A. Burtt, 791–852. New York: Random House: 1939.

Berkowitz, Peter. "Other People's Mothers, The Utilitarian Horrors of Peter Singer." *New Republic* (January 10, 2000): 27–37. http://www.peterberkowitz.com/otherpeoplesmothers.htm.

Catechism of the Catholic Church. 2nd edition. Translated by the United States Conference of Catholic Bishops. Washington, D.C.: USCCB, 1997.

Chesterton, G. K. *St. Francis of Assisi*. Nashville, Tenn.: Sam Torode Books Arts, 2010.

Colosi, Peter J. "What's Love Got to Do with It: The Ethical Contradictions of Peter Singer." 2005. http://www.catholiceducation.org/en/health/euthanasia-and-assisted-suicide/what-s-love-got-to-do-with-it-the-ethical-contradictions-of-peter-singer.html.

——. "The Uniqueness of Persons in the Life and Thought of Karol Wojtyła/Pope John Paul II, with Emphasis on His Indebtedness to Max Scheler." In *Karol Wojtyla's Philosophical Legacy*, edited by Nancy Mardas Billias, Agnes B. Curry, and George F. McLean, 61–99. Washington, D.C.: Council for Research in Values and Philosophy, 2008.

——. "John Paul II and Christian Personalism vs. Peter Singer and Utilitarianism: Two Radically Opposed Conceptions of the Nature and Meaning of Suffering." *Ethics Education* 15, no. 1 (2009): 20–41.

——. "John Paul II and Max Scheler on the Meaning of Suffering." *Logos: A Journal of Catholic Thought and Culture* 12, no. 3 (Summer 2009): 17–32.

——. "Christian Personalism vs. Contemporary Utilitarianism: The Cognitive Dimension of Love and Its Relation to Moral Decision Making." In *El Amor a La Verdad: Toda Verdad y en Todas Las Cosas. Ensayos en Honor de Josef Seifert, a Sus 65 Años de Edad/The Love of Truth, Every Truth and in Every Thing, Essays in Honor of Josef Seifert on His 65th Birthday*, edited by Carlos A. Casanova, 391–406. Santiago de Chile: Pontificia Universidad Católica de Chile, 2010.

——. "What's Love Got to Do with It: The Ethical Contradictions of Peter Singer." http://www.catholiceducation.org/en/health/euthanasia-and-assisted-suicide/what-s-love-got-to-do-with-it-the-ethical-contradictions-of-peter-singer.html.

Congregation for the Doctrine of the Faith. *Donum Vitae, Instruction on Respect for Human Life in Its Origin and on the Dignity of Procreation*. February 22, 1987. http://www.vatican.va/roman_curia/congregations/cfaith/documents/rc_con_cfaith_doc_19870222_respect-for-human-life_en.html.

——. *Responses to Certain Questions of the United States Conference of Catholic Bishops Concerning Artificial Nutrition and Hydration*. August 1, 2007. http://www.vatican.va/roman_curia/congregations/cfaith/documents/rc_con_cfaith_doc_20070801_risposte-usa_en.html.

——. *Dignitas Personae, Instruction on Certain Bioethical Questions*. September 8, 2008. http://www.vatican.va/roman_curia/congregations/cfaith/documents/rc_con_cfaith_doc_20081208_dignitas-personae_en.html.

Craven, Lyndsay, Helen A. Tuppen, Gareth D. Greggains, et al. "Pronuclear Transfer in Human Embryos to Prevent Transmission of Mitochondrial DNA Disease." *Nature* 465 (May 6, 2010): 82–85.

Crosby, John F. *The Selfhood of the Human Person*. Washington, D.C.: The Catholic University of America Press, 1996.

——. *Personalist Papers*. Washington, D.C.: The Catholic University of America Press, 2004.

————. "The Human Person as *Gottsucher* in the Thought of Max Scheler." In *El Amor a La Verdad: Toda Verdad y en Todas Las Cosas. Ensayos en Honor de Josef Seifert, a Sus 65 Años de Edad/The Love of Truth, Every Truth and in Every Thing, Essays in Honor of Josef Seifert on His 65th Birthday*, edited by Carlos A. Casanova, 261–75. Santiago de Chile: Pontificia Universidad Católica de Chile, 2010.

de Lubac, Henri. *At the Service of the Church: Henri de Lubac Reflects on the Circumstances that Occasioned His Writings*. Translated by Anne Elizabeth Englund. San Francisco: Ignatius Press, 1989.

de Saint-Exupéry, Antoine. *The Little Prince*. Translated by Katherine Woods. London: Piccolo Books, 1974.

Habermas, Jürgen, and Joseph Ratzinger. *The Dialectics of Secularization*. San Francisco: Ignatius Press, 2006.

Henderson, Mark. "Babies with Three Parents May Be Key to Preventing Genetic Disorders." *Times Online* (London), April 15, 2010. http://www.thetimes.co.uk/tto/science/genetics/article2477217.ece.

John Paul II, Pope. *Redemptor Hominis, The Redeemer of Man*. Encyclical Letter. March 4, 1979.

————. *Salvifici Doloris, On the Christian Meaning of Human Suffering*. Apostolic Letter. February 11, 1984.

————. *Letter to Families*. February 2, 1994. http://www.vatican.va/holy_father/john_paul_ii/letters/1994/documents/hf_jp-ii_let_02021994_families_en.html.

————. *Evangelium Vitae, On the Value and Inviolability of Human Life*. Encyclical Letter. March 25, 1995.

————. *Fides et Ratio, On the Relationship between Faith and Reason*. Encyclical Letter. September 14, 1998.

————. "To the Participants in the International Congress on 'Life-Sustaining Treatments and Vegetative State: Scientific Advances and Ethical Dilemmas'." March 20, 2004. http://w2.vatican.va/content/john-paul-ii/en/speeches/2004/march/documents/hf_jp-ii_spe_20040320_congress-fiamc.html.

————. *Man and Woman He Created Them: A Theology of the Body*. Translated by Michael Waldstein. Boston: Pauline Books and Media, 2006.

Kagan, Shelly. *The Limits of Morality*. Oxford: Clarendon Press, 1989.

Kass, Leon. "Defending Human Dignity." In *Human Dignity and Bioethics: Essays Commissioned by the President's Council on Bioethics*, 297–331. Washington, D.C.: President's Council on Bioethics, 2008.

Koterski, Joseph. "Boethius and the Theological Origins of the Concept of Person." *American Catholic Philosophical Quarterly* 78, no. 2 (Spring 2004): 203–24.

McDonough, Richard. "The Abuse of the Hypocrisy Charge in Politics." *Public Affairs Quarterly* 23, no. 4 (October 2009): 296–98.

Miller, Joshua. "Scheler on the Twofold Source of Personal Uniqueness." *American Catholic Philosophical Quarterly* 79, no. 1 (Winter 2005): 163–81.

Neuhaus, Richard John. "A Curious Encounter with a Philosopher from Nowhere." *First Things* 120 (February 2002): 77–82.

Noone, Timothy B. "Editor's introduction." *American Philosophical Quarterly* 85, no. 1 (Winter 2011): 1–6.

Pascal, Blaise. *Pascal's Pensées*. Translated by Martin Turnell. London: Harvill Press, 1962.

Pellegrino, Edmund D. "The Catholic Physician in an Era of Secular Bioethics." *Linacre Quarterly* 78, no. 1 (February 2011): 13–28.

Plato. *The Republic of Plato*. Translated by Allan Bloom. New York: Basic Books, 1991.

Pontifical Council for Justice and Peace. *Compendium of the Social Doctrine of the Church*. Vatican City: Libreria Editrice Vaticana, 2004.

Prentice, David. "UK Scientists Clone 3-Parent Embryos." *Family Research Council Blog*, April 15, 2010. http://www.frcblog.com/2010/04/uk-scientists-clone-3-parent-embryos.

Quinton, Anthony. *Utilitarianism*. London: Duckworth, 1989.

Ratzinger, Joseph Cardinal. "Concerning the Notion of Person in Theology." *Communio* 17 (Fall 1990): 439–54.

————. *Christianity and the Crisis of Cultures*. Translated by Brian McNeil. San Francisco: Ignatius Press, 2006.

Scheler, Max. *Formalism in Ethics and Non-Formal Ethics of Values*. Translated by Manfred S. Frings and Roger L. Funk. Evanston, Ill.: Northwestern University Press, 1973.

Schönborn, Christoph. *God's Human Face*. Translated by Lothar Krauth. San Francisco: Ignatius Press, 1994.

Seifert, Josef. *Essere e Persona*. Milan: Vita e Pensiero, 1989.

———. "The Right to Life and the Fourfold Root of Human Dignity." In *The Nature and Dignity of the Human Person as the Foundation of the Right to Life*, edited by Juan de Djos Vial Correa and Elio Sgreccia, 194–215. Vatican City, Libreria Editrice Vaticana, 2003.

———. "Is the Right to Life or Is Another Right the Most Fundamental Human Right—The 'Urgrundrecht'? Human Dignity, Moral Obligations, Natural Rights and Positive Law." *Journal of East-West Thought* 3, no. 4 (Winter 2013): 11–31. http://www.cpp.edu/~jet/Documents/JET/Jet9/Seifert11-31.pdf.

Singer, Peter. *The Expanding Circle*. Oxford: Clarendon Press 1981.

———. *Practical Ethics*. Cambridge: Cambridge University Press, 1993.

———. *Unsanctifying Human Life*. Edited by Helga Kuse. Oxford: Blackwell Publishers, 2002.

———. "Outsiders: Our Obligations to Those Outside Our Borders." In *The Ethics of Assistance*, edited by Dean Chatterjee, 11–32. Cambridge: Cambridge University Press, 2004.

Smith, Wesley J. *Forced Exit: The Slippery Slope from Assisted Suicide to Legalized Murder*. Dallas, Tex.: Spence Publishing, 2003.

Specter, Michael. "The Dangerous Philosopher." *The New Yorker*, September 6, 1999: 46–55.

Teresa of Calcutta, Mother. Essay for the Architects of Peace Project. https://legacy.scu.edu/ethics/architects-of-peace/Teresa/essay.html.

Thomas Aquinas. *Summa theologiae*. Translated by the Fathers of the English Dominican Province. New York: Benzinger Brothers, 1947.

Vatican Council II. *Gaudium et Spes, Pastoral Constitution on the Church in the Modern World*. December 7, 1965.

Vatican Radio. "Pope Benedict XVI Answers Questions on Special Television Broadcast." April 22, 2011. http://en.radiovaticana.va/storico/2011/04/22/pope_benedict_xvi_answers_questions_on_special_television_broadcast/en1-480959.

von Hildebrand, Dietrich. *The Heart: An Analysis of Human and Divine Affectivity*. South Bend, Ind.: St. Augustine's Press, 2006.

Wang, Stephen. "The Distortion of Language in Bioethical Debate." *Bridges and Tangents Blog*. March 11, 2011. http://bridgesandtangents.wordpress.com/2011/03/15/the-distortion-of-language-in-bioethical-debate.

White, John R. "St. Bonaventure and the Problem of Doctrinal Development." *American Philosophical Quarterly* 85, no. 1 (Winter 2011), 177–202.

Wojtyła, Karol. *The Acting Person*. Translated by Andrzej Potocki. Dordrecht: D. Reidel Publishing Company, 1979.

———. "Über die Möglichkeit eine christliche Ethik in Anlehnung an Max Scheler zu schaffen." In *Primat des Geistes: Philosophische Schriften*, edited by Juliusz Stroynowski, 35–197. Stuttgart: Seewald Verlag, 1980.

———. *Love and Responsibility*. San Francisco: Ignatius Press, 1993.

———. "Subjectivity and the Irreducible in the Human Being." In *Person and Community: Selected Essays*, translated by Theresa Sandok, OSM, 209–17. New York: Peter Lang, 1993.

———. *Valuazioni sulla Possibilità di Costruire l'Etica Cristiana sulle Basi del Sistema di Max Scheler*. In *Metafisica della Persona, Tutte le Opere Filosofiche e Saggi Integrative*. Edited by Giovanni Reale and Tadeusz Styczeń. Translated by Sandro Bucciarelli, 263–449. Milan: Bompiani, 2003.

Weigel, George. *Witness to Hope: The Biography of Pope John Paul II*. New York: Harper Collins, 1999.

Reverend Philip G. Bochanski

3. PASTORAL CARE OF THE SICK AND DYING

At the very heart of Christianity is the person Jesus of Nazareth, God, the Second Person of the Holy Trinity, who became man in the course of human history. Among the many realities brought to humanity and revealed through Jesus is, of course, his deep compassion for every person, especially those he encountered who were sick and dying. As the mystical body of Christ, the Church continues his ministry to the sick and dying; her sacramental formulation for this service is the subject of Father Bochanski's chapter. In it he begins with the image of the Good Shepherd and traces elements of pastoral care of the sick and dying to their biblical foundations. He then discusses the ministers who provide care to the sick and dying, which in reality is the call of everyone. Next he shows us the nature of pastoral care, but before explaining its various forms, he first tells us what it is not. At the end of the chapter, Father Bochanski shows how the four effects of the Anointing of the Sick, as enumerated in the *Catechism*, correspond to the four fruits of good pastoral care for the sick and dying. It is important for health-care practitioners to recognize the spiritual dimension of persons who are sick and dying, and to understand the complementary role that pastoral care shares with medical care. For those involved with day-to-day medical care of patients, this chapter provides a refreshing view of the richness of Catholic pastoral care.—*Editors*

Introduction

Over the course of many centuries, particularly since the reforms of the sixteenth-century Council of Trent, the standard text for priests and bishops in the practical exercise of their ministry has been the *Rituale Romanum*, the Roman Ritual. Through all its various editions, its basic structure has remained intact, including the chapter "On the Sacrament of Extreme Unction" (*De Sacramento Extremae Unctionis*), which is followed by penitential psalms and litanies to be prayed with dying persons and then by the section titled "On the Visitation and Care of the Sick" (*De Visitatione et Cura Infirmorum*).

One of the first works undertaken by the Second Vatican Council, which met from 1962 to 1965, was an effort "to impart an ever increasing vigor to the Christian life of the faithful . . . [by] undertaking the reform and promotion of the liturgy."[1] This reform included a revision of the *Rituale* and its division into a number of liturgical books for the celebration of the sacraments. The section dealing with extreme unction underwent several name changes before it was reissued in 1972 as *Ordo Unctionis Infirmorum eorumque pastoralis curae* (Order of the Anointing of the Sick and Their Pastoral Care).

First, as the council itself noted,

"extreme unction," which may also and more fittingly be called "anointing of the sick," is not a sacrament for those only who are at the point of death. Hence, as soon as any one of the faithful begins to be in danger of death from sickness or old age, the fitting time for him to receive this sacrament has certainly already arrived.[2]

Accordingly, the title of the ritual was changed, and now begins *Ordo Unctionis Infirmorum*, the "Order of the Anointing of the Sick." This makes a statement about what the Church believes the Lord calls her to do:

Heal the sick (Mt 10:8)! The Church has received this charge from the Lord and strives to carry it out by taking care of the sick as well as by accompanying them with her prayer of intercession. She believes in the life-giving presence of Christ, the physician of souls and bodies. This presence is particularly active through the sacraments, and in an altogether special way through the Eucharist, the bread that gives eternal life and that St. Paul suggests is connected with bodily health (cf. 1 Cor 11:30).

However, the apostolic Church has its own rite for the sick, attested to by St. James: "Is any among you sick? Let him call for the priests of the Church and let them pray over him, anointing him with oil in the name of the Lord; and the prayer of faith will save the sick man, and the Lord will raise him up; and if he has committed sins, he will be forgiven" (Jas 5:14–15). Tradition has recognized in this rite one of the seven sacraments.[3]

The second change in the title was more subtle, but no less important. Where the previous *Rituale* mentioned the "visitation and care of the sick," the new liturgical book describes this ministry as "pastoral care" (*pastoralis curae*). The use of this terminology, at once so familiar and so nebulous to most people in modern health-care settings, may seem neither significant nor novel at first glance. However, the Catholic physician will be both enlightened and challenged by carefully considering the specifically *pastoral* nature of care for the sick and dying, along with the scriptural and doctrinal meaning of such care. The physician who realizes just what it means to care for a patient in the name of the Good Shepherd and who follows the Shepherd's example is enabled to love as Christ loves and to extend the redemptive power of Christ's passion, death, and resurrection to those who share in his suffering.

---

1. Vatican Council II, *Sacrosanctum Concilium, Constitution on the Sacred Liturgy*, December 4, 1963, no. 1.

2. Ibid., no. 73.

3. *Catechism of the Catholic Church*, 2nd ed., trans. United States Conference of Catholic Bishops (Washington, D.C.: USCCB, 1997), nos. 1509–1510.

The Good Shepherd

From the beginning of his public ministry, Jesus Christ went about through Galilee and Judea working miraculous signs, including healing many people who were sick.[4] The *Catechism of the Catholic Church* tells us: "Christ's compassion toward the sick and his many healings of every kind of infirmity are a resplendent sign that 'God has visited his people' (Lk 7:16) and that the Kingdom of God is close at hand."[5] These healings are not simply acts of power to impress simple minds, but signs of his divinity meant to lead people to faith, "so that the works of God might be made visible through [them]" (Jn 9:3).

Christ likewise gave authority to his apostles to heal the sick in his name, both during his public ministry (Mk 6:7, 13) as they were preparing towns to receive him, as well as after his resurrection (Mk 16, 18), when they were sent out to proclaim the gospel. Throughout the history of the Church, this has been the experience of missionaries "speaking out boldly for the Lord, who confirmed the word about his grace by granting signs and wonders to occur through their hands" (Acts 14:3). So it is no surprise that the first specific "act" that Luke relates following the dramatic events and preaching of Pentecost morning is the miraculous healing of the infirm man by the apostles Peter and John at the Beautiful Gate of the Temple (Acts 3:1ff.). Both of the apostles were accustomed to exercising the healing power entrusted to them by Christ, and, filled with the Holy Spirit for the sake of spreading the gospel, they had a newfound zeal and urgency for putting that power to good use.

But these apostles were not the same men who had been sent out two by two several years earlier, to cast out demons in the name of Jesus of Nazareth and to anoint the sick with oil for their healing. They had been transformed by the events of his passion, death, and resurrection, and by the part they had to play in those events. Peter in particular had been given a special responsibility as a result of that pivotal week's events. Walking along the beach with the risen Lord, Peter was invited to undo his threefold denial of Christ with a triple affirmation of loyalty and friendship. In response to his profession of love, he hears the command to "feed my lambs.... Tend my sheep.... Feed my sheep" (Jn 21:15–17).

Simon Peter is called to be not only an apostle but also a shepherd—in Latin, *pastor*. He who once fled like a hireling who sees the wolf coming (see Jn 10:12) is now commanded to model himself after the "Good Shepherd [who] lays down his life for the sheep" (Jn 10:11). Recognizing the responsibility that the Lord has shared with him and his fellow elders, Peter later exhorts his coworkers in the pastoral ministry: "As a witness to the sufferings of Christ, and one who has a share in the glory to be revealed: Tend the flock of God in your midst" (1 Pt 5:2).

That this pastoral ministry will involve caring for the sick seems obvious from the Lord's general command to all of his disciples to practice the works of mercy. In

---

4. Mt 4:23–25; Mk 1:32–34; Lk 6:17–19; etc.
5. *Catechism of the Catholic Church*, no. 1503.

a parable replete with images of the Divine Shepherd and his flocks, it becomes clear that "[Christ's] compassion toward all who suffer goes so far that he identifies himself with them"[6] and that he demands no less of those who would claim to be his followers: "I was hungry and you gave me food, ... ill and you cared for me.... Whatever you did for one of these least brothers of mine, you did for me" (Mt 25:35–36, 40). This parable was addressed primarily to the apostles; Matthew includes it among several sayings pronounced by the Lord "as he was sitting on the Mount of Olives, [and] the disciples approached him privately" (Mt 24:2–3). But it is clear that these admonitions are addressed to the whole flock, not only to its leaders.

Yet another, more ancient Scripture passage, relating God's words to the prophet Ezekiel, may provide deeper insights into the specifically pastoral nature of the ministry to the sick entrusted to the apostles. These words were directed to the Israelites who had been exiled to Babylon in the sixth century before Christ:

Son of man, prophesy against the shepherds of Israel. Thus says the Lord God: "Woe to the shepherds of Israel who have been pasturing themselves! Should not shepherds, rather, pasture sheep? You have fed off their milk, worn their wool, and slaughtered the fatlings, but the sheep you have not pastured." (Ezek 34:1–3)

The Lord goes on to charge the shepherds with a specific act of neglect, one usually associated in those days not with public leaders but rather with domestic responsibility. "You did not strengthen the weak," he says, "nor heal the sick nor bind up the injured" (Ezek 34:4). The results of this neglect are devastating:

You did not bring back the strayed nor seek the lost, but you lorded it over them harshly and brutally. So they were scattered for lack of a shepherd, and became food for all the wild beasts. My sheep were scattered and wandered over all the mountains and high hills; my sheep were scattered over the whole earth, with no one to look after them or to search for them. (Ezek 34:4–6)

As he has done several times before in salvation history, the Lord decides on a solution to his people's plight:

Thus says the Lord God: I swear I am coming against these shepherds.... I myself will look after and tend my sheep. As a shepherd tends his flock when he finds himself among his scattered sheep, so will I tend my sheep. I will rescue them from every place where they were scattered when it was cloudy and dark.... I myself will pasture my sheep; I myself will give them rest, says the Lord God. The lost I will seek out, the strayed I will bring back, the injured I will bind up, the sick I will heal ... shepherding them rightly. (Ezek 34:10–12, 15–16.)

The Lord thus heals the most dramatic effect of suffering, the reality that links physical, emotional, and spiritual suffering to the mystery of evil and the consequence of original sin: the fact that suffering is *isolating*. The sick and suffering sheep were already in pain, and this reality in some degree set them apart from their family members and neighbors who were well and thus able to go about their regular duties. The prophet's rebuke, however, charges that the neglect of the leaders, who shirked their

---

6. *Catechism of the Catholic Church*, no. 1503.

responsibility to lead and feed those unable to care for themselves, left the suffering sheep further scattered and more isolated. The Lord God steps in to both lead and feed his people. Throughout this passage, God is promising to care for and shepherd his people in his own name: to bring them back, to bind them up, and, by doing so, to heal them.

In the process, he provides a model for the ministry of pastoral care, which is no less necessary in our own day. "How can we forget," Pope John Paul II wrote, "all those who at health-care facilities—hospitals, clinics, leprosariums, centers for the disabled, nursing homes—or in their own dwellings undergo the Calvary of sufferings which are often neglected, not always suitably relieved, and sometimes even aggravated by a lack of adequate support?"[7] We should not for an instant undervalue the immense contribution of the medical arts and sciences to the treatment and alleviation of physical and mental illness in its myriad forms. But pastoral care of the sick and dying acknowledges another reality: the causes of human suffering come from a deeper source than science can discover, and its effects cause deeper wounds than medicine can cure. "The field of human suffering is much wider, more varied, and multi-dimensional," says John Paul II in *Salvifici Doloris*; "Suffering is something which is still wider than sickness, more complex and at the same time still more deeply rooted in humanity itself."[8] The Good Shepherd still appoints his shepherds to work alongside physicians and nurses who treat the body, in order to carry out the work of binding and healing these "more deeply rooted" spiritual wounds.

The Ministers of Pastoral Care

To consider the ministry of serving the sick in the name of the Good Shepherd, it is proper to begin with the question, "Who are the shepherds?" The very words associated with this topic—"ministry," "shepherds," "pastoral care"—make it clear that service to the sick and the dying is part of the work of the Church, and a particular responsibility of the bishops, together with the priests who assist them in the sacramental ministry. At the same time, we read in *Pastoral Care of the Sick*:

If one member suffers in the Body of Christ, which is the Church, all the members suffer with that member (1 Cor 12:26). For this reason, kindness shown toward the sick and works of charity and mutual help for the relief of every kind of human want are held in special honor. Every scientific effort to prolong life and every act of care of the sick, on the part of any person, may be considered a preparation for the Gospel and a sharing in Christ's healing ministry. It is thus especially fitting that all baptized Christians share in this ministry of mutual charity within the Body of Christ by doing all that they can to help the sick return to health, by showing love for the sick, and by celebrating the sacraments with them. Like the other sacraments, these too have a community aspect, which should be brought out as much as possible when they are celebrated.[9]

---

7. Pope John Paul II, Message for the First World Day of the Sick (1993), no. 2.

8. Pope John Paul II, *Salvifici Doloris, On the Christian Meaning of Human Suffering*, Apostolic Letter, February 11, 1984, no. 5.

9. Sacred Congregation for the Sacraments and Divine Worship, *Pastoral Care of the Sick: Rites of Anoint-*

The Church therefore encourages all its members to participate in the ministry of caring for the sick, each according to his or her ability, in a spirit of collaboration. Within the particular sphere of pastoral care there are various dimensions, and it is valuable to consider each of them in turn.

Bishops

The wide-ranging daily work of the bishops often precludes their direct involvement with visiting the sick in hospital or home settings on a regular basis. Nevertheless, the importance of the bishop to the ministry of pastoral care cannot be overlooked, particularly when one recalls the role of the shepherd to lead the flock and bind it together as one. He is required to forge a connection with the pastoral care of the sick members of his flock, a connection made visible in various ways.

The sacramental sign associated with the Anointing of the Sick is the unction itself. Ordinarily, the Oil of the Sick used for the sacrament is blessed by the diocesan bishop in an annual ceremony known as the Chrism Mass, which takes place on Holy Thursday (or another day in Holy Week) and is concelebrated by as many priests of the diocese as possible. In this way, the bishop, who cannot be physically present at every anointing, symbolizes his pastoral care of all of the sick through the priests who collaborate with him in their ministry around the diocese throughout the year.

In addition, "the diocesan bishop has the responsibility of supervising those celebrations at which many sick persons may come together to receive the sacrament" of the Anointing of the Sick.[10] The bishop is also called to provide appropriate opportunities to catechize the faithful on the sacraments and on the nature of Christian suffering. He is further charged with overseeing Catholic hospitals and health-care institutions in his diocese and appointing their chaplains; they in turn are charged to work in collaboration with him. "In order to make the witness of love practical," Pope John Paul II wrote,

those involved in the pastoral care of the sick must act in full communion among themselves and with their bishops. This is of particular importance in Catholic hospitals, which in responding to modern needs are called upon to reflect ever more clearly in their policies the values of the Gospel, as the Magisterium's social and moral guidelines insist. This requires united involvement on the part of Catholic hospitals in every sector, including that of finance and administration.[11]

One of the Greek verbs that the prophet Ezekiel uses to describe the Lord's care for his people—*episkepsomai*, "I will tend"—is also used by Christ in the parable of the Last Judgment, when he says to those on his right, "I was sick and you cared for [*epeskepsasthe*] me" (Mt 25:36). The same verb is the root of the Greek noun *episkopos*—in Latin, *episcopus*—that is, bishop. The Divine Author of the Scripture uses

---

ing and Viaticum (1983), nos. 32–33. For an account of the history of this work, see the section below, "The Forms of Pastoral Care."

10. Ibid., no.17.

11. Pope John Paul II, Message for the Eleventh World Day of the Sick (2003), no. 3.

the same word to name those who will lead the Church to describe the healing care he expects his disciples to show one another, and to illuminate the nature of the shepherd's love for his people.

Priests

In their pastoral work, the bishops are assisted by the ministry of priests; the general introduction to *Pastoral Care of the Sick* specifically names "pastors and their assistants, chaplains of health-care facilities, and superiors of clerical religious institutes,"[12] who have a special responsibility for pastoral care of the sick. "Every priest [*sacerdos*] and a priest alone validly administers the anointing of the sick,"[13] according to the Code of Canon Law. Because the priest is the irreplaceable celebrant of this sacrament and of Confession, and is (along with the deacon) the ordinary minister of Holy Communion, his regular, committed involvement is essential to any authentic plan to reintegrate those isolated by physical and spiritual suffering into the life of the Church. The deep significance of this sacramental ministry of healing and reconciliation must not be overlooked. The U.S. Conference of Catholic Bishops tells us, "Priests are not simply functionaries, workers, or professionals," to be called in at a particular point along a patient's spectrum of care. "Who they are sacramentally, their way of being, is as crucial, if not more so, than their particular functioning."[14] The priest acts *in persona Christi*, "in the person of Christ," the Shepherd who says through the prophet, "I am coming," who has come "to seek and to save what was lost" (Lk 19:10).

Priests, by virtue of their share in the teaching office of the Church, have, in addition to the sacramental ministry, a responsibility to proclaim the "Gospel of Life" to those to whom they minister. In doing so, they not only relieve the suffering of the sick but also help them to understand more deeply their situation in light of the teaching of Christ and the Church. Priests are called to impart this teaching, first of all, by modeling Christian charity, as described in *Pastoral Care of the Sick*:

Priests, particularly pastors ... should remember that it is their duty to care for the sick by personal visits and other acts of kindness. Especially when they give the sacraments, priests should stir up the hope of those present and strengthen their faith in Christ who suffered and is glorified. By bringing the Church's love and the consolation of faith, they comfort believers and raise the minds of others to God.[15]

Moreover, in light of their own intellectual and doctrinal formation, priests must provide solid catechesis to the faithful, helping them above all to prepare for the reception of the sacraments. "In this way," we read in *Pastoral Care of the Sick*, "[the sick] will understand more fully what has been said about the anointing of the sick

---

12. *Pastoral Care of the Sick*, no. 16.

13. *Code of Canon Law*, new English trans., trans. Canon Law Society of America (Washington, D.C.: Canon Law Society of America, 1998), can. 1003, §1. The term *sacerdos* includes bishops and priests (*presbyters*).

14. United States Conference of Catholic Bishops, *The Basic Plan for the Ongoing Formation of Priests* (2001), II.E, http://www.usccb.org/beliefs-and-teachings/vocations/priesthood/priestly-life-and-ministry/national-plan-for-the-ongoing-formation-of-priests.cfm.

15. *Pastoral Care of the Sick*, no. 35.

and about viaticum, and the celebration of these sacraments will nourish, strengthen, and manifest faith more effectively."[16] Once again, the priest's responsibility as pastor—as shepherd—to draw the faithful to a deeper understanding is paramount. He is not simply distributing a talisman but is nourishing the flock; not merely dropping in on a client, but as is the case many times, reaching out in order to draw the individual back into the life of the community. *Pastoral Care of the Sick* tells us, "The prayer of faith which accompanies the celebration of the sacrament is nourished by the profession of this faith,"[17] a faith proclaimed by the whole Church.

This profession of faith finds its living expression in the consistent application of Church teaching, and so the pastoral teaching office of the priest also requires him to speak honestly and directly on matters of doctrine and morality. He will find opportunities to do so in his contact with the sick, both in encouraging those who are ill to live holy lives and be converted, and in helping the sick and their caregivers face ethical choices in treatment and care, especially at the end of life. Regarding the first responsibility, a former edition of the *Rituale Romanum* was firm in its admonition:

Let him be so well prepared when he makes a sick call, that he will always be enabled to speak to the person in convincing terms, using especially examples from the lives of the saints, a practice which proves most beneficial. Moreover, he will admonish the sick to place all confidence in God, to repent of sin, to implore the divine mercy, to bear patiently the pains of illness, believing them to be a fatherly visitation from God and conducive to salvation, a means for reforming his life.[18]

When the priest is dealing with questions of medical ethics, preparation is no less necessary. He must not simply rely on a course or two in the seminary but must do his best to keep informed of developments in medicine and in the teaching of the Church. He should also be familiar with the *Ethical and Religious Directives for Catholic Health Care Services,* which is published by the United States Conference of Catholic Bishops and regularly updated.[19] All of this presupposes a solid foundation during the priest's initial seminary formation and a commitment to ongoing formation on the part of both the individual priest and the diocese. "Proper attention," Pope John Paul II insisted, "should be given to the pastoral aspect of health care in the formation of priests and religious. For it is in care for the sick more than in any other way that love is made concrete and a witness of hope in the Resurrection is offered."[20]

16. Ibid., no. 36.

17. Ibid.

18. *Rituale Romanum: De Visitatione et Cura Infirmorum*, no. 7, quoted in *The Roman Ritual in Latin and English*, vol. 1, *The Sacraments and Processions*, trans. and ed. Rev. Philip T. Weller (Milwaukee Wisc.: Bruce, 1952), 375.

19. United States Conference of Catholic Bishops, *Ethical and Religious Directives for Catholic Health Care Services*, 5th ed. (Washington, D.C.: USCCB, 2009).

20. Pope John Paul II, Message for the Eleventh World Day of the Sick (2003), no. 5.

Deacons

The pastoral ministry of priests is supported and enriched by the collaboration of deacons, who also share in the sacrament of Holy Orders, which the Congregation for the Clergy tells us "brings about in the one who receives it a specific conformation to Christ, Lord and servant of all."[21] The important ministry of deacons must not be reduced to their being simply "other ministers" of Holy Communion and of blessings, who can fill in when priests are not available. They can and often do take on these roles, as well as more formal roles in organized pastoral care teams, and so what has been said above about the initial and ongoing formation of priests applies as well to deacons. But the diaconal ministry also has its own particular contribution to make to the life of the Christian community.

The apostles themselves ordained the first deacons to carry out works of charity, literally gathering, feeding, and tending to the needs of widows and the elderly. In this way, the pastoral ministry itself was enriched and safeguarded, and the weakest members of the community were assured of the concern of the Twelve (cf. Acts 6:1–6). The service of deacons to the sick, particularly to the housebound members of a parish, gives witness to the constant concern of the Church for the weakest of her members—the deacons are sent, not as hired employees of the parish, but as ordained collaborators with the bishop, to represent the shepherd to each member of his flock. "Permanent" deacons—that is, those who, married or celibate, live in the world and have secular occupations—become a special bridge between the community and the bishop, and between the pastor and his flock, as they live among the people and take special note of the needs of their neighbors. In all of this, they carry out not only works of charity but also the mission of evangelization, giving witness to the truth of the gospel that Christ has come to draw all people to himself, to raise up the fallen and heal all wounds.

Consecrated Men and Women

The ministry to the sick provided by ordained clergy—bishops, priests, and deacons—is supported and enriched by the dedicated collaboration of countless consecrated men and women, who dedicate their lives in service to the Church through their vows of poverty, chastity, and obedience. The one Church is blessed with an enormous diversity of institutes of consecrated life and societies of apostolic life, many of them entrusted by their founders with special charisms for serving the poor, the sick, and the dying. Indeed, many religious congregations were founded for the specific purpose of providing practical and pastoral care to the sick and the dying; in some cases they were the only health-care providers for the communities they served. In addition to hands-on care, many religious have been—individually or corporately—founders and

---

21. Congregation for Clergy and Congregation for Catholic Education, *Basic Norms for the Formation of Permanent Deacons*, February 22, 1998, no. 5.

administrators of hospitals, nursing homes, and other health-care institutions, and some maintain that role, although modern systems of reimbursement and administration make this increasingly difficult.

The contribution of consecrated men and women to the ministry of pastoral care is specified by the very nature of their vocation, by the unique purpose of their consecration. By professing the evangelical counsels of poverty, chastity, and obedience, religious take on a role of service toward the Church. Their profession is, according to the Second Vatican Council's *Lumen Gentium*,

a sign which can and ought to attract all the members of the Church to an effective and prompt fulfillment of the duties of their Christian vocation.... The people of God have no lasting city here below, but look forward to one that is to come. Since this is so, the religious state, whose purpose is to free its members from earthly cares, more fully manifests to all believers the presence of heavenly goods already possessed here below.... The religious state clearly manifests that the Kingdom of God and its needs, in a very special way, are raised above all earthly considerations. Finally it clearly shows all men both the unsurpassed breadth of the strength of Christ the King and the infinite power of the Holy Spirit marvelously working in the Church.[22]

How is this "sign value" connected with the pastoral ministry, the shepherding role of healing the sick, tending and feeding them? The answer lies in the inherent tendency of the injured to be afraid of the shepherd—the instinct of the creature in pain to pull away from the one who is trying to heal it. Those who have handed themselves over to Christ by a total consecration, who have put their trust and security in him alone, may give others the courage to do the same. Furthermore, the witness of consecrated religious who have embraced the evangelical counsels in a radical way is a call to conversion and a challenge to all the faithful, even to the shepherds, to live more fully committed lives of detachment, purity, and humility.

Lay Members of Christ's Faithful

Finally, the responsibility for pastoral care of the sick rests, at some point, on every member of the faithful, as every human being is subject to the reality of suffering, illness, and mortality. The lay members of Christ's faithful, it must be remembered, have a special vocation to fulfill—a specifically secular vocation, as *Lumen Gentium* described it:

The laity, by their very vocation, seek the kingdom of God by engaging in temporal affairs and by ordering them according to the plan of God. They live in the world, that is, in each and in all of the secular professions and occupations. They live in the ordinary circumstances of family and social life, from which the very web of their existence is woven. They are called there by God that, by exercising their proper function and led by the spirit of the Gospel, they may work for the sanctification of the world from within as a leaven. In this way they may make Christ known to others, especially by the testimony of a life resplendent in faith, hope, and charity. Therefore, since they are tightly bound up in all types of temporal affairs,

---

22. Vatican Council II, *Lumen Gentium, Dogmatic Constitution on the Church*, November 21, 1964, no. 44.

it is their special task to order and to throw light upon these affairs in such a way that they may come into being and then continually increase according to Christ to the praise of the Creator and the Redeemer.[23]

The ministry of pastoral care provided by the laity to their sick brothers and sisters, therefore, is true ministry, carried out not sacramentally but according to the nature of this secular vocation—that is, according to the laity's responsibility, entrusted to them by Christ, to sanctify the world from within. It is also truly pastoral, in the sense of drawing together, feeding and leading the flock of Christ, although here the ministry is not that of the shepherd but rather "sheep to sheep," as it were. The pastoral aspect of ministry by one member of the flock to another involves the power of witnessing, of one person's ability to speak to another about his or her experience of God's love, mercy, and power to heal. It is difficult for a wounded, isolated individual to trust even the Good Shepherd, much less those other shepherds who try to serve in his name. When a trusted companion can give reassurance and consolation, the sick person can more easily accept the invitation to the sacraments and to spiritual healing and reintegration.

The Family

The Church points out that various groups of the lay faithful have specific contributions to make in this regard. Not surprisingly, Pope John Paul II points first to the "domestic church," the *family*. It is not always easy for the sick, especially the elderly, to be cared for in their own homes or by their own families. Nevertheless, the Holy Father points out that the sacrifices this may involve bring great blessings upon the caregivers as well as the sick:

While inviting the ecclesiastical and civil community to assume responsibility for the difficult situations in which many families find themselves, under the burden imposed by the illness of a relative, I remind you that the Lord's command to visit the sick is addressed first of all to the relatives of the ill. When carried out in a spirit of loving self-donation and supported by faith, prayer, and the sacraments, the care of sick relatives can be transformed into an irreplaceable therapeutic instrument for the ill and become an occasion for everyone to discover precious human and spiritual values.[24]

Similarly, *Pastoral Care of the Sick* has this to offer:

The family and friends of the sick and those who take care of them in any way have a special share in this ministry of comfort. In particular, it is their task to strengthen the sick with words of faith and by praying with them, to commend them to the suffering and glorified Lord, and to encourage them to contribute to the well-being of the people of God by associating themselves willingly with Christ's passion and death.[25]

The Synod of Bishops, meeting in 2015 to discuss "The Vocation and Mission of the Family in the Church and in the Contemporary World," dedicated a chapter of

---

23. Ibid., no. 31.
24. Pope John Paul II, Message for the Sixth World Day of the Sick (1998), no. 8.
25. *Pastoral Care of the Sick*, no. 34.

its final report to issues of "inclusion" in the family. The report highlighted the particular challenges faced by families whose members are elderly, are sick, or have special needs, and urged that the Church provide "special pastoral attention" to them.[26] And it also recognized the blessings that elderly or infirm members bring to the family itself, not least of which is the opportunity to "render the Church and society an invaluable witness of their faithfulness to the gift of life."[27] By caring for family members with special needs, the synod suggests,

the family has the opportunity to discover, together with the Christian community, new approaches, new ways of acting, a different manner in understanding and identifying the family and in welcoming and caring for the mystery of the fragility of human life. People with disabilities are a gift for the family and an opportunity to grow in love, mutual aid and unity.[28]

The presence of the sick in the home is also an opportunity for each family member to deepen his or her life of prayer. "For our loved ones who suffer because of illness we ask first for their health," Pope Francis writes. "But love animated by faith makes us ask for them something greater than physical health: we ask for peace, a serenity in life that comes from the heart and is God's gift . . . which the Father never denies to those who ask him for it with trust."[29] Especially as the illness progresses, and the possibility of a physical healing and restoration becomes more remote, this lesson on the real object of prayer for the sick is a difficult but necessary one. Of course, the peace and serenity sought for the sick person can often take root, not just in the sick, but in the whole household, and provide a real consolation that outlasts the temporary moment of suffering and death.

Catholic Health-Care Professionals

Although this chapter focuses principally on the subject of pastoral care, that focus does not suggest a diminished importance for the broad spectrum of medical care that is provided by Catholic physicians, nurses, and allied health professionals. Indeed, from the Church's perspective, the opposite is true. The popes speak often about the opportunities Catholic health workers encounter to give witness to gospel values, to be evangelizers and Good Samaritans in the midst of their daily work—in a word, to provide truly pastoral care to their patients.

"Since a Catholic health care institution is a community of healing and compassion," insists the *Ethical and Religious Directives,* "the care offered is not limited to the treatment of a disease or bodily ailment but embraces the physical, psychological, social, and spiritual dimensions of the human person."[30] Catholics in health care need not compartmentalize professional knowledge and practice from their lives

---

26. Synod of Bishops, Fourteenth Ordinary General Assembly, Final Report of the Synod of Bishops to the Holy Father, Pope Francis, October 24, 2015, no. 20.

27. Ibid., no. 21.

28. Ibid.

29. Pope Francis, Message for the Twenty-Fourth World Day of the Sick (2016).

30. USCCB, *Ethical and Religious Directives*, part 2, intro.

of faith; the two are intimately connected. "The medical expertise offered through Catholic health care is combined with other forms of care to promote health and relieve human suffering."[31]

The hectic pace of modern institutions and practices may not seem to leave much time for pastoral involvement, but attitudes of charity make a great impact and reorient patients toward the sacraments and the Church. "How much there is of the Good Samaritan," Pope John Paul II wrote, "in the profession of the doctor, or the nurse, or others similar! Considering its 'evangelical' content, we are inclined to think here of a vocation rather than simply a profession."[32] It was this same pope who established the annual observance of the World Day of the Sick, noting in one of his annual messages for the occasion that "an organized health-care apostolate is part of the evangelizing task."[33]

The *Ethical and Religious Directives* highlight the importance of collaboration between hospital professionals and the leaders of local parishes for the provision of pastoral care. Because "technological advances in medicine have reduced the length of hospital stays dramatically," it notes,

the pastoral care of patients, especially administration of the sacraments, will be provided more often than not at the parish level, both before and after one's hospitalization. For this reason, it is essential that there be very cordial and cooperative relationships between the personnel of pastoral care departments and the local clergy and ministers of care.[34]

Thus far we have discussed pastoral care in general and idealized terms, which should not be confused with unrealistic or unattainable goals: Christians must always strive for the ideal revealed in the Word made flesh. Nonetheless, some specific characteristics have emerged. Rooted in the biblical notion of leading the people of God, pastoral care seeks out those who are isolated by physical, mental, or emotional pain, extending an invitation to reintegration with the community of believers, the Church. Because it also involves feeding the flock, pastoral care, through charitable encounters and especially through offering the sacraments, strengthens with God's grace those who are weakened by suffering. And because the Church's ministers must watch over the flock, pastoral care bears witness to the healing presence of the Good Shepherd, who comes to seek out and save the lost sheep and lays down his life for them. "Priests, deacons, religious, and laity exercise diverse but complementary roles" as they give testimony to the power of Christ working through them and their ministry.[35]

---

31. Ibid.

32. John Paul II, *Salvifici Doloris*, no. 29.

33. Pope John Paul II, Address to the Fourth Plenary Assembly of the Pontifical Commission for Latin America, June 23, 1995, no. 8, quoted in Pope John Paul II, Message for the Fourth World Day of the Sick (1996), no. 2.

34. USCCB, *Ethical and Religious Directives*, part 2, intro.

35. Ibid.

The Limits of Pastoral Care

Before we consider the various elements of pastoral care, it may be helpful to begin by examining what pastoral care *is not*. In this way one may avoid the temptation to take too much upon oneself; one may recognize that, in terms of healing, "there are different forms of service but the same Lord . . . different workings but the same God who produces all of them in everyone" (1 Cor 12:5–6). Because pastoral care has a unique contribution to make to the spiritual health and well-being of the individual, an appreciation of the proper limits of ministers and their responsibilities enhances a correct understanding of the ministry and safeguards a proper autonomy of the pastoral minister in providing care.

Pastoral Care Is Not Psychotherapy

Outwardly, the setting in which many pastoral ministers encounter patients, whether at home or in hospitals or other institutions resembles in many ways a counseling session. The loneliness and isolation inherent in illness, coupled with the fear, anxiety, and questions that disease can provoke in patients, prompts a great desire in many patients to talk with the visiting pastoral minister and to discuss many personal issues. Clergy and other pastoral ministers with various degrees of preparation and certification may indeed have been formally trained in pastoral counseling; still, the pastoral care visit is in itself a different encounter from a psychological consultation or counseling session. Pastoral ministers, especially those with little or no counseling training, must be very careful to distinguish between the two; and all pastoral ministers should be prepared to refer persons with emotional or behavioral issues to trained professionals. To attempt to handle serious issues without proper qualifications is to do the sick person a disservice.

Pastoral Care Is Not Identical with Medical Ethics

It has already been noted that the pastoral minister's responsibility to lead the people of God involves faithfully proclaiming the gospel and applying the truths of the faith to the situations and decisions of daily life. This is particularly true for members of the clergy. Few decisions are more difficult or urgent than those surrounding the care of seriously ill and dying persons. For this reason, those involved in pastoral care have a special responsibility to keep informed of advances in medical science and to understand Church teaching regarding the ethics of medical decision making. Pastoral care ministers should be able to communicate the teaching of the Church in a sensitive, clear way to patients and their families, in order to assist them in making decisions consistent with the moral law. Often these decisions must be made under a great deal of stress and in very trying circumstances; the compassion of the pastoral minister in "speaking the truth in love" (Eph 4:15) is a great gift in this time of need.

It is simply not possible, however, for every parish priest, hospital chaplain, or pastoral visitor, however well intentioned or well read, to be an expert in moral theology. One ought not to pretend to have answers to such serious questions when one is unsure, nor rush to compile an answer in order to have something to say. There is no shame in a pastoral minister's admitting to a patient or his or her family that a particular issue is complicated. Ministers must not hesitate to call upon moral theologians and ethicists in order to obtain the best possible answers to questions that arise in the course of their ministry to the sick. Again, failing, out of expediency or pride, to refer a case to an expert is a disservice to the patient.

The difficult case may also arise in which a pastoral minister may be obliged to question the opinion of doctors or an ethics committee regarding whether a particular course of treatment is morally acceptable. Maintaining a clear understanding of roles in this case—humbly acknowledging that the pastoral minister is not taking over medical care or hospital policy but is speaking as someone interested in the patient's spiritual and moral well-being—will permit a constructive dialogue concerning the truth and avoid confrontation.

Pastoral Care of the Dying Is Not Identical with Hospice Care

For many centuries, the sacrament of the Anointing of the Sick was known colloquially as the "Last Rites," a term that even today lives in popular speech and understanding. As a result, in many cases a priest is not called to attend to a sick person and offer the sacraments until all medical means to save the person's life have been exhausted and the patient is imminently dying. In such cases, it is usually too late for the patient to participate consciously in the sacramental celebration. We may be thankful, though, that the rise of modern hospice care, which attends not only to palliative relief of pain but also to pastoral care of the dying person, provides opportunities for the fuller participation of the dying in the celebration of the sacraments.

In this regard, however, the pastoral minister must retain a certain autonomy vis-à-vis the hospice care provider. It may be necessary, for example, to discuss honestly with the patient and his or her family whether the pain medication suggested by the hospice clouds the patient's mental faculties to such an extent that praying or participating in the sacramental rites becomes difficult or impossible. In such cases the patient may be willing to accept a certain degree of suffering—which is a relative, not an absolute, evil—for its redemptive value and for the sake of being able to communicate clearly with God and with loved ones.

Such a conversation seems to be anticipated by the *Ethical and Religious Directives*. "Patients should be kept as free of pain as possible so that they may die comfortably and with dignity," reads directive 61, while adding that "since a person has the right to prepare for his or her death while fully conscious, he or she should not be deprived of consciousness without a compelling reason." This is a decision that health care professionals, particularly those coming from a secular perspective, may not always understand or support, but which a pastoral minister may find it necessary to defend on the patient's behalf. Once again, a clear distinction of roles allows a pastoral minister to raise the suggestion without giving the appearance of trying to take over the patient's care and thus provoking a defensive reaction from the hospice provider.

The Forms of Pastoral Care

Among the rituals revised following the Second Vatican Council was the *Ordo Unctionis Infirmorum eorumque pastoralis curae* (the "Order of the Anointing of the Sick and Their Pastoral Care," 1972), first issued in a provisional English translation in 1973. In 1982, the U.S. Catholic Bishops approved an expanded compilation, titled *Pastoral Care of the Sick: Rites of Anointing and Viaticum*. This edition reordered and expanded some sections of the *Ordo Unctionis*, incorporating prayers and Scripture readings from other liturgical books, to provide a handbook for pastoral ministers "in a format ... as suitable as possible for pastoral use."[36] This section will follow the outline of *Pastoral Care of the Sick*, to explain briefly the various forms of pastoral care ministry.

Visits to the Sick

In the older *Rituale Romanum*, a section titled "Visits to the Sick" formed the latter part of the chapter dedicated to care of the infirm. In the new liturgical books, visits come first. In the Latin *Ordo Unctionis*, the subject of visits is dealt with mostly in the rubrics—that is, in the small-print introductory remarks—aside from readings and prayers, which are provided in an appendix. In the English *Pastoral Care of the Sick*, two special sections are provided at the front of the book, each with a short Liturgy of the Word, arranged with readings, the Lord's Prayer, and a selection of concluding prayers to be chosen according to the condition of the sick person.

The importance of the visit as an expression of compassion and solidarity is central to the nature of pastoral care as *pastoral*. We have already identified its model as the Good Shepherd, who "came to seek and to save what was lost" (Lk 19:10). The pastoral minister's willingness to "be with" the suffering person is of great importance in overcoming the isolation inherent in suffering. "Pastoral care encompasses the full range of spiritual services, including a listening presence; help in dealing with powerlessness, pain, and alienation; and assistance in recognizing and responding to God's will with greater joy and peace."[37]

Often, simply being present with someone who is suffering is enough to bring relief and to help the person draw closer to the saving mystery of Christ's redeeming love. "*Suffering and being at the side of the suffering*: whoever lives these two situations in faith comes into particular contact with the sufferings of Christ and is allowed to share 'a very special particle of the infinite treasure of the world's Redemption,'" John Paul II tells us.[38] The *Rituale*'s advice to the pastor may well be applied to every pas-

---

36. *Pastoral Care of the Sick*, no. 38f.
37. USCCB, *Ethical and Religious Directives*, part 2, intro.
38. Pope John Paul II, Message for the Fourth World Day of the Sick, no. 5 (emphasis in original), quoting John Paul II, *Salvifici Doloris*, no. 27.

toral minister: "Immediately upon learning that one of his parishioners is ill, without waiting to be summoned, he ought to visit him of his own accord; and this not only once but frequently throughout the duration of the illness."[39] This advice can seem burdensome or even unrealistic in the midst of the many responsibilities of parish or family life: "Occasionally our world forgets the special value of time spent at the bedside of the sick," Pope Francis notes, "since we are in such a rush; caught up as we are in a frenzy of doing, of producing, we forget about giving ourselves freely."[40] But "time spent with the sick is holy time" he says, that rewards both the visited and the visitor.[41]

Moreover, the presence of the pastoral minister in the home or the hospital room of the sick person is a reminder of the presence of the Church and of the patient's enduring connection with the Body of Christ. This reminder may serve, where it is needed, as an invitation and encouragement toward reintegration; always it can serve as a challenge to the infirm to recall their responsibilities toward the community. "The minister should encourage the sick person to offer his or her sufferings in union with Christ and to join in prayer for the Church and the world," the liturgical rubrics advise.[42] This admonition to pray is not at all vague, and it is by no means patronizing. It is based on a firm belief that "the Lord hears the cry of the poor" (Ps 34:7) and of those who suffer, and that there are others whose needs are greater even than one's own; for example, "people suffering in a particular disaster."[43]

An often significant aspect of this "presence of the Church" during the pastoral visit is the opportunity it provides for the pastoral minister to call the sick person to conversion. The pastoral visit can encourage the patient to consider his or her spiritual condition in light of physical circumstances and to approach the Church for healing, especially through the sacrament of Reconciliation. The mystery of suffering is inseparable from the mystery of sin, and often enough the inescapable reality of physical limitation reminds a person of his own mortality and makes him aware of his need for God's mercy. "This is an extremely important aspect of suffering," Pope John Paul II insists:

It is profoundly rooted in the entire Revelation of the Old and above all the New Covenant. Suffering must serve for conversion, that is, for the rebuilding of goodness in the subject, who can recognize the divine mercy in this call to repentance. The purpose of penance is to overcome evil, which under different forms lies dormant in man. Its purpose is also to strengthen goodness both in man himself and in his relationships with others and especially with God.[44]

All the rites associated with pastoral care of the sick and dying note the importance of the sacrament of Reconciliation, although they often suggest that it be celebrated at another time, distinct from the celebration of Anointing or Viaticum.

---

39. *Rituale Romanum: De Visitatione et Cura Infirmorum*, no. 1, quoted in Weller, *The Roman Ritual*, 375.
40. Pope Francis, Message for the Twenty-Third World Day of the Sick (2015), no. 4.
41. Ibid., no. 3.
42. *Pastoral Care of the Sick*, no. 56.
43. Ibid.
44. John Paul II, *Salvifici Doloris*, no. 12.

When a pastoral visit is conducted by a priest, it is natural enough for him to offer the sacrament to the patient, at least from time to time. The *Ethical and Religious Directives* stress the importance of providing and publicizing opportunities for Confession in the hospital or nursing home setting.[45]

Pastoral ministers should likewise encourage the sick to make contact with their parish priest or hospital chaplain to celebrate the sacrament on a regular, frequent basis.[46] It is easier to broach this subject when the pastoral visitor has a personal rapport with the sick person, as it requires a certain pastoral sensitivity. A great deal of patience is also necessary, along with an understanding of what the Pontifical Council for the Family calls "the pastoral 'law of gradualness' . . . [which] consists of requiring a *decisive break* with sin together with a *progressive path* towards total union with the will of God and with his loving demands."[47]

Pastoral Care of the Sick: Rites of Anointing and Viaticum includes two sections on visits: the first is presented in general terms, and the newly composed second chapter contains prayers for "Visits to a Sick Child." As *Salvifici Doloris* tells us, "human suffering . . . intimidates";[48] it "remains a mystery [and] we are conscious of the insufficiency and inadequacy of our explanations."[49] This is all the more true for children, who have a much more limited understanding of why they are sick or in pain, let alone why they must suffer. For this reason, the Church encourages pastoral ministers to "help sick children to understand that the sick are very special in the eyes of God because they are suffering as Christ suffered and because they can offer their sufferings for the salvation of the world."[50] Pope Benedict XVI points out the need to extend sensitive pastoral care to the families of sick children:

Since the sick child belongs to a family that frequently shares in his or her suffering with serious hardship and difficulties, Christian communities cannot but also feel duty-bound to help families afflicted by the illness of a son or daughter. After the example of the "Good Samaritan," it is necessary to bend over the people so harshly tried and offer them the support of their concrete solidarity. In this way the acceptance and sharing of suffering is expressed in the practical support of sick children's families, creating in them an atmosphere of serenity and hope and making them feel that they are in the midst of a larger family of brothers and sisters in Christ.[51]

Special care must be taken for children in danger of death who have not yet completed the sacraments of initiation. "Newly born infants in danger of death, including those miscarried, should be baptized if this is possible."[52] While requests for baptism

---

45. See USCCB, *Ethical and Religious Directives,* dir. 13.

46. See ibid., dir. 14.

47. Pontifical Council for the Family, *Vademecum for Confessors Concerning Some Aspects of the Morality of Conjugal Life* (1997), no. 3.9, emphasis in original, http://www.vatican.va/roman_curia/pontifical_councils/family/documents/rc_pc_family_doc_12021997_vademecum_en.html.

48. John Paul II, *Salvifici Doloris,* no. 4.

49. Ibid., no. 13.

50. *Pastoral Care of the Sick,* no. 64.

51. Pope Benedict XVI, Message for the Seventeenth World Day of the Sick (2009).

52. USCCB, *Ethical and Religious Directives,* dir. 17.

are typically referred to the chaplain of the institution or the parish priest, "in case of emergency, if a priest or a deacon is not available, anyone can validly baptize"; one who has performed such an emergency baptism should notify the chaplain that the baptism has taken place.[53] "When a Catholic who has been baptized but not yet confirmed is in danger of death, any priest may confirm the person."[54]

Holy Communion for the Sick

In Holy Communion, the pastoral nature of care becomes more outwardly visible, not only because the ministry is explicitly sacramental, but also because the Blessed Sacrament is the "true food" (Jn 6:55) with which the Good Shepherd and his pastoral ministers feed the hungry members of his flock. Again, *Pastoral Care of the Sick* provides two relevant formulas: the first deals with Holy Communion "in ordinary circumstances" (that is, when a full liturgical celebration may be carried out), and the second in the more restrictive conditions of a hospital or other institution.

The basic pattern followed "in ordinary circumstances" resembles a typical celebration of a Liturgy of the Word. It is celebrated by a priest or deacon or, with appropriate permission, by an Extraordinary Minister of Holy Communion. The minister greets the sick person, then places the vessel (called a pyx) containing the sacred Host on a table, prepared if possible with a cloth. The liturgy begins with a penitential rite, which may include sprinkling with holy water, and the Liturgy of the Word. This is followed by the Lord's Prayer and the reception of Holy Communion. After a period of silent prayer, the minister leads a spoken prayer and concludes the rite with the final blessing. In a hospital or other busy institution, the rite may be shortened—if, for example, the number of patients to be visited by one pastoral minister allows only a few moments with each patient. In such a case only the greeting, the Lord's Prayer, and the invitation to Communion ("Behold the Lamb of God . . ." / "Lord, I am not worthy . . .") are said with each patient.

The introduction to the chapter on the Communion of the Sick speaks of "the faithful who are ill" being "deprived of their rightful and accustomed place in the Eucharistic community."[55] It thus views the bringing of Holy Communion to the sick not merely as a duty and an obligation on the part of the pastoral minister, but as a sign of the community's support:

Priests with pastoral responsibilities should see to it that the sick or the aged, even though not seriously ill or in danger of death, are given every opportunity to receive the Eucharist frequently, even daily, especially during the Easter season. . . . In bringing communion to [the sick] the minister of communion represents Christ and manifests faith and charity on behalf of the whole community toward those who cannot be present at the Eucharist. For the sick the reception of communion is not only a privilege but also a sign of support and concern shown by the Christian community for its members who are ill.[56]

---

53. Ibid.
54. Ibid., dir. 18.
55. *Pastoral Care of the Sick*, no. 73.
56. Ibid., nos. 72–73.

As a practical matter, it is important to note that the discipline of the Church permits that "sick people who are unable to receive communion under the form of bread may receive it under the form of wine alone."[57] Specific regulations apply in this regard:

If the wine is consecrated at a Mass not celebrated in the presence of the sick person, the Blood of the Lord is kept in a properly covered vessel and is placed in the tabernacle after Communion. The Precious Blood should be carried to the sick in a vessel which is closed in such a way as to eliminate all danger of spilling. If some of the Precious Blood remains, it should be consumed by the minister, who should also see to it that the vessel is properly purified.[58]

This pastoral provision regarding the Precious Blood may prove useful in several ways. The first is perhaps familiar from Sunday Mass: by receiving the Precious Blood, those who suffer from celiac disease or other gluten intolerance may receive Holy Communion without receiving the sacred host. It is also possible to administer Holy Communion in this way to those who would otherwise be unable to receive it because they cannot take solid food by mouth. Patients who can take liquids by cup, spoon, or straw, and are able to swallow safely, may be given the Precious Blood in this manner, provided they can do so without risk of spilling it, and provided that the vessels and instruments employed are reserved for this purpose and are properly purified after use.

In addition to stressing the importance of bringing the Eucharist to the sick, the Church also makes it very clear that the adoration and reception of the Eucharist are sources of strength for those working in pastoral ministry. In the Eucharist, the paschal mystery of Christ—the fullness of his suffering, death, and Resurrection—is made present and is shared with those who believe in him, and only in the context of that mystery is the redemptive value of human suffering revealed. All ministry to the sick must find its reference point in the Eucharist, as Pope Benedict points out:

Jesus Christ redeemed the world through his suffering, death, and Resurrection, and he wanted to remain with us as the "bread of life" on our earthly pilgrimage.... We are thus encouraged to commit ourselves ... [personally] to helping our brethren, especially those in difficulty, because the vocation of every Christian is truly that of being, together with Jesus, bread that is broken for the life of the world. It thus appears clear that it is specifically from the Eucharist that pastoral care in health must draw the necessary spiritual strength to come effectively to man's aid and to help him to understand the salvific value of his own suffering.[59]

So also does Pope John Paul II:

The command of the Lord at the Last Supper: "Do this in memory of me," besides referring to the breaking of bread, also alludes to the body given and the blood poured out by Christ for us (cf. Lk 22:19–20), in other words, to the gift of self for others. A particularly significant expression of this gift of self lies in service to the sick and suffering. Hence those who dedicate themselves to this service will always find in the Eucharist an unfailing source of strength and a stimulus to ever renewed generosity.[60]

57. Ibid., no. 74.
58. Ibid.
59. Pope Benedict XVI, Message for the Sixteenth World Day of the Sick (2008), nos. 3–4.
60. Pope John Paul II, Message for the Tenth World Day of the Sick (2002), no. 3.

The Sacrament of the Anointing of the Sick

The new ritual book's centerpiece is the sacrament that the *Catechism* tells us is "especially intended to strengthen those who are being tried by illness, the Anointing of the Sick."[61] The roots of this sacrament are "alluded to indeed by Mark,"[62] and made most explicit in the Letter of James:

> Is anyone among you sick? He should summon the priests of the church, and they should pray over him and anoint him with oil in the name of the Lord, and the prayer of faith will save the sick person, and the Lord will raise him up. If he has committed any sins, he will be forgiven. (Jas 5:14–15)

The ritual book envisions several possible scenarios in which the celebration of the sacrament may take place. A full complement of prayers and readings is provided for occasions when the anointing can take place during the celebration of Mass, either during a communal celebration in a parish or institution (such as a Catholic nursing home), or in a sick room in a private home. A slightly shorter form is provided for those occasions when the sacramental liturgy is celebrated fully outside the context of Mass. An abbreviated ritual is provided for use in hospitals and other busy institutions when, either because of large numbers of patients or the pressing demands of their medical care, a priest can spend only a few moments with each person. Finally, a rite for emergencies includes only the essential elements for a valid celebration of the sacrament, when circumstances limit time with or access to a seriously injured or dying person.

In addition to the typical elements of Act of Penitence, Liturgy of the Word, and Communion Rite, the Liturgy of Anointing comprises several important signs that speak to the nature of the celebration. The first is the "prayer of faith" to which St. James refers in his letter, signified by the litany which begins the Liturgy of Anointing:

> The community, asking God's help for the sick, makes its prayer of faith in response to God's word and in a spirit of trust. The entire Church is made present in this community—represented by at least the priest, family, friends, and others—assembled to pray for those to be anointed. If they are able, the sick persons should also join in this prayer.[63]

Next, the priest places his hands on the head of the person to be anointed. "This is the *epiclesis* proper to this sacrament,"[64] the *Catechism* explains, using a Greek term that means a "calling down" of the Holy Spirit. "With this gesture the priest indicates that this particular person is the object of the Church's prayer of faith.... The laying on of hands is also an invocation: the Church prays for the coming of the Holy Spirit upon the sick person."[65]

---

61. *Catechism of the Catholic Church*, no. 1511.
62. Ibid. See Mk 6:13.
63. *Pastoral Care of the Sick*, no. 105.
64. *Catechism of the Catholic Church*, no. 1519.
65. *Pastoral Care of the Sick*, no. 106.

Finally, the sick person is anointed with oil, which "signifies healing, strengthening, and the presence of the Spirit."[66] This oil, blessed by the bishop during the Chrism Mass on the preceding Holy Thursday, recalls the bishop's pastoral concern for every member of his flock each time the sacrament is celebrated. The Church provides the priest celebrating the sacrament with the faculty to bless new oil in case of emergency or other genuine necessity.

Pastoral ministers should be aware of the Church's teaching regarding the appropriate time for receiving the Anointing of the Sick, and they should help the sick understand this teaching. The *Catechism* summarizes it in this way:

The Anointing of the Sick "is not a sacrament for those only who are at the point of death. Hence, as soon as anyone of the faithful begins to be in danger of death from sickness or old age, the fitting time for him to receive this sacrament has certainly already arrived.

If a sick person who received this anointing recovers his health, he can in the case of another grave illness receive this sacrament again. If during the same illness the person's condition becomes more serious, the sacrament may be repeated. It is fitting to receive the Anointing of the Sick just prior to a serious operation. The same holds for the elderly whose frailty becomes more pronounced.[67]

It is necessary, then, to safeguard the nature of the sacrament by avoiding either of two extremes. On the one hand, the Sacrament of the Sick should not be relegated to the last moments—it is no longer "Extreme Unction" or "Last Rites." A person should be encouraged to request anointing early on in an illness for many reasons: not only because he or she will be able to participate more fully in celebrating the ritual, but because of the sacrament's many spiritual effects on the soul. In addition, receiving the sacrament early in the course of serious illness or before a serious operation prevents the patient from becoming too isolated in illness. It is much better to intervene early and with the grace of the sacraments and the charity of the Church than to allow someone to struggle alone for many weeks, months, or years, only to discover this grace when they have exhausted all other avenues of support.

The other extreme, administering the sacrament to those who do not require it, is equally to be avoided. Although the Church no longer waits until someone is at the point of death, both doctrine and law still reserve the sacrament to "those of the faithful whose health is seriously [*periculose*] impaired by sickness or old age."[68] In making such distinctions, the Church is not setting up a scale of heroism, placing value on some levels of suffering and not on others. She is, however, testifying to the fact that not all suffering is harmful, and that a certain amount of pain may be patiently borne, with Christ's help, for the sake of penance and the good of one's soul. "Illness," the *Catechism* insists, "can make a person more mature, helping him discern in his life what is not essential so that he can turn toward that which is. Very often illness provokes a search for

---

66. Ibid., no. 107.

67. *Catechism of the Catholic Church*, nos. 1514–15, quoting Vatican Council II, *Sacrosanctum Concilium*, no. 73. Cf. USCCB, *Ethical and Religious Directives*, dir. 15.

68. *Pastoral Care of the Sick*, no. 8.

God and a return to him."[69] In this case, it is prayer for perseverance and conversion, and not the Anointing of the Sick, which provides the help the sick person needs.

In such instances, of course, great discretion is necessary on the part of the pastoral minister. Not all—perhaps not most—serious or dangerous illnesses are externally evident; thus, the pastoral minister must inquire in a very delicate manner, respecting the person's privacy, exactly why the person is requesting the sacrament. Generally speaking, in a hospital setting, the patient's admission to a particular inpatient service will give the priest or pastoral minister a good sense of the condition's seriousness without much need for direct inquiry. The question arises more often in the setting of a parish communal anointing service, particularly when some of the congregants are not personally known to the celebrant. Practical steps in such a situation might include asking that those intending to receive the sacrament make themselves known before the Mass and sit together in one part of the church, rather than coming up spontaneously at the Liturgy of the Anointing. In addition, clear catechesis on what constitutes a "serious illness" can be provided beforehand in the church bulletin or from the lectern before the Mass. These and similar measures promote both respect for the nature of the sacrament and sensitivity to those striving to understand both Church teaching and the nature of their own sufferings.

Pastoral sensitivity is also required when the priest arrives to find that the person whom he was called to anoint has already drawn his or her last breath. As the rubrics for the rite indicate,

> when a priest has been called to attend a person who is already dead, he is not to administer the sacrament of anointing. Instead, he should pray for the dead person, asking that God forgive his or her sins and graciously receive him or her into the kingdom. It is appropriate that he lead the family and friends, if they are present, in some of the prayers suggested at the end of the "Commendation of the Dying." ... Sometimes the priest may find it necessary to explain to the family of the person who has died that sacraments are celebrated for the living, not for the dead, and that the dead are effectively helped by the prayers of the living.[70]

However, the exact moment of death may be difficult to determine, even in a merely physical sense (as will be discussed in another chapter of this book), and the Church takes into consideration that doubt may arise over whether a person is actually dead: that is, whether the soul has separated from the body. Thus, canon law directs that "this sacrament is to be administered in a case of doubt whether the sick person ... is dead."[71] It should be noted that this is a pastoral decision, not strictly speaking a medical one: the general introduction to *Pastoral Care of the Sick* states that the sacrament should be conferred "if *the priest* is doubtful whether the sick person is dead,"[72] while the introduction to the "Rite for Emergencies" says that "if *the priest* has reason to believe that the person is still living, he anoints him or her."[73] What is sought here is moral certainty,

---

69. *Catechism of the Catholic Church*, no. 1501
70. *Pastoral Care of the Sick*, no. 263.
71. *Code of Canon Law*, can. 1005.
72. *Pastoral Care of the Sick*, no. 15, emphasis added.
73. Ibid., no. 263, emphasis added.

rather than absolute certainty, and it is ordinarily sufficient for the priest to observe that commonly observable signs of physical death—such as *pallor, rigor, livor,* or *algor mortis*—have not yet set in to justify conferring the sacrament conditionally.[74]

Pastoral Care of the Dying—General Considerations

Pastoral Care of the Sick: Rites of Anointing and Viaticum next addresses the reality that "the Christian community has a continuing responsibility to pray for and with the person who is dying."[75] This is the point at which the physician may turn to the pastoral care minister and say, in essence, "I've done all I can, Father. It's your turn." Unfortunately, this attitude, spoken or unspoken, may pose a major challenge at this juncture in pastoral care: convincing the patient and those around him or her that speaking of death and beginning to prepare for it is not an admission of defeat. Rather, these steps acknowledge the reality that life in this world must come to an end if life in the next world is to begin.

The old *Rituale* advised the pastor to speak clearly to his parishioners about the reality of death, and it pointed out that some people do not want to admit that a loved one is mortal:

Whenever the condition of the sick person becomes critical, the pastor should warn him not to be deceived in any way, whether by the devil's wiles, or by the insincere assurances of the physician or false encouragement of relatives and friends, so as to delay the timely concern for his soul's welfare. On the contrary, he should be urged to receive with due speed and devotion the holy sacraments, while his mind is still sound and his sense intact, casting aside that false and pernicious procrastination which has already brought many to everlasting punishment and daily continues to do so through the illusions of the devil.[76]

C. S. Lewis, in his witty and insightful book *The Screwtape Letters*, writes from the perspective of the Devil, who advises his nephew, a junior tempter, to keep his new "patient" away from places like the battlefield, where he might be prepared for death:

How much better for us if *all* humans died in costly nursing homes amid doctors who lie, nurses who lie, friends who lie, as we have trained them, promising life to the dying, encouraging the belief that sickness excuses every indulgence, and even, if our workers know

---

74. The generally accepted definition of moral certainty is that proposed by Pope Pius XII in an allocution to the Roman Rota: "There is an absolute certainty, in which every possible doubt concerning the truth of the fact and the non-existence of the opposite is totally excluded.... [M]*oral certainty* ... on the positive side, is characterized by the fact that it excludes every founded or reasonable doubt ... [while] on the negative side, there still exists the absolute possibility of the contrary.... In any case, this certainty should be understood as an objective certainty, that is, based on objective reasons; not as a purely subjective certainty, founded on sentiment, or on merely subjective opinion as to this or that, or even perhaps personal credulity, recklessness or inexperience. One does not have such objectively founded moral certainty if there are reasons to the contrary that a sane, serious and competent judgment would declare, at least in some way, worthy of attention, and which in consequence would make it so that the contrary would be qualified as not only absolutely possible, but even more, in some way probable" (Pius XII, *Discorso al Tribunale della Sacra Romana Rota*, October 1, 1942, nos. 1, 3; translation mine).

75. *Pastoral Care of the Sick*, no. 163.

76. *Rituale Romanum: De Visitatione et Cura Infirmorum*, no. 10, quoted in Weller, *The Roman Ritual*, 377.

their job, withholding all suggestion of a priest lest it should betray to the sick man his true condition![77]

Both of these passages urge the pastoral minister to be honest with a dying person about his condition, primarily from a negative viewpoint: if he does not know he is dying, he will not have time to repent and confess his sins, and so he may run the risk of condemnation. This is, of course, a real and serious concern. There is also, however, a positive reason that pastoral care involves a healthy appreciation for the reality of death. The Good Shepherd lays down his life for the sheep, in order to take it up again (see Jn 10:15, 18). In his Resurrection, he gives life to all those who believe in him, and this is the source of hope for every Christian. Pastoral ministers who speak compassionately yet unflinchingly of death *and* resurrection give witness to the power of Christ to conquer all things, even sickness and death itself.

Thanks to faith in Christ's victory over death, [the Christian] trustingly awaits the moment when the Lord "will transfigure our mortal body to conform it to his glorious body, by virtue of the power he has to subject all things to himself" (Phil 3:21).

Unlike those who "lack hope" (cf. 1 Thes 4:13), the believer knows that the time of suffering represents an occasion for new life, grace, and resurrection. He expresses this certainty through therapeutic dedication, a capacity for accepting and accompanying, and sharing in the life of Christ communicated in prayer and the sacraments. To take care of the sick and dying, to help the *outward man* that is decaying so that the *inward man* may be renewed day by day (cf. 2 Cor 4:16)—is this not to cooperate in that *process of resurrection* which the Lord has introduced into human history with the Paschal Mystery and which will be fully consummated at the end of time? Is this not to account for the hope (cf. 1 Pt 3:15) which has been given to us? In every tear which is dried, there is already an announcement of the last times, a foretaste of the final plenitude (cf. Rv 21:4 and Is 25:8).[78]

An examination of the ritual books reveals the wealth of spiritual gifts the Church has reserved for those who are dying: touching prayers and passages from Scripture, grace-filled signs and moments provided to strengthen a person on the journey from this life to the next. It is a matter of justice and charity to make all of these gifts available to the dying person at the earliest possible moment; this requires an honest assessment of the patient's condition and a willingness to approach him or her with compassion. For this reason, the Church advises her children not to be afraid of death and encourages them to ask their families and doctors to deal plainly with them. The "Model Living Will" proposed by the Pennsylvania Catholic Conference, for example, contains this important clause:

I ask that if I fall terminally ill, I be told so I might prepare myself for death. If I am unable to understand, communicate, or make decisions for myself, I direct that a Catholic priest be contacted to attend to my spiritual needs so I may receive the Sacraments of Reconciliation and the Anointing of the Sick, Viaticum, and be supported by prayer.[79]

---

77. C. S. Lewis, *The Screwtape Letters* (San Francisco: HarperCollins, 2001), 23–24.

78. Pope John Paul II, Message for the Sixth World Day of the Sick (1998), no. 9, emphasis in original.

79. Pennsylvania Catholic Conference, *Combined Living Will and Health Care Power of Attorney* (2008), pt. III.

Viaticum: Holy Communion for the Dying

With its name derived from the Latin for "with you on the way" ([*in*] *via tecum*), this special celebration of Holy Communion with a dying person is described in *Pastoral Care of the Sick* as "food for the passage through death to eternal life ... signifying that the Christian follows the Lord to eternal glory and the banquet of the heavenly kingdom."[80] The Church desires that, whenever possible, Viaticum be administered within the celebration of Mass; the Church thus permits this Mass to be celebrated in the sick person's home, hospital room, or similar setting, presuming that the liturgy will be simplified as necessary to meet the conditions. Because of this preference for celebrating Viaticum within Mass, the ordinary minister of Viaticum is the parish priest of the sick person, or the chaplain of a health-care institution. "In case of necessity ... any priest or deacon may give Viaticum, or if no ordained minister is available, any member of the faithful who has been duly appointed."[81]

Certain distinctive elements mark the celebration of Viaticum. One is the renewal of baptismal promises by the dying person, which takes place after the homily. *Pastoral Care of the Sick* explains: "Through the baptismal profession at the end of earthly life, the one who is dying uses the language of his or her initial commitment.... In the context of Viaticum, it is a renewal and fulfillment of initiation into the Christian mysteries, Baptism leading to the Eucharist."[82] At the sign of peace, "the minister and all who are present embrace the dying Christian. In this and in other parts of the celebration, the sense of leave-taking need not be concealed or denied, but the joy of Christian hope, which is the comfort and strength of the one near death, should also be evident."[83] When Holy Communion is administered, after the words, "The Body of Christ," the celebrant adds, "May the Lord Jesus Christ protect you and lead you to eternal life." These words are meant to serve "as an indication that the reception of the Eucharist by the dying Christian is a pledge of resurrection and food for the passage through death."[84] At the end of the rite, the priest may bestow the apostolic pardon, which imparts a plenary indulgence at the time that death approaches.[85]

In the ritual for Viaticum, as with many of the rituals for the dying, pastoral ministry takes on a new dimension, beyond the element of feeding the sheep with the food of eternal life and shepherding them in the Lord's name. Now the sheep's destination is much more definite and much closer to hand; the pastoral minister is preparing to hand the sheep over definitively into the hands of the Good Shepherd. This task is accomplished through the final task of pastoral care to the dying person: the prayers of commendation.

---

80. *Pastoral Care of the Sick*, no. 175.
81. Ibid., no. 29.
82. Ibid., no. 179.
83. Ibid., no. 180.
84. Ibid., no. 181.
85. Pope Paul VI, *Indulgentiarum Doctrina*, *The Revision of Sacred Indulgences*, Apostolic Constitution, January 1, 1967, norm 18.

Commendation of the Dying

Pastoral Care of the Sick teaches: "In Viaticum the dying person is united with Christ in his passage out of this world to the Father. Through the prayers for the commendation of the dying … the Church helps to sustain this union until it is brought to fulfillment after death."[86] While the Viaticum itself may be described as a "moment," the patient's passage through death is a process that may occur over the course of hours, days, or weeks. Different people in the dying person's life—family, friends, pastoral ministers, clergy—will be involved in this process in different ways and to varying degrees. All of them may benefit from the prayers provided in the ritual books for the commendation, or handing over, of the dying person to God.

The process of dying, which comes to all of us, can be a great struggle on several fronts. "God did not make death," the Book of Wisdom insists, "nor does he rejoice in the destruction of the living" (1:13); therefore, death itself is naturally repulsive to the human spirit. Moreover, spiritual tradition has always identified the "hour of death" as a time of particular temptation, when Satan tries to turn even the most devout human souls away from the Lord at the last moment, attempting to frighten them with a remembrance of past sins or despair at the judgment that awaits, in order to shake their faith in God. It does happen that patients with attachments to persons or things in the world struggle to hold on to earthly life, even as God calls them out of this world to the next. In other instances, the patient's loved ones find it difficult to "let go," seeking to compel the dying person to cling to earthly life for the sake of the surviving family members. In the midst of this tumult of emotion, the commendation prayers seek to "help Christians to embrace death in mysterious union with the crucified and risen Lord, who awaits them in the fullness of life."[87]

These prayers take various forms; many of them consist of texts from the Sacred Scriptures, especially the Psalms. Litanies are also provided, which call on the saints or offer short prayers of supplication. These are useful because they allow for one person to lead the prayers and others to participate with a short, repetitive response. The dying person, and others who are overcome with emotion, may find it easiest to take part in this kind of prayer. Specific prayers of commendation, to be prayed "when the moment of death seems near," address the dying person directly,[88] offering courage to go to God without fear. In the words of *Pastoral Care of the Sick*,

These texts are intended to help the dying person, if still conscious, to face the natural human anxiety about death by imitating Christ in his patient suffering and dying. The Christian

---

86. Ibid., no. 212.

87. Ibid., no. 163.

88. "Go forth, Christian soul, from this world / in the name of God the almighty Father, who created you, / in the name of Jesus Christ, Son of the living God, who suffered for you, / in the name of the Holy Spirit, who was poured out upon you, / Go forth, faithful Christian! / May you live in peace this day, / may your home be with God in Zion, / with Mary, the virgin Mother of God, / with Joseph and all the angels and saints." (*Catechism of the Catholic Church*, no. 1020, citing *Order of Christian Funerals*, "Prayer of Commendation").

will be helped to surmount his or her fear in the hope of heavenly life and resurrection through the power of Christ, who destroyed the power of death by his own dying.[89]

The pastoral minister who prays with the dying person's family likewise gives comfort and pastoral care to those who are grieving their loved one's passing. "Even if the dying person is not conscious, those who are present will draw consolation from these prayers and come to a better understanding of the paschal character of Christian death,"[90] says *Pastoral Care of the Sick*. For the same reason, the prayers of commendation are immediately followed by prayers for the dead and for those who mourn. If the pastoral minister has been with the family throughout the process of dying, he or she may lead these prayers with them immediately. Otherwise, when the minister is called to the hospital or home, it is appropriate to begin by gathering the loved ones in the presence of the deceased's body and leading them in prayers for the dead. Many of the prayers contained in the book *Pastoral Care of the Sick* are the same as those used in the funeral liturgies of the Church.

The Fruits of Pastoral Care

The second section of the *Catechism*—"The Celebration of the Christian Mystery"—is a comprehensive discussion of the seven sacraments. Here the *Catechism* outlines the history and theology of each sacrament, its recipient and its minister, the requirements for its valid celebration, and its various effects. The four effects of the Anointing of the Sick outlined in this section might also be seen as four fruits of effective pastoral ministry. When ministry to the sick is carried out in imitation of Christ and according to his plan, it aims to produce these effects in the sick person. It is an essential point of theology, however, to note that these effects are caused directly by the Holy Spirit only through a valid celebration of the sacrament.

A Particular Gift of the Holy Spirit

The *Catechism* tells us:

The first grace of this sacrament is one of strengthening, peace, and courage to overcome the difficulties that go with the condition of serious illness or the frailty of old age. This grace is a gift of the Holy Spirit, who renews trust and faith in God and strengthens against the temptations of the evil one, the temptation to discouragement and anguish in the face of death."[91]

Here the pastoral responsibility to feed and strengthen Christ's flock in his name becomes clear. Every sacrament configures the one who receives it to Christ in a particular way; that is, it transforms the person to become more like Christ in some aspect of his life and ministry.[92] The sacrament of the Anointing of the Sick imparts to the

---

89. Paul VI, *Indulgentiarum Doctrina*, no. 215.
90. Ibid.
91. *Catechism of the Catholic Church*, no. 1520.
92. See *Catechism of the Catholic Church*, no. 1129.

sick person the gift of the Holy Spirit, who descended upon Christ at his Baptism and anointed him with power and strength. "This assistance from the Lord by the power of his Spirit is meant to lead the sick person to healing of the soul, but also of the body if such is God's will."[93]

Union with the Passion of Christ

The *Catechism* continues: "By the grace of this sacrament the sick person receives the strength and the gift of uniting himself more closely to Christ's Passion: in a certain way he is consecrated to bear fruit by configuration to the Savior's redemptive Passion."[94] The paradox of this second effect of the sacrament makes it at once almost unbearably beautiful and excruciatingly difficult to accept. A person who is enduring physical pain, even a person of great faith and holiness, often finds it difficult to make sense of his or her own condition; and the patient may already feel powerless in the face of illness. "Our first response may at times be one of rebellion," Pope Francis admits. "Why has this happened to me? We can feel desperate, thinking that all is lost, that things no longer have meaning."[95] To have to confront also Christ's apparent weakness under the weight of his cross, and to be expected to take the beaten, humiliated Crucified One as a model of strength, may at first seem too much to bear. Pastoral ministers, as shepherds of the flock, must bear witness to the truth of faith: that the apparent defeat of the cross was actually the ultimate victory.

Those who share in Christ's sufferings have before their eyes the Paschal Mystery of the Cross and Resurrection, in which Christ descends, in a first phase, to the ultimate limits of human weakness and impotence: indeed, he dies nailed to the Cross. But if at the same time in this weakness there is accomplished his *lifting up*, confirmed by the power of the Resurrection, then this means that the weaknesses of all human sufferings are capable of being infused with the same power of God manifested in Christ's Cross. In such a concept, *to suffer* means to become particularly *susceptible*, particularly *open to the working of the salvific powers of God*, offered to humanity in Christ. In him God has confirmed his desire to act especially through suffering, which is man's weakness and emptying of self, and he wishes to make his power known precisely in this weakness and emptying of self.[96]

In this way, those who are configured to Christ in the Sacrament of the Sick, and all who through pastoral care are led to accept their sufferings in union with him, have a share in the redemptive value of his suffering, as well as in his victory. As the *Catechism* says: "Suffering, a consequence of original sin, acquires a new meaning; it becomes a participation in the saving work of Jesus."[97]

---

93. Ibid., no. 1520.
94. Ibid., no. 1521.
95. Francis, Message for the Twenty-Fourth World Day of the Sick, no. 3.
96. John Paul II, *Salvifici Doloris*, no. 23, emphasis in original.
97. *Catechism of the Catholic Church*, no. 1521.

An Ecclesial Grace

We read further in the *Catechism*, "The sick who receive this sacrament, 'by freely uniting themselves to the passion and death of Christ,' 'contribute to the good of the People of God.'"[98] Apart from ministry in hospitals and skilled nursing facilities, much pastoral care takes place in the rather mundane setting of parish homes, in visits to elderly people whose physical limitations prevent them from attending church. The complaints of many of these "shut-ins" center not around their physical aches and pains, but around feelings of isolation and uselessness—that they are unable to contribute to family, neighborhood, and parish life as they once did. The insight of the *Catechism* in this regard is particularly gratifying. The Sacrament of the Sick imparts an "ecclesial grace," meaning that it "re-churches" the sick, so to speak; it reintegrates them into the Body of Christ by incorporating their prayers, needs, and sacrifices into the life and the work of the Church community. This is, as we have seen, the characteristic principle of pastoral care, and the purpose of its tending and caring nature, drawing the flock together and binding up the People of God.

The *Catechism* states:

By celebrating this sacrament the Church, in the communion of saints, intercedes for the benefit of the sick person; and he, for his part, through the grace of this sacrament, contributes to the sanctification of the Church and to the good of all men for whom the Church suffers and offers herself through Christ to God the Father.[99]

One cannot underestimate the contribution that the sick themselves make to the ministry of pastoral care. In many ways they are the real teachers, the real ministers, as they demonstrate patience and prompt those who care for them to grow in holiness and compassion. Pope John Paul II, who himself was a hero in his acceptance of suffering, spoke eloquently in this regard:

Dear people who are sick ... yours is a mission of most lofty value for both the Church and society. "You that bear the weight of suffering occupy the first places among those whom God loves" ... Manage to be generous witnesses to this privileged love through the gift of your suffering, which can do so much for the salvation of the human race.[100]

The Holy Spirit ... transforms the soul of countless sick people.... Even when they do not obtain the gift of bodily health, they are able to receive another that is much more important: the conversion of heart, source of peace and interior joy. This gift transforms their existence and makes them apostles of the Cross of Christ, standard of hope, even amid the hardest and most difficult trials.[101]

With this attitude of deep sharing, the Church reaches out to life's injured in order to offer them Christ's love through the many forms of help that "creativity in charity" suggests to her.

---

98. Ibid., no. 1522, quoting Vatican Council II, *Lumen Gentium*, no. 11.2.

99. *Catechism of the Catholic Church*, no. 1522.

100. Pope John Paul II, Message for the Fifth World Day of the Sick (1997), no. 4, quoting John Paul II, Homily, Liturgy of the Word for the Sick and Suffering, Tours, September 21, 1996, no. 2.3.

101. Pope John Paul II, Message for the Twelfth World Day of the Sick (2004), no. 3.

She repeats to each one: Courage, God has not forgotten you. Christ suffers with you. And by offering up your sufferings, you can collaborate with him in the redemption of the world.[102]

A Preparation for the Final Journey

"The Anointing of the Sick completes our conformity to the death and Resurrection of Christ, just as Baptism began it,"[103] says the *Catechism*. It is natural for someone at the end of life to revisit the events of his earthly days and to consider the brevity of life in this world. The *Catechism* offers a similar revisiting, but this one ponders the connection between the anointing of the sick and the anointings at baptism and confirmation, important events in the life of the soul; as both bodily and spiritual life had a beginning in this world, so both are coming to an end. In doing so, the *Catechism* makes clear that only the sacramental grace that comes from the Holy Spirit can enable the Christian to face death with hope, fortitude, and confidence in eternal life. "This last anointing fortifies the end of our earthly life like a solid rampart for the final struggles before entering the Father's house."[104]

Likewise, the sacrament's connection with Baptism recalls the nature of pastoral care to the sick and dying, its origin, its limits, and its goal. Pastoral care ministers go about their work not in their own name, but in the name of the Good Shepherd, tending his flock at his command. He has formed his people and consecrated them in Baptism; those who lead the flock must not "pasture themselves," as he warned the shepherds through the prophet, but must truly pasture the sheep. When they have tended the flock, leading and nourishing them rightly, then the shepherds must hand the sheep back to the Good Shepherd, who will bring them back into the sheepfold, where "there will be one flock, one Shepherd" (Jn 10:16).

Conclusion

To some degree, every human being has considered the problem of suffering and pain, of illness and disease, and has asked the same question: "Why?" Why did God make us, if it was only to suffer? Why did God create a world in which suffering would be possible? Why would a good God allow innocent people—innocent children!—to undergo such terrible pain, such senseless suffering? This age-old dilemma has faced every generation and has tested the faith of many a soul.

The answer lies in the understanding that everything is a gift; at the heart of things, every single part of existence is dependent on God's free, generous choice to give of himself to his creation. In a mysterious and profound way, God's complete self-giving, made most visible in the sacrifice of Christ who was "obedient to death,

---

102. Pope John Paul II, Message for the Thirteenth World Day of the Sick (2005), no. 5, quoting John Paul II, *Novo Millennio Ineunte*, Apostolic Letter at the Close of the Great Jubilee of the Year 2000, January 6, 2001, no. 50.

103. *Catechism of the Catholic Church*, no. 1523.

104. Ibid.

even death on a cross" (Phil 2:8), is the resolution of every doubt, the healing of every wound, the relief of every suffering, and the end of every pain.

The pastoral care minister, who nourishes the sick with the Word of God and the sacraments, who tends to their needs in Jesus' name, and who leads suffering souls back to the heart of the Church, is privileged to bear witness to Christ's self-gift to the world. Pastoral ministers must never forget that theirs is a delegated authority: as shepherds, they serve on behalf of Jesus, the Good Shepherd. He does not need their assistance to accomplish his will, but he is pleased that they collaborate in building up his kingdom and carrying out his work. Whether clergy, religious, or laity, physicians, family members, or even the sick themselves, all who reach out with love to the least of Christ's brethren show compassion to Christ himself. They in turn receive, not only the reward of their labors, but a share in the paschal mystery through which he redeemed the world.

Bibliography

Benedict XVI, Pope. Message for the Sixteenth World Day of the Sick (2008).

———. Message for the Seventeenth World Day of the Sick (2009).

Catechism of the Catholic Church. 2nd edition. Translated by the United States Conference of Catholic Bishops. Washington, D.C.: USCCB, 1997.

Code of Canon Law. New English translation. Translated by the Canon Law Society of America. Washington, D.C.: Canon Law Society of America, 1998.

Congregation for the Clergy and Congregation for Catholic Education, *Basic Norms for the Formation of Permanent Deacons.* February 22, 1998.

Francis, Pope. Message for the Twenty-Third World Day of the Sick. 2015.

———. Message for the Twenty-Fourth World Day of the Sick. 2016.

John Paul II, Pope. *Salvifici Doloris, On the Christian Meaning of Human Suffering.* Apostolic Letter. February 11, 1984.

———. Message for the First World Day of the Sick. 1993.

———. Message for the Fourth World Day of the Sick. 1994.

———. Address to the Fourth Plenary Assembly of the Pontifical Commission for Latin America. June 23, 1995.

———. Message for the Fifth World Day of the Sick. 1997.

———. Message for the Sixth World Day of the Sick. 1998.

———. Message for the Tenth World Day of the Sick. 2002.

———. Message for the Eleventh World Day of the Sick. 2003.

———. Message for the Twelfth World Day of the Sick. 2004.

———. Message for the Thirteenth World Day of the Sick. 2005.

Lewis, C. S. *The Screwtape Letters.* San Francisco: HarperCollins, 2001.

Paul VI, Pope. *Indulgentiarum Doctrina, The Revision of Sacred Indulgences.* Apostolic Constitution. January 1, 1967.

Pennsylvania Catholic Conference. *Combined Living Will and Health Care Power of Attorney.* 2008.

Pius XII, Pope. *Discorso al Tribunale della Sacra Romana Rota.* October 1, 1942.

Pontifical Council for the Family. *Vademecum for Confessors Concerning Some Aspects of the Morality of Conjugal Life.* 1997. http://www.vatican.va/roman_curia/pontifical_councils/family/documents/rc_pc_family_doc_12021997_vademecum_en.html.

Sacred Congregation for the Sacraments and Divine Worship. *Pastoral Care of the Sick: Rites of Anointing and Viaticum.* Translated by the International Commission on English in the Liturgy. New York: Catholic Book Publishing Co., 1983.

Synod of Bishops. Fourteenth Ordinary General Assembly, Final Report of the Synod of Bishops to the Holy Father, Pope Francis. October 24, 2015.

United States Conference of Catholic Bishops. *The Basic Plan for the Ongoing Formation of Priests.* 2001. http://www.usccb.org/beliefs-and-teachings/vocations/priesthood/priestly-life-and-ministry/national-plan-for-the-ongoing-formation-of-priests.cfm.

———. *Ethical and Religious Directives for Catholic Health Care Services.* 5th edition. Washington, D.C.: USCCB, 2009.

Vatican Council II. *Sacrosanctum Concilium, Constitution on the Sacred Liturgy.* December 4, 1963.

———. *Lumen Gentium, Dogmatic Constitution on the Church.* November 21, 1964.

Weller, Philip T., trans. and ed. *The Roman Ritual in Latin and English.* Vol. 1, *The Sacraments and Processions.* Milwaukee, Wisc.: Bruce, 1952.

PART II

WITNESS IN PRACTICE:
THE CLINICAL CONTEXT

Kathleen M. Raviele

4. REPRODUCTIVE HEALTH AND THE PRACTICE OF GYNECOLOGY

Moral alternatives for women's health problems, spacing the births of their children, and infertility treatment, though not as widely discussed as contraceptives, sterilization, and in vitro fertilization, are available to the Catholic physician and patient. These alternatives respect the dignity of the human person, the totality of the human person as an ensouled body, and the integrity of marriage in both its unitive and its procreative aspects. Whereas contraceptives have unwanted side effects and complications, natural methods of fertility awareness help in diagnosis with no adverse effects. Here Dr. Raviele explores alternative treatments for polycystic ovary syndrome, ovarian cysts, abnormal uterine bleeding, and dysmenorrhea. On the topic "Counseling the Adolescent Patient," she examines the American Congress of Obstetricians and Gynecologists opinion on the matter, and reminds us that in taking a neutral position toward an adolescent's sexual activity, a physician is, in effect, affirming that activity. The spiritual works of mercy are difficult but necessary in this situation; promoting chastity shows care and concern for the adolescent. Other topics in this chapter are genetic testing, ectopic pregnancies, early induction of labor, complications from abortion, emergency contraception in cases of rape, and endometriosis. Even when the life of the mother is at grave risk, there are alternatives that do not directly attack the child. Respect for the dignity and life of both the mother and the new human life is at the center of moral treatment. Infertility is another topic presented in this chapter, and Dr. Raviele indicates that most forms of assisted reproductive technology, though they do in fact produce a child, do nothing to solve the physical problem of infertility itself; at the same time, they separate the unitive and procreative aspects of marriage. Approaching countless gynecologic problems with an abiding view of the sanctity of human life and the dignity of the human being is an essential part of practicing medicine in truth and love.—*Editors*

Background

Upon completion of medical school and residency training in obstetrics and gynecology, family practice, or pediatrics, physicians have been thoroughly trained in the use of contraception, sterilization, and even abortion to treat the health problems of the adolescent and adult woman. It can be difficult, though, to find alternative treatments that would allow them to practice in accordance with their faith. The purpose of this chapter is to discuss some of the moral dilemmas encountered in caring for a woman's reproductive health and the health of her unborn child and to offer sound alternative solutions to the common practice of treating all women's health problems, from acne to headaches to abnormal bleeding, with hormonal contraceptives. Treatments for these problems, other than oral contraceptives, can be difficult to find. Also, Catholic patients, desiring to follow their consciences in difficult pregnancies, infertility, and the spacing of children, may have difficulty finding a physician who shares their values or at least respects their desires to avoid contraception, abortion, in vitro fertilization, and sterilization, and can offer a different clinical perspective. It is the author's hope that this chapter will arm patients and physicians with some concrete suggestions for handling these situations without violating Catholic teaching and their consciences. Further, it provides the etiology and treatment of many conditions in obstetrics and gynecology that are fraught with moral dilemmas, and it suggests explanations a physician can share with patients when offering other treatments for diseases or conditions that are commonly treated with hormonal contraception. Ultimately the physician will be providing the best care for the patient by working up the abnormality and treating the root cause rather than covering it up with synthetic hormones.

Let us first look at the moral teachings on marriage and the conjugal act in order to understand why the Church has always taught that using a contraceptive device, drug, or action during sexual intercourse is morally wrong. The Church calls us to be responsible parents, able to provide food and shelter for our children and to educate them. This is different from the common misunderstanding that Catholics are to have as many children as possible. The Church teaches that "Sacred Scripture and the Church's traditional practice see in large families a sign of God's blessing and the parents' generosity."[1] The Church also teaches responsible parenthood. Catholics are called to *both* generosity *and* responsibility.

"Married couples should regard it as their proper mission to transmit human life and to educate their children; they should realize that they are thereby cooperating with the love of God the Creator and are, in a certain sense, its interpreters. They will fulfill this duty with a sense of human and Christian responsibility."

A particular aspect of this responsibility concerns the regulation of procreation. For just reasons, spouses may wish to space the births of their children. It is their duty to make certain

---

1. *Catechism of the Catholic Church* (New York: Doubleday, 1997), no. 2373.

that their desire is not motivated by selfishness but is in conformity with the generosity appropriate to responsible parenthood.[2]

As Catholic physicians, we are called to treat women with respect for their dignity as human persons and to support and protect their reproductive systems, as well as the dignity and integrity of the marital act. "The acts in marriage by which the intimate and chaste union of the spouses takes place are noble and honorable; the truly human performance of these acts fosters the self-giving they signify and enriches the spouses in joy and gratitude."[3] Children are the fruit of the marital act and are a gift, not a right, for the couple. Because couples share in the creative power of God, the Magisterium has always taught that "each and every marriage act [must] remain ordered per se to the procreation of human life."[4]

The Book of Genesis reveals the truths about the nature of marriage between a man and a woman and about married love. God blessed Adam and Eve and commanded them to "be fertile and multiply" (Gn 1:28).[5] This revealed one aspect of married love—it was to be procreative; that is, a man and a woman would cooperate with God to bring new life into the world within marriage.

The second aspect was revealed in that Eve came out of the side of Adam, to be his equal partner in life; when the couple unites in the marital act, they are no longer two people, they become "one body." Therefore, the union of our bodies in sexual relations has two meanings, the unitive and the procreative: the completion and fulfillment of each other in love, and the creation of a new human being that has never lived before, and will never live again, as the fruit of that love. That is why the Church has taught from the time of Christ that sexual relations outside of marriage are illicit. With regard to family planning, the Church teaches that the unitive and procreative aspects of the marital act are to be respected, as this respects the language of the couple's bodies. Church teaching states that "every action which, whether in anticipation of the conjugal act, or in its accomplishment, or in the development of its natural consequences, proposes, whether as an end or as a means, to render procreation impossible" is intrinsically evil.[6]

Therefore, the means by which we space our children have to respect the integrity and true meaning of the marital act. When couples have to space children or even avoid any further pregnancies for serious health or financial reasons, they can learn one of the scientifically sound methods of fertility awareness or natural family planning (NFP) and practice abstinence during the fertile window if they want to avoid pregnancy. The woman's chart can assist the physician in diagnosing the cause of gynecological disorders, whether hormonal or structural. Therefore it is advisable that the physician become an expert in all the methods of natural family planning

---

2. *Catechism of the Catholic Church*, nos. 2367–68; quoting Vatican Council II, *Gaudium et Spes*, no. 50.

3. *Catechism of the Catholic Church*, no. 2362.

4. Pope Paul VI, *Humanae Vitae, Of Human Life* (Boston: Pauline Books and Media, 1968), no. 11.

5. Quote is taken from the New Revised Standard Version.

6. Paul VI, *Humanae Vitae*, no. 14.

and even make NFP classes available to patients. It is of great benefit to a physician or other health-care provider to go through training in how to teach one of the methods of NFP. "Catholic health institutions may not promote or condone contraceptive practices but should provide, for married couples and the medical staff who counsel them, instruction both about the Church's teaching on responsible parenthood and in methods of natural family planning."[7] Because of their medical expertise, physicians can be credible promoters of fertility awareness programs.

Now we will discuss some of the serious complications of contraceptives that are frequently minimized or overlooked when counseling women. Even if a physician or patient cannot be won over by the moral arguments presented, understanding the serious side effects of these products can be the beginning of questioning their use.

Oral contraceptives (OCs) are the most common form of birth control in the United States; 17 percent of women ages 15 to 44 years of age are current users. More than 10 million women in the United States and 100 million women worldwide are users of OCs. In developed nations, 80 percent of women have been on OCs at some time in their lives. This reality makes it very difficult to find an unexposed population that can be compared with current users in research on side effects or serious complications of OCs.

Hormonal contraception became possible first with the discovery in the 1930s of the effects of the female hormone progesterone after ovulation and then with the hormone's isolation from Mexican yams in the 1940s. In 1951 the first synthetic progestin was produced and in 1960 the Food and Drug Administration (FDA) approved the first synthetic hormonal contraceptive, containing both synthetic estrogen and a progestin. It was first placed on the U.S. drug market in 1963, and by 1965 it had become the most commonly used method of contraception. A predictable sequela of this new control over one's fertility was the U.S. Supreme Court's legalization of abortion on demand in 1973 for the "failure" of contraception. (Even today 40 percent of unplanned pregnancies occur while contraception is being used.)[8] By the late 1970s package inserts of OCs contained warnings that these drugs carried the risk of thromboses and cancer.

The primary use of hormonal contraceptives today is the prevention of pregnancy, but there are many secondary uses. These include heavy or irregular periods, endometriosis, polycystic ovary syndrome, dysmenorrhea, acne, and premenstrual syndrome, among others. Most oral contraceptives contain 10–40 mcg of ethinyl estradiol, a

---

7. United States Conference of Catholic Bishops (USCCB), *Ethical and Religious Directives for Catholic Health Care Services*, 5th ed. (Washington, D.C.: USCCB, 2009), dir. 52.

8. Note that the feminist movement claims that contraception—backed up, when it fails, by abortion—is fundamental to a woman's right to equality with men and to attaining happiness through educational and economic achievement. However, the origin of contraception and making sexual intercourse sterile unless the couple is "planning" to have a child was based on population control and eugenics, which promoted having more children from the upper class and the educated and fewer children from developing nations and the uneducated. A thorough analysis of this eugenic background of the birth control revolution can be found in Angela Franks, *Margaret Sanger's Eugenic Legacy: The Control of Female Fertility* (Jefferson, N.C.: McFarland, 2005).

synthetic estrogen, and a synthetic progestin. There have been several generations of progestins developed over the decades. A first generation progestin is norethindrone; a second generation progestin is levonorgestrel; a third generation includes desogestrel and gestodene; and the fourth generation progestin is drospirenone. It is important to distinguish among the four generations when discussing complications of OCs, particularly in the area of thrombotic events.

The mechanisms of action of OCs include the prevention of ovulation by suppression of the pituitary and its production of follicle stimulating hormone (FSH); thickening of cervical mucus; and, as a back-up, impeding the development of a normal endometrial lining necessary for successful implantation, should ovulation and fertilization take place. The seven days off the drug for a withdrawal menses allow adequate production of FSH so that ovulation occurs in 10 percent of cycles; in those instances, the endometrial effects prevent the continuation of a clinically detectable pregnancy and are thereby causing the loss of an early human life.[9] This effect can be minimized if the woman does not stop the drug for more than three days.

The many unpleasant side effects of OCs include weight gain, decreased libido, chronic vaginal discharge, a lighter or absent menstrual flow (which is the goal in many cases), irregular bleeding, headaches, depression, breast pain and/or masses, increased blood pressure, and an increased possibility of seizures.[10] However, there are several life-threatening complications that are often not discussed or emphasized with the patient.

When evaluating studies on serious side effects of OCs it is important to understand how to interpret the risk, if there is one. Studies may give comparisons based on relative risk (RR), which is the probability of an event occurring in an exposed group versus an unexposed group. This term is usually applied to randomized controlled trials and cohort studies. Case-control studies discuss risk based on the odds ratio (OR) or the odds of a disease among exposed individuals divided by the odds of disease among the unexposed.

Hormonal contraceptives increase the risk of ischemic stroke and ischemic heart disease in current users. These two conditions are the leading causes of death for women in the United States and worldwide, accounting for 30 percent of all deaths. There is a twofold increased risk of ischemic stroke in women currently on OCs as compared with nonusers.[11] Their use is justified in otherwise healthy women because during pregnancy and in the postpartum period, women have a threefold to eightfold risk of ischemic stroke. However, pregnancy and the postpartum period last 44 weeks, whereas a woman may be on OCs for many years or even her entire reproductive life.

9. See A. R. Baerwald, O. A. Olatunbosun, and R. A. Pierson, "Effects of Oral Contraceptives Administered at Defined Stages of Ovarian Follicular Development," *Fertility and Sterility* 86 (2006): 27–35.

10. See A. G. Herzog, "Differential Impact of Antiepileptic Drugs on the Effects of Contraceptive Methods on Seizures: Interim Findings of the Epilepsy Birth Control Registry," *Seizure* 28 (May 2015): 71–75, doi: 10.1016/j.seizure.2015.02.011.

11. See R. Peragallo Urrutia et al., "Risk of Thromboembolic Events with Oral Contraceptive Use," *Obstetrics and Gynecology* 122 (2013): 380–89.

In a multicenter study conducted by the World Health Organization (WHO), a fivefold increased risk of acute myocardial infarction (MI) was found in OC users compared to nonusers.[12] The risk is higher among women who smoke or are hypertensive. The risk of myocardial infarction in hypertensive users of OCs carries an OR of 6 to 68 over normotensive nonusers.[13] In most cases, patients—many of them taking these drugs for non-life-threatening conditions—are not aware of these increased risks.

It was known from the beginning that OCs carried an increased risk of thrombosis.[14] Oral contraceptives affect many coagulation factor proteins (including decreased protein S and antithrombin) that are involved in hemostasis; their effects can lead to a prothrombotic state. It is well known that changes in coagulation parameters, reduced blood flow, and damage to the vessel wall all lead to venous or arterial thrombosis and then the resultant heart disease, stroke, venous thrombosis, pulmonary embolus, and even death.[15] Women who have risk factors for thrombosis—such as antithrombin deficiency, protein S or C deficiencies, factor V Leiden mutation, the prothrombin 20210A mutation, lupus anticoagulant, and antiphosphalipid syndrome—should never be placed on OCs containing synthetic estrogen. A careful family history for thromboembolic events should always be taken before considering these drugs for medical reasons.

There is an abundance of literature on the increased risk of thromboembolic events associated with the use of hormonal contraceptives, but we will focus on some of the largest studies. A Danish cohort study looked at thromboembolic events in women aged 15 to 44 years in Denmark from 2001 until 2009.[16] The study is unique because in Denmark there is a linkage between four national registries, which include prescriptions, hospital discharge diagnoses, surgical codes, births, and abortions. Every citizen in the country has a 10-digit unique identifier. A total of 10.4 million women-years were studied and 3.3 million women-years on OCs. These women had no known personal history of heart disease or cancer. The researchers found the risk of a venous thromboembolic event or pulmonary embolus (VTE/PE) in an OC nonuser was 3.01/10,000 women-years. The risk for OC users was 6.29/10,000 women-years. The risk improved with lower estrogen dosages and longer duration of use; the highest risk was observed for OCs containing third- and fourth-generation progestins. There was no increased risk with progestin-only OCs or progestin IUDs.

A follow-up study published in 2011 compared the risk of VTE/PE with the type of progestin contained in the OCs. The relative risk of VTE/PE increased with

12. See F. R. Rosendaal, F. M. Helmerhorst, and J. P. Vandenbroucke, "Female Hormones and Thrombosis," *Arteriosclerosis, Thrombosis and Vascular Biology* 22 (2002): 201–10.

13. See K. M. Curtis et al., "Combined Oral Contraceptive Use among Women with Hypertension: A Systematic Review," *Contraception* 73 (2006): 179–88.

14. See P. M. Sandset et al., "Mechanisms of Thrombosis Related to Hormone Therapy," *Thrombosis Research* 123, Suppl. 2 (2009): S70–S73.

15. See J. Rosing, J. Curvers, and G. Tans, "Oral Contraceptives, Thrombosis and Haemostasis," *European Journal of Obstetrics and Gynecology and Reproductive Biology* 95 (2001): 193–97.

16. See Ø. Lidegaard et al., "Hormonal Contraception and Risk of Venous Thromboembolism," *British Medical Journal* 339 (2009): b2890, doi:10.1136/bmj.b2890.

third- and fourth-generation progestins. With levonorgestrel (2nd generation) the RR was 2.9; with desogestrel and gestodene (3rd generation) the RR was 6.6 and 6.2, respectively; and with drospirenone (4th generation) the RR was 6.4.[17] In the third study published on the Danish data, the investigators compared OCs with other hormone-containing contraceptives. In nonusers they found a VTE/PE risk of 2.1/10,000 women years. For those on a levonorgestrel OCs (2nd generation) the RR was 2.9 for a VTE/PE; for the norelgestromin/ethinyl estradiol patch, the RR was 7.9; for the etonorgestrel/ethinyl estradiol vaginal ring the RR was 6.5. The risk was still elevated with an etonorgestrel subcutaneous implant at an RR of 1.4; with the levonorgestrel intrauterine device (IUD), the risk decreased to an RR of .6.[18] In comparison, the arthritis medication rofecoxib was voluntarily withdrawn from the market in 2004 when the VIOXXTM Gastrointestinal Outcomes Research (VIGOR) trial showed a fourfold increased risk of MI over naproxen and the Adenomatous Polyp Prevention on VIOXX (APPROVe) trial showed a RR of 1.92 of MI or stroke over placebo.

In addition to the above serious risks, the International Agency for Research on Cancer of the World Health Organization (WHO) declared oral contraceptives to be Group I carcinogens, increasing a woman's risk of breast (44 percent), liver (50 percent) and cervical cancer (100 percent).[19] Endometrial cancer risk was reduced with longer duration of use and persisted for 15 years after discontinuation, as did ovarian cancer risk, which persisted for at least 20 years.

Teens are being encouraged to use contraception that does not rely on remembering to take a pill daily. Long-acting medroxyprogesterone acetate is administered as an injection every three months; it is highly effective at preventing ovulation but has annoying side effects such as irregular bleeding, weight gain, headaches, depression, hair loss, and acne. When used for more than two years, it causes osteoporosis. Young women are also being encouraged to use a long-acting reversible contraceptive (LARC) such as a levonorgestrel IUD or a copper IUD, which can be left in the uterus for five years or ten years, respectively. These devices work primarily by endometrial thinning and inflammation. They prevent implantation, and they do not prevent ovulation. Serious side effects include perforation of the uterus (which requires a major surgery to remove the device) and pelvic inflammatory disease (which could result in permanent sterility). More than 2 million women in the United States currently use an IUD. The woman has no control over its removal. The other LARC is the etonorgestrel subcutaneous implant, which has significant abnormal bleeding associated with its use, as well as headaches, weight gain, acne, and breast pain; it can be left in for up to five years and requires a minor surgery for removal.

17. See Ø. Lidegaard et al., "Risk of Venous Thromboembolism from Use of Oral Contraceptives Containing Different Progestogens and Oestrogen Doses: Danish Cohort Study, 2001–2009," *British Medical Journal* 343 (2011): d6423, doi: 10.1136/bmj.d6423.

18. See Ø. Lidegaard et al., "Venous Thrombosis in Users of Non-Oral Hormonal Contraception: Follow-Up Study, Denmark 2001–10," *British Medical Journal* 344 (2012): e2990, doi: 10.1136/bmj.e2990.

19. See V. Cogliano et al., WHO International Agency for Research on Cancer, "Carcinogenicity of Combined Oestrogen-Progesterone Contraceptives and Menopausal Treatment," *Lancet Oncology* 6 (2005): 552–53.

Prescriptions for oral contraceptives constitute a large part of a gynecologist's daily practice, so it can appear to be impossible to practice medicine as a gynecologist without prescribing hormonal contraceptives. However, foregoing the prescription of oral contraceptives opens up a whole new world of alternative therapies that get to the root of the problem without covering up the symptoms. Patients will seek out physicians knowledgeable in natural family planning for these therapies, as many women have contraindications to hormonal contraceptives or experience side effects when taking them. Most physicians have only a switch in formulation to offer, so their patients will look for alternative treatments. Other women will come to NFP-only physicians from a pro-life standpoint, after learning of the potential for post-fertilization effects on the embryo, should conception occur with a breakthrough ovulation.[20] Still other patients will seek out their help from a desire to avoid synthetic hormones as the standard treatment for most women's problems. An NFP-only practice is a "niche" medical practice.

We will now discuss how to manage a woman's fertility without the pill and with alternative treatments for conditions commonly treated by hormonal contraceptives. We will also discuss alternative managements for gynecologic conditions that do not interfere with the couple's fertility.

Case Studies

Case 1. Polycystic Ovary Syndrome

J. D. is a 31-year-old single woman, gravida 0 para 0, with a long history of irregular cycles. She has facial hair, which requires shaving, she weighs 174 pounds, her height is 61 inches, and she has a family history of diabetes. She has avoided gynecologists because she is not sexually active and the last physician she saw wanted to put her on oral contraceptives.

Polycystic ovary syndrome (PCOS) affects 5 to 7 percent of women of childbearing age today in the United States, or 3 million women.[21] The symptoms are typically weight gain, hirsutism, acne, oligomenorrhea, irregular bleeding, and infertility. Seventy-five percent of patients have insulin resistance, also known as prediabetes or metabolic syndrome,[22] which leads to obesity, overt diabetes, infertility, hypercholesterolemia, hypertension, and uterine cancer. The Rotterdam criteria for diagnosing PCOS require two out of three signs being present: eight or fewer cycles per year, a hyperandrogen state as determined by blood work or facial hair and acne, or classical polycystic ovaries diagnosed by ultrasound.[23] Laboratory evaluation includes:

---

20. See W. L. Larimore and J. B. Stanford, "Postfertilization Effects of Oral Contraceptives and Their Relationship to Informed Consent," *Archives of Family Medicine* 9 (1999): 126–33.

21. See A. M. Clark et al., "Weight Loss in Obese Infertile Women Results in Improvement in Reproductive Outcome for All Forms of Fertility Treatment," *Human Reproduction* 13 (1998): 1502–5.

22. See D. S. Guzick, "Polycystic Ovary Syndrome," *Obstetrics and Gynecology* 103 (2004): 181–93.

23. See F. J. Broekmans et al., "PCOS according to the Rotterdam Consensus Criteria: Change in Preva-

fasting glucose, fasting insulin, HgbA1c, fasting lipid screen, total testosterone, and DHEAS, in patients with masculinization. The patient should have serum levels of prolactin, LH, and FSH levels drawn on day 3 of her cycle, and a pelvic ultrasound looking for 12 or more follicles in an ovary that measure 2–9 mm in diameter or an ovarian volume greater than 10 cm³. Although oral contraceptives are typically given to women with this condition to regulate their cycles, this medication will worsen the glucose intolerance, contribute to weight gain, and increase the LDL cholesterol while decreasing the HDL cholesterol.

In all women with prediabetes or insulin resistance, the first action should be an increase in exercise combined with dietary changes that restrict calories to induce a weight loss of 10 percent of the woman's body weight. These women do best with a low carbohydrate diet that emphasizes vegetables, fruit, meat and fish, and limited complex carbohydrates. The beneficial effect of change in diet on the patient's risk for diabetes is comparable to medication.[24] If this fails, she can be started on oral agents that improve peripheral insulin resistance, such as metformin. This drug rarely causes hypoglycemia and may assist in weight loss and a return to normal cycles. Doses should be in the range of 1500 to 2000 mg per day, in gradually increasing doses to avoid intestinal side effects. For example, begin with metformin extended-release 750 mg at dinner for two weeks and then increase to twice daily with food.

If the woman is not cycling regularly, she can receive a withdrawal period with bioidentical progesterone 200 to 400 mg per day beginning on day 16 of her cycle for 10 days, or three days after ovulation if she is charting her fertility using a fertility awareness method. Progesterone does have side effects such as dizziness and premenstrual symptoms. These effects may be reduced by using the product vaginally and taking vitamin B6 at 200 mg/day while the patient is on the medication. The progesterone will not prevent ovulation. A synthetic progestin, such as medroxyprogesterone acetate at 10 mg/day, may be used during the same time by a woman who is not sexually active.

Facial hair and acne can be treated with spironolactone, which acts as a diuretic and aldosterone antagonist, and also binds to the androgen receptor as an antagonist. It works by the inhibition of ovarian and adrenal steroidogenesis, competition for androgen receptors in hair follicles, and direct inhibition of 5-α-reductase activity. The usual dose is 25–100 mg, twice a day to avoid symptoms of orthostatic hypotension. However, 20 percent of women will develop menstrual irregularities on the drug. Dietary restrictions of dairy products, sugar, high-fructose corn syrup, and high-glycemic carbohydrates may also improve the acne.

---

lence among WHO-II Anovulation and Association with Metabolic Factors," *British Journal of Obstetrics and Gynecology* 113 (2006): 1210–17.

24. See Diabetes Prevention Program Research Group, "Reduction in the Incidence of Type-2 Diabetes with Lifestyle Intervention or Metformin," *New England Journal of Medicine* 346 (2002): 393–403.

Case 2. Ovarian Cysts

T. G. is a 41-year-old married woman with a two-week history of right lower quadrant pain and spotting before this period. She has a known history of small fibroids and generally bleeds heavily for two days each menstrual cycle, changing a pad an hour and sometimes soiling her clothes. Her Hgb is 11, and she is on no vitamins or iron. Pelvic exam reveals a 10-week-sized uterus and fullness in the right adnexa compatible with an ovarian cyst. Pelvic ultrasound shows an 11 cm fibroid uterus with a 4.5 cm simple cyst in the right ovary.

Functional ovarian cysts are a common gynecological problem among women of reproductive age and can be associated with pain and irregular bleeding, but most are benign and self-limited. Large ovarian cysts may require surgical removal. As the use of oral contraceptives seemed to reduce the risk of ovarian cysts, it has been standard practice since the 1970s to treat women with oral contraceptives to resolve ovarian cysts without surgery. A previous tubal ligation increases a woman's risk for an ovarian cyst, as does the use of drugs to induce ovulation.

In a recent review of the literature on the use of oral contraceptives to treat functional cysts, David Grimes et al. found there was no benefit in using oral contraceptives and that most resolved in two to three months.[25] Thomas Hilgers has found that progesterone in oil, 200 mg given intramuscularly, disrupts estrogen dominance in follicular cysts and dissolves luteal cysts, thus reducing pain symptoms.[26] A follow-up ultrasound on day 5 of the next cycle will often show resolution. In patients who have recurrent ovarian cysts, cyclic oral, sustained-release progesterone can be administered, 200 mg by mouth daily or b.i.d., on day 16–25 of the cycle or on the third day after the peak of mucus, third day of temperature rise, or third day after the LH surge for 10 days. If the cysts do not resolve and they are 5 cm or greater or are symptomatic, laparoscopy is indicated.

Case 3. Abnormal Uterine Bleeding

D. H. is a 17-year-old single woman who presented, after treatment elsewhere with OCs, with menorrhagia and chronic anemia and a hemoglobin of 9.0. The patient described flooding with her periods and cramps, changing pads more often than one per hour. Ultrasound was normal, hypothyroid profile, prolactin, CBC, and an evaluation for von Willebrand's disease were all negative. She was treated with cyclic progesterone and antibiotics for possible endometritis. One severe episode that could not be stopped with hormone treatment necessitated a dilation and curettage (D&C) and blood transfusion.

---

25. See David A. Grimes et al., "Oral Contraceptives for Functional Ovarian Cysts," *Cochrane Database of Systematic Reviews* 2009, Issue 2: Art. No. CD006134.

26. See Thomas W. Hilgers, *The Medical and Surgical Practice of NaProTECHNOLOGY* (Omaha, Neb.: Pope Paul VI Institute Press, 2004), 382–86.

Finally, after trying several non-steroidal anti-inflammatories (NSAIDs), her bleeding became normal on meclofenamate sodium 100 mg three times daily during her period.

Normal menstrual bleeding is cyclic menstruation every 28 (± 7 days) days lasting 4 to 7 days and not exceeding 60 ml per cycle. Frequently, bleeding patterns outside these normal values are treated with OCs, even without further evaluation. Irregular bleeding, defined as an unusually heavy period of more than a pad an hour, or bleeding outside the seven days of a period, can be pregnancy related or caused by a malignancy of the cervix, endometrium, myometrium, ovary, or fallopian tube.

Polymenorrhea is defined as periods closer than 21 days from day 1 to the last day before the next period begins. Oligomenorrhea is a cycle lasting more than 35 days. Menorrhagia occurs with periods where the bleeding exceeds 80 ml/cycle; typically women experiencing this condition will describe changing a pad or tampon every hour for a day or more. Intermenstrual bleeding is bleeding that occurs outside the seven days of menstrual flow.[27]

The source of the bleeding abnormality should always be ascertained before treatment, and the likely causes vary by age. An adolescent would be more likely to have anovulation or a bleeding disorder. A reproductive-age woman could have abnormal bleeding that is hormonal or pregnancy related; caused by a structural abnormality such as a fibroid, polyp, or adenomyosis; or caused by cervical cancer. A peri-menopausal woman could have a hormonal problem that is secondary to dysfunctional ovulation, endometrial hyperplasia, or cancer.

Evaluation includes a careful history and physical examination; labs should include a CBC, TSH, prolactin, pregnancy test if indicated, Pap smear, and pelvic ultrasound. If the woman is charting using a fertility awareness program, review of the charts to determine the timing of the bleeding and adequacy of the length of the luteal phase, as well as whether ovulation is occurring is extremely helpful in the workup and management of the patient. Women over age 40 may need an endometrial biopsy to rule out endometrial hyperplasia or endometrial cancer, and suspicions of an endometrial polyp will prompt a hysteroscopy and D&C.

If a hormonal problem, either secondary to thyroid disease or caused by a progesterone deficiency, is the cause of the abnormal bleeding, those hormones should be replaced. Bioidentical progesterone in doses of 200 to 400 mg/day is given three days after ovulation for ten days each month or days 16–25 of the woman's cycle, if she is not ovulating. Treatment for menorrhagia includes several nonsteroidal, anti-inflammatory drugs (NSAIDs) such as mefenamic acid, 250 mg every six hours on the heavy days of the period, and meclofenamate sodium, 100 mg three times daily with food. Tranexamic acid, an anti-fibrinolytic drug, is also highly effective at decreasing heavy bleeding with a period.

27. See Linda M. Szymanski and Kimberly B. Fortner, "Abnormal Uterine Bleeding," in *The Johns Hopkins Manual of Gynecology and Obstetrics*, 3rd ed., ed. Kimberly B. Fortner et al. (Baltimore: Lippincott Williams and Wilkins, 2006), 417.

If fibroids are present and are the cause of the abnormal bleeding, uterine artery embolization or surgical removal of the fibroids should be considered.

Laser ablation of the endometrium, as a minimally invasive method of treating abnormal uterine bleeding in women who had completed their families, was introduced in 1981. It utilizes an Nd:YAG laser through the hysteroscope. Subsequent energy sources such as cryosurgery, radiofrequency electricity, microwaves, and thermal balloons were also introduced for endometrial ablation. This procedure was designed for women with normal endometrium who had failed medical therapy, but currently is used in women without anemia who have not necessarily had medical therapy. It is investigational in women past menopause. Preoperative evaluation should include endometrial sampling and pelvic ultrasound, or saline sonohysterography or hysteroscopy, to rule out intracavitary pathology. Patients with endometrial hyperplasia or endometrial cancer are not candidates for endometrial ablation. Studies on the effectiveness of endometrial ablation versus hysterectomy show patient satisfaction with endometrial ablation is high, but patient satisfaction from subsequent amenorrhea is highest after hysterectomy.[28] In clinical trials of resectoscopic endometrial ablation, 24–36 percent of patients had either a repeat ablation or a hysterectomy by four years after the procedure.[29]

Complications of the resectoscopic procedure include distention media fluid overload, endometritis (2 percent), uterine trauma such as cervical laceration or uterine perforation, and injury to intrabdominal organs or blood vessels, burns to the vagina or vulva, failure to diagnose a subsequent endometrial malignancy, postablation tubal ligation syndrome (10 percent) with intermittent pelvic pain, and pregnancy. Pregnancies after an ablation carry a high rate of complications such as prematurity, placenta accreta, and malpresentation.[30] Women are strongly encouraged to undergo a sterilization procedure at the time of an ablation, which would violate Catholic teaching. There is no medical reason to undergo a bilateral tubal ligation as it does not treat a medical condition. Contraindications to an ablation include a large endometrial cavity that exceeds the limitations of the device used, submucus leiomyomata greater than or equal to 3 cm, endometrial hyperplasia or cancer, a recent pregnancy, and a thinned area of myometrium due to a previous cesarean section, myomectomy, or a previous ablation.

As Catholic physicians, we should be performing this procedure only in women who cannot conceive, such as those who have had a previous sterilization or are in their late 40s and unlikely to conceive. The procedure does not correct the underlying pathology; it merely alleviates the symptoms of heavy bleeding by creating an abnor-

28. See N. Dwyer, J. Hutton, and G. M. Stirrat, "Randomized Controlled Trial Comparing Endometrial Resection with Abdominal Hysterectomy for the Surgical Treatment of Menorrhagia," *British Journal of Obstetrics and Gynaecology* 100 (1993): 237–43.

29. See Aberdeen Endometrial Ablation Trials Group, "A Randomized Trial of Endometrial Ablation versus Hysterectomy for the Treatment of Dysfunctional Uterine Bleeding: Outcome at Four Years," *British Journal Obstetrics and Gynaecology* 106 (1999): 360–66.

30. See A. A. Hare and K. S. Olah, "Pregnancy Following Endometrial Ablation: A Review Article," *Journal of Obstetrics and Gynaecology* 25 (2005): 108–14.

mally thin endometrium, which is now inhospitable to an implanting blastocyst. The abnormal endometrium would then be responsible for embryonic loss or, if implantation does occur, significant maternal and fetal complications.

Another commonly recommended treatment for abnormal bleeding caused by adenomyosis, leiomyomata, or endometriosis is the insertion of a levonorgestrel intrauterine system (LNG IUS, Mirena). The device is a T-shaped intrauterine device (IUD) containing 52 mg of levonorgestrel; it releases 20 mcg/day until, by five years after insertion, it is releasing 10 mcg/day. The drug has a profoundly thinning effect on the endometrium, which makes the glands inactive and therefore inhospitable to implantation. It also thickens cervical mucus, but the majority of cycles are ovulatory.[31] Despite the intention to treat abnormal bleeding, this device would still allow ovulation and possibly fertilization to take place but would prevent successful implantation, so it should not be used in women who are sexually active. By contrast, oral contraceptives containing first generation progestogens, taken for all but three days a month, would not be likely to result in ovulation and subsequent fertilization and would thus achieve the same desired effect as the Mirena IUS without bringing about the undesired one.

Case 4. Dysmenorrhea

L. C. is a 15-year-old girl with menarche age 10, who was placed on oral contraceptives for 6 months for dysmenorrhea. She required ibuprofen at 400 mg four times daily to control her cramps the first three days of her period. There was no family history of endometriosis. She developed an aplastic anemia and symptoms of rheumatoid arthritis that were supported by lab studies, and her mother discontinued treatment with oral contraceptives. They sought a second opinion for control of her dysmenorrhea.

Oral contraceptives are commonly prescribed for the treatment of dysmenorrhea in young women, as the pain can be severe in 15 percent of adolescent girls and leads to repetitive short-term absenteeism from school. Dysmenorrhea is common, affecting 50 percent of women, and its etiology is the increased production of prostaglandins in the secretory endometrium at the end of the cycle, which increase uterine tone and produce more severe contractions of the uterus.[32] As a result, the non-steroidal, anti-inflammatory drugs (NSAIDs) have been very useful in treating this disorder due to their inhibition of COX enzyme activity. They should be started before the period begins and taken at prescribed intervals throughout the days of the cycle that are normally painful. The drugs should be continued for up to six months before abandoning this therapy, using different formulations if necessary. In addition, vitamin B1

31. See M. I. Rodriguez et al., "Intrauterine Progestins, Progesterone Antagonists, and Receptor Modulators: A Review of Gynecologic Applications," *American Journal of Obstetrics and Gynecology* 202 (2010): 420–28.

32. See N. E. Wiqvist et al., "The Patho-Physiology of Primary Dysmenorrhea, *Research Clinical Forums* 1 (1979): 47–54.

at 100 mg/day and magnesium at 500 mg/day have been shown to ameliorate symptoms. Sometimes, short-term narcotic use is needed to control the pain. Oral contraceptives are routinely used for this purpose, because they convert the endometrium to an early proliferative phase endometrium, thus bringing about decreased production of prostaglandins. If the patient does not respond to NSAIDs, laparoscopy should be considered to rule out endometriosis as the cause of the pain, even in a teenager.

Case 5. Counseling the Adolescent Patient

A. G. is a 14-year-old girl brought to the office for an exam, if necessary, for irregular cycles. During the history, it becomes apparent that the relationship between the mother and daughter is strained. The mother expresses concern that the daughter has found some friends of whom she does not approve. She has been caught lying about where she is and whether the parents are home. The physician suggests to the mother that she go to the waiting room while the child is examined. When alone, the girl denies any sexual contact but says she is dating a 19-year-old boy. On examination, she has an unusual vaginal discharge. Subsequent cervical cultures come back positive for gonorrhea. The physician calls the mother and informs her of the test results and the need for treatment, as well as a repeat test in two weeks. A referral to an adolescent/family counselor is made, and the physician notifies the mother that this will be reported to the state department of family and children's services as a case of child sexual abuse.

The American Congress of Obstetricians and Gynecologists (ACOG), in Committee Opinion number 480, titled "The Initial Reproductive Visit," states that at a medical visit for a child 13 to 15 years old, an age-appropriate discussion, without the parent being present, be conducted with the child, regarding the following topics: pubertal development, normal menses, timing of routine exams, healthy eating habits, sexually transmitted infections (STIs), pregnancy prevention, sexual orientation and gender identity, substance abuse and use, and date-rape prevention.[33] The aim of this counseling, they allege, is to assist the child in avoiding the consequences of sexual activity outside of marriage. Methods of contraception and the treatment or prevention of STIs should be presented in a neutral fashion by the physician, as a supporter of the "choices" the child is making, according to ACOG. The physician is encouraged to develop a confidential relationship with the child on issues of sexuality, not disclosing information to the parents unless the child discloses "any evidence of or risk of bodily harm to herself or others." State laws can be reviewed through the state medical society or through the research arm of Planned Parenthood (that is, the Guttmacher Institute) with regard to the obligation of a health-care provider to report sexual abuse of minors and age of legal consent for minors. By law, a parent

---

33. See the American Congress of Obstetricians and Gynecologists (ACOG), "The Initial Reproductive Health Visit," Committee Opinion no. 460 (2010).

must give permission for health care in all other areas for a child under the age of 18 and has to give consent for a child to marry under the age of 18. However, the parent knows the child best and presumably has the best interests of the child in mind. Despite these realities, groups have worked to gradually erode the parents' control over a child's care in what is euphemistically called "reproductive health" by emancipating children to obtain contraceptives, seek an abortion, and receive treatment of sexually transmitted diseases without parental consent or knowledge.

A neutral attitude toward the adolescent's sexual activity is actually an affirmation of that activity. By providing contraceptives as the means to continue that behavior and avoid its consequences, a physician is condoning that behavior with formal cooperation. We must remember the words of Jesus Christ when he talked about sin: "Whoever causes one of these little ones who believe in me to sin, it would be better for him if a great millstone were put around his neck and he were thrown into the sea" (Mk 9:42).[34] Counseling by the physician for a return to chastity, with or without a parent present, is difficult but necessary, as the health consequences associated with adolescent sexual activity are great. Physicians are generally respected by their patients, so words of encouragement to them to be chaste will be heard and remembered, even if not acted upon by the girl at that time. Included in the discussion can be mode of dress and choices of books, media, and friends. Drug or alcohol use should also be explored with the child. Often it helps to have short brochures from a chastity speaker on hand to give her in follow-up. Remind them that the only practice that prevents pregnancy and the acquisition of STIs with 100 percent effectiveness is abstinence and chaste behavior. Sexual activity in the adolescent patient causes considerable disruption in the relationships in the family. There are possible long-term consequences of sexually transmitted diseases, which may render the girl infertile or even result in her contracting a fatal disease such as HIV; and her emotional and spiritual well-being as well as school performance may suffer. In most cases, however, fear of acquiring an STI does not deter a girl from sexual activity.

Ethical Dilemmas

The field of obstetrics has several areas that present ethical dilemmas to the Catholic physician and patient. These include genetic testing, management of ectopic pregnancies, induction of labor prior to term, emergency contraception in cases of rape, and abortion for fetal or maternal indications. Care of the neonate is not in the purview of this chapter. Let's consider some of these situations.

Genetic Testing

At the time of the patient's first visit, either as a gynecologic patient or as an obstetrical patient, an accurate and complete family history for genetic diseases should be

---

34. New American Bible.

taken. All physicians should have the ability to provide both basic genetic risk identi-fication and counseling. Couples who have a risk of conceiving a child with a genetic abnormality, based on a previously affected child, maternal age, or other family mem-bers with genetic disorders, should be counseled about their risk for a child with a genetic defect, and if appropriate, be tested for carrier status. They should be referred if necessary for more in-depth genetic counseling if it is beyond the knowledge of the health-care provider. According to the *Ethical and Religious Directives for Catholic Health Care Services,*

> genetic counseling may be provided in order to promote responsible parenthood and to pre-pare for the proper treatment and care of children with genetic defects, in accordance with Catholic moral teaching and the intrinsic rights and obligations of married couples regard-ing the transmission of life.[35]

Although any woman could conceive a child with Down syndrome, the risk of autosomal trisomy occurs more frequently after age 35. At age 25 the risk is 1:1,340, age 30 it is 1:940, age 35 it is 1:353, age 40 it is 1:85, and age 45 it is 1:35.[36] Currently the American Congress of Obstetricians and Gynecologists recommends that all preg-nant women, regardless of age, be offered serum screening for chromosomal defects or neural tube defects in the first trimester with ultrasound determination of gesta-tional age and measurement of the nuchal translucency or serum screening alone in the second trimester. The risk to the baby of genetic testing and chromosomal analysis depends upon the procedure. Chorionic villus sampling (CVS) is performed at 10 to 12 weeks' gestation either transcervically or transabdominally. The procedure carries a risk of miscarriage of 1:100 to 1:200; if done before 10 weeks, it can be complicated by leakage of amniotic fluid, infection, or fetal limb defects.[37] Amniocentesis is per-formed in the 15th to 20th week of pregnancy and carries a risk of fetal loss of 1:200 to 1:400, through injury of the baby or umbilical cord, leakage of amniotic fluid, or infection.[38] The risk for the procedure should not exceed the risk of an abnormality. Some couples want to know ahead of time that the baby has a chromosomal abnor-mality or neural tube defect so they can prepare themselves emotionally, but most of-ten this information is obtained to prevent the child from coming to term. Although as physicians we are obligated to perform the test to obtain the information for the mother, it cannot be to facilitate an abortion, should the baby be abnormal.

In the instruction *Dignitas Personae* (On Certain Bioethical Questions), the issue of preimplantation genetic testing is addressed. Unlike the genetic testing discussed above, this testing is performed on embryos created through in vitro fertilization

---

35. USCCB, *Ethical and Religious Directives*, dir. 54.

36. See March of Dimes, "Birth Defects: Down Syndrome" (2009), http://www.marchofdimes.com/baby/birthdefects_downsyndrome.html.

37. See R. S. Olney et al., "Chorionic Villus Sampling and Amniocentesis: Recommendations for Prenatal Counseling," *Morbidity and Mortality Weekly Report* (*MMWR*) 44 (1995): 1–12, http://www.cdc.gov/mmwr/preview/mmwrhtml/00038393.htm.

38. See Francisco Rojas, Elizabeth Wood, and Karin Blakemore, "Preconception Counseling and Prenatal Care," in *The Johns Hopkins Manual of Gynecology and Obstetrics*, ed. Fortner et al., 73.

prior to their being transferred into the uterus. The testing is done to assure that the embryos are free of defects or are of the desired sex. The document states:

Unlike other forms of prenatal diagnosis, in which the diagnostic phase is clearly separated from any possible later elimination and which provide therefore a period in which a couple would be free to accept a child with medical problems, in this case the diagnosis before implantation is immediately followed by the elimination of an embryo suspected of having genetic or chromosomal defects, or not having the sex desired, or having other qualities not wanted. Preimplantation diagnosis—connected as it is with artificial fertilization, which is itself always intrinsically illicit—is directed toward the *qualitative selection and consequent destruction of embryos*, which constitutes an act of abortion.[39]

Management of Ectopic Pregnancies

The incidence of ectopic pregnancy was reported as 2 percent of pregnancies in 1992. Ectopic pregnancy is the leading cause of maternal death in the first trimester and is responsible for 9 percent of all pregnancy-related deaths.[40] The majority of ectopic pregnancies occur in the fallopian tube, but they can also occur in the abdomen, the ovary, the cervix, or the cornual portion of the uterus. Predisposing factors include: maternal age greater than 40, more than three previous miscarriages, history of pelvic inflammatory disease, previous tubal surgery, previous ectopic pregnancy, adhesions from endometriosis or pelvic surgery, two or more previous abortions, infertility, and the use of assisted reproductive technologies.[41] One third of all pregnancies after a tubal ligation are ectopic. The classical presentation occurs at six to eight weeks after the last normal menstrual period, with abnormal bleeding, unilateral pelvic pain, and/or an adnexal mass. Often the patient does not realize she is pregnant, as she may have had what appeared to be a period at the usual time. Unless the patient presents with symptoms indicating a rupture of the ectopic pregnancy with a hematoperitoneum (which necessitates immediate surgery), serial ultrasounds, serial progesterone levels, and quantitative β-hCG levels will assist in the diagnosis so that treatment can be instituted before the fallopian tube ruptures. The differential diagnosis includes a threatened abortion, a normal intrauterine pregnancy, an ectopic pregnancy, or a blighted ovum. The presence of a sac in the uterus with a β-hCG level of 1500–2000 mIU/ml (the discriminatory zone) confirms an intrauterine pregnancy. The absence of a sac in the uterus by vaginal ultrasound at the discriminatory zone of β-hCG should be rechecked in 48 hours with a repeat β-hCG, as it may be a twin pregnancy or a spontaneous abortion. The absence of a sac in the uterus, fluid in the cul de sac, a dilated fallopian tube, or the presence of a sac in the fallopian tube with possible cardiac activity, are indicative of an ectopic pregnancy at a β-hCG level of 2000 mIU/ml.

39. Congregation for the Doctrine of the Faith, *Dignitas Personae, Instruction on Certain Bioethical Questions* (Vatican City, Vatican: Libreria Editrice Vaticana, 2008), no. 22.

40. See K. T. Barnhart, I. Katz, A. Hummel, and C. R. Gracia, "Presumed Diagnosis of Ectopic Pregnancy," *Obstetrics and Gynecology* 100 (2002): 505–10.

41. See J. Bouyer et al., "Risk Factors for Ectopic Pregnancy: a Comprehensive Analysis Based on a Large Case-Control, Population-Based Study in France," *American Journal of Epidemiology* 157 (2003): 185–94.

Serum progesterone levels greater than or equal to 20 ng/ml confirm a normal pregnancy, whereas a level less than 5 ng/ml confirms an abnormal pregnancy. Most ectopic pregnancies have progesterone levels between 10 ng/ml and 20 ng/ml.[42] A rise in β-hCG of less than 53 percent in 48 hours confirms an ectopic pregnancy with 99 percent sensitivity.[43]

There are four possible managements of ectopic pregnancy. Expectant management may be carried out for the patient who is asymptomatic and has declining β-hCG levels that start out at less than 200 mU/ml. Of these patients, 88 percent will resolve without treatment.[44] The other three treatments are dependent on whether the ectopic pregnancy has ruptured with a hematoperitoneum or is unruptured. Patients who have a ruptured ectopic pregnancy classically present in shock with severe abdominal pain, possible shoulder pain, some vaginal bleeding, and signs of acute blood loss secondary to the hematoperitoneum. Surgical treatment, either by laparoscopy or laparotomy, with partial or complete salpingectomy is still the treatment of choice for a ruptured ectopic pregnancy.

The ethical dilemma occurs when the patient presents with an unruptured ectopic pregnancy. Removal of the portion of the damaged fallopian tube where the ectopic pregnancy resides, even if an embryo is present, is ethical under the principle of double effect.[45] The action of removing a damaged part of the fallopian tube is a good action as it prevents further ectopic pregnancies on that side and saves the mother from certain hemorrhage and possible death. The bad effect of ending the embryo's life with an indirect abortion is not intended and does not bring about the good effect for the mother. There is no hope for survival of the child in the tube, so it is less proportionate than the good effect for the mother. This is covered in directive 47 of the *Ethical and Religious Directives*:

Operations, treatments, and medications that have as their direct purpose the cure of a proportionately serious pathological condition of a pregnant woman are permitted when they cannot be safely postponed until the unborn child is viable, even if they will result in the death of the child.[46]

However, directive 48 states: "In case of extrauterine pregnancy, no intervention is morally licit which constitutes a direct abortion."[47] A direct abortion is defined in directive 45 as "the directly intended termination of pregnancy before viability or the directly intended destruction of a viable fetus."[48]

42. See T. G. Stovall et al., "Serum Progesterone and Uterine Curettage in Differential Diagnosis of Ectopic Pregnancy," *Fertility and Sterility* 57 (1992): 456–57.

43. See K. T. Barnhart et al., "Symptomatic Patients with an Early Viable Intrauterine Pregnancy: HCG Curves Redefined," *Obstetrics and Gynecology* 104 (2004): 50–55.

44. See J. Korhonen, U. H. Stenman, and P. Ylotalo, "Serum Human Chorionic Gonadotropin Dynamics during Spontaneous Resolution of Ectopic Pregnancy," *Fertility and Sterility* 63 (1994): 632–36.

45. For an explanation of the principle of double effect, see ch. 1, section titled "On the Four Principles of Medical Ethics," par. 5, above.

46. USCCB, *Ethical and Religious Directives*, dir. 47.

47. Ibid., dir. 48.

48. Ibid., dir. 45.

Two newer treatments for an unruptured ectopic pregnancy actually attack the embryo directly: these treatments remove the embryo and trophoblastic tissue either surgically from the tube by a linear salpingostomy, or chemically with the administration of methotrexate, without removing the damaged portion of tube. Subsequent pregnancy rates are the same after either a salpingostomy or partial salpingectomy, despite blocking the tube on the side of the ectopic with a partial salpingectomy.[49] Failure rates of salpingostomy for a persistent ectopic pregnancy range from 2 to 20 percent.[50] If there is a live embryo present in the tube, these two treatments would constitute a direct abortion of the embryo. So are these treatments ever licit?

Two ethical arguments, which have been put forth by Christopher Kaczor and Rev. Martin Rhonheimer, defend the permissibility of salpingostomy or methotrexate for the treatment of ectopic pregnancies. Their arguments were refuted by M. A. Anderson et al. in an article published in 2011.[51] Kaczor said the action of removing the embryo from the tube was not an evil action, as the embryo could be moved somewhere else. However, that is not what happens. The authors of the 2011 article countered that with a linear salpingostomy an action is taken that directly kills the embryo. Kaczor also justified the use of methotrexate in ectopic pregnancies, as it would stop further damage to the fallopian tube caused by the trophoblastic tissue. Anderson et al. concluded that it would be licit to administer methotrexate if the embryo was dead, but if it was dying such administration would be illicit. Rhonheimer's moral justification for these treatments was that, as the action was intended to save the life of the mother and as the embryo had no chance for survival in its ectopic location, it did not have the right to be immune from being killed. Anderson et al. countered that the right to life of the embryo and its protection from being directly killed by a linear salpingostomy or methotrexate were true justice.

However, it is justified to use these treatments to end the ectopic pregnancy and save the life of the mother provided there is no live embryo present, just as, in the case of a missed abortion in which the baby has died but the woman has not passed the products of conception, one would be perfectly justified in performing a D&C. According to a review article on the ethics of treating ectopic pregnancies, A. Pivarunas cited several articles that show that a live embryo is present in only 14 to 17.8 percent of ectopic pregnancies.[52] Therefore, in the majority of cases of ectopic pregnancy, a live embryo is not present. But, how can that be determined with some degree of certainty? Obviously if cardiac activity is seen in the tubal mass, a live embryo is present, and the treatment should be a partial salpingectomy. In a study by D. Brown and P. Doubilet, cardiac activity is seen by ultrasound in about 20 percent of ectopic preg-

49. See S. J. Ory et al., "Fertility after Ectopic Pregnancy," *Fertility and Sterility* 60 (1993): 231–35.

50. See D. L. Fylstra, "Tubal Pregnancy: A Review of Current Diagnosis and Treatment," *Obstetrical and Gynecological Survey* 53 (1998): 320–28.

51. M. A. Anderson et al., "Ectopic Pregnancy and Catholic Morality: A Response to Arguments in Favor of Salpingostomy and Methotrexate," *National Catholic Bioethics Quarterly* 11, no. 1 (Spring 2011): 667–84.

52. See A. R. Pivarunas, "Ethical and Moral Considerations in the Treatment of Ectopic Pregnancy," *Linacre Quarterly* 70 (2003): 195–209.

nancies.[53] Pivarunas also stated that in a patient with an ectopic with a progesterone level less than 5 ng/ml *and* β-hCG levels that rise less than 25 percent over 48 hours, embryonic death has occurred and treatment with either partial salpingectomy, salpingostomy, or methotrexate would be appropriate. The decision to use methotrexate should never be made based on a single set of lab values or a single ultrasound. The single-dose regimen of methotrexate is 50 mg/sq m on day 1, followed by drawing serum β-hCG levels between days 4 and 7. There should be a 15 percent decrease in the levels. Levels should be followed weekly until they return to non-pregnant levels. If the decrease of 15 percent is not seen between days 4 and 7, the dose is repeated, and the levels are followed in the same way. Absolute contraindications to the use of methotrexate are breastfeeding, a compromised immune system, liver disease, blood dyscrasias, peptic ulcer disease, active pulmonary disease, and kidney disease.[54] Failures are more likely to occur with rupture of the ectopic pregnancy if the sac is larger than 3.5 cm and there is cardiac activity, which would be an absolute contraindication for physicians who want to provide the patient with the best treatment that does not constitute a direct abortion.

Case 6. Early Induction of Labor

M. R. is a 36-year-old woman, gravida 2 para 1001, with a previous cesarean section for cephalopelvic disproportion, who learns at 18 weeks' gestation that the child she is carrying has Trisomy 13. After receiving the explanation that this is a lethal anomaly, and not wanting to experience another cesarean for a child who may not live beyond the newborn period, she asks if the baby could be delivered early, at 22 weeks' gestation, to avoid a cesarean.

The *Ethical and Religious Directives* state in directive 49: "For a proportionate reason, labor may be induced after the fetus is viable."[55] This means that for a clinically significant reason, in the case of either disease in the mother or a condition affecting both mother and child, or illness in the infant, labor can be induced before term, or 37 or greater weeks' gestation from the last menstrual period. Some of those reasons for the mother may include severe preeclampsia, hypertension, a malignancy, cardiac disease, or premature rupture of membranes with chorioamnionitis. For the fetus, it may be hydrops fetalis, hydrocephalus, oligohydramnios, or other evidence of fetal distress and intrauterine growth retardation. The consideration about when to induce labor or do an elective cesarean weighs the gravity of the medical condition versus the risk to the baby from early delivery.

A baby is considered premature if delivery occurs prior to 37 weeks, and survival of the baby depends on the gestational age. Delivery at 23 weeks has a 17 percent

53. See D. Brown and P. Doubilet, "Transvaginal Sonography for Diagnosing Ectopic Pregnancy: Positivity Criteria and Performance Characteristics," *Journal of Ultrasound in Medicine* 13 (1994): 259–66.

54. See ACOG, "Medical Management of Ectopic Pregnancy," *ACOG Practice Bulletin*, no. 94 (2008).

55. USCCB, *Ethical and Religious Directives*, dir. 49.

chance of survival, at 24 weeks a 39 percent chance of survival, and at 25 weeks a 50 percent chance of survival.[56] Delivery at 24 weeks is considered the limit of viability. Even if the child survives, however, he or she faces significant risks, including apnea, retinopathy of prematurity, cerebral palsy, intraventricular hemorrhage, hypoxic-ischemic encephalopathy, and developmental disabilities. These children invariably have respiratory distress syndrome with subsequent chronic lung disease, hypoglycemia, necrotizing enterocolitis, sepsis, feeding problems, and jaundice. Only 20 percent of these children will survive without disabilities, whereas 46 percent have severe or moderate disabilities such as cerebral palsy, vision or hearing loss, or learning disabilities; another 34 percent are mildly disabled.[57] In addition, elective induction in a nulliparous woman between 37 and 41 weeks' gestation is associated with increased rates of cesarean section, postpartum hemorrhage, neonatal resuscitation, and longer hospital stays.[58] In all cases of decision making for early delivery for fetal reasons, the risks to the mother must be proportionate to the benefit to the child. When early delivery is considered for maternal reasons, the risk to the baby must be proportionate to the benefit to the mother, as they have equal dignity and value as human persons.

Therefore, to avoid undue morbidity for the child, all attempts must be made to get the pregnancy to 34 weeks' gestation. In the situation of premature rupture of membranes, a complication of pregnancy that places both the mother and the baby at risk for sepsis, the management depends on the gestational age. Patients at 34 to 36 weeks' gestation are induced to delivery. At 32 to 33 weeks the risk of prematurity for the baby is greater than the risk of infection, so they are managed expectantly, with Group B Streptococcal prophylaxis, possible corticosteroids, and antibiotics to prolong latency. At 24 to 31 weeks' gestation, they are managed expectantly with the same treatment as 32 to 33 weeks and also possible tocolysis if labor ensues.[59]

A major bioethical dilemma comes with premature rupture of membranes at less than 24 to 26 weeks' gestation. A recent review of 11 studies showed a 21 percent perinatal survival rate at this gestational age.[60] An induction of labor should be carried out only if the mother is becoming septic as a result of the premature rupture of membranes. An induction of labor is not intended to end the life of the child but to treat the underlying sepsis by delivery, so even if the child should die as a result of the induction, there is no bioethical problem because this would fall under the principle of double effect. The action of inducing labor is not evil, and the induction is not in-

56. See Quint Boenker Preemie Survival Foundation, "Premature Birth Statistics," http:/preemiesurvival.org/info/index.html.

57. See H. N. Simhan and S. N. Caritas, "Prevention of Preterm Delivery," *New England Journal of Medicine* 357 (2007): 477–87.

58. See J. H. Vardo, L. L. Thornburg, and J. C. Glantz, "Maternal and Neonatal Morbidity among Nulliparous Women Undergoing Elective Induction of Labor," *Journal of Reproductive Medicine* 56 (2011): 25–30.

59. See ACOG, "Premature Rupture of Membranes," *ACOG Practice Bulletin*, no. 80 (Washington, D.C.: ACOG, 2007).

60. See H. Dewan and J. M. Morris, "A Systematic Review of Pregnancy Outcome following Preterm Rupture of Membranes at a Previable Gestational Age," *Australia New Zealand Journal of Obstetrics and Gynaecology* 41 (2001): 389–94.

tended to attack the baby directly but to deliver the infected products of conception that put both the mother and baby at risk. The delivery of the baby is intended by a good means (induction of labor). Lastly, the risk to the mother is great, so the induction must be carried out.

The same principles can be applied in cases of maternal pregnancy-induced hypertension. This condition affects 5 to 8 percent of pregnancies and is most common in first pregnancies.[61] The decision to deliver the baby takes into account the degree of maternal disease and the gestational age and condition of the baby. The criteria for diagnosing preeclampsia include a blood pressure of 140 mm systolic or greater and/or 90 mm diastolic or greater after 20 weeks' gestation in a previously normotensive woman, and proteinuria of 0.3 g or more in a 24-hour urine specimen.[62] As long as the mother's disease is controlled with bed rest and possibly anti-hypertensives, and her laboratory values do not indicate the development of severe preeclampsia, expectant management until 37 weeks is appropriate. However, if the woman develops severe pregnancy induced hypertension (defined as a BP of 160 systolic or 110 diastolic or higher on two occasions six or more hours apart, proteinuria of 5 g or more in a 24-hour period or 3+ protein on two urine samples 4 hours apart, oliguria of 500 ml in 24 hours, cerebral or visual disturbances, pulmonary edema or cyanosis, epigastric pain, impaired liver function, thrombocytopenia, or intrauterine growth retardation), then the patient needs to be delivered. If the baby is preterm, this should be accomplished in a tertiary-care setting with consultation from a maternal-fetal medicine specialist as well as a neonatologist.[63]

Some conditions are unique for risk to the mother, such as the development of a cancer, an automobile accident rendering her comatose, or a preexisting medical condition that is worsened by the pregnancy. Breast cancer is the most common cancer in a pregnant woman, occurring in 1 out of 3,000 pregnancies. It was frequently recommended that a woman diagnosed with breast cancer in the first trimester have an abortion, but termination of pregnancy does not change the outcome for the woman and is no longer a therapeutic option.[64] Procedures for staging and treating the woman have to be modified to avoid harm to the baby from radiation, as nuclear scans and MRIs cannot be performed in pregnancy since they can lead to fetal damage. Surgery is the primary treatment for breast cancer and can be performed at any time. Radiation should be postponed until the patient has delivered. Chemotherapy can be given in the second and third trimesters without harm to the fetus.[65] Women diagnosed

61. See F. G. Cunningham et al., "Hypertensive Disorders in Pregnancy," in *Williams Obstetrics*, 21st ed. (New York: McGraw-Hill, 2001), 567–618.

62. Data from National High Blood Pressure Education Program Working Group on High Blood Pressure in Pregnancy, "Report of the National High Blood Pressure Education Program Working Group on High Blood Pressure in Pregnancy," *American Journal of Obstetrics and Gynecology* 183 (2000): S1–S22.

63. See ACOG, "Diagnosis and Management of Preeclampsia and Eclampsia," *ACOG Practice Bulletin* no. 33 (Washington, D.C.: ACOG, 2002).

64. See H. S. Rugo, "Management of Breast Cancer Diagnosed during Pregnancy," *Current Treatment Options in Oncology* 4 (2003): 165–73.

65. See H. M. Kuerer et al., "Conservative Surgery and Chemotherapy for Breast Carcinoma during Pregnancy," *Surgery* 131 (2002): 108–10.

with breast cancer in pregnancy may have a worse survival rate, but this could be due to a delay in the diagnosis, not because of the pregnancy.[66] Women who have had breast cancer are usually told to avoid pregnancy for two years after the diagnosis, primarily to watch for an early recurrence.[67]

Cardiac disease in the mother complicates 1 to 4 percent of pregnancies in women without preexisting heart disease and is a major cause of non-obstetric maternal morbidity in pregnancy.[68] Pregnancy increases maternal blood volume by 40 to 50 percent, partly because of the estrogen-mediated activation of the renin-aldosterone axis. There is also an increase in red blood cell mass, but this is less than the blood volume, so most women have a decrease in their hemoglobin. By 20 to 24 weeks' gestation, cardiac output increases by 30 to 50 percent, peaking by 27 weeks. The increase in cardiac output is caused by an increased preload from the increased blood volume, reduced afterload (because of the fall in systemic vascular resistance), and an increased maternal heart rate. Delivery results in increased maternal blood pressure and blood loss. The relief of vena caval compression once the baby delivers results in an increased venous return, increased cardiac output, and diuresis.[69] It is important that preconception counseling be provided for women with known heart disease, so that both the maternal and the fetal risks and the mother's long-term survival rate are understood. The four risk factors that will determine her outcome should she get pregnant include a previous cardiac event; cyanosis (or the New York Heart Association class III and IV heart failure); left heart obstruction; and systemic ventricular dysfunction.[70]

Pulmonary hypertension (PH), also called Eisenmenger's syndrome, is a rare, progressive condition, which when associated with pregnancy carries a significant mortality rate to the mother, estimated to be 30 to 56 percent;[71] it is also a contraindication to pregnancy. The standard recommendation has been to terminate the pregnancy because of the risk to the mother of sudden death. The causes of PH can vary; they include pulmonary arterial hypertension, which is idiopathic or associated with a congenital heart defect such as an atrial septal or ventricular septal defect or systemic sclerosis; PH in association with left heart disease; PH in association with lung disease; chronic thromboembolic pulmonary hypertension; and miscellaneous causes.[72] Pulmonary arterial hypertension is caused by a proliferation of the intima

---

66. See W. T. Yang et al., "Imaging of Breast Cancer Diagnosed and Treated with Chemotherapy during Pregnancy," *Radiology* 239 (2006): 52–60.

67. See J. A. Petrek, "Pregnancy Safety after Breast Cancer," *Cancer* 74 (1994): 528–31.

68. See S. C. Siu et al., "Risk and Predictors for Pregnancy-Related Complications in Women with Heart Disease," *Circulation* 96 (1997): 2789–94.

69. See S. Davidson and E. M. Graham, "Cardiopulmonary Disorders of Pregnancy," in *The Johns Hopkins Manual of Gynecology and Obstetrics*, ed. Fortner et al., 192–203.

70. See S. C. Siu et al., "Prospective Multicenter Study of Pregnancy Outcomes in Women with Heart Disease," *Circulation* 104 (2001): 515–21.

71. See B. M. Weiss et al., "Outcome of Pulmonary Vascular Disease in Pregnancy: A Systematic Overview from 1978 through 1996," *Journal of the American College of Cardiology* 31 (1998): 1650–57.

72. See G. Simmoneau et al., "Updated Clinical Classification of Pulmonary Hypertension," *Journal of the American College of Cardiology* 54 (2009): S43–54.

and media of the pulmonary arterial system with resultant increased pulmonary vascular resistance. Chronic thromboembolic pulmonary hypertension results from an obstruction in pulmonary blood flow caused by chronic pulmonary emboli. All of these variants result in a right ventricle that cannot tolerate an increased afterload (which leads to right heart failure) and cannot adjust to an increase in cardiac output or the large fluid shifts that especially occur at delivery.[73] The most frequent time for sudden death is immediately postpartum due to blood loss and diuresis, but cardiac decompensation can occur at any time during the pregnancy. The cardiovascular changes described above that normally occur in pregnancy worsen the pulmonary hypertension resulting in right heart failure, liver enlargement, and thromboses.

Over the past ten years, new drugs have been introduced that have greatly improved the treatment of PH, namely prostacyclin analogues, phosphodiesterase inhibitors, and endothelin-receptor antagonists. A multidisciplinary approach with a management team of cardiologists, intensivists, obstetricians, anesthesiologists, and neonatologists has succeeded in reducing the maternal mortality to 25 percent.[74] Important features of care include anticoagulation before and after delivery, the avoidance of general anesthesia, cardiac monitoring including central venous catheters and arterial lines in labor that monitor the right atrial pressure, and the use of vasodilators such as intravenous epoprostenol.[75] No deleterious effects have been seen on the mother or infant from these agents.

In a recent retrospective review in the *British Journal of Obstetrics and Gynecology*,[76] nine women with PH during ten pregnancies chose to continue their pregnancies. The authors described a unique management program that used frequent monitoring, early nebulized targeted therapy, escalation of targeted therapy when the patient's condition worsened, and elective cesarean delivery under regional anesthesia at 34 weeks' gestation. The patients were cared for through a pulmonary vascular disease unit. The outcomes were excellent with this aggressive multidisciplinary approach, as all women and babies survived pregnancy and delivery. Four women required intravenous prostanoid therapy, all women were delivered between 26 and 37 weeks' gestation by cesarean section, of which nine out of ten were planned deliveries. One of the nine women, who on her own discontinued therapy, died four weeks postpartum.

Although pregnancy still carries a very significant risk to the mother with PH—and should be avoided by learning a modern method of natural family planning and using only the post-ovulatory phase for intercourse—there are encouraging new treatments for this serious disease that help both the mother and the unborn child. If in treating the mother, the baby dies, the treatment is nevertheless justified under the principle of double effect. It was not the intention that the baby die with the

73. See D. G. Kiely et al., "Improved Survival in Pregnancy and Pulmonary Hypertension Using a Multiprofessional Approach," *British Journal of Obstetrics and Gynecology* 117 (2010): 565–74.
74. See E. Bedard, K. Dimopoulos, and M. A.Gatzoulis, "Has There Been Any Progress Made on Pregnancy Outcomes among Women with Pulmonary Hypertension?" *European Heart Journal* 30 (2009): 256–65.
75. See R. Stewart et al., "Pregnancy and Primary Pulmonary Hypertension: Successful Outcome with Epoprostenol Therapy," *Chest* 153 (2001): 1037–47.
76. Kiely et al., "Improved Survival in Pregnancy and Pulmonary Hypertension."

treatment. The standard medical recommendation for this condition has been to terminate the pregnancy in the first trimester. This can never be justified, as directive 45 of the *Ethical and Religious Directives* states:

Abortion (that is, the directly intended termination of pregnancy before viability or the directly intended destruction of a viable fetus) is never permitted. Every procedure whose sole immediate effect is the termination of pregnancy before viability is an abortion, which, in its moral context, includes the interval between conception and implantation of the embryo. Catholic health care institutions are not to provide abortion services.[77]

Likewise, Catholic doctors should never perform a direct abortion, even in cases of rape, incest, or to save the life of the mother. A suction dilation and evacuation procedure (D&E) on the pregnant uterus in the presence of a live fetus is a direct attack on the fetus. The fetus does not die as a result of treatment for the mother, but at the hand of the doctor performing the abortion. Some have attempted to justify this as a removal of the placenta, which they say is aggravating the woman's condition, but a dilation and evacuation of a gravid uterus in the presence of a live fetus is the deliberate killing of an innocent human being.[78]

In cases of nonlethal anomalies in the baby, for example, Down syndrome (trisomy 21), or structural defects, such as spina bifida, hydrocephalus, or omphalocele, a mother may want to have the baby aborted or have a second-trimester abortion by labor induction, out of emotional distress at having a child with anomalies. This is never in the best interest of the child, who has dignity as a human person regardless of a disability. It is so important to provide the parents with sound counseling, as frequently the prognosis for the child is portrayed in only negative terms. It can never be justified to abort the baby or to deliver prior to 37 weeks' gestation because of emotional stress for the mother. The family needs support through the pregnancy, delivery, and neonatal period.

In cases of lethal anomalies in the baby such as trisomy 13, trisomy 18, anencephaly, renal agenesis, and others, the decision to deliver the baby before 37 weeks cannot be made on the basis that the child will die anyway or that the situation is too stressful for the family to wait.[79] Likewise, in Case 6 presented above, early delivery in the second trimester because the mother will need repeat cesareans if she is not induced and the baby is going to die anyway puts the baby at a disproportionate risk from the induction compared to minimal indications for the mother if not induced early. If the mother develops severe preeclampsia or significant polyhydramnios, then there is a significant risk for the mother of continuing the pregnancy and a proportionate reason for induction for both mother and child. The child's life is not any less valuable because of the disability. In all these cases, the decision making starts first with

---

77. USCCB, *Ethical and Religious Directives*, dir. 45.

78. See USCCB, *The Distinction between Direct Abortion and Legitimate Medical Procedures* (Washington, D.C.: USCCB, 2010).

79. On anencephaly, see USCCB, "Moral Principles Concerning Infants with Anencephaly," September 19, 1996, http://www.usccb.org/issues-and-action/human-life-and-dignity/end-of-life/moral-principles-concerning-infants-with-anencephaly.cfm.

the risk to the mother of continuing the pregnancy. If there is not a great risk to her health, the pregnancy should follow its natural course to the end.[80]

Case 7. Induced Abortion and Its Complications

A. H. is a 32-year-old married elementary school teacher who telephones the doctor about an unexpected pregnancy at 6 weeks. Her physician cared for her through her two previous pregnancies and deliveries. She says she wants an abortion and a tubal ligation, because she and her husband wanted only two children and this child is inconvenient. When her physician tells her she does not perform abortions, that this is a child just like her other two children, and that having an abortion will harm her relationship with her husband, she asks for a referral to the safest place to have an abortion. The physician refuses to give a recommendation for abortion to the patient.

The *Catechism of the Catholic Church* states:

Human life must be respected and protected absolutely from the moment of conception. From the first moment of his existence, a human being must be recognized as having the rights of a person—among which is the inviolable right of every innocent being to life. "Before I formed you in the womb I knew you, and before you were born I consecrated you."[81]

This was a teaching of the Church from its inception: "You shall not kill the embryo by abortion and shall not cause the newborn to perish."[82]

The Church also states that formal cooperation in an abortion, that is, a "willing participation on the part of the cooperative agent in the sinful act of the principle agent,"[83] is grounds for excommunication because it "is gravely contrary to the moral law": "every innocent human individual" has an "inalienable right to life."[84]

Human life is sacred because from its beginning it involves "the creative action of God" and it remains forever in a special relationship with the Creator, who is its sole end. God alone is the Lord of life from its beginning until its end: no one can, in any circumstance, claim for himself the right to destroy directly an innocent human being.[85]

Anyone who procures a completed abortion, performs or actively assists in an abortion, or pressures a woman into having an abortion incurs the automatic penalty of excommunication. In this way, the Church "makes clear the gravity of the crime com-

---

80. See P. Cataldo and T. M. Goodwin, "Early Induction of Labor," in *Catholic Healthcare Ethics*, 2nd ed., ed. Edward J. Furton, Peter J. Cataldo, and Albert S. Moraczewski, OP (Philadelphia: The National Catholic Bioethics Center, 2009), 111–18.

81. *Catechism of the Catholic Church*, no. 2270.

82. *Didache* (c. 100), 2, 2 (SCh 248, 148). Quoted in the *Catechism of the Catholic Church*, no. 2271.

83. National Catholic Bioethics Center, "Formal and Material Cooperation," *Ethics and Medics* 20, no. 6 (June 1995): 1–2.

84. *Catechism of the Catholic Church*, nos. 2271, 2273.

85. Congregation for the Doctrine of the Faith, *Donum Vitae, Instruction on Respect for Human Life in Its Origin and on the Dignity of Procreation*, February 22, 1987, intro., no. 5 (quoting Pope John XXIII, *Mater et Magistra*, Encyclical Letter, May 15, 1961, no. 194), http://www.vatican.va/roman_curia/congregations/cfaith/documents/rc_con_cfaith_doc_19870222_respect-for-human-life_en.html.

mitted, the irreparable harm done to the innocent who is put to death, as well as to the parents and the whole of society."[86] In the United States, with the legalization of abortion in 1973, most of the bishops in the country gave to the priests of their dioceses the faculty to lift the penalty of excommunication through the sacrament of Reconciliation. Pope Francis extended that faculty to every Catholic priest in the world for the period of the Extraordinary Jubilee Year of Mercy, December 8, 2015, until November 20, 2016; and then in his apostolic letter *Misericordia et Misera*, he gave this faculty permanently to all priests.[87]

Abortion was made legal in the United States on January 22, 1973, by the U.S. Supreme Court under the right to privacy of the woman to choose to end a pregnancy. Janet Smith has an excellent treatise on the right to privacy.[88] At the time of the Supreme Court's decision, we did not have the sophisticated obstetrical ultrasound that we have today, nor the clear biological evidence showing scientifically when a human life begins.[89] There is no mandatory reporting of abortions or their complications in the United States, and it is estimated that there are 1.3 million abortions in this country each year, with 82 percent of them occurring in unmarried women.[90] African-American women have abortions at three times the rate of Caucasian women in the United States. Also, complications from abortions are not reported in the United States to any central government agency, so it is impossible to confirm either the claim that legal abortion is safe or the actual numbers of abortions being performed. The short-term complications of induced abortion include hemorrhage, infection, retained products of conception, uterine perforation, and cervical laceration. A failure to document products of conception, that is, the fetus, at the time of the abortion could result in the rupture of an undiagnosed ectopic pregnancy.

Medical abortion is carried out by the self-administration of 200 mg of mifepristone, which blocks the progesterone and glucocorticoid receptors, followed in two days with 800 mcg of misoprostol, a prostaglandin. The procedure was approved in the United States up to 49 days from the last menstrual period, but it is done consistently up to 70 days. Although these medical abortions are not being tracked in the United States, there have been some studies comparing the safety of this medical procedure to the safety of a surgical abortion. I. M. Spitz et al. studied the failure rate for medical abortions based on gestational age.[91] Mifepristone administered at 49 days or less failed 8 percent of the time. When given at 50 to 56 days, it failed 17 percent of the

86. *Catechism of the Catholic Church*, no. 2272.

87. Pope Francis, *Misericordia et Misera*, Apostolic Letter, November 20, 2016, no. 12, https://w2.vatican.va/content/francesco/en/apost_letters/documents/papa-francesco-lettera-ap_20161120_misericordia-et-misera.html.

88. Janet E. Smith, *The Right to Privacy* (Philadelphia: National Catholic Bioethics Center and Ignatius Press, 2008).

89. See M. L. Condic, *When Does Human Life Begin?* (Thornwood, N.Y.: Westchester Institute for Ethics and the Human Person, 2008).

90. See L. B. Finer and S. K. Henshaw, "Abortion Incidence and Service in the United States in 2000," *Perspectives in Sexual Reproductive Health* 35 (2003): 6–15.

91. See I. M. Spitz et al., "Early Pregnancy Termination with Mifepristone and Misoprostol in the United States," *New England Journal of Medicine* 338 (1998): 1241–47.

time and at 57 to 63 days, 23 percent of women failed to abort completely. In a prospective study of 178 women undergoing a medical abortion as compared with 199 undergoing a surgical abortion, and followed for two weeks post-procedure, investigators found the medical abortions failed 18.3 percent of the time and the woman required a D&C as compared with 4.7 percent of surgical abortions that required a repeat D&C for continued bleeding.[92] Those having medical abortions reported bleeding for longer periods of time, with more pain and more nausea and vomiting than those having surgical abortions. The largest study on outcomes of medical abortions, however, has come out of Finland, where women register to have an abortion and vital statistics are cross-checked with emergency room visits and death certificates.[93] All women undergoing induced abortion between 2000 and 2006 were reviewed. These included 22,368 undergoing medical abortions and 20,251 women undergoing a surgical abortion. All were followed for six weeks post-procedure. Those having a medical abortion had four times the risk of complications (20 percent) as compared with a 5.6 percent rate of complications in those who had a surgical abortion, including hemorrhage and a follow-up D&C procedure. The researchers expressed concern over this complication rate, because medical abortions were on the rise, with 64 percent of all abortions in Finland in 2007 being done with mifepristone; hence, they predicted a rise in maternal morbidity from abortion.

A study published in 2002 by J. Bouyer et al. demonstrated that a prior medical abortion was associated with an increased risk of a subsequent ectopic pregnancy, with an adjusted odds ratio of 2.5; they found no such association after a surgical abortion.[94]

In the first four years of use of mifepristone in the United States (2000–2004), 607 adverse events were reported to the Food and Drug Administration,[95] which included hemorrhage requiring blood transfusion, unplanned surgery, and ruptured undiagnosed ectopic pregnancies; and there were 7 cases of septic shock due to *Clostridium sordelli* resulting in 6 maternal deaths. As mifepristone blocks both the progesterone and glucocorticoid receptors and interferes with the controlled release and functioning of cortisol and cytokines, it has been proposed that the resultant suppression of the immune system makes the woman more vulnerable to an overwhelming uterine infection after medical abortion.[96]

G. Delgado and M. L. Davenport published a series of case reports of six women who had ingested mifepristone at the abortion facility and then sought help in reversing the medical abortion that would ensue.[97] In each case, the second drug, misopro-

92. See J. T. Jensen et al., "Outcomes of Suction Curettage and Mifepristone Abortion in the United States," *Contraception* 59 (1999): 153–59.

93. See M. Niinimaki et al., "Immediate Complications after Medical Compared with Surgical Termination of Pregnancy," *Obstetrics and Gynecology* 114 (2009): 795–804.

94. See Bouyer et al., "Risk Factors for Ectopic Pregnancy."

95. See M. M. Gary and D. J. Harrison, "Analysis of Severe Adverse Events Related to the Use of Mifepristone as an Abortifacient," *The Annals of Pharmacotherapy* 40 (2006): 191–97.

96. See R. P. Miech, "Pathophysiology of Mifepristone-Induced Septic Shock Due to *Clostridium sordellii*," *Annals of Pharmacotherapy* 39 (2005): 1483–88.

97. G. Delgado and M. L. Davenport, "Progesterone Use to Reverse the Effects of Mifepristone," *Annals of Pharmacotherapy* 46, no. 12 (December 2012): e36. doi: 10.1345/aph.1R252.

stol, had not been ingested. In four of the six cases, the abortion was stopped and the women went on to deliver full term infants without complications or birth defects. A website was established at www.AbortionPillReversal.com for women to find a physician near them who could treat them with progesterone to reverse the effects of mifepristone. Now being collected is a registry of cases that use a protocol of intra-muscular progesterone in oil 200 mg as soon as possible, repeated daily for the next two days, then every other day for up to two weeks. The patient then receives weekly intramuscular progesterone until 12 weeks of pregnancy. An ultrasound should be performed within 72 hours to document a live fetus. If progesterone in oil is not available, the patient can receive oral progesterone 400mg twice daily until the end of the first trimester. Alternatively, the oral capsules can be used vaginally, to minimize side effects of fatigue and dizziness.

There are three consistent, long-term complications of abortion that are ignored by the medical field, all of which can be averted by the woman delivering at term. These complications should be an important part of informed consent when a woman is considering terminating a pregnancy.

The first is the increased risk of premature delivery subsequent to an abortion. There is overwhelming evidence from at least 122 statistically significant studies from 1963 until January 2011, worldwide, demonstrating a significantly increased risk of a subsequent premature delivery in women who have had an abortion. The Institute of Medicine published a report in 2006 on causes of preterm birth at less than 37 weeks' gestation in the United States.[98] They found that the incidence of preterm birth in 2004 was 12.5 percent, which represented an increase of 30 percent since 1981, with a cost of $26 billion a year to society. The highest rates of prematurity were in African-American women at 17.8 percent, compared with white women at 11.5 percent. In the report's appendix on page 519, they listed prior first-trimester abortion as an "immutable" risk factor for premature delivery. When they looked at early premature births at less than 32 weeks, they found that African-American women had three times the incidence as compared with white women. According to the Centers for Disease Control, African-American women have three times the rate of abortions compared with white women.[99]

In B. Rooney and B. C. Calhoun's meta-analysis of 49 studies, they found at least a 95 percent confidence in an increased risk of preterm birth, low birth weight, or second-trimester spontaneous abortion in women with a previous induced abortion.[100] Although the risk of preterm delivery increases with each previous induced abortion, it decreases with each full term delivery. In a study out of Germany, these investigators found an odds ratio (OR) of 2.5 for an extremely premature birth (EPB)

98. Institute of Medicine of the National Academies, Committee on Understanding Premature Birth and Assuring Healthy Outcomes, *Preterm Birth: Causes, Consequences, and Prevention*, ed. Richard E. Behrman and Adrienne Stith Butler (Washington, D.C.: National Academies Press, 2006).

99. L. T. Strauss et al., "Abortion Surveillance-United States, 2003," *MMWR* 55 (2006): 1–32, http://www.cdc.gov/mmwr/preview/mmwrhtml/ss5511a1.htm.

100. B. Rooney and B. C. Calhoun, "Induced Abortion and Risk of Premature Births," *Journal of American Physicians and Surgeons* 8 (2003): 46–49.

at less than 32 weeks' after one abortion, an OR of 5.2 for an EPB after two induced abortions, and an OR of 8.0 for an EPB with three or more abortions.[101] The odds ratio is the ratio of the odds of an event occurring in one group to the odds of it occurring in another group.

Rooney and Calhoun concluded that these increased risks of subsequent premature delivery could be attributed to an incompetent cervix, especially after a dilation and evacuation procedure, uterine adhesions, or infection after the abortion. They stated: "The evidence meets four of the criteria for determining causality: (1) the abortions preceded the premature births; (2) the association is strong; (3) there is a dose-response relationship; and (4) the association is plausible."[102] Because of the increased morbidity for the premature infant and the enormous cost to society, it is important that women choosing an abortion be informed of these risks.

In a subsequent article by Calhoun et al. the cost of these preventable premature deliveries was calculated. Induced abortion increased the rate of EPB (less than 32 weeks) for an additional 22,917 cases, with a yearly neonatal unit cost of more than $1.2 billion, and 1,096 additional cases of cerebral palsy in the babies who weighed less than 1500 grams at birth.[103]

The EUROPOP study, published in 2004, was a case-control study of data collected from 1994 to 1997 from ten European nations.[104] Those women who had had one or more abortions had a 50 percent increased risk of delivering a subsequent child at 22 to 32 weeks. If they separated out the women who had had two or more abortions, it rose to an 80 percent increased risk. They controlled for all the other social and economic factors that could have caused the increase. In an analysis of the EPIPAGE study from France of outcomes of infants born prior to 33 weeks in 1997 in a case-control dataset from several maternity centers across France, whose data were not included in the EUROPOP study,[105] the results showed that those women who had undergone one or more induced abortions had a 50 percent greater chance of delivering a baby at 22 to 32 weeks. A history of two or more abortions increased the risk by 160 percent, and a history of one abortion increased the risk of delivering at 22 to 27 weeks by 70 percent. Induced abortion is a preventable cause of subsequent premature births.

The second long-term sequel to abortion is its psychological effect on the woman. Despite the growing body of evidence of increased rates of suicide, depression, substance abuse, and difficulties with intimate partner bonding and maternal-child

101. J. A. Martius et al., "Risk Factors Associated with Preterm (<37+0 weeks) and Early Preterm (<32+0 weeks): Univariate and Multi-Variate Analysis of 106,345 Singleton Births from 1994 Statewide Perinatal Survey of Bavaria," *European Journal of Obstetric and Gynecologic Reproductive Biology* 80 (1998): 183–89.

102. Rooney and Calhoun, "Induced Abortion and Risk of Premature Births," 47.

103. B. C. Calhoun et al., "Cost Consequences of Induced Abortion as an Attributable Risk for Preterm Birth and Impact on Informed Consent," *Journal of Reproductive Medicine* 52 (2007): 929–37.

104. P. Ancel et al., "History of Induced Abortion as a Risk Factor for Preterm Birth in European Countries: Results of the EUROPOP Survey," *Human Reproduction* 19 (2004): 734–40.

105. C. Moreau et al., "Previous Induced Abortions and the Risk of Very Preterm Delivery: Results of the EPIPAGE Study," *British Journal of Obstetrics and Gynecology* 112 (2005): 430–37.

bonding, the American Psychological Association's Mental Health and Abortion Task Force concluded in August 2008: "The best scientific evidence published indicates that among adult women who have an unplanned pregnancy, the relative risk of mental health problems is no greater if they have a single elective first-trimester abortion or deliver that pregnancy."[106] The studies have not shown that to be the case, and this can be readily ascertained anecdotally in medical practice, as patients voluntarily share the guilt they feel from a past abortion. A major landmark study on this came from Finland in 1997; it investigated the results of a register linkage study of patients who obtained a certificate to have an abortion from 1987 to 1994 with subsequent deaths from suicide.[107] The study included 9,192 women ages 15 to 49 who died during that time. They found that when women who had an abortion were compared with women who delivered at term, the women who aborted were 3.5 times more likely to die within a year from all causes, which included suicide, accidents, homicide, unknown causes, and natural causes. When suicide alone was selected out of the data set, a woman who had a full-term delivery had half the risk of suicide of the general population. If a woman had had an abortion, she had a six times increased risk of suicide compared with a woman who had delivered at term, and her risk peaked near the expected due date of the baby she had aborted.

David Fergusson (who describes himself as "pro-choice") and fellow researchers in New Zealand reviewed the national data on women from the ages of 15 to 25 who had an abortion as compared with women who had no pregnancies or delivered at term.[108] They controlled for confounding variables in a longitudinal study over 25 years. Their results showed those who had abortions had "elevated rates of subsequent mental health problems, including depression, anxiety, suicidal behaviors, and substance use disorders." Of women who had aborted, 27 percent reported suicidal ideation, which was four times greater than women who had never been pregnant and three times higher than women who delivered at term. Of women who had aborted, 42 percent reported major depression and 39 percent suffered from anxiety disorders by age 25.

N. P. Mota et al., in a study from Canada based on a nationally representative sample, found that women who had an abortion had a 59 percent increased risk of suicidal ideation, a 61 percent increased risk for mood disorders, and a 261 percent and 142 percent increased risk for alcohol abuse and drug abuse, respectively, compared with women who had not had an abortion.[109] Suicide is a sentinel event for depression, and several studies have shown an increased risk of depression or bipolar disorder after an abortion. P. K. Coleman et al. reported a 40 percent increase for

---

106. American Psychological Association, Task Force on Mental Health and Abortion, "Report of the Task Force on Mental Health and Abortion" (Washington, D.C.: American Psychological Association, 2008), 4.

107. M. Gissler et al., "Pregnancy-Associated Deaths in Finland 1987–1994: Definition Problems and Benefits of Record Linkage," *Acta Obstetrica et Gynecologica Scandinavica* 76 (1997): 651–57.

108. D. M. Fergusson, L. J. Horwood, and E. M. Ridder, "Abortion in Young Women and Subsequent Mental Health," *Journal of Child Psychology and Psychiatry* 47 (2006): 16–24.

109. N. P. Mota et al., "Associations between Abortion, Mental Disorders, and Suicidal Behaviors in a Nationally Representative Sample," *The Canadian Journal of Psychiatry* 55 (2010): 239–46.

medical claims for neurotic depression in women who aborted versus women who delivered.[110] In a 2009 study by Coleman et al., women who aborted had a 167 percent increased risk of developing bipolar disorder and 45 percent increased risk of depression.[111] They also found an increased risk of panic disorders, panic attacks, post-traumatic stress disorders, and agoraphobia in women who aborted when compared with women who had not been pregnant. Risk of alcohol abuse and drug abuse increased 120 percent and 79 percent respectively in women who aborted.

The effect of abortion on the father of the child and other family members has not been researched satisfactorily.

As clinicians, we should review the obstetrical history in a nonjudgmental way in any woman with psychological symptoms such as those described above. Often the patient is ashamed to admit to having had an abortion, especially when she knows you do not refer for abortion. Be ready to mirror the mercy of God as you explore whether an abortion in her past may be contributing to your patient's panic attacks twenty years later, and be prepared to refer her to a therapist who will help her work through her grief, or to Project Rachel or other healing retreat for post-abortion treatment and healing. Women have a difficult time forgiving themselves for an abortion, and we can play a key role in getting them the help they need. In the words of Blessed Madeleine Delbrêl: "It is our duty to know the concrete and particular conditions in which their salvation is being played out. It is our mission to make them feel the presence of God through us. This is the temporal service we are required to perform for which there is no one else to take our place."[112]

The last serious long-term complication of abortion, frequently denied by the secular medical community and by the politics of abortion, is the increased risk of breast cancer after an abortion. This can be physiologically explained by the normal development of the breast and by the fact that the best protection against the development of breast cancer is to have the first pregnancy end in a full-term delivery by the age of 30.

The human breast is composed of 15 to 20 lobulated masses of glandular tissue, with fibrous tissue connecting the lobes and fatty tissue in between. Each lobe is made up of lobules of alveoli, which make up the milk glands, blood vessels, and lactiferous ducts. At birth, the breast is made up of Type I lobules, which are primarily lactiferous ducts and a few alveoli. Type I lobules are susceptible to carcinogens such as benzopyrene in cigarette smoke, those in alcohol, or a metabolite of estrogen such as catechol estrogen quinine. At puberty, with the rise in estrogen, the lactiferous ducts sprout and branch, and the ends form small spheroidal masses which later develop into true alveoli. These are Type II lobules, which are also susceptible to carcinogens, as both Type I and Type II lobules replicate their DNA rapidly. Early in pregnancy, under the

110. P. K. Coleman et al., "State-Funded Abortions vs. Deliveries: A Comparison of Outpatient Mental Health Claims over Four Years," *American Journal of Orthopsychiatry* 72 (2002): 141–52.

111. P. K. Coleman et al., "Induced Abortion and Anxiety, Mood, and Substance Abuse Disorders: Isolating the Effects of Abortion in the National Comorbidity Survey," *Journal of Psychiatric Research* 43 (2009): 770–76.

112. Madeleine Delbrêl, *We, the Ordinary People of the Streets*, trans. David Louis Schindler Jr. and Charles F. Mann (Grand Rapids, Mich.: William B. Eerdmans, 2000), 196.

influence of estrogen levels 2,000 times higher than normal, there is hypertrophy of the ductular-lobular-alveolar system of the immature Type II lobules. But it is not until 32 weeks' gestation that the lobules mature into Type III lobules, which are resistant to carcinogens.[113] After delivery, the precipitous fall in estrogen and progesterone makes the lobules responsive to prolactin, and lactation is initiated in what are now Type IV lobules, which also are resistant to carcinogens. Based on this understanding of breast development, we would expect that a woman exposed to carcinogens such as cigarette smoke or (before a full-term pregnancy) to the synthetic estrogen in birth control pills, or a woman who had an induced abortion, or one who delivered prematurely before 32 weeks, or who went on hormone replacement in menopause and had never delivered a baby, would have an increased risk of breast cancer.

A study published in 1994 by J. R. Daling et al. of the Fred Hutchinson Research Center looked at 845 white women diagnosed with breast cancer between January 1983 and April 1990 from three counties in Washington State, comparing them with 961 women, all born after 1944, who had not developed breast cancer.[114] The researchers looked at reproductive events that may have contributed to the breast cancer. Their results showed that

among women who had been pregnant at least once, the risk of breast cancer in those who had experienced an induced abortion was 50 percent higher than among other women (95 percent CI = 1.2–1.9). While this increased risk did not vary by the number of induced abortions or by the history of a completed pregnancy, it did vary according to the age at which the abortion occurred and the duration of that pregnancy. Highest risks were observed when the abortion was done at ages younger than 18 years—particularly if it took place after 8 weeks' gestation—or at 30 years of age or older. No increased risk of breast cancer was associated with a spontaneous abortion (RR = 0.9; 95 percent CI = 0.07–1.2).[115]

If the woman was younger than 18 at the time of the abortion, her relative risk (RR) of subsequent breast cancer was 2.5. If the abortion was done on any woman at 9 to 12 weeks' gestation, the RR was 1.9. Daling et al. found the greatest risk for developing breast cancer was in women less than 18 years old who underwent an abortion between 9 and 24 weeks' gestation (RR 9). In the women with a family history of breast cancer who fit into this category, all twelve of them developed breast cancer by age 45. The researchers recommended that in studies on risk for breast cancer, induced abortion be examined as a risk factor. Dolle et al. also found a relative risk of 1.4 of developing any type of breast cancer with a previous history of abortion.[116]

K. E. Innes and T. E. Byers in 2004 reported on a matched case-control study of 2,522 women aged 22 to 55 years diagnosed with breast cancer in New York State between 1978 and 1995, who had completed one pregnancy one year or more before

---

113. See Angela Lanfranchi and Joel Brind, *Breast Cancer: Risks and Prevention* (Poughkeepsie, N.Y.: Breast Cancer Prevention Institute, 2005).

114. J. R. Daling et al., "Risk of Breast Cancer among Young Women: Relationship to Induced Abortion," *Journal of the National Cancer Institute* 86 (1994): 1584–92.

115. Ibid., 1584.

116. J. M. Dolle et al., "Risk Factors for Triple-Negative Breast Cancer in Women under the Age of 45 Years," *Cancer Epidemiologic Biomarkers and Prevention* 18 (2004): 1157–66.

the diagnosis and were matched with 10,052 primiparous women.[117] Women who delivered before 32 weeks' gestation carried an increased risk of breast cancer with an adjusted odds ratio (OR) of 2.1.

M. DeSilva et al. matched 100 women with breast cancer with 203 controls of the same age and parity.[118] They looked at prolonged breastfeeding and other factors in the development of breast cancer. If a woman breastfed more than 24 months during her life, she had a significantly reduced risk of breast cancer compared with those women who did not, but they found that an abortion in the past increased the woman's risk with an OR of 3.42 for the development of breast cancer, as did exposure to passive smoking (OR = 2.96).

As of November 2014, a total of 73 studies looked at the risk of breast cancer after abortion; 57 of them have found a positive correlation, and 34 of them were statistically significant. Studies that do not show an association may include a cohort of women who did not have an abortion after their first pregnancy, or they may include women who were not of reproductive age when abortion was legalized in that country, or they may include a cohort of women who were not followed long enough. A continuous analysis of all the studies, which looks at the link between induced abortion and breast cancer, can be reviewed at www.bcpinstitute.org.

Emergency Contraception

There probably is no drug more politicized than levonorgestrel (LNG), marketed as Plan B in the United States, as an "emergency contraceptive." Despite studies showing that ease of access to LNG did not reduce unplanned pregnancy or abortion rates, the FDA approved its sale over the counter in August 2006.[119] No other pharmaceutical-grade hormone is available without a doctor's prescription in the United States. In addition, pharmacists, physicians, and Catholic hospitals have had inordinate pressure placed upon them to dispense this drug, despite their concerns that the drug is preventing pregnancy by a post-fertilization effect in some cases.[120]

Rape

It is estimated that 683,000 women in the United States are victims of attempted rape, rape, or sexual assault each year, according to the National Women's Study.[121] Sexual

---

117. K. E. Innes and T. E. Byers, "First Pregnancy Characteristics and Subsequent Breast Cancer Risk among Young Women," *International Journal of Cancer* 112 (2004): 306–11.

118. M. DeSilva et al., "Prolonged Breastfeeding Reduces Risk of Breast Cancer in Sri Lankan Women: A Case-Control Study," *Cancer Epidemiology* 34 (2010): 267–73.

119. See T. R. Raine et al., "Direct Access to Emergency Contraception through Pharmacies and Effect on Unintended Pregnancy and STIs," *Journal of the American Medical Association* 293 (2005): 54–62; E. G. Raymond et al., "Impact of Increased Access to Emergency Contraceptive Pills," *Obstetrics and Gynecology* 108 (2006): 1098–106.

120. See T. J. Davis, "Plan B and the Rout of Religious Liberty," *Ethics and Medics* 32, no. 12 (December 2007), 1–4.

121. D. G. Kilpatrick, C. N. Edmunds, and A. K. Seymour, *Rape in America* (New York: National Victim Center, 1992), 2.

assaults occur across all ages and socioeconomic groups, with the very young, the disabled, and the elderly being more vulnerable to attack. The legal definition of rape includes: the use of physical force, deception, intimidation, or the threat of bodily harm; lack of consent or inability to give consent due to age, mental or physical impairment, or impaired state of consciousness; and oral, vaginal, or rectal penetration with a penis, finger, or object. The study revealed that one out of eight adult women has experienced a completed rape in their lifetime, 29 percent as children under the age of 11, 32 percent between the ages of 11 and 17, and 22 percent between the ages of 18 and 24. Only 26 percent of women who have been assaulted seek medical care in an emergency room; frequently, medical care is sought because of bodily injury.[122] In order for forensic evidence to be gathered, the woman would have to be seen within 72 hours of the assault, and preferably within 6 hours.[123]

The usual care in treating rape victims in secular facilities, aside from documenting and treating injuries, is to test the woman by serum and culture for sexually transmitted illnesses (STIs) and to perform a pregnancy test to determine if she is pregnant from a previous sexual encounter, not the assault. She is treated prophylactically with antibiotics as though having acquired an STI, with follow-up testing in two weeks. She is also given emergency contraception, generally LNG, against the possibility that a child was conceived through the assault.

Sexual assault is extremely traumatic, and these women need be treated with the utmost compassion and care. It is preferable to have a support person with her, such as a family member or rape counselor; and follow-up psychological counseling and multidisciplinary support is critical, as post-traumatic stress disorder is common after a sexual assault. For this reason, directive 36 of the *Ethical and Religious Directives* explains that rape would be a special circumstance in which a contraceptive could be used to avoid pregnancy as a result of the rape, but with the caveat that it must not interfere with an already-conceived human life:

Compassionate and understanding care should be given to a person who is the victim of sexual assault. Health-care providers should cooperate with law enforcement officials and offer the person psychological and spiritual support as well as accurate medical information. A woman who has been raped should be able to defend herself against a potential conception from the sexual assault. If, after appropriate testing, there is no evidence that conception has occurred already, she may be treated with medications that would prevent ovulation, sperm capacitation, or fertilization. It is not permissible, however, to initiate or to recommend treatments that have as their purpose or direct effect the removal, destruction, or interference with the implantation of a fertilized ovum.[124]

---

122. See J. McFarlane et al., "Intimate Partner Assault against Women: Frequency, Health Consequences, and Treatment Outcome," *Obstetrics and Gynecology* 105 (2005): 99–108.

123. See ACOG, *Précis: An Update in Obstetrics and Gynecology: Primary and Preventive Care*, 3rd ed. (Washington, D.C.: ACOG, 2004).

124. USSCB, *Ethical and Religious Directives*, dir. 36.

The national rape-related pregnancy rate is estimated to be 5 percent per rape in women between the ages of 12 and 45 years.[125] Fifty percent of women who conceive as a result of a rape undergo an abortion. In contrast to secular institutions, Catholic health-care systems and physicians had declined in the past to provide emergency contraception because of the endometrial effects of the Yuzpe regimen, which consists of two combined oral contraceptives taken within 72 hours of the rape, and repeated in 12 hours, and which clearly had post-fertilization effects. However, LNG has been touted by its proponents as working primarily as an anovulant; resultant pressure has been exerted on Catholic physicians and hospitals to use it in cases of rape.

The most important requirement of an emergency contraceptive is that it be highly effective in preventing a clinically detectable pregnancy when given after an act of intercourse during the fertile time. The drug is of greater value the longer after the act of intercourse it can be given and still be effective. To be effective, the method has to disrupt crucial events in the establishment of a pregnancy, as the time in the woman's cycle in which it is given will vary.[126] There is a six-day fertile phase in the woman's cycle when pregnancy can occur, corresponding to the maximum amount of time of sperm survival of five days and of oocyte survival of 24 hours.[127] Therefore, in order to achieve high efficacy, emergency contraceptives have to act not only to prevent ovulation and fertilization, but also to disrupt the period of early embryonic development prior to implantation, or the implantation process itself, that is post-fertilization. In order to understand the mechanisms of action of Plan B, it is first important to understand the process of establishing a pregnancy.

The Process of Conception and Implantation

The menstrual cycle begins with the first day of the period. Through a complex system of positive and negative feedback of blood levels of estrogen and progesterone in the ovaries, and follicle-stimulating hormone (FSH) and luteinizing hormone (LH) from the pituitary gland in the brain, one of the developing follicles in the ovary, containing an oocyte, is prepared for ovulation. This "dominant" follicle produces a surge of estrogen that triggers a rapid rise in LH and FSH; ovulation occurs 24 to 36 hours later. After ovulation the follicle develops into the corpus luteum, which produces progesterone to maintain a possible pregnancy until the placenta is adequately developed. The point at which ovulation occurs in the cycle varies; it can be as early as day 10 of the cycle or as late as day 24 or later. If conception occurs, fertilization takes place in the ampullary portion of the fallopian tube. The sperm present in the tube have undergone capacitation, which allows them to become more motile, and they are transformed by the acrosome reaction, which allows one of the sperm to fertilize the oocyte.

125. See M. M. Holmes et al., "Rape-Related Pregnancy: Estimates and Descriptive Characteristics from a National Sample of Women," *American Journal of Obstetrics and Gynecology* 175 (1996): 320–25.

126. See H. Von Hertzen and P. F. A. VanLook, "Research on New Methods of Emergency Contraception," *Family Planning Perspectives* 28 (1996): 52–57.

127. See A. J. Wilcox, C. R. Weinberg, and D. D. Baird, "Timing of Sexual Intercourse in Relation to Ovulation: Effects on the Probability of Conception, Survival of the Pregnancy and Sex of the Baby," *New England Journal of Medicine* 333 (1995): 1517–21.

Immediately, the early conceptus, or zygote, has total dependence on its maternally inherited cytoplasm. Any deficiency in oocyte maturation will result in impaired or failed early development and pregnancy loss. Over 3.5 days, the embryo travels through the fallopian tube and arrives in the uterus at the blastocyst stage at 4.5 days. Upon arrival in the uterus, the conceptus "communicates" with the mother and signals its presence to the maternal pituitary-ovarian axis so the corpus luteum is maintained and progesterone dominates to support the pregnancy. The blastocyst floats in the uterus, bathed by uterine secretions, from which it draws oxygen and substrates required for continued growth and survival. Prior to implantation, the conceptus develops its own vascular system, exchanging essential metabolites and distributing them throughout its tissues, until at 7 to 9 days after conception, it attaches to the endometrial lining of the uterus and implantation has occurred. If the endometrium is either in the pre-receptive or refractory phase, the endometrium resists attachment by the blastocyst. In order to survive, the early development and transport of the conceptus must be coordinated precisely with the changing receptivity of the uterus.[128]

Blood samples taken from pregnant women 8 to 12 days after fertilization show rising levels of human chorionic gonadotropin (β-hCG), the protein giving a positive pregnancy test. It is produced by the implanting blastocyst as early as 6 to 7 days after fertilization. It binds to LH receptors in the ovary, helping to sustain the pregnancy.

The Effectiveness of LNG

Plan B (LNG-EC) is 1.5 mg of levonorgestrel, a synthetic progestogen, given in a single dose or a split dose in a 24-hour period. This same drug is used in smaller doses in a mini-pill oral contraceptive, Microlut, which contains 0.03 mg of levonorgestrel. LNG-EC is equivalent to a 50-day supply of this oral contraceptive, but instead is taken in 24 hours. The World Health Organization (WHO) conducted a multi-center trial comparing the efficacy and side effects of LNG with the Yuzpe regimen (100 mg of ethinyl estradiol and 1 mg norgestrel given twice at 12-hour intervals) if given within 72 hours of coitus. It was estimated that LNG prevented 85 percent of the expected pregnancies and the Yuzpe regimen prevented 57 percent.[129] A more recent multicenter study by WHO compared three different regimens for emergency contraception: (1) two doses of 0.75 mg levonorgestrel; (2) a single dose of 1.5 mg of levonorgestrel; and (3) 10 mg of mifepristone (RU-486) given within 120 hours of coitus.[130] Even five days after intercourse, all three regimens appeared to prevent 58 to 63 percent of the expected pregnancies.

The effectiveness of short-term LNG-EC in disrupting ovulation has been studied and is dependent on the timing of administration in the menstrual cycle. M. Durand et al. found that ovulation was suppressed in 80 percent of women receiving the drug on day 10 of the cycle, when that day was four days or more before the LH

---

128. See M. H. Johnson, *Essential Reproduction* (Oxford: Blackwell Science, 2007), 168–221.

129. See Guzick, "Polycystic Ovary Syndrome."

130. See H. Von Hertzen and G. Piaggio, "Levonorgestrel and Mifepristone in Emergency Contraception," *Steroids* 68 (2003): 1107–13.

surge.[131] Women who received LNG-EC within 3 days of the onset of the LH surge, all ovulated; however, they had deficient progesterone production and a shorter luteal phase. Likewise, all women who received the drug at the time of the serum LH surge or 48 hours later ovulated. Unlike with the Yuzpe regimen, Durand et al. could not find any histological change in the endometrium to explain its mechanism of action in those who ovulated. A recent article by G. Noé et al. confirmed that LNG-EC did not effectively prevent ovulation, when the exact time of ovulation was known by serum levels of estradiol, LH, progesterone, and by ultrasound.[132] They found that 63.7 percent of women were given the drug outside the fertile window and could not have gotten pregnant anyway. Of the 72 remaining women given the drug in the five days leading up to ovulation, 79 percent ovulated, which made the authors conclude: "This suggests that other mechanisms than suppression of ovulation prevent pregnancy in these women."

In another study, D. Hapangama et al. also found that 8 out of 12 women given LNG-EC on or before the day of the LH surge ovulated and had normal cycle lengths.[133] They stated that if LNG-EC worked only by interfering with ovulation, its effectiveness would be only 42 percent, so it must work by other mechanisms of action.

Novikova et al. reported on the effectiveness of LNG-EC given before or after ovulation.[134] A group of 99 women, in six family-planning clinics, who sought LNG-EC for sexual intercourse that had occurred up to 120 hours earlier had blood drawn for LH, estradiol, and progesterone at the time they presented, then were given a single dose of LNG-EC of 1.5 mg. The investigators relied on the woman's self-report of the first day of their last menstrual period and their cycle history of 21 to 35 days, recognizing that this can be unreliable data. They concluded that this single set of hormonal data was 80 percent accurate in determining the day of the cycle relative to ovulation, whereas menstrual history was accurate only 39 percent of the time. The pregnancy rate was 3 percent and occurred in those women who took LNG-EC two days after ovulation. There were no pregnancies in women who took LNG-EC two or more days before ovulation. They concluded that LNG-EC had no effect on post-ovulatory events, but they did no studies looking at hormonal levels after giving LNG-EC.

In a study by Tirelli et al., bleeding patterns were studied in women given LNG-EC either in the follicular phase (from the beginning of the cycle up to 2 days before expected ovulation), in the periovulatory phase (day of ovulation ± 1 day), or in the lu-

131. M. Durand et al., "On the Mechanisms of Action of Short-term Levonorgestrel Administration in Emergency Contraception," *Contraception* 64 (2001): 227–34.

132. G. Noé et al., "Contraceptive Efficacy of Emergency Contraception with Levonorgestrel Given before or after Ovulation," *Contraception* 81 (2010): 414–20.

133. D. Hapangama, A. F. Glasier, and D. T. Baird, "The Effects of Peri-ovulatory Administration of Levonorgestrel on the Menstrual Cycle," *Contraception* 63 (2001): 123–29.

134. N. Novikova et al., "Effectiveness of Levonorgestrel Emergency Contraception Given before or after Ovulation: A Pilot Study," *Contraception* 75 (2007): 112–18. The study was funded by the Family Planning Foundation, FPA Health, Sydney.

teal phase (more than 1 day post ovulation).[135] The women all had self-reported cycle lengths of 24 to 34 days, and their time in the cycle was based on their history of the last menstrual period, which is notoriously unreliable. Bleeding patterns after giving LNG-EC were ascertained in follow-up telephone interviews. The researchers found that if the drug was taken in the follicular phase by history, the cycle was shortened by 10.9 ± 1.0 days, but there was no effect on cycle length if it was taken in the peri-ovulatory phase or luteal phase. Eight women were selected to take the drug between days 11 to 13 of the cycle and were followed with hormone studies and ultrasound. The researchers claimed that LNG-EC prevented ovulation in 7 of the 8 women, but their cycles were shortened by 15.0 ± 1 days, so they were in the follicular phase and could have been women with longer cycles who were still remote from ovulation.

With regard to sperm function, W. S. B. Yeung et al. showed that LNG-EC affected sperm function only in high concentrations and therefore was unlikely to play a significant role in inhibiting sperm function in its effect.[136] A study by investigators in Brazil found no effect on the development of the acrosomal reaction in sperm in the uterus 36 to 60 hours after coitus and 24 to 48 hours after LNG-EC administration, or on the number of sperm in the uterus.[137] The investigators concluded that a single dose of 1.5 mg levonorgestrel does not impair the quality of cervical mucus and sperm penetration or its ability to fertilize an oocyte.

Many studies have been conducted to understand better the morphologic and biochemical factors present in a receptive endometrium and the conditions in which a blastocyst may successfully implant. There has to be a carefully timed and balanced stimulation of estrogen and progesterone. Specific factors, regulated by these two hormones, chiefly progesterone, are markers of a receptive endometrium. These include leukemia inhibitory factor, glycodelin, prostaglandins, integrins, and vascular endothelial growth factors as well as others.[138] Medical research continues to be carried out to develop drugs to block these factors by using antiprogestins, such as mifepristone (RU-486), and to prevent successful implantation or disrupt a previously implanted human life.

In a study done by C. Meng et al., endometrial tissue was obtained from 12 women aged 22 to 40 with proven fertility.[139] The samples were obtained 4 or 5 days after the LH surge, which was documented by urinary LH. The samples were cultured an additional 5 days and were then exposed to levonorgestrel or mifepristone, now at 9 or 10 days after the LH surge. The levonorgestrel did not affect the expression of

135. A. Tirelli, A. Cagnacci, and A. Volpe, "Levonorgestrel Administration in Emergency Contraception: Bleeding Pattern and Pituitary Function," *Contraception* 77 (2008): 328–32.

136. W. S. B. Yeung et al., "The Effects of Levonorgestrel on Various Sperm Functions," *Contraception* 66 (2002): 453–57.

137. J. A. A. de Nascimento et al., "*In Vivo* Assessment of the Human Sperm Acrosome Reaction and the Expression of Glycodelin-A in Human Endometrium after Levonorgestrel-Emergency Contraceptive Pill Administration," *Human Reproduction* 22 (2007): 2190–95.

138. See H. Achache and A. Revel, "Endometrial Receptivity Markers, the Journey to Successful Embryo Implantation," *Human Reproduction Update* 12 (2006): 731–46.

139. C. Meng et al., "Effect of Levonorgestrel and Mifepristone on Endometrial Receptivity Markers in a Three-Dimensional Human Endometrial Cell Culture Model," *Fertility and Sterility* 91 (2009): 256–64.

the markers that were studied when administered in the implantation window, but mifepristone blocked those markers by binding to the progesterone receptors, thus preventing implantation. It is reassuring to know that if Plan B is given at the time of implantation of a conceptus that occurred 7 to 9 days earlier, it will not disrupt implantation at that time in the cycle.

Therefore, if LNG-EC does not consistently prevent ovulation unless it is given four or more days before the LH surge, if it does not thicken cervical mucus, if it is does not affect sperm motility or the ability of the sperm to fertilize an oocyte, and if it does not alter the histology of the endometrium, what is its mechanism of action? The answer may be found in the complex, immunohistochemistry of the endometrium that allows successful implantation.

Durand et al. studied serum glycodelin-A concentration in serum and the endometrium in the last week of the luteal phase when implantation of the blastocyst is occurring.[140] Glycodelin-A is a major secretory progesterone-regulated glycoprotein of the human endometrium. It is absent during the periovulatory phase, because it suppresses sperm function, and is expressed only in the late luteal phase. In the late luteal phase, it inhibits the mother's immune cells, playing a part in the feto-maternal defense mechanism. Glycodelin-A is also a potent inhibitor of the binding of the sperm to the zona pellucida of the oocyte. Durand et al. concluded that LNG administered prior to the LH surge does not always prevent ovulation, but it has a deleterious effect on progesterone production by the corpus luteum, which is needed to sustain the pregnancy. It also causes an early rise in serum glycodelin-A, as well as significantly lower levels in the late luteal phase (when implantation is taking place) than is seen in controls. Decreased levels found in the endometrium confirmed this. Glycodelin-A inhibits the natural killer cells present at the implantation site. Decreased endometrial levels of glycodelin-A may weaken the immuno-suppressive environment that allows the blastocyst to implant without being "recognized" by the mother as a foreign body. In a follow-up to this study, Durand et al. found increased levels of glycodelin-A in serum and uterine washings after LNG-EC was administered pre-ovulatory;[141] this increased level of glycodelin-A could inhibit fertilization, but it has not been shown to do so.

The argument that LNG-EC works only by preventing ovulation is not consistent with the effectiveness of the drug, especially if it is given 72 hours after intercourse, when ovulation and fertilization may have already taken place. If the drug were perfectly effective at preventing fertilization when given within 24 hours of intercourse, it would be only 59 percent effective; when given 72 hours later, only 16 percent effective.[142] This does not agree with reported studies of 85 percent effectiveness. Therefore, LNG-EC must have post-fertilization effects.

140. M. Durand et al., "Late Follicular Phase Administration of Levonorgestrel as an Emergency Contraceptive Changes the Secretory Pattern of Glycodeline in Serum and Endometrium during the Luteal Phase of the Menstrual Cycle," *Contraception* 71 (2005): 451–57.

141. M. Durand et al., "Hormonal Evaluation and Midcycle Detection of Intrauterine Glycodelin in Women Treated with Levonorgestrel as in Emergency Contraception," *Contraception* 82 (2010): 526–33.

142. See R. T. Mikolajczyk and J. B. Stanford, "Levonorgestrel Emergency Contraception: A Joint Analysis of Effectiveness and Mechanism of Action," *Fertility and Sterility* 88 (2007): 565–71.

Some articles have contradicted the findings of these large, well-done studies by Durand and Noé, but the contradictory studies are limited, either because of their small sample size,[143] or because of the timing of administration of the drug (on the day of the LH surge or later).[144] It has also been proposed that in the women who ovulate, the ovum may be dysfunctional because lower LH levels result in an egg that is not capable of being fertilized.[145] Proponents of this theory rely on *in vitro* studies that did not test with high doses of progesterone, whereas the administration of LNG-EC is high dose.[146] In a study of Macaque monkeys given synthetic progesterone prior to ovulation, the LH surge was blunted but 40 percent of the oocytes achieved fertilization and early embryonic development.[147]

In summary, LNG-EC prevents ovulation 80 percent of the time when given four or more days before the LH surge. It does not prevent ovulation if given within three days of the LH surge or at the time of ovulation. It has no significant effect on sperm motility or on the ability of the sperm to fertilize the oocyte; since it does not thicken the cervical mucus, it does not prevent sperm from penetrating the cervix and thus achieving access to the uterine cavity. It does not affect the histology of the endometrium. LNG-EC's effectiveness appears to be in its alteration of the balance of progesterone-mediated factors needed to be present at the time of implantation. Administering this drug at a time when a woman is most likely to conceive—that is, within three days of the LH surge and at the time of ovulation—gives the woman a large bolus of a progesterone-like drug that sets off events in the endometrium that would have occurred later in the woman's cycle, thus potentially disrupting successful implantation. Pregnancy tests are done before administering a drug to a woman to make sure she is not already pregnant from a previous cycle, not from the assault. Further, when urinary LH levels indicate that ovulation has occurred, and that administration of the drug, therefore, will not prevent ovulation, the drug could affect implantation. Therefore, levonorgestrel cannot be administered to a female rape victim without a strong possibility of it affecting the development and successful implantation of a new human life.

Other Emergency Contraceptives

Another emergency contraceptive, ulipristal acetate, a selective progesterone receptor modulator, has received FDA approval. This drug is related to mifepristone and can be assumed to have effects beyond the prevention of ovulation. In a single dose

143. See L. Marions et al., "Effect of Emergency Contraception with Levonorgestrel or Mifepristone on Ovarian Function," *Contraception* 69 (2004): 373–77.

144. See W. A. Palomino et al., "A Single Midcycle Dose of Levonorgestrel Similar to Emergency Contraceptive Does Not Alter the Expression of the L-Selectin Ligand or Molecular Markers of Endometrial Receptivity," *Fertility and Sterility* 94, no. 5 (2010): 1589–94.

145. See N. P. G. Austriaco, "Levonorgestrel, Luteinizing Hormone Levels, and Oocyte Quality," letter to the editor, *National Catholic Bioethics Quarterly* 14, no. 2 (2014): 201–3.

146. See W. M. Verpoest et al., "Relationship between Mid-Cycle Luteinizing Hormone Surge Quality and Oocyte Fertilization," *Fertility and Sterility* 73, no. 1 (2000): 75–77.

147. Sherri M. Borman et al., "Progesterone Promotes Oocyte Maturation, but Not Ovulation, in Nonhuman Primate Follicles Without a Gonadotropin Surge," *Biology of Reproduction* 71, no. 1 (July 2004): 366–73.

of 30 mg, it is effective in preventing ovulation when given prior to the LH surge or after the surge begins but before the peak of LH and can be used up to 120 hours after intercourse.[148] However, this drug competes with progesterone for binding to its receptors, and it can be assumed it will have other effects that prevent survival of the blastocyst or prevent implantation.

Lastly, a nonhormonal emergency contraceptive that has been proposed is meloxicam, a selective cyclooxygenase-2 (COX-2) inhibitor. This drug is used to treat rheumatoid arthritis and may be taken inadvertently in pregnancy but is usually discontinued once pregnancy is detected or if the woman is experiencing infertility. Disruption of the COX-2 enzyme, which regulates the formation of prostacyclins, prostaglandins, and thromboxane, can lead to failure in ovulation, fertilization, implantation, and decidualization in female mice. These effects are not related to disruption of gonadotropins or estrogen or progesterone.[149] In a study of 22 volunteers in a single center, in a double blind crossover study, the effects on ovulation with two doses of meloxicam were assessed in sterilized women. If meloxicam was given daily (at 15 mg/day) for five days, dysfunctional ovulation occurred in 50 percent of cycles. When the dose was increased to 30 mg/day for five days, dysfunctional ovulation occurred in 90.9 percent of the cycles. There was no change in LH, estradiol, progesterone levels, or cycle lengths.[150] Although the action of this drug is more in keeping with the intention to prevent ovulation, the drug also could, through nonhormonal means, disrupt implantation. If it were to be administered in cases of rape, a progesterone level indicating ovulation had not occurred would allow it to be used more in keeping with the intention to prevent ovulation, not to disrupt a developing conceptus.

Preventing Conception, Not Implantation

In the recent document *Dignitas Personae*, the Congregation for the Doctrine of the Faith speaks to the use of emergency contraception:

Alongside methods of preventing pregnancy which are properly speaking, contraceptive, that is, which prevent conception following from a sexual act, there are other technical means which act after fertilization, when the embryo is already constituted, either before or after implantation in the uterine wall. Such methods are *interceptive* if they interfere with the embryo before implantation, and *contragestative* if they cause the elimination of the embryo once implanted.

In order to promote wider use of interceptive methods, it is sometimes stated that the way in which they function is not sufficiently understood. It is true that there is not always complete knowledge of the way that different pharmaceuticals operate, but scientific studies indicate that *the effect of inhibiting implantation is certainly present*, even if this does not

---

148. See V. Brache et al., "Immediate Pre-Ovulatory Administration of 30 mg Ulipristal Acetate Significantly Delays Follicular Rupture," *Human Reproduction* 25 (2010): 2256–63.

149. See H. Lim et al., "Multiple Female Reproductive Failures in Cyclooxygenase 2-deficient Mice," *Cell* 91 (1997): 197–208.

150. See C. Jesam et al., "Suppression of Follicular Rupture with Meloxicam, a Cyclooxygenase-2 Inhibitor: Potential for Emergency Contraception," *Human Reproduction* 25 (2010): 368–73.

mean that such interceptives cause an abortion every time they are used, also because conception does not occur after every act of sexual intercourse. It must be noted, however, that anyone who seeks to prevent the implantation of an embryo which may possibly have been conceived and who therefore requests or prescribes such a pharmaceutical, generally intends an abortion.[151]

As Catholic physicians, we are justified in protecting a woman from the consequences of a rape, including conception, only if we can prevent ovulation or the sperm reaching the oocyte to fertilize it. In most cases when it is administered in the fertile window, LNG does not prevent ovulation. Ulipristal acetate clearly has post-fertilization and abortifacient effects. Meloxicam is more effective as an anovulant, but it too can prevent the survival and implantation of the blastocyst if it is administered after ovulation and fertilization have taken place. The next emergency contraceptive most likely will be low-dose mifepristone, because of its low incidence of side effects and high degree of efficacy in disrupting implantation. It is unlikely that any drug will be found to inhibit ovulation post-coitally that does not have a post-fertilization effect. According to the *Catechism of the Catholic Church*: "Human life must be respected and protected absolutely from the moment of conception. From the first moment of existence, a human being must be recognized as having the rights of a person—among which are the inviolable right of every innocent being to life."[152] Regardless of the circumstances under which a human life is conceived, even in a sexual assault, physicians do not have the right to disrupt the normal progression of that life.

Case 8. Treatment of Endometriosis

G. M. is a 28-year-old married woman, gravida 0 para 0, on OCs for acne until three years ago. She described her periods off the pill as lasting 12 or 13 days with spotting for several days before and after her period. She denied dysmenorrhea or dyspareunia but had some nausea before her period. Thyroid function and prolactin levels were normal but a progesterone level 7 days after ovulation was low at 4.8 ng/ml. She was started on vaginal progesterone capsules, to begin on the third day of temperature rise, but the bleeding was not corrected. On ultrasound she was found to have what appeared to be a bicornuate uterus, which was confirmed by hysterosalpingogram. She also had a small 1.5 cm cyst on the left ovary as well as a 1.1 cm mass described as a possible dermoid. She was referred to a reproductive endocrinologist for surgical repair prior to attempting pregnancy. Unexpectedly, she was found to have Stage III endometriosis and a thick intrauterine septum. The septum was resected, and the endometriosis, which involved the bladder flap, cul-de-sac, and bilateral broad ligaments, with adhesions of the left ovary to the pelvic sidewall, was ablated with laser. Two small endometriomas on the left ovary were removed.

---

151. Congregation for the Doctrine of the Faith, *Dignitas Personae*, no. 23, emphasis in original.
152. *Catechism of the Catholic Church*, no. 2270.

Endometriosis is defined as the presence of endometrial tissue in an extrauterine location. The endometrial glands and stroma are most commonly present in the ovaries (44 percent of occurrences), the cul de sac and vesicouterine space (34 percent), the uterosacral ligaments (20 percent), and the pelvic peritoneum (22 percent).[153] It also can occur outside of the pelvis on the vagina or cervix, the appendix, in an abdominal incision scar, and in the pleural and pericardial spaces. It is a common disease, with 5 to 10 percent of women of reproductive age affected, or 3 to 6 million American women.[154] In patients presenting with infertility, 30 to 50 percent will be found to have endometriosis; in women presenting with chronic pelvic pain, 50 percent will have endometriosis, including adolescents who go to surgery.[155] A detailed medical history and the timing of symptoms is important in suspecting the diagnosis, as women will report severe dysmenorrhea, pain with ovulation that often extends to the period, dyspareunia, bleeding before and after a period, bladder symptoms, and gastrointestinal symptoms around the menses. Family history is valuable also, as the history of a first-degree relative with endometriosis increases a woman's risk by seven times.[156] No specific gene has been identified, so the inheritance is probably multifactorial. The risk is low (1 percent) for developing cancer in endometriosis.[157] There is no evidence in controlled prospective studies that endometriosis is associated with recurrent pregnancy loss,[158] or that surgical or medical treatment of endometriosis prevents miscarriage.[159]

The first theory for the development of endometriosis was proposed by J. A. Sampson in the 1920s; he theorized that the disease was caused by the retrograde flow of menstrual blood during the period and implantation of the endometrial cells.[160] However, retrograde menstruation occurs in 90 percent of women, yet only 10 percent of women develop the disorder. Women with cervical stenosis or an imperforate hymen are more likely to have the disease, due to obstruction of the outflow of the menstrual blood. It is more common in women with short cycles, and it is estrogen-dependent, resolving after menopause. Aromatase, an enzyme necessary for the production of estrogen, is present in endometriosis implants but not in normal endometrial tissue, and is induced by prostaglandin E2 (PGE2).[161] As only a

---

153. See J. S. Hesla and J. A. Rock, "Endometriosis," in *TeLinde's Operative Gynecology*, ed. J. A. Rock and H. W. Jones III (Philadelphia: Lippincott William and Wilkins, 2003), 595–638.

154. See E. Attar and S. E. Bulun, "Aromatase Inhibitors: The Next Generation of Therapeutics for Endometriosis?" *Fertility and Sterility* 85 (2006): 1307–18.

155. See H. S. Taylor, "Endometriosis: New Insights and Novel Treatments," *ACOG Update* 36 (2011): 1–10.

156. See S. E. Bulun, "Endometriosis," *New England Journal of Medicine* 360 (2009): 268–79.

157. See D. W. Cramer and S. A. Missmer, "The Epidemiology of Endometriosis," *Annals of the New York Academy of Science* 955 (2002): 11–22, discussion 34–36, 396–406.

158. See R. Matorras et al., "Endometriosis and Spontaneous Abortion Rate: A Cohort Study in Infertile Women," *European Journal of Obstetrical and Gynecological Reproductive Biology* 77 (1998): 101–5.

159. See S. Marcoux et al., "Laparoscopic Surgery in Infertile Women with Minimal or Mild Endometriosis," *New England Journal of Medicine* 337 (1997): 217–22.

160. See J. A. Sampson, "Peritoneal Endometriosis Due to Menstrual Dissemination of Endometrial Tissue into the Pelvic Cavity," *American Journal of Obstetrics and Gynecology* 14 (1927): 422–69.

161. See S. E. Bulun et al., "Aromatase and Endometriosis," *Seminars in Reproductive Medicine* 22 (2004): 45–50.

small percentage of women with retrograde menstruation acquire this disorder, there must be other explanations for its development. Theories include immunologic factors that may play a role in the attachment and proliferation of endometrial cells. Studies have shown that activated macrophages produce vascular endothelial growth factor (VGEF), a potent angiogenic growth factor contributing to vascularization of the implants.[162] These macrophages also produce increased levels of migration inhibitory factor (MIF) in endometriosis, which in turn results in increased proinflammatory cytokines, leading to an inflammatory milieu.[163] Natural killer cells would normally clear this inflammation, but they appear to have decreased activity in this condition. Secretion of proteins from the implants leads to adhesions. Suppression of the pro-inflammatory cytokines, which are elevated in the peritoneal fluid of these patients, is the main mechanism of action in several treatments for the symptoms of endometriosis.

Another theory for the development of endometriosis is coelomic metaplasia of the peritoneal cells or other cells in the body, perhaps in response to inflammation. Endometriosis has been reported in the lungs, in the brain, and even in men, so this may occur with differentiation of multipotent stem cells. There may also be lymphatic and vascular spread of endometrial cells.[164]

The clinical exam is often normal in these patients, but nodularity along the uterosacral ligaments, thickening of the rectovaginal septum, an ovarian mass or a fixed, retroverted uterus are a good indication of endometriosis. A pelvic ultrasound should be performed, looking for endometriomas in the ovaries. A definitive diagnosis is made with laparoscopy by an obstetrician-gynecologist experienced in the treatment of endometriosis and preservation of the woman's fertility. The extent of disease should be staged by the classification of the American Society of Reproductive Medicine.[165] These include Stage I (minimal disease), superficial lesions and filmy adhesions; Stage II (mild disease), includes the above plus deep lesions in the cul-de-sac; Stage III (moderate disease), includes the above plus endometriomas in the ovaries and more adhesions; and Stage IV (severe disease), includes the above plus large endometriomas and extensive adhesions.

An expert panel of practicing gynecologists from the United States, along with experts on developing consensus guidelines, produced a consensus statement for the management of chronic pelvic pain from endometriosis in 2002.[166] They began by stating that other causes for the pain needed to be ruled out, including potential food allergens such as dairy, gluten, corn, and soy. Nonsteroidal anti-inflammatory

162. See T. Harada, T. Iwabe, and N. Terkawa, "Role of Cytokines in Endometriosis," *Fertility and Sterility* 76 (2001): 1–10.

163. See N. G. Mahutte et al., "Elevations in Peritoneal Fluid Macrophage Migration Inhibitory Factor are Independent of the Depth of Invasion or Stage of Endometriosis," *Fertility and Sterility* 82 (2004): 97–101.

164. See Taylor, "Endometriosis: New Insights and Novel Treatments."

165. American Society for Reproductive Medicine, "Revised American Society for Reproductive Medicine Classification of Endometriosis: 1996," *Fertility and Sterility* 67 (1997): 817–21.

166. J. C. Gambone et al., "Consensus Statement for the Management of Chronic Pelvic Pain and Endometriosis: Proceedings of an Expert-Panel Consensus Process," *Fertility and Sterility* 78 (2002): 961–72.

drugs (NSAIDs) should be used as the first-line medical treatment for the cyclic pain of endometriosis. Often the patient will come in using over-the-counter doses of an NSAID, but prescription strength doses or changing the NSAID may be more effective at relieving her pain.

Oral contraceptives are recommended as the second line treatment for pelvic pain and dysmenorrhea. Directive 53 of the *Ethical and Religious Directives for Catholic Health Care Services* states:

Direct sterilization of either men or women, whether permanent or temporary, is not permitted in a Catholic health-care institution. Procedures that induce sterility are permitted when their direct effect is the cure or alleviation of a present and serious pathology and a simpler treatment is not available.[167]

If it is necessary to use oral contraceptives, it should be for as short a period of time as possible, and they should be given continuously, without a seven-day break or, if abnormal bleeding occurs, taken with three days off instead of seven. Studies have shown that the pregnancy rate with oral contraceptives is 4 to 10 percent, depending on the population of users.[168] Regarding the results of taking time off the pill: In a study by A. R. Baerwald et al., half of patients developed a follicle of 10 mm, 7 percent got to 14 mm, and 7 percent got to nearly 18 mm in the seven days off a 30 mcg oral contraceptive, which could mean as high as a 10 percent ovulation rate per cycle.[169] Pregnancy rates in fact are lower than that, because of thickening of cervical mucus and endometrial effects, which prevent implantation. The suppression of FSH and prevention of follicular development are the result of the dosage of estrogen in the pill; therefore, higher ovulation rates could be anticipated using the 20 mcg pills. Ovulatory activity is much less likely to happen if the time off the pill is shortened. In deciding to use OCs for the symptoms of endometriosis, the serious side effects of OCs should be kept in mind, as well as increased temptation for sexual activity before marriage when on OCs.

Depot-medroxyprogesterone acetate (another contraceptive), 150 mg IM, is also approved for the treatment of pain from endometriosis and is given every three months for one year. It effectively suppresses the LH surge and causes atrophy and decidualization of endometrial tissue, but it is associated with weight gain, breakthrough bleeding, and depression, as well as osteoporosis with long-term use. It appears to be as effective as the gonadotropin-releasing hormone agonist in relieving the pain symptoms of endometriosis.[170]

Danazol is a synthetic androgen, a derivative of 17α-ethinyl-testosterone, which inhibits ovarian steroidogenesis in the corpus luteum, suppresses the LH surge, and

167. USCCB, *Ethical and Religious Directives*, dir. 53.

168. See J. Endrikat et al., "Double-Blind Multicenter Comparison of Efficacy, Cycle Control, and Tolerability of a 23-Day versus a 21-Day Low Dose Oral Contraceptive Regimen Containing 20 mcg Ethinyl Estradiol and 75 mcg Gestodene," *Contraception* 64 (2001): 99–105.

169. Baerwald, Olatunbosun, and Pierson, "Effects of Oral Contraceptives."

170. See P. Vercellini, "Progestins for Symptomatic Endometriosis: A Critical Analysis of the Evidence," *Fertility and Sterility* 68 (1997): 393–401.

creates a low estrogen environment, inhibiting the growth of endometriosis.[171] Typically, the drug is begun on the woman's period, at oral doses of 400 to 800 mg/day, and is continued for six months. Pain symptoms are improved by two months, but tend to recur after the drug is stopped. Side effects include deepening of the woman's voice, hirsutism, acne, hot flashes, and other signs of virilization. Patients need to avoid pregnancy while on this drug. However, in a study by S. Razzi et al., low-dose, vaginal danazol of 200 mg/day, inserted in a capsule at bedtime for 12 months, was studied in women with recurrent, deeply infiltrating endometriosis.[172] Dysmenorrhea, dyspareunia, and pelvic pain were significantly decreased by three months of treatment and disappeared by six months of treatment without systemic effects. Women continued to have regular cycles, and there was a reduction of nodularity in the rectovaginal septum. This dosage can be made by a compounding pharmacy in a methylcellulose capsule. The authors of the study recommended this regimen, rather than multiple surgeries, to control symptoms.

Gonadotropin-releasing hormone agonists (GnRH-a), such as depot leuprolide acetate (3.75 mg/month for six months), also are effective for the treatment of pain from endometriosis; they are comparable to oral danazol, according to the consensus statement, which cites several articles.[173] It is recommended that patients receive add-back therapy of norethindrone, 5 mg/day from the start of therapy, to prevent hot flashes and osteoporosis. Patients have to avoid pregnancy while using this drug. Use of this drug for six months post-operatively improves pain relief 24 months after surgery with ablation of the implants in 70 percent of women as compared to 23 percent who had surgery alone.[174]

As mentioned above, it has been proposed that inflammatory processes in the peritoneal fluid have been the cause of the clinical symptoms of endometriosis, which are chronic or intermittent pain and adhesions resulting in infertility.[175] In a study by A. A. Murphy et al., 25 women with endometriosis had strong evidence for a pro-oxidant environment in the peritoneal fluid.[176] They had a higher concentration of lipid peroxidation markers, which could lead to increased adhesions of the endometrial cells to the peritoneum. These patients exhibited oxidative stress. They also had significantly lower levels of vitamin E in the peritoneal fluid than controls. J. Mier-Cabrera et al. found that women with endometriosis had a lower intake of the

171. See D. L. Olive and E. A. Pritts, "Treatment of Endometriosis," *New England Journal of Medicine* 345 (2001): 266–75.

172. S. Razzi et al., "Efficacy of Vaginal Danazol Treatment in Women with Recurrent Deeply Infiltrating Endometriosis," *Fertility and Sterility* 88 (2007): 789–94.

173. See Gambone et al., "Consensus Statement for the Management of Chronic Pelvic Pain and Endometriosis."

174. Ibid.

175. See J. Halme, S. Becker, and S. Haskill, "Altered Maturation and Function of Peritoneal Macrophages: Possible Role in Pathogenesis of Endometriosis," *American Journal of Obstetrics and Gynecology* 156 (1987): 783–89.

176. A. A. Murphy et al., "Lysophosphatidyl Choline, a Chemotactic Factor for Monocytes/T-Lymphocytes Is Elevated in Endometriosis," *Journal of Clinical Endocrinology and Metabolism* 83 (1998): 2110–13.

anti-oxidant vitamins A, C, E, zinc, and copper than women who did not have endometriosis.[177] They demonstrated that placing these women on a diet high in fruits and
vegetables, as well as seeds, increased their peripheral concentrations of vitamins A, C,
and E by three months. S. Ziaei et al. prescribed 500 units of vitamin E to 50 girls with
primary dysmenorrhea and compared them with 50 controls.[178] The girls on vitamin
E had significantly reduced pain by two months of therapy. In a study presented at
the American Society for Reproductive Medicine by Nino Kavtaradze in 2003 and
reported in *Ob-Gyn News*, investigators at Emory University placed 46 patients with
endometriosis on 1200 IU of vitamin E daily and 1000 mg of vitamin C daily. They
were able to demonstrate by laparoscopy a reduction in inflammatory markers in the
peritoneal fluid by two months. There was a significant improvement in chronic pain
by two months in 43 percent of women, improvement in dysmenorrhea in 37 percent,
and improved dyspareunia in 24 percent, compared with controls.[179]

Surgical treatment of endometriosis plays an important role in the treatment of
pain in a woman of childbearing age. The consensus panel concluded that either laparoscopic surgery or laparotomy with excision or ablation of the endometriosis was effective for pain relief. They found that uterosacral nerve ablation was not of any benefit, but that presacral neurectomy was beneficial for midline pain relief. Removal of
endometriomas or other cysts associated with endometriosis, rather than fenestration
and ablation, is more effective for pain relief. If the patient with endometriosis comes
to hysterectomy, her ovaries should also be removed, as 31 percent will require another
operation to remove the ovaries if they are left in place at the time of hysterectomy.[180]

A review of the literature by P. P. Yeung et al. from articles in MEDLINE (the bibliographical database of the U.S. National Library of Medicine) from 1966 to 2009
on laparoscopic surgery for endometriosis drew some important conclusions.[181] First,
patients experiencing infertility due to endometriosis are best treated with surgery, as
medical therapy does not improve pregnancy rates. Second, there is significant benefit from surgery in women with Stage I and Stage II endometriosis for infertility,
up to the age of 39. Unlike surgery for pain, where it is beneficial to follow up the
surgery with medical therapy for six months, the researchers concluded that medical
treatment after laparoscopy does not improve fecundity. In women who have an en-
dometrioma, the cyst should be excised, rather than fenestrated and coagulated, for
improved pregnancy rates. As far as preventing post-operative adhesions, Interceed
barrier is an oxidized regenerated cellulose compound that does not require suturing

177. J. Mier-Cabrera et al., "Women with Endometriosis Improved Their Peritoneal Antioxidant Markers after the Application of a High Antioxidant Diet," *Reproductive Biology and Endocrinology* 7 (2009), doi:
10.1186/1477-7827-7-54.

178. S. Ziaei et al., "A Randomized Placebo-Controlled Trial to Determine the Effect of Vitamin E in
Treatment of Primary Dysmenorrhea," *British Journal of Obstetrics and Gynecology* 108 (2001): 1181–83.

179. Nino Kavtaradze et al., "Vitamin E and C Supplementation Reduces Endometriosis Related Pelvic
Pain," *Fertility and Sterility* 80, Supplement 3 (September 2003): S221–22.

180. See A. B. Namnoum et al., "Incidence of Symptom Recurrence after Hysterectomy for Endometriosis," *Fertility and Sterility* 64 (1995): 898–902.

181. P. P. Yeung, J. Shwayder, and R. P. Pasic, "Laparoscopic Management of Endometriosis: Comprehensive Review of Best Evidence," *Journal of Minimally Invasive Gynecology* 16 (2009): 269–81.

and is flexible. It is highly effective at preventing adhesions as long as it is applied after hemostasis is attained. The solution Adept, or 4 percent icodextrin, is also highly effective at preventing post-operative adhesions, which is critical in the surgical treatment of endometriosis with infertility.

Case 9. Management of Infertility

P. C. is a 42-year-old, gravida 1 para 0010, engaged woman who comes in for a second opinion for secondary infertility. She is scheduled to have a myomectomy and bilateral salpingectomies to treat her infertility, followed by in vitro fertilization; and she is having second thoughts. Evaluation by the reproductive endocrinologist revealed bilateral hydrosalpinges with no tubal spillage and numerous fibroids, including a submucosal fibroid. Her anti-mullerian hormone level is 0.89. She shares that her fiancé had an affair with another woman last year, but she thinks they may still get married. You counsel her that children have the right to a mother and father committed to each other for life and that they should be conceived in an act of love between a husband and a wife, not in the laboratory. It appears her relationship with her fiancé is on shaky ground; they need to decide if they will commit to marriage or not. In addition, her advanced age and significant structural abnormalities of the uterus make it unlikely that in vitro will succeed, even at great personal expense. Although she is not Catholic, she shares that she has been thinking about the situation in just this way.

In 1988, the Congregation for the Doctrine of the Faith issued an instruction titled *Donum Vitae*, which established some fundamental principles to be followed in managing patients with infertility. All evaluations and treatments should respect three fundamental goods: "the right to life and physical integrity of every human being from conception to natural death; the unity of marriage, which means reciprocal respect for the right within marriage to become a father or mother only together with the other spouse"; and that "the procreation of a human person be brought about as the fruit of the conjugal act specific to the love between spouses."[182] Therefore, all tests and treatments for infertility have to respect those three principles.

Infertility is defined as twelve months of random acts of intercourse during the fertile time without conception. Infertility affects about 15 percent of couples in the United States. The prevalence has not changed since 1965, but the percentage of couples with primary infertility, or no previous pregnancy, has increased.[183] The main causes of infertility include male factor; ovulatory disorders including polycystic ovary syndrome, decreased ovarian reserve, tubal damage, or adhesions; endometriosis; uterine abnormalities; cervical mucus abnormalities; systemic disease; and unknown.

182. Congregation for the Doctrine of the Faith, instruction *Donum Vitae* (1988), nos. 87, 92.
183. See R. O. Burney, D. J. Schust, and M. W. M. Yao, "Infertility," in *Berek and Novak's Gynecology*, ed. J. S. Berek (Philadelphia: Lippincott Williams and Wilkins, 2007), 1185–87.

Male factor is the cause of the couple's infertility in 40 percent of cases and is evaluated with a semen analysis after 48 to 72 hours of abstinence. As masturbation is usually recommended to obtain a specimen but is "an intrinsically and gravely disordered action,"[184] a satisfactory specimen should be obtained by the couple having marital relations using a sheath that contains no lubricant or spermicidal, with several pinholes poked in the end of the sheath to avoid a contraceptive intent. The World Health Organization determined that a normal semen analysis consists of (a) volume of >2 ml; (b) concentration of 20 million or more sperm per ml; (c) sperm motility of >50 percent or >25 percent rapidly progressive; and (d) sperm morphology >15 percent normal forms. Men with abnormal results should be referred to a urologist for further evaluation.

Female factors are the cause of the couple's infertility in 40 percent of cases, a combination of both male and female factors account for 10 percent of infertility, and in 10 percent of cases, no cause can be found. In the female, ovulatory abnormalities account for 40 percent of infertility, 40 percent is due to tubal factors or peritoneal factors such as endometriosis, 5 percent of cases are due to inadequate cervical mucus, and in 10 to 15 percent of cases, the woman has a systemic disease.[185]

The evaluation of the couple may be completed in one menstrual cycle. A careful history should be taken, with attention to exercise and diet, a previous history of appendicitis, pelvic inflammatory disease, and symptoms of masculinization or galactorrhea. In the menstrual history, it is very important to determine the amount of bleeding with the period, whether there is spotting pre- or post-menses, whether the patient has pain with ovulation or for several days on her period, and the length and regularity of the menstrual cycle. If she is charting a method of natural family planning, it is valuable to identify ovulation by a peak with the cervical mucus, a temperature rise or a urinary LH surge, and to identify a normal luteal phase. Physical examination with careful attention to palpation of the thyroid, checking for signs of masculinization, cervical cultures for chlamydia, gonorrhea, ureaplasma urealyticum, and mycoplasma hominis should be performed as well as a Pap smear.

The evaluation of the woman includes a serum FSH, LH, and estradiol on day 3, a hysterosalpingogram on day 7 to 10, with the couple abstaining in that cycle until the hysterosalpingogram is completed to avoid disrupting an early pregnancy, a pelvic ultrasound early in the cycle, a postcoital test day 12 to 14 to assess the quality of cervical mucus, and documentation of ovulation with LH testing by reliable urinary sticks, an estrone/LH monitor, or temperature rise. Postcoital tests can be used to evaluate cervical mucus during the fertile window, but because of the widespread use of intrauterine insemination (which bypasses the cervix) postcoital tests have fallen into disuse. The two approaches do seem to be equally effective in pregnancy outcomes;[186] since our goal is to optimize all conditions so the woman can achieve

---

184. *Catechism of the Catholic Church*, no. 2352.

185. See Burney, Schust, and Yao, "Infertility," 1186–93.

186. See S. G. Oei et al., "Effectiveness of the Postcoital Test: Randomized Controlled Trial," *British Medical Journal* 317 (1998): 502–55.

a pregnancy through marital relations, it is important to evaluate cervical mucus. The test is done one to two days before ovulation. The couple has intercourse, and the woman is seen within eight hours. Mucus is aspirated from the cervical canal and viewed microscopically. Sperm should be present with at least one sperm moving actively in a forward direction per high-power field. The mucus should be clear and stretch at least one inch, and when left to dry on the slide should show a ferning pattern. A serum progesterone should be obtained seven days after ovulation (normal is 10 ng/ml or higher), together with a T4, TSH, and prolactin. If these tests reveal suboptimal cervical mucus, the treatments described below for this condition can be used.

If a cervical factor is present—decreased cervical mucus during the fertile window, including poor quality mucus and inflammation on the postcoital test—it is worthwhile to treat the woman with oral guaifenesin and an antibiotic such as ampicillin during the fertile window, according to Thomas Hilgers, based on personal experience, but there are no published studies.[187] There is no treatment for cervical factor caused by a previous cone biopsy where much of the endocervical canal was removed, with resultant infertility.

The age of the woman can play a major role in infertility. A woman's fertility peaks at age 25, declines at age 30; and by the age of 40, one third of women can no longer achieve a pregnancy.[188] For a woman consulting a physician about infertility who is 32 years or older, an assessment of ovarian reserve with a clomiphene citrate challenge test (CCCT) and an anti-mullerian hormone level should be done. Clomiphene citrate (100 mg) is given days 5 to 9 of the cycle, after obtaining FSH and estradiol levels on day 3, followed by serum FSH and estradiol levels on day 10. An FSH level on day 3 of 11.1 mIU/ml or more is predictive of decreased ovarian reserve, and a combined FSH level of 26 mIU/ml or higher after clomiphene is also predictive of infertility caused by this form of ovarian failure, particularly in women over 40.[189] Anti-mullerian hormone is produced by the ovarian granulosa cells of the preantral and small antral follicles; that hormone inhibits the growth of the primordial follicles, and its level declines with age. A normal anti-mullerian level, which can be done any time in the cycle, is 1.0 ng/ml or greater. Levels less than 0.7 ng/ml are associated with a low ovarian reserve.[190] Women with polycystic ovary syndrome (PCOS) have high levels of anti-mullerian hormone (over 3.0 ng/ml) because they have multiple small follicles in the ovary.

If tubal patency is present, the semen analysis is normal, and the problem appears to be ovulatory dysfunction, a course of clomiphene citrate can be carried out for a

187. See Hilgers, *The Medical and Surgical Practice of NaProTECHNOLOGY*, 620–22.
188. See C. Tietze, "Reproductive Span and Role of Reproduction among Hutterite Women," *Fertility and Sterility* 8 (1957): 89–97.
189. See A. H. Watt et al., "The Prognostic Value of Age and Follicle-Stimulating Hormone Levels in Women over Forty Years of Age Undergoing In Vitro Fertilization," *Journal of Assisted Reproductive Genetics* 17 (2000): 264–68.
190. See Richard Sherbahn, "Anti-Mullerian Hormone Testing of Ovarian Reserve," http://www.advancedfertility.com/amh-fertility-test.htm.

maximum of six ovulatory cycles. Clomiphene citrate at 50 to 150 mg/day is taken orally beginning days 2 to 5 of the cycle for five days. A serum progesterone is drawn between day 21 and day 23 of the cycle, or seven days after ovulation; an adequate response is 15 mg/ml or greater. The dose is increased by 50 mg each cycle until an adequate response is achieved or doses of 150 mg have been reached without a response. Women with side effects, such as blurry vision, pain, bloating, or vasomotor symptoms, can be tried on 25 mg/day for five days. Clomiphene acts as an estrogen antagonist, is safe, generally produces one egg each cycle, is inexpensive, and does not require a lot of high-tech monitoring. By the third cycle of use, as many as 80 percent of couples will achieve a pregnancy.[191] Approximately 73 percent of women with PCOS will ovulate with clomiphene, and 36 percent will achieve a pregnancy.[192] Women with PCOS may benefit from dexamethasone treatment as an adjunct to clomiphene. Dexamethasone at a dose of 0.5 mg/day or 2 mg daily for ten days starting the day of the clomiphene has improved fertility rates.[193] Disadvantages of clomiphene include a 5 to 7 percent chance of multiple births, usually twins; and it may decrease cervical mucus. If ovulation does not occur, human chorionic gonadotropin (hCG), 5,000 to 10,000 IU, can be given to stimulate the LH surge if a dominant follicle develops but ovulation is not occurring.[194]

Women with PCOS and insulin resistance and a body mass index greater than 28 kg/m² should be placed on metformin together with clomiphene; this achieves an 89 percent ovulation rate compared with 12 percent with clomiphene alone.[195] However, the live birth rate is not significantly different with metformin and clomiphene versus clomiphene alone.[196] Women with PCOS who fail to respond to doses of clomiphene of up to 200 mg/day in conjunction with metformin may respond to laparoscopic ovarian diathermy or ovarian drilling. Studies show a significant decrease in LH, testosterone, and DHEAS, and a reduced LH to FSH ratio, as well as a return of ovulation in 73 percent of women after ovarian drilling.[197] This procedure replaces the older procedure, ovarian wedge resection, which causes pelvic adhesions and contributes to infertility.

Luteal phase defect is somewhat controversial, and histologic dating of the endometrium has not been shown to correlate with successful implantation. However, there are many factors that are mediated by progesterone and that are necessary for

---

191. See E. A. Rybak and E. E. Wallach, "Infertility and Assisted Reproductive Technologies," in *The Johns Hopkins Manual of Gynecology and Obstetrics*, ed. Fortner et al., 389.

192. See R. Homburg, "Oral Agents for Ovulation Induction: Clomiphene Citrate versus Aromatase Inhibitors," *Human Fertility* 11 (2008): 17–22.

193. See J. Brown et al., "Clomiphene and Anti-oestrogens for Ovulation Induction in PCOS," *Cochrane Database System Review* 2009, Issue 4: Art. No. CD002249.

194. See Burney, Schust, and Yao, "Infertility," 1210–15.

195. See J. E. Nestler et al., "Effects of Metformin on Spontaneous and Clomiphene-Induced Ovulation in the Polycystic Ovary Syndrome," *New England Journal of Medicine* 338 (1998): 1876–80.

196. See R. S. Legro et al., "Clomiphene, Metformin, or Both for Infertility in the Polycystic Ovary Syndrome," *New England Journal of Medicine* 356 (2007): 551–66.

197. See A. Felemban, S. I. Tan, and T. Tulandi, "Laparoscopic Treatment of Polycystic Ovaries with Insulated Needle Cautery: A Reappraisal," *Fertility and Sterility* 73 (2000): 266–69.

implantation. In cases of unexplained infertility and repeated pregnancy losses, luteal phase defect may play a key role. The various treatments for it have been evaluated in the assisted reproductive technologies (ART) literature. In the early years of ART, luteal support was provided with hCG injections post ovulation; however, the standard of care now is progesterone. The current treatment is vaginal progesterone in oil capsules, 200 mg three times daily, or 90 mg in a bioadhesive gel vaginally daily, or progesterone in oil 50 mg intramuscularly daily, beginning three days after the LH surge.[198]

Patients with hypogonadotropic hypogonadal ovarian dysfunction have low gonadotropin levels and do not respond to ovulation induction. This condition is usually caused by inadequate calorie intake, eating disorders, excessive exercise, or emotional stress. These patients should be encouraged to decrease exercise, increase calorie intake, gain weight, and seek professional help.

Laparoscopy as part of the infertility evaluation has fallen into disuse; however, tubal or peritoneal factors are the cause of 40 percent of infertility that is caused by the female factor. If there is no explanation for the infertility, if the woman has symptoms that could be the result of endometriosis, or if the history and hysterosalpingogram indicate a tubal factor, laparoscopy should be performed by a gynecologist skilled at treating endometriosis and pelvic adhesions. However, as it is the most invasive and expensive treatment, it is reserved for the final step in the evaluation. If laparoscopy is performed and endometriosis is present, treatment of Stage I or II endometriosis with excision or ablation increases the woman's cumulative probability of pregnancy from 17.7 percent after a diagnostic laparoscopy alone to 30.7 percent with treatment of the endometriosis.[199] There is no benefit to medical therapy for endometriosis after laparoscopic treatment of endometriosis in the infertile patient.[200]

Patient selection is important for tubal corrective surgery. If it is being performed to reverse a tubal ligation, pregnancy rates are 47 percent after sterilization done with unipolar cautery, 67 percent after Fallope ring sterilization, and 75 percent after a Pomeroy tubal ligation, as long as the final length of the tube is 4 cm or greater.[201] There is an approximately 28 percent pregnancy rate after either laparoscopic fimbrioplasty or neosalpingostomy, and the rate of ectopic pregnancy is 4 percent.[202]

Why is laparoscopy seldom performed any more for infertility? It is generally thought that if the hysterosalpingogram is normal, there are no tubal or peritoneal factors causing the infertility, and laproscopy, therefore, would be unnecessary. How-

198. See P. W. Zarutskie and J. A. Phillips, "A Meta-Analysis of the Role of Administration of Luteal Phase Support in Assisted Reproductive Technology: Vaginal versus Intramuscular Progesterone," *Fertility and Sterility* 92 (2009): 163–69.

199. See Marcoux et al., "Laparoscopic Surgery in Infertile Women with Minimal or Mild Endometriosis."

200. See Yeung, Shwayder, and Pasic, "Laparoscopic Management of Endometriosis."

201. See S. J. Silber and R. Cohen, "Microsurgical Reversal of Female Sterilization: The Role of Tubal Length," *Fertility and Sterility* 33 (1980): 598–601.

202. See J. M. Kasia et al., "Laparoscopic Fimbrioplasty and Neosalpingostomy: Experience of the Yaounde General Hospital, Cameroon (Report of 194 Cases)," *European Journal of Obstetrics and Gynecological Reproductive Biology* 73 (1997): 71–77.

ever, a retrospective review found that 21 to 68 percent of infertile patients with a normal hysterosalpingogram will have abnormalities by laparoscopy.[203] If laproscopy is performed and adhesions, for example, are found, release of peritubal adhesions has been shown to raise the cumulative pregnancy rate at a year from 11 percent to 32 percent.[204] However, after the introduction of ART in 1978, it was found that in vitro fertilization was able to achieve pregnancy in a third of patients by bypassing damaged tubes, peritoneal inflammation or adhesions from endometriosis, low sperm counts, and cervical factors, making laparoscopy unnecessary.

All methods of ART involve the retrieval of oocytes from the woman after superovulation. These procedures include in vitro fertilization (IVF), intracytoplasmic sperm injection (ICSI), gamete intrafallopian transfer (GIFT), zygote intrafallopian transfer (ZIFT), and use of donor oocytes and cryopreserved embryos. Nationwide ART statistics from the 2002 National Fertility Clinic data gave a 34.3 percent pregnancy rate and a 28.3 percent live birth rate in the use of fresh embryos conceived with nondonor eggs.[205] Much of the increased morbidity in the pregnancies after IVF comes from multiple gestations (44 percent of conceptions are twins, and 9 percent triplets or higher) and prematurity; but even in singleton IVF pregnancies, there is an increased risk of preterm delivery and infants who are small for their gestational age. Ovarian hyperstimulation syndrome is the major short-term complication for the woman, occurring in a mild form in 25 percent of women; in 2 percent of women, severe forms occur that can be fatal.[206] Use of IVF is also associated with increased likelihood of adverse perinatal outcomes, including preeclampsia, gestational hypertension, placental abruption, placenta previa, and increased risk of cesarean delivery.[207] In addition to the risk to the mother and child of IVF when pregnancy is successful, it is estimated that 80 percent of embryos created by IVF are sacrificed, so for every two children conceived, eight children are lost.[208]

Any infertility treatment we, as Catholic physicians, undertake—or for which we refer the patient—that enhances, but does not replace, the marital act to achieve a pregnancy would be legitimate. *Dignitas Personae* states:

Techniques which assist procreation "are not to be rejected on the grounds that they are artificial. As such, they bear witness to the possibilities of the art of medicine. But they must be given a moral evaluation in reference to the dignity of the human person, who is called to realize his vocation from God to the gift of love and the gift of life."[209]

---

203. See, for example, S. L. Corson, A. Cheng, and J. N. Gutmann, "Laparoscopy in the 'Normal' Infertile Patient: a Question Revisited," *Journal of the American Association of Gynecologic Laparoscopists* 7 (2000): 317–24.

204. See T. Tulandi et al., "Treatment-Dependent and Treatment-Independent Pregnancy among Women with Periadnexal Adhesions," *American Journal of Obstetrics and Gynecology* 162 (1990): 354–57.

205. See Rybak and Wallach, "Infertility and Assisted Reproductive Technologies," 388–89.

206. See B. J. Van Voorhis, "Outcomes from Assisted Reproductive Technology," *Obstetrics and Gynecology* 107 (2006): 183–200.

207. See T. Shevell et al., "Assisted Reproductive Technology and Pregnancy Outcome," *Obstetrics and Gynecology* 106 (2005): 1039–45.

208. Congregation for the Doctrine of Faith, *Dignitas Personae*, no. 14, note 27.

209. Ibid., no. 12, quoting Congregation for the Doctrine of the Faith, *Donum Vitae*, Introduction, no. 3.

Although intrauterine insemination is not strictly speaking ART, it separates the marital act from procreation, whether the insemination is homologous or heterologous, and therefore is illicit. The combination of clomiphene citrate and intrauterine insemination is more effective than clomiphene citrate alone at achieving pregnancy, but it replaces the marital act with a laboratory procedure. Semen is collected from the man through masturbation and is processed to remove seminal factors that would cause a reaction in the woman when it is introduced into the endometrial cavity. As the Congregation for the Doctrine of the Faith instructed: "Homologous artificial insemination within marriage cannot be admitted except for those cases in which the technical means is not a substitute for the conjugal act, but serves to facilitate and to help so that the act attains its natural purpose."[210]

Catholic obstetrician-gynecologists need to become well versed in the management of infertility and, if possible, become skilled at treating endometriosis and tubal disease laparoscopically. Otherwise, their patients will very shortly be tempted to engage in ART or insemination. If a tubal factor is present and can be corrected, treating the tubal disease may give the couple an opportunity to achieve pregnancy on their own, and repeatedly.

Living the Catholic Faith in Your Practice

Case 10. Testifying for Culture of Life Legislation

Dr. C. is a pro-life gynecologist and is contacted the week before a hearing in the health and human services committee of her state senate to respond to the criticisms the state ob-gyn society has for a bill restricting late-term abortions. The archdiocesan pro-life coordinator provides her with the bill and scientific resources to justify the bill. The physician clears her schedule that following Monday afternoon to provide expert testimony. When they arrive for the committee hearing, there are eight pro-abortion ob-gyns prepared to testify against the bill.

Who? . . . ME?

When asked to testify on a bill that promotes the culture of life, or to oppose a bill that promotes the culture of death, just say "yes"—you may be the only one to do it! Clear your calendar unless it is impossible, but make it a priority. One effective medical expert can make all the difference in the passage of the legislation.

The first important step is to study the bill. Never testify about a bill you have not read. Make sure you agree with the aspects that you will be supporting. If you disagree with aspects of it, discuss this with the legislator or group requesting your testimony ahead of time.

---

210. *Dignitas Personae,* no. 12. While most ART are unacceptable when analyzed with the help of *Dignitas Personae* and *Donum Vitae,* GIFT and intrauterine insemination (IUI) have not been definitively addressed by the Magisterium. For arguments for and against, see Peter Cataldo, "Reproductive Technologies," in *Catholic Healthcare Ethics,* 2nd ed., ed. Edward J. Furton, Peter J. Cataldo, and Albert S. Moraczewski, OP (Philadelphia: National Catholic Bioethics Center, 2009), 107–8.

Prepare your testimony, research your facts carefully, and type out your testimony, with references, if necessary. Know how much time you will have to speak, and stay within the limits of your allotted time. Rehearse giving the testimony ahead of time. Make sure everything you say is factual, clear, and respectful.

Clear your schedule for the time you are testifying. Make sure your personal appearance conveys professionalism and authority. Wear a business suit, and look your best. Be clear as to where you are going, park in a lot with unlimited time, and arrive early. Don't forget to pray beforehand for the outcome of the hearing, and have others praying for you during the hearing.

When you arrive, notify the group that you are representing of your arrival. You usually have to sign in to speak at a hearing. Make sure you are not the first to speak, so you can hear the concerns of the opposition and be able to answer them. Remember that you are the medical authority and the legislators are usually attorneys. Always show respect for the members of the committee and for your opponents. Address the chairman and members of the committee and state that you are speaking in support of or in opposition to bill such-and-such. Avoid all slang or crass language with your testimony. As you give your testimony, speak slowly, clearly, and succinctly. Be prepared to answer questions from the committee. A rushed testimony will be ineffective. Remain in the room to listen to the other testimony and the comments of the legislators. This will be educational for you. Never make noises or loud comments while others are speaking.

After the committee hearing is over, sit down with the group you have represented and go over the testimony, the arguments of the opposition, and the comments and questions by the legislators. If the bill has passed in your favor, do what you can to make sure it is implemented the way it was intended, and thank God!

Natural Family Planning in My Practice?

So you have had a change of heart and have decided to follow Church teaching in your practice, which means not providing contraception, sterilization, or abortion, and not referring for those practices. Where do you begin to make the transition? If you are in a group practice, sit down with your office staff and partners and explain the change in your practice of medicine. In some cases, you may have to leave and begin another practice. If possible, stay in your same town as you already have built up a patient practice, and many of those patients will still come to see you. Develop a brochure that states your new position, and develop a statement for patients when they call for appointments to avoid in-office conflicts. Advertise your new practice to the community, particularly in the Catholic publications, as it not only will attract like-minded patients but is a tool for evangelization. Your stand will have an effect on others and may influence others in health care to do the same.

Contact your diocesan family life office and see what resources are already available. Contact NFP instructors within your diocese and make them aware of your practice and willingness to accept referrals for medical evaluation if so desired by an individual or couple. Offer to help them promote NFP in marriage prep classes, RCIA programs, priest retreats, young adult programs, and baptismal classes. Offer to give talks to medical groups on natural family planning and its medical applications.

Next, become educated in at least one method of NFP. It helps to learn several methods of NFP, as your patients will come with charts from all the methods, and each should be treated with respect. Pope Paul VI Institute offers a medical consultant program which educates doctors in alternative treatments for gynecologic conditions that do not resort to oral contraceptives. If possible and your schedule allows it, become a teacher of one of the USCCB-approved programs.[211] It is extremely helpful to experience the difficulties of the couples as they learn a new method, and this will greatly enhance your understanding of NFP and the doctor-patient relationship. Become knowledgeable about Catholic bioethics and study Church documents pertaining to the life issues, some of which have been cited in this chapter.

Lastly, make sure you have a strong prayer life. Catholic physicians are in a spiritual battle and need to have on all the armor of the Church. Pray daily and, if possible, say the Rosary. Frequent the sacraments with monthly confession and daily Mass. Read Sacred Scripture each day and other spiritual works, and, if possible, find a priest to provide you with regular spiritual direction. As you start your day, pray to the Holy Spirit to guide you in all you say and do, and expect miracles as you carry out the work of the Divine Physician.

Bibliography

Aberdeen Endometrial Ablation Trials Group. "A Randomized Trial of Endometrial Ablation versus Hysterectomy for the Treatment of Dysfunctional Uterine Bleeding: Outcome at Four Years." *British Journal of Obstetrics and Gynaecology* 106 (1999): 360–66.

Achache, H., and A. Revel. "Endometrial Receptivity Markers, the Journey to Successful Embryo Implantation." *Human Reproduction Update* 12 (2006): 731–46.

American Congress of Obstetricians and Gynecologists (ACOG). "Diagnosis and Management of Preeclampsia and Eclampsia," *ACOG Practice Bulletin* no. 33. Washington, D.C.: ACOG, 2002.

———. *Précis: An Update in Obstetrics and Gynecology: Primary and Preventive Care.* 3rd edition. Washington, D.C.: ACOG, 2004.

———. "Premature Rupture of Membranes." *ACOG Practice Bulletin*, no. 80. Washington, D.C.: ACOG, 2007.

———. "Medical Management of Ectopic Pregnancy," *ACOG Practice Bulletin*, no. 94. Washington, D.C.: ACOG, 2008.

———. "The Initial Reproductive Health Visit." Committee Opinion no. 460. Washington, D.C.: ACOG, 2010.

American Psychological Association, Task Force on Mental Health and Abortion. "Report of the Task Force on Mental Health and Abortion." Washington, D.C.: American Psychological Association, 2008.

American Society for Reproductive Medicine. "Revised American Society for Reproductive Medicine Classification of Endometriosis: 1996." *Fertility and Sterility* 67 (1997): 817–21.

Ancel, P., N. Lelong, E. Papiernik, M. J. Saurel-Cubizolles, M. Kaminski; EUROPOP. "History of In-

---

211. See ch. 5 below by Richard Fehring, "Fertility Care Services."

duced Abortion as a Risk Factor for Preterm Birth in European Countries: Results of the EURO-POP Survey." *Human Reproduction* 19 (2004): 734–40.

Anderson, M. A., R. L. Fastiggi, D. E. Hargroder, J. C. Howard Jr., and C. W. Kischer. "Ectopic Pregnancy and Catholic Morality: A Response to Arguments in Favor of Salpingostomy and Methotrexate." *National Catholic Bioethics Quarterly* 11, no. 1 (Spring 2011): 667–84.

Attar, E., and S. E. Bulun. "Aromatase Inhibitors: The Next Generation of Therapeutics for Endometriosis?" *Fertility and Sterility* 85 (2006): 1307–18.

Austriaco, N. P. G. "Levonorgestrel, Luteinizing Hormone Levels, and Oocyte Quality." Letter to the editor. *National Catholic Bioethics Quarterly* 14, no. 2 (2014): 201–3.

Baerwald, A. R., O. A. Olatunbosun, and R. A. Pierson. "Effects of Oral Contraceptives Administered at Defined Stages of Ovarian Follicular Development." *Fertility and Sterility* 86 (2006): 27–35.

Barnhart, K. T., I. Katz, A. Hummel, and C. R. Gracia. "Presumed Diagnosis of Ectopic Pregnancy." *Obstetrics and Gynecology* 100 (2002): 505–10.

Barnhart, K. T., M. D. Sammel, P. F. Rinaudo, L. Zhou, A. C. Hummel, and W. Guo. "Symptomatic Patients with an Early Viable Intrauterine Pregnancy: HCG Curves Redefined." *Obstetrics and Gynecology* 104 (2004): 50–55.

Bedard, E., K. Dimopoulos, and M. A. Gatzoulis. "Has There Been Any Progress Made on Pregnancy Outcomes among Women with Pulmonary Hypertension?" *European Heart Journal* 30 (2009): 256–65.

Borman, Sherri M., Charles L. Chaffin, Kristine M. Schwinof, Richard L. Stouffer, and Mary B. Zelinski-Wooten. "Progesterone Promotes Oocyte Maturation, but Not Ovulation, in Nonhuman Primate Follicles without a Gonadotropin Surge." *Biology of Reproduction* 71, no. 1 (July 2004), 366–73.

Bouyer, J., J. Coste, T. Shojaei, J. L. Pouly, H. Fernandez, L. Gerbaud, and N. Job-Spira. "Risk Factors for Ectopic Pregnancy: A Comprehensive Analysis Based on a Large Case-Control, Population-Based Study in France." *American Journal of Epidemiology* 157 (2003): 185–94.

Brache, V., L. Cochon, C. Jesam, R. Maldonado, A. M. Salvatierra, D. P. Levy, E. Gainer, and H. B. Croxatto. "Immediate Pre-Ovulatory Administration of 30 mg Ulipristal Acetate Significantly Delays Follicular Rupture." *Human Reproduction* 25 (2010): 2256–63.

Broekmans, F. J., E. A. Knauff, O. Valkenburg, J. S. Laven, M. J. Eijkemans, and B. C. Fauser. "PCOS according to the Rotterdam Consensus Criteria: Change in Prevalence among WHO-II Anovulation and Association with Metabolic Factors." *British Journal of Obstetrics and Gynecology* 113 (2006): 1210–17.

Brown, D., and P. Doubilet. "Transvaginal Sonography for Diagnosing Ectopic Pregnancy: Positivity Criteria and Performance Characteristics." *Journal of Ultrasound in Medicine* 13 (1994): 259–66.

Brown, J., C. Farquhar, J. Beck, C. Boothroyd, and E. Hughes. "Clomiphene and Anti-oestrogens for Ovulation Induction in PCOS." *Cochrane Database of Systematic Reviews* 2009, Issue 4: Art. No. CD002249.

Bulun, S. E. "Endometriosis." *New England Journal of Medicine* 360 (2009): 268–79.

Bulun, S. E., Z. Fang, G. Imir, B. Gurates, M. Tamura, B. Yilmaz, D. Langoi, S. Amin, S. Yang, and S. Deb. "Aromatase and Endometriosis." *Seminars in Reproductive Medicine* 22 (2004): 45–50.

Burney, R. O., D. J. Schust, and M. W. M. Yao. "Infertility." In *Berek and Novak's Gynecology*, edited by J. S. Berek, 1185–87. Philadelphia: Lippincott Williams and Wilkins, 2007.

Calhoun, B. C., E. Shadigian, and B. Rooney. "Cost Consequences of Induced Abortion as an Attributable Risk for Preterm Birth and Impact on Informed Consent." *Journal of Reproductive Medicine* 52 (2007): 929–37.

Cataldo, Peter. "Reproductive Technologies." In *Catholic Healthcare Ethics*, 2nd edition, edited by Edward J. Furton, Peter J. Cataldo, and Albert S. Moraczewski, OP, 107–8. Philadelphia: National Catholic Bioethics Center, 2009.

Cataldo, P., and T. M. Goodwin. "Early Induction of Labor." In *Catholic Healthcare Ethics*, 2nd edition, edited by Edward J. Furton, Peter J. Cataldo, and Albert S. Moraczewski, OP, 111–18. Philadelphia: The National Catholic Bioethics Center, 2009.

Catechism of the Catholic Church. New York: Doubleday, 1997.

Clark, A. M., B. Thornley, L. Tomlinson, C. Galletley, and R. J. Norman. "Weight Loss in Obese Infertile Women Results in Improvement in Reproductive Outcome for All Forms of Fertility Treatment." *Human Reproduction* 13 (1998): 1502–5.

Cogliano, V., Y. Grosse, R. Baan, K. Straif, B. Secretan, and F. El Ghissassi;. WHO International Agency for Research on Cancer. "Carcinogenicity of Combined Oestrogen-Progesterone Contraceptives and Menopausal Treatment." *Lancet Oncology* 6 (2005): 552–53.

Coleman, P. K., C. T. Coyle, M. Shuping, and V. M. Rue. "Induced Abortion and Anxiety, Mood, and Substance Abuse Disorders: Isolating the Effects of Abortion in the National Comorbidity Survey." *Journal of Psychiatric Research* 43 (2009): 770–76.

Coleman, P. K., D. C. Reardon, V. M. Rue, and J. Cougle. "State-Funded Abortions vs. Deliveries: A Comparison of Outpatient Mental Health Claims over Four Years." *American Journal of Orthopsychiatry* 72 (2002): 141–52.

Condic, M. L. *When Does Human Life Begin?* Thornwood, N.Y.: Westchester Institute for Ethics and the Human Person, 2008.

Congregation for the Doctrine of the Faith. *Donum Vitae, Instruction on Respect for Human Life in Its Origin and on the Dignity of Procreation.* February 22, 1987.

———. *Dignitas Personae, Instruction on Certain Bioethical Questions.* Vatican City, Vatican: Libreria Editrice Vaticana, 2008.

Corson, S. L., A. Cheng, and J. N. Gutmann. "Laparoscopy in the 'Normal' Infertile Patient: A Question Revisited." *Journal of the American Association of Gynecologic Laparoscopists* 7 (2000): 317–24.

Cramer, D. W., and S. A. Missmer. "The Epidemiology of Endometriosis." *Annals of the New York Academy of Science* 955 (2002): 11–22; discussion, 34–36, 396–406.

Cunningham, F. G., N. F. Gant, K. J. Levine, L. C. Gilstrap III, J. C. Hauth, and K. D. Wenstrom, eds. "Hypertensive Disorders in Pregnancy." In *Williams Obstetrics,* 21st edition, 567–618. New York: McGraw-Hill, 2001.

Curtis, K. M., A. P. Mohllajee, S. L. Martins, and H. B. Peterson. "Combined Oral Contraceptive Use among Women with Hypertension: A Systematic Review." *Contraception* 73 (2006): 179–88.

Daling, J. R., K. E. Malone, L. F. Voigt, E. White, and N. S. Weiss. "Risk of Breast Cancer among Young Women: Relationship to Induced Abortion." *Journal of the National Cancer Institute* 86 (1994): 1584–92.

Davidson, S., and E. M. Graham. "Cardiopulmonary Disorders of Pregnancy." In *The Johns Hopkins Manual of Gynecology and Obstetrics,* edited by Fortner et al., 192–203.

Davis, T. J. "Plan B and the Rout of Religious Liberty." *Ethics and Medics* 32, no. 12 (December 2007), 1–4.

Delbrêl, Madeleine. *We, the Ordinary People of the Streets.* Translated by David Louis Schindler Jr., and Charles F. Mann. Grand Rapids, Mich.: William B. Eerdmans Publishing Co., 2000.

Delgado, G., and M. L. Davenport. "Progesterone Use to Reverse the Effects of Mifepristone." *Annals of Pharmacotherapy* 46, no. 12 (December 2012): e36. doi: 10.1345/aph.1R252.

de Nascimento, J. A. A., M. Seppälä, A. Perdigão, X. Espejo-Arce, M. J. Munuce, L. Hautala, R. Koistinen, L. Andrade, and L. Bahamondes. "*In Vivo* Assessment of the Human Sperm Acrosome Reaction and the Expression of Glycodelin-A in Human Endometrium after Levonorgestrel-Emergency Contraceptive Pill Administration." *Human Reproduction* 22 (2007): 2190–95.

DeSilva, M., U. Senarath, M. Gunatilake, and D. Lokuhetty. "Prolonged Breastfeeding Reduces Risk of Breast Cancer in Sri Lankan Women: A Case-Control Study." *Cancer Epidemiology* 34 (2010): 267–73.

Dewan, H., and J. M. Morris. "A Systematic Review of Pregnancy Outcome following Preterm Rupture of Membranes at a Previable Gestational Age." *Australia New Zealand Journal of Obstetrics and Gynaecology* 41 (2001): 389–94.

Diabetes Prevention Program Research Group. "Reduction in the Incidence of Type-2 Diabetes with Lifestyle Intervention or Metformin." *New England Journal of Medicine* 346 (2002): 393–403.

Dolle, J. M., J. R. Daling, E. White, L. A. Brinton, D. R. Doody, P. L. Porter, and K. E. Malone. "Risk Factors for Triple-Negative Breast Cancer in Women under the Age of 45 Years." *Cancer Epidemiologic Biomarkers and Prevention* 18 (2004): 1157–66.

Durand, M., M. del Carmen Cravioto, E. G. Raymond, O. Durán-Sánchez, M. de la Luz Cruz-Hinojosa, A. Castell-Rodríguez, R. Schiavon, and F. Larrea. "On the Mechanisms of Action of Short-term Levonorgestrel Administration in Emergency Contraception." *Contraception* 64 (2001): 227–34.

Durand, M., R. Koistinen, M. Chirinos, J. L. Rodríguez, E. Zambrano, M. Seppälä, and F. Larrea. "Hormonal Evaluation and Midcycle Detection of Intrauterine Glycodelin in Women Treated with Levonorgestrel as in Emergency Contraception." *Contraception* 82 (2010): 526–33.

Durand, M., M. Seppälä, C. Cravioto Mdel, H. Koistinen, R. Koistinen, J. González-Macedo, and F. Larrea. "Late Follicular Phase Administration of Levonorgestrel as an Emergency Contraceptive Changes the Secretory Pattern of Glycodeline in Serum and Endometrium during the Luteal Phase of the Menstrual Cycle." *Contraception* 71 (2005): 451–57.

Dwyer, N., J. Hutton, and G. M. Stirrat. "Randomized Controlled Trial Comparing Endometrial Resection with Abdominal Hysterectomy for the Surgical Treatment of Menorrhagia." *British Journal of Obstetrics and Gynaecology* 100 (1993): 237–43.

Endrikat, J., M. Cronin, C. Gerlinger, A. Ruebig, W. Schmidt, and B. Düsterberg. "Double-Blind Multicenter Comparison of Efficacy, Cycle Control, and Tolerability of a 23-Day versus a 21-Day Low Dose Oral Contraceptive Regimen Containing 20 mcg Ethinyl Estradiol and 75 mcg Gestodene." *Contraception* 64 (2001): 99–105.

Felemban, A., S. I. Tan, and T. Tulandi. "Laparoscopic Treatment of Polycystic Ovaries with Insulated Needle Cautery: A Reappraisal." *Fertility and Sterility* 73 (2000): 266–69.

Fergusson, D. M., L. J. Horwood, and E. M. Ridder. "Abortion in Young Women and Subsequent Mental Health." *Journal of Child Psychology and Psychiatry* 47 (2006): 16–24.

Finer, L. B., and S. K. Henshaw. "Abortion Incidence and Service in the United States in 2000." *Perspectives in Sexual Reproductive Health* 35 (2003): 6–15.

Fortner, Kimberly B., Linda M. Szymanski, Harold E. Fox, and Edward E. Wallach, eds. *The Johns Hopkins Manual of Gynecology and Obstetrics*. 3rd edition. Baltimore: Lippincott Williams and Wilkins, 2006.

Franks, Angela. *Margaret Sanger's Eugenic Legacy: The Control of Female Fertility*. Jefferson, N.C.: McFarland, 2005.

Fylstra, D. L. "Tubal Pregnancy: A Review of Current Diagnosis and Treatment." *Obstetrical and Gynecological Survey* 53 (1998): 320–28.

Gambone, J. C., B. S. Mittman, M. G. Munro, A. R. Scialli, and C. A. Winkel; Chronic Pelvic Pain/Endometriosis Working Group. "Consensus Statement for the Management of Chronic Pelvic Pain and Endometriosis: Proceedings of an Expert-Panel Consensus Process." *Fertility and Sterility* 78 (2002): 961–72.

Gary, M. M., and D. J. Harrison. "Analysis of Severe Adverse Events Related to the Use of Mifepristone as an Abortifacient." *Annals of Pharmacotherapy* 40 (2006): 191–97.

Gissler, M., R. Kauppila, J. Meriläinen, H. Toukomaa, and E. Hemminki. "Pregnancy-Associated Deaths in Finland 1987–1994: Definition Problems and Benefits of Record Linkage." *Acta Obstetrica et Gynecologica Scandinavica* 76 (1997): 651–57.

Grimes, David A., L. B. Jones, L. M. Lopez, K. F. Schulz. "Oral Contraceptives for Functional Ovarian Cysts." *Cochrane Database of Systematic Reviews* 2009, Issue 2: Art. No. CD006134.

Guzick, D. S. "Polycystic Ovary Syndrome." *Obstetrics and Gynecology* 103 (2004): 181–93.

Halme, J., S. Becker, and S. Haskill. "Altered Maturation and Function of Peritoneal Macrophages: Possible Role in Pathogenesis of Endometriosis." *American Journal of Obstetrics and Gynecology* 156 (1987): 783–89.

Hapangama, D., A. F. Glasier, and D. T. Baird. "The Effects of Peri-ovulatory Administration of Levonorgestrel on the Menstrual Cycle." *Contraception* 63 (2001): 123–29.

Harada, T., T. Iwabe, and N. Terkawa. "Role of Cytokines in Endometriosis." *Fertility and Sterility* 76 (2001): 1–10.

Hare, A. A., and K. S. Olah. "Pregnancy Following Endometrial Ablation: A Review Article." *Journal of Obstetrics and Gynaecology* 25 (2005): 108–14.

Herzog, A. G. "Differential Impact of Antiepileptic Drugs on the Effects of Contraceptive Methods on Seizures: Interim Findings of the Epilepsy Birth Control Registry." *Seizure* 28 May (2015): 71–75. doi: 10.1016/j.seizure.2015.02.011.

Hesla, J. S., and J. A. Rock. "Endometriosis." In *TeLinde's Operative Gynecology*, edited by J. A. Rock and H. W. Jones III, 595–638. Philadelphia: Lippincott William and Wilkins, 2003.

Hilgers, Thomas W. *The Medical and Surgical Practice of NaProTECHNOLOGY*. Omaha, Neb.: Pope Paul VI Institute Press, 2004.

Holmes, M. M., H. S. Resnick, D. G. Kilpatrick, and C. L. Best. "Rape-Related Pregnancy: Estimates and Descriptive Characteristics from a National Sample of Women." *American Journal of Obstetrics and Gynecology* 175 (1996): 320–25.

Homburg, R. "Oral Agents for Ovulation Induction: Clomiphene Citrate versus Aromatase Inhibitors." *Human Fertility* 11 (2008): 17–22.

Innes, K. E., and T. E. Byers. "First Pregnancy Characteristics and Subsequent Breast Cancer Risk among Young Women." *International Journal of Cancer* 112 (2004): 306–11.

Institute of Medicine of the National Academies, Committee on Understanding Premature Birth and Assuring Healthy Outcomes. *Preterm Birth: Causes, Consequences, and Prevention*. Edited by Richard E. Behrman and Adrienne Stith Butler. Washington, D.C.: National Academies Press, 2006.

Jensen, J. T., S. J. Astley, E. Morgan, and M. D. Nichols. "Outcomes of Suction Curettage and Mifepristone Abortion in the United States." *Contraception* 59 (1999): 153–59.

Jesam, C., A. M. Salvatierra, J. L. Schwartz, and H. B. Croxatto. "Suppression of Follicular Rupture with Meloxicam, a Cyclooxygenase-2 Inhibitor: Potential for Emergency Contraception." *Human Reproduction* 25 (2010): 368–73.

Johnson, M. H. *Essential Reproduction*. Oxford: Blackwell Science, 2007.

Kasia, J. M., J. Raiga, A. S. Doh, J. M. Biouele, J. L. Pouly, F. Kwiatkowski, T. Edzoa, and M. A. Bruhat. "Laparoscopic Fimbrioplasty and Neosalpingostomy: Experience of the Yaounde General Hospital, Cameroon (Report of 194 Cases)." *European Journal of Obstetrics and Gynecological Reproductive Biology* 73 (1997): 71–77.

Kavtaradze, Nino, Celia E. Dominguez, John A. Rock, Sampath Parthasarathy, and Ana A. Murphy. "Vitamin E and C Supplementation Reduces Endometriosis-Related Pelvic Pain." *Fertility and Sterility* 80, Supplement 3 (September 2003), S221–22.

Kiely, D. G., R. Condliffe, V. Webster, G. H. Mills, I. Wrench, S. V. Gandhi, and K. Selby. "Improved Survival in Pregnancy and Pulmonary Hypertension Using a Multiprofessional Approach." *British Journal of Obstetrics and Gynecology* 117 (2010): 565–74.

Kilpatrick, D. G., C. N. Edmunds, and A. K. Seymour. *Rape in America*. New York: National Victim Center, 1992.

Korhonen, J., U. H. Stenman, and P. Ylotalo. "Serum Human Chorionic Gonadotropin Dynamics during Spontaneous Resolution of Ectopic Pregnancy." *Fertility and Sterility* 63 (1994): 632–36.

Kuerer, H. M., K. Gwyn, F. C. Ames, and R. L. Theriault. "Conservative Surgery and Chemotherapy for Breast Carcinoma during Pregnancy." *Surgery* 131 (2002): 108–10.

Lanfranchi, Angela, and Joel Brind. *Breast Cancer: Risks and Prevention*. Poughkeepsie, N.Y.: Breast Cancer Prevention Institute, 2005.

Larimore, W. L., and J. B. Stanford. "Postfertilization Effects of Oral Contraceptives and Their Relationship to Informed Consent." *Archives of Family Medicine* 9 (1999): 126–33.

Legro, R. S., H. X. Barnhart, W. D. Schlaff, et al. "Clomiphene, Metformin, or Both for Infertility in the Polycystic Ovary Syndrome," *New England Journal of Medicine* 356 (2007): 551–66.

Lidegaard, Ø., E. Løkkegaard, A. L. Svendsen, and C. Agger. "Hormonal Contraception and Risk of Venous Thromboembolism." *British Medical Journal* 339 (2009): b2890. doi:10.1136/bmj.b2890.

Lidegaard, Ø., L. H. Nielsen, C. W. Skovlund, and E. Løkkegaard. "Venous Thrombosis in Users of Non-Oral Hormonal Contraception: Follow-Up Study, Denmark 2001–10." *British Medical Journal* 344 (2012): e2990. doi: 10.1136/bmj.e2990.

Lidegaard, Ø., L. H. Nielsen, C. W. Skovlund, F. E. Skjeldestad, and E. Løkkegaard. "Risk of Venous Thromboembolism from Use of Oral Contraceptives Containing Different Progestogens and Oestrogen Doses: Danish Cohort Study, 2001–2009." *British Medical Journal* 343 (2011): d6423. doi: 10.1136/bmj.d6423.

Lim, H., B. C. Paria, S. K. Das, J. E. Dinchuk, R. Langenbach, J. M. Trzaskos, and S. K. Dey. "Multiple Female Reproductive Failures in Cyclooxygenase 2-deficient Mice." *Cell* 91 (1997): 197–208.

Mahutte, N. G., I. M. Matalliotakis, A. G. Goumenou, G. E. Koumantakis, S. Vassiliadis, and A. Arici. "Elevations in Peritoneal Fluid Macrophage Migration Inhibitory Factor Are Independent of the Depth of Invasion or Stage of Endometriosis." *Fertility and Sterility* 82 (2004): 97–101.

Marcoux, S., R. Maheux, and S. Bérubé. "Laparoscopic Surgery in Infertile Women with Minimal or Mild Endometriosis." *New England Journal of Medicine* 337 (1997): 217–22.

Marions, L., S. Z. Cekan, M. Bygdeman, and K. Gemzell-Danielsson. "Effect of Emergency Contraception with Levonorgestrel or Mifepristone on Ovarian Function." *Contraception* 69 (2004): 373–77.

Martius, J. A., T. Steck, M. K. Oehler, and K. H. Wulf. "Risk Factors Associated with Preterm (<37+0 weeks) and Early Preterm (<32+0 weeks): Univariate and Multi-Variate Analysis of 106,345 Singleton Births from 1994 Statewide Perinatal Survey of Bavaria." *European Journal of Obstetric and Gynecologic Reproductive Biology* 80 (1998): 183–89.

Matorras, R., F. Rodríguez, G. Gutierrez de Terán, J. I. Pijoan, O. Ramón, and F. J. Rodríguez-Escudero. "Endometriosis and Spontaneous Abortion Rate: A Cohort Study in Infertile Women." *European Journal of Obstetrical and Gynecological Reproductive Biology* 77 (1998): 101–5.

McFarlane, J., A. Malecha, K. Watson, J. Gist, E. Batten, I. Hall, and S. Smith. "Intimate Partner Sexual Assault against Women: Frequency, Health Consequences, and Treatment Outcomes." *Obstetrics and Gynecology* 105 (2005): 99–108.

Meng, C., K. L. Andersson, U. Bentin-Ley, K. Gemzell-Danielsson, and P. G. Lalitkumar. "Effect of Levonorgestrel and Mifepristone on Endometrial Receptivity Markers in a Three-Dimensional Human Endometrial Cell Culture Model." *Fertility and Sterility* 91 (2009): 256–64.

Miech, R. P. "Pathophysiology of Mifepristone-Induced Septic Shock Due to *Clostridium sordellii*." *The Annals of Pharmacotherapy* 39 (2005): 1483–88.

Mier-Cabrera, J., T. Aburto-Soto, S. Burrola-Méndez, L. Jiménez-Zamudio, M. C. Tolentino, E. Casanueva, and C. Hernández-Guerrero. "Women with Endometriosis Improved Their Peritoneal Antioxidant Markers after the Application of a High Antioxidant Diet." *Reproductive Biology and Endocrinology* 7 (2009). doi: 10.1186/1477-7827-7-54.

Mikolajczyk, R. T., and J. B. Stanford. "Levonorgestrel Emergency Contraception: A Joint Analysis of Effectiveness and Mechanism of Action," *Fertility and Sterility* 88 (2007): 565–571.

Moreau, C., M. Kaminski, P. Y. Ancel, J. Bouyer, B. Escande, G. Thiriez, P. Boulot, et al. "Previous Induced Abortions and the Risk of Very Preterm Delivery: Results of the EPIPAGE Study." *British Journal of Obstetrics and Gynecology* 112 (2005): 430–37.

Mota, N. P., M. Burnett, and J. Sareen. "Associations between Abortion, Mental Disorders, and Suicidal Behaviors in a Nationally Representative Sample." *Canadian Journal of Psychiatry* 55 (2010): 239–46.

Murphy, A. A., N. Santanam, A. J. Morales, and S. Parthasarathy. "Lysophosphatidyl Choline, a Chemotactic Factor for Monocytes/T-Lymphocytes Is Elevated in Endometriosis." *Journal of Clinical Endocrinology and Metabolism* 83 (1998): 2110–13.

Namnoum, A. B., T. N. Hickman, S. B. Goodman, D. L. Gehlbach, and J. A. Rock. "Incidence of Symptom Recurrence after Hysterectomy for Endometriosis." *Fertility and Sterility* 64 (1995): 898–902.

National Catholic Bioethics Center. "Formal and Material Cooperation." *Ethics and Medics* 20, no. 6 (June 1995): 1–2.

National High Blood Pressure Education Program Working Group on High Blood Pressure in Pregnancy. "Report of the National High Blood Pressure Education Program Working Group on High Blood Pressure in Pregnancy." *American Journal of Obstetrics and Gynecology* 183 (2000): S1–S22.

Nestler, J. E., D. J. Jakubowicz, W. S. Evans, and R. Pasquali. "Effects of Metformin on Spontaneous and Clomiphene-Induced Ovulation in the Polycystic Ovary Syndrome." *New England Journal of Medicine* 338 (1998): 1876–80.

Niinimaki, M., A. Pouta, A. Bloigu, M. Gissler, E. Hemminki, S. Suhonen, and O. Heikinheimo. "Immediate Complications after Medical Compared with Surgical Termination of Pregnancy." *Obstetrics and Gynecology* 114 (2009): 795–804.

Noé, G., H. B. Croxatto, A. M. Salvatierra, V. Reyes, C. Villarroel, C. Muñoz, G. Morales, and A. Retamales. "Contraceptive Efficacy of Emergency Contraception with Levonorgestrel Given before or after Ovulation." *Contraception* 81 (2010): 414–20.

Novikova, N., E. Weisberg, F. Z. Stanczyk, H. B. Croxatto, and I. S. Fraser. "Effectiveness of Levonorgestrel Emergency Contraception Given before or after Ovulation: A Pilot Study." *Contraception* 75 (2007): 112–18.

Oei, S. G., F. M. Helmerhorst, K. W. Bloemenkamp, F. A. Hollants, D. E. Meerpoel, and M. J. Keirse. "Effectiveness of the Postcoital Test: Randomized Controlled Trial." *British Medical Journal* 317 (1998): 502–55.

Olive, D. L., and E. A. Pritts. "Treatment of Endometriosis." *New England Journal of Medicine* 345 (2001): 266–75.

Olney, R. S., C. A. Moore, M. J. Khoury, D. Erickson, L. D. Edmonds, L. D. Botto, H. K. Atrash. "Chorionic Villus Sampling and Amniocentesis: Recommendations for Prenatal Counseling." *Morbidity and Mortality Weekly Report (MMWR)* 44 (1995): 1–12. http://www.cdc.gov/mmwr/preview/mmwrhtml/00038393.htm.

Ory, S. J., E. Nnadi, R. Herrmann, P. S. O'Brien, and L. J. Melton, III. "Fertility after Ectopic Pregnancy." *Fertility and Sterility* 60 (1993): 231–35.

Palomino, W. A., P. Kohen, and L. Devoto. "A Single Midcycle Dose of Levonorgestrel Similar to Emergency Contraceptive Does Not Alter the Expression of the L-Selectin Ligand or Molecular Markers of Endometrial Receptivity." *Fertility and Sterility* 94, no. 5 (2010): 1589–94.

Paul VI, Pope. *Humanae Vitae, Of Human Life* [Encyclical Letter. July 25, 1968]. Boston: Pauline Books and Media, 1968.

Peragallo Urrutia, R. P., R. R. Coeytaux, A. J. McBroom, et al. "Risk of Thromboembolic Events with Oral Contraceptive Use." *Obstetrics and Gynecology* 122 (2013): 380–89.

Petrek, J. A. "Pregnancy Safety after Breast Cancer." *Cancer* 74 (1994): 528–31.

Pivarunas, A. R. "Ethical and Moral Considerations in the Treatment of Ectopic Pregnancy." *Linacre Quarterly* 70 (2003): 195–209.

Raine, T. R., C. C. Harper, C. H. Rocca, R. Fischer, N. Padian, J. D. Klausner, and P. D. Darney. "Direct Access to Emergency Contraception through Pharmacies and Effect on Unintended Pregnancy and STIs." *Journal of the American Medical Association* 293 (2005): 54–62.

Raymond, E. G., F. Stewart, M. Weaver, C. Monteith, and B. Van Der Pol. "Impact of Increased Access to Emergency Contraceptive Pills." *Obstetrics and Gynecology* 108 (2006): 1098–1106.

Razzi, S., S. Luisi, F. Calonaci, A. Altomare, C. Bocchi, and F. Petraglia. "Efficacy of Vaginal Danazol Treatment in Women with Recurrent Deeply Infiltrating Endometriosis." *Fertility and Sterility* 88 (2007): 789–94.

Rosendaal, F. R., F. M. Helmerhorst, and J. P. Vandenbroucke. "Female Hormones and Thrombosis." *Arteriosclerosis, Thrombosis and Vascular Biology* 22 (2002): 201–10.

Rodriguez, M. I., M. Warden, and P. D. Darney. "Intrauterine Progestins, Progesterone Antagonists, and Receptor Modulators: A Review of Gynecologic Applications." *American Journal of Obstetrics and Gynecology* 202 (2010): 420–28.

Rojas, Francisco, Elizabeth Wood, and Karin Blakemore. "Preconception Counseling and Prenatal Care." In *The Johns Hopkins Manual of Gynecology and Obstetrics*, edited by Fortner et al., 58–74.

Rooney, B., and B. C. Calhoun. "Induced Abortion and Risk of Premature Births." *Journal of American Physicians and Surgeons* 8 (2003): 46–49.

Rosing, J., J. Curvers and G. Tans. "Oral Contraceptives, Thrombosis and Haemostasis." *European Journal of Obstetrics and Gynecology and Reproductive Biology* 95 (2001): 193–97.

Rugo, H. S. "Management of Breast Cancer Diagnosed during Pregnancy." *Current Treatment Options in Oncology* 4 (2003): 165–73.

Rybak, E. A., and E. E. Wallach. "Infertility and Assisted Reproductive Technologies." In *The Johns Hopkins Manual of Gynecology and Obstetrics*, edited by Fortner et al., 389.

Sampson, J. A. "Peritoneal Endometriosis Due to Menstrual Dissemination of Endometrial Tissue into the Pelvic Cavity." *American Journal of Obstetrics and Gynecology* 14 (1927): 422–69.

Sandset, P. M., E. Høibraaten, A. L. Eilertsen, and A. Dahm. "Mechanisms of Thrombosis related to Hormone Therapy." *Thrombosis Research* 123, Suppl. 2 (2009): S70–S73.

Shevell, T., F. D. Malone, J. Vidaver, T. F. Porter, D. A. Luthy, C. H. Comstock, G. D. Hankins, et al. "Assisted Reproductive Technology and Pregnancy Outcome." *Obstetrics and Gynecology* 106 (2005): 1039–45.

Silber, S. J., and R. Cohen. "Microsurgical Reversal of Female Sterilization: the Role of Tubal Length." *Fertility and Sterility* 33 (1980): 598–601.

Simhan, H. N., and S. N. Caritas. "Prevention of Preterm Delivery." *New England Journal of Medicine* 357 (2007): 477–87.

Simmoneau, G., I. M. Robbins, M. Beghetti, et al. "Updated Clinical Classification of Pulmonary Hypertension." *Journal of the American College of Cardiology* 54 (2009): S43–S54.

Siu, S. C., M. Sermer, J. M. Colman, et al. "Prospective Multicenter Study of Pregnancy Outcomes in Women with Heart Disease." *Circulation* 104 (2001): 515–21.

Siu, S. C., M. Sermer, D. A. Harrison, et al. "Risk and Predictors for Pregnancy-Related Complications in Women with Heart Disease." *Circulation* 96 (1997): 2789–94.

Smith, Janet E. *The Right to Privacy.* Philadelphia: National Catholic Bioethics Center and Ignatius Press, 2008.

Spitz, I. M., C. W. Bardin, L. Benton, and A. Robbins. "Early Pregnancy Termination with Mifepristone and Misoprostol in the United States." *The New England Journal of Medicine* 338 (1998): 1241–47.

Stewart, R., D. Tuazon, G. Olson, and A. G. Duarte. "Pregnancy and Primary Pulmonary Hypertension: Successful Outcome with Epoprostenol Therapy." *Chest* 153 (2001): 1037–47.

Stovall, T. G., F. W. Ling, S. A. Carson, and J. E. Buster. "Serum Progesterone and Uterine Curettage in Differential Diagnosis of Ectopic Pregnancy," *Fertility and Sterility* 57 (1992): 456–457.

Strauss, L. T., S. B. Gamble, W. Y. Parker, D. A. Cook, S. B. Zane, and S. Hamdan. "Abortion Surveillance—United States, 2003," *MMWR* 55 (2006): 1–32. http://www.cdc.gov/mmwr/preview/mmwrhtml/ss5511a1.htm.

Szymanski, Linda M., and Kimberly B. Fortner. "Abnormal Uterine Bleeding." In *The Johns Hopkins Manual of Gynecology and Obstetrics*, edited by Fortner et al., 417–27.

Taylor, H. S. "Endometriosis: New Insights and Novel Treatments." *ACOG Update* 36 (2011): 1–10.

Tietze, C. "Reproductive Span and Role of Reproduction among Hutterite Women." *Fertility and Sterility* 8 (1957): 89–97.

Tirelli, A., A. Cagnacci, and A. Volpe. "Levonorgestrel Administration in Emergency Contraception: Bleeding Pattern and Pituitary Function." *Contraception* 77 (2008): 328–32.

Tulandi, T., J. A. Collins, E. Burrows, J. F. Jarrell, R. A. McInnes, W. Wrixon, and C. W. Simpson. "Treatment-Dependent and Treatment-Independent Pregnancy among Women with Periadnexal Adhesions." *American Journal of Obstetrics and Gynecology* 162 (1990): 354–57.

United States Conference of Catholic Bishops (USCCB). "Moral Principles Concerning Infants with Anencephaly." September 19, 1996. http://www.usccb.org/issues-and-action/human-life-and-dignity/end-of-life/moral-principles-concerning-infants-with-anencephaly.cfm.

——. *Ethical and Religious Directives for Catholic Health Care Services.* 5th edition. Washington, D.C.: USCCB, 2009.

——. *The Distinction between Direct Abortion and Legitimate Medical Procedures.* Washington, D.C.: USCCB, 2010.

Van Voorhis, B. J. "Outcomes from Assisted Reproductive Technology." *Obstetrics and Gynecology* 107 (2006): 183–200.

Vardo, J. H., L. L. Thornburg, and J. C. Glantz. "Maternal and Neonatal Morbidity among Nulliparous Women Undergoing Elective Induction of Labor." *Journal of Reproductive Medicine* 56 (2011): 25–30.

Vercellini, P. "Progestins for Symptomatic Endometriosis: A Critical Analysis of the Evidence." *Fertility and Sterility* 68 (1997): 393–401.

Verpoest, W. M., D. J. Cahill, C. R. Harlow, and M. G. Hull. "Relationship between Mid-Cycle Luteinizing Hormone Surge Quality and Oocyte Fertilization." *Fertility and Sterility* 73, no. 1 (2000): 75–77.

Von Hertzen, H., and G. Piaggio. "Levonorgestrel and Mifepristone in Emergency Contraception." *Steroids* 68 (2003): 1107–13.

Von Hertzen, H., and P. F. A. VanLook. "Research on New Methods of Emergency Contraception." *Family Planning Perspectives* 28 (1996): 52–57.

Watt, A. H., A. T. Legedza, E. S. Ginsburg, R. L. Barbieri, R. N. Clarke, and M. D. Hornstein. "The Prognostic Value of Age and Follicle-Stimulating Hormone Levels in Women over Forty Years of Age Undergoing In Vitro Fertilization." *Journal of Assisted Reproductive Genetics* 17 (2000): 264–68.

Weiss, B. M., L. Zemp, B. Seifert, and O. M. Hess. "Outcome of Pulmonary Vascular Disease in Pregnancy: A Systematic Overview from 1978 through 1996." *Journal of the American College of Cardiology* 31 (1998): 1650–57.

Wilcox, A. J., C. R. Weinberg, and D. D. Baird. "Timing of Sexual Intercourse in Relation to Ovulation: Effects on the Probability of Conception, Survival of the Pregnancy and Sex of the Baby." *New England Journal of Medicine* 333 (1995): 1517–21.

Wiqvist, N. E., B. Lindblom, and L. Wilhelmsson. "The Patho-Physiology of Primary Dysmenorrhea." *Research Clinical Forums* 1 (1979): 47–54.

Yang, W. T., M. J. Dryden, K. Gwyn, G. J. Whitman, and R. Theriault. "Imaging of Breast Cancer Diagnosed and Treated with Chemotherapy during Pregnancy." *Radiology* 239 (2006): 52–60.

Yeung, W. S. B., P. C. Chiu, C. H. Wang, Y. Q. Yao, and P. C. Ho. "The Effects of Levonorgestrel on Various Sperm Functions." *Contraception* 66 (2002): 453–57.

Yeung, P. P., J. Shwayder, and R. P. Pasic. "Laparoscopic Management of Endometriosis: Comprehensive Review of Best Evidence." *Journal of Minimally Invasive Gynecology* 16 (2009): 269–81.

Zarutskie, P. W., and J. A. Phillips. "A Meta-Analysis of the Role of Administration of Luteal Phase Support in Assisted Reproductive Technology: Vaginal versus Intramuscular Progesterone." *Fertility and Sterility* 92 (2009): 163–69.

Ziaei, S., S. Faghihzadeh, F. Sohrabvand, M. Lamyian, and T. Emamgholy. "A Randomized Placebo-Controlled Trial to Determine the Effect of Vitamin E in Treatment of Primary Dysmenorrhea." *British Journal of Obstetrics and Gynecology* 108 (2001): 1181–83.

Richard J. Fehring

5. FERTILITY CARE SERVICES

The Catholic Church calls married couples to responsible parenthood; this includes both openness to new human life and the avoidance of pregnancy when serious reasons present themselves. Natural methods of family planning respect the dignity of the person and the integrity of the sexual act. They treat fertility as a natural process rather than a disease. Natural family planning (NFP) works with a woman's menstrual cycle; it uses awareness of fertile and infertile times to achieve or avoid pregnancy and allows married couples, through their awareness, to respect and maintain both the unitive and the procreative aspects of the sexual act. In this chapter, Dr. Fehring points out that the benefits of using NFP are "a better understanding of fertility, increased communication, self-mastery of sexual desires, greater generosity toward new human life, and openness to God's will." He also explores the history of fertility awareness methods, their scientific basis, and their efficacy. He discusses some medical side benefits of tracking fertility: it can reveal abnormalities and is an aid in the assessment and treatment of infertility. Daily discussion of fertility enhances communication between spouses. Periods of abstinence, while difficult at times, also provide opportunities for the couple to develop nonsexual expressions of intimacy, thereby enhancing mutual respect and married life. The teaching and use of NFP is an effective way of promoting the culture of life.—*Editors.*

For legitimate reasons of responsible parenthood, married couples may limit the number of their children by natural means. The Church cannot approve contraceptive interventions that "either in anticipation of the marital act, or in its accomplishment or in the development of its natural consequences, have the purpose, whether as an end or a means, to render procreation impossible." Such interventions violate "the inseparable connection, willed by God . . . between the two meanings of the conjugal act: the unitive and procreative meaning." (pt 4, intro.)

Catholic health institutions may not promote or condone contraceptive practices but should provide, for married couples and the medical staff who counsel them, instruction both about the Church's teaching on responsible parenthood and in methods of natural family planning. (dir. 54)

USCCB, *Ethical and Religious Directives for Catholic Health Care Services*

Introduction

The *Ethical and Religious Directives for Catholic Health Care Services* of the United States Conference of Catholic Bishops indicate that Catholic hospitals should not offer contraception services for family planning purposes. Furthermore, the directives state that the medical staff should both provide natural family planning services and explain the Church's teaching on these matters[1]—two important responsibilities. Therefore, it behooves Catholic physicians and other Catholic health professionals to be knowledgeable about these methods, to be able to offer them when requested, to promote them as the only moral way to plan families, and to be ready to explain (and defend) the Church's teaching on the use of contraception and NFP.

Most Catholic couples do not use NFP as a means of avoiding pregnancy or for facilitating the transmission of new life,[2] and most Catholic physicians do not provide or know how to provide NFP services.[3] There are many reasons for this, but the most common is that health-care providers and potential users have tended to find NFP methods ineffective, hard to use, and difficult to provide or teach.[4] Furthermore, difficult medical situations often arise in which the physician might be reluctant to prescribe, and the patient would be reluctant to depend on, NFP methods. Some common examples include a medical condition in which pregnancy would be detrimental or even life-threatening, or a case that involves a patient who takes a medication that would jeopardize either her life or that of her unborn baby should she become pregnant.

However, from a health perspective, NFP should be viewed as good health care, rather than as something forced upon Catholic health-care providers. Human fertility is a natural process, not a disease. NFP is a healthy and holy means of family planning that respects the human person and maintains the integrity of the sexual act and its procreative nature. It does not block, suppress with drugs, or destroy with surgery the reproductive system. It is a means by which women's health and the health of the

---

1. See United States Conference of Catholic Bishops (USCCB), *Ethical and Religious Directives for Catholic Health Care Services*, 5th ed. (Washington, D.C.: USCCB, 2009), dir. 52.

2. See J. Ohlendorf and R. Fehring, "The Influence of Religiosity on Contraceptive Use among US Catholic Women," *Linacre Quarterly* 74 (2007): 135–44.

3. See R. J. Fehring, "Physician and Nurse's Knowledge and Use of Natural Family Planning," *Linacre Quarterly* 63 (1995): 22–28.

4. See J. B. Stanford, P. B Thurman, and J. C. Lemaire, "Physicians' Knowledge and Practices Regarding Natural Family Planning," *Obstetrics and Gynecology* 94 (1999): 672–78; also R. Fehring, L. Hanson, and J. Stanford, "Nurse-Midwives' Knowledge and Promotion of Lactational Amenorrhea and Other Natural Family Planning Methods for Child Spacing," *Journal of Nurse Midwifery and Women's Health* 46 (2001): 68–73.

marital relationship can be enhanced. Physicians and other health-care professionals who provide modern NFP services should not be apologetic or feel that they are providing a substandard form of health care.

Natural family planning is simply a method of monitoring and understanding the fertile and infertile times of a woman's menstrual cycle, and using that knowledge to either achieve or avoid pregnancy. If a couple wishes to become pregnant, they have intercourse during the fertile time of the menstrual cycle; if they wish to avoid pregnancy, they avoid intercourse during the fertile time.

NFP is also referred to as "fertility awareness" or "fertility appreciation"; the latter term is sometimes preferred by those who also teach the use of barrier contraception (condoms, spermicides, and/or diaphragms) during the fertile phase of the menstrual cycle. Strictly speaking, however, any use of contraceptive methods such as condoms during the fertile time of the menstrual cycle, or the use of withdrawal, is not natural family planning.

From a philosophical and religious perspective, NFP differs from contraception in that it does nothing against conception or the nature of the marital act. NFP allows intercourse to remain integrated and whole, and to maintain its dual meaning as both a love-producing (unitive) and a potentially life-giving (procreative) act, as the Creator intended it to be. "What God has put together, let no man separate" (Mt 19:6; Mk 10:9).[5]

Philosophy of Natural Family Planning

Sexuality is an integral and good part of human life and marriage. When used in an ordered, or proper, way, sexuality is life-giving and serves to integrate and unify human relationships. When used improperly, or in a disordered way, sexuality retards human growth, destroys relationships, and places individuals at high risk for disease and even death. For an unmarried person, sexuality is ordered when expressed in a modest and chaste (non-genital) way. Sexuality is also ordered when expressed chastely and physically between a man and woman who are married to each other, and when it is an expression of love that is open to the possibility of new human life. An act of intercourse between a husband and wife is a true expression of love when there is a total giving of self, which includes giving and receiving the gift of fertility.[6] Any act of suppressing, blocking, or destroying the gift of fertility, or destroying new human life once begun, is an act against love and life.

Although couples are called to be generous to new life, there are times during married life when spacing or limiting the number of children is prudent and responsible.[7] A married couple should discern this responsibility in a prayerful and selfless

---

5. See also Pope John Paul II, *Familiaris Consortio, The Role of the Christian Family in the Modern World* [*Apostolic Exhortation, November 22, 1981*] (Boston: Daughters of St. Paul, 1981), no. 32.

6. See John Paul II, *Familiaris Consortio*, no. 32.

7. See Pope Paul VI, *Humanae Vitae, Of Human Life,* Encyclical Letter, July 25, 1968 (Boston: Pauline Books, 1968); also Pope Pius XII, "Address to Italian Catholic Union of Midwives," October 29, 1951, in

way, within the context of the couple's duties to God, themselves, their family, and society. Serious reasons for spacing or limiting children could include issues related to physical or psychological health, economic or financial constraints, or social considerations.[8]

When a married couple has discerned a need to space or limit children, they must still remain true to love, to the integrity of the sexual act, and to the gift of fertility. Natural family planning is a means by which a couple learns how to monitor the woman's monthly cycle and to interpret the natural signs that tell them when the woman is fertile and when she is not. If the couple has serious reasons to avoid pregnancy, they then periodically abstain from intercourse and genital contact during the fertile times of the cycle. During these times, couples are challenged to express their intimacy in non-genital ways. These may include intellectual activities, like sharing a good book, or talking and listening to each other's needs, desires, and fears. The couple may build spiritual closeness through prayer, or share physical closeness by walking together or just holding each other. Although this may be difficult and at times seem impossible, God does not ask the impossible, and he will be with the couple in a special way through their difficult times.

The practice of NFP and periodic abstinence, far from harming married love, actually confers upon married life a higher human value.[9] Couples who practice chastity within marriage and use NFP reap such benefits as a better understanding of fertility, increased communication, self-mastery of sexual desires, greater generosity toward new human life, and openness to God's will. These effects were all predicted by Pope Paul VI and have been validated in quantitative and qualitative studies (see "Marital Dynamics of Using NFP" below).

Scientific and Physiological Base

A 1995 study published in the *New England Journal of Medicine* confirmed that there is only a six-day window of fertility in the menstrual cycle: the day of ovulation and the five preceding days.[10] Subsequent research established that the most fertile days of this window are the two days before ovulation, and that the fertile phase varies from cycle to cycle. Other studies have indicated that the most common length of the fertile phase is only three days; that the fertile window occurs most frequently between days 8 and 20 of the menstrual cycle; and that the probability of pregnancy with an act of intercourse during the fertile window decreases as a woman ages.[11]

Natural Family Planning: Nature's Way—God's Way, ed. Anthony Zimmerman (Milwaukee, Wisc.: DeRance, 1980), 229–30.

8. See Paul VI, *Humanae Vitae*, no. 21.

9. See ibid.

10. See A. J. Wilcox, C. R. Weinberg, and D. D. Baird, "Timing of Sexual Intercourse in Relation to Ovulation: Effects on the Probability of Conception, Survival of the Pregnancy, and Sex of the Baby," *New England Journal of Medicine* 333 (1995): 1517–21.

11. See D. B. Dunson et al., "Day-Specific Probabilities of Clinical Pregnancy Based on Two Studies with Imperfect Measures of Ovulation," *Human Reproduction* 14 (1999): 1835–39; A. J. Wilcox et al., "The Timing

The six-day length of the fertile phase in the menstrual cycle makes sense, since the human egg, once released from the follicle at ovulation, lives only 12 to 24 hours and most likely is fertilizable only in the first 12 hours. We also know that the lifespan of sperm is between three and five days, provided they are in a receptive environment with the proper nutrients and pH level.[12] The vagina is essentially a hostile environment for sperm, as it is too acidic for sperm to survive more than a few minutes.[13] However, during the three to five days leading up to ovulation, women of reproductive age produce mucus from their cervix that provides the appropriate pH and nourishment for sperm and is essential for sperm transport and capacitation.

A number of physiological factors combine to create the fertile window and allow fertilization to take place. At the beginning of each menstrual cycle, follicle-stimulating hormone (FSH) is released from the anterior portion of the pituitary gland; this hormone stimulates the ovaries to develop a group of immature, or antral, follicles, each containing an undeveloped human egg within.[14] As the follicles develop and enlarge, they release the hormone estrogen. However, only a few follicles will mature and grow to the point of ovulation. Usually, only one follicle-egg complex, termed the dominant follicle, grows to complete maturity at a size of 18 to 24 mm, releasing higher levels of estrogen and proceeding to ovulation. The higher estrogen levels affect the woman's body to facilitate the possible fertilization of the egg, or oocyte.

The opening of the woman's cervix (the os of the uterus) is essentially tight and closed except during the fertile window. Estrogen from the developing follicles softens the cells of the cervix, opening the os wider and elevating the cervix's position within the woman's body. At the time of ovulation and the peak of estrogen production, the os is soft and open. The columnar cells lining the passage of the canal from the os into the body of the uterus (the endocervical canal) are also stimulated by estrogen to produce mucus. The mucus at first is minimal, cloudy, and rather thick, but as estrogen levels increase, the mucus thins and becomes more watery and profuse. At the peak of fertility, the mucus is abundant, liquid, and slippery, made up primarily of water (more than 90 percent) with glycogen bonds that hold the water in a gel-like state. The mucus at this stage of fertility also contains carbohydrates and

---

of the 'Fertile Window' in the Menstrual Cycle: Day Specific Estimates from a Prospective Study," *British Medical Journal* 321 (2000): 1259–62; D. B. Dunson, B. Columbo, and D. D. Baird, "Changes with Age in the Level and Duration of Fertility in the Menstrual Cycle," *Human Reproduction* 17 (2002): 1399–1403; R. Fehring and M. Schneider, "Variability of the Fertile Phase of the Menstrual Cycle," *Fertility and Sterility* 90 (2008): 1232–35.

12. See L. Speroff and M. Fritz, "Regulation of the Menstrual Cycle", ch. 6, and "Sperm and Egg Transport, Fertilization, and Implantation," ch. 7 in *Clinical Gynecologic Endocrinology and Infertility*, 7th ed. (Philadelphia: Lippencott Williams and Wilkins, 2005).

13. See K. S. Moghissi, "Cervical Mucus Changes and Ovulation Prediction and Detection," *Journal of Reproductive Medicine* 31 Supp. (1986): 748–53; E. Odeblad, "Cervical Mucus and Their Functions," *Journal of the Irish Colleges of Physicians and Surgeons* 26 (1997): 27–32; S. Palter and D. Olive, "Reproductive Physiology," in *Novak's Gynecology*, ed. S. J. Berek (Philadelphia: Lippincott Williams and Wilkins, 2002), 149–74.

14. See E. Clubb and J. Knight, *Fertility* (Exeter, U.K.: David and Charles, 1999), 28–30; L. J. Heffner, and D. J. Schust, "The Menstrual Cycle," in *The Reproduction System at a Glance*, 4th ed. (Malden, Mass.: Wiley Blackwell, 2014), 36–37.

salts that neutralize the vagina's acidic environment and nourish sperm.[15] The cervical mucus at this time literally pours from the soft and open os. The estrogen increase also stimulates another reproductive hormone, luteinizing hormone, or LH, which surges to prepare the follicle for release of the mature egg.

After ovulation, LH converts, or luteinizes, the cells of the follicle, at which time the follicle is called the corpus luteum. The corpus luteum produces large amounts of the hormone progesterone, which readies the uterine lining for possible implantation of a new embryonic human life. Progesterone also raises the woman's body temperature by about 0.5 degree Fahrenheit and serves to dry up the cervical mucus and tighten and close the cervical os. The dried mucus produces a mucus plug that prevents sperm or bacteria from entering the uterus. If an egg released at the time of ovulation is not fertilized by the man's sperm, the corpus luteum is eventually reabsorbed and the levels of progesterone and estrogen drop off. As progesterone levels drop, the lining of the uterus is no longer hormonally supported and is sloughed off in menses. The onset of the menstrual period marks a new menstrual cycle, even though the FSH levels are already increasing and follicular development is taking place. Menses occurs about nine to seventeen days after the day of ovulation.

Natural Signs of Human Fertility

NFP is essentially the use of naturally occurring signs of fertility to estimate the beginning, peak, and end of the fertile window, and the tracking of the fertile window's variability from menstrual cycle to menstrual cycle. For NFP to be effective and useful, it must also track fertility during the various stages of the woman's reproductive life and during special reproductive circumstances, such as breastfeeding and perimenopause. The traditional signs of fertility include changes in basal body temperature, in the characteristics of cervical mucus, in the cervix, and in female reproductive hormones secreted in the urine.[16] Users and providers of NFP also use calendar-based methods to estimate the fertile phase of the menstrual cycle, alone or in combination with other markers of fertility.

Basal body temperature (BBT) measures the post-ovulatory increase in the woman's body temperature (between 0.2 and 1 degree Fahrenheit) that is a result of increased progesterone production.[17] This temperature rise, or shift, becomes a natural physiological marker that ovulation has recently taken place. A woman determines

15. See M. Menarguez, L. M. Pastor, and E. Odeblad, "Morphological Characterization of Different Human Cervical Mucus Types Using Light and Scanning Electron Microscopy," *Human Reproduction* 18 (2004): 1782–89; Moghissi, "Cervical Mucus Changes and Ovulation Prediction and Detection"; Odeblad, "Cervical Mucus and Their Functions"; R. Fehring, "Accuracy of the Peak Day of Cervical Mucus as a Biological Marker of Fertility," *Contraception* 66 (2002): 231–35.

16. See Clubb and Knight, *Fertility*, 33.

17. See M. L. Barron and R. J. Fehring, "Basal Body Temperature Assessment: Is It Useful to Couples Seeking Pregnancy?" *MCN: American Journal of Maternal Child Nursing* 30 (2005): 290–96; J. J. McCarthy, and H. E. Rockette, "A Comparison of Methods to Interpret the Basal Body Temperature Graph," *Fertility and Sterility* 39 (1983): 640–46.

her BBT shift by taking her temperature every morning before rising. When she observes a sustained shift in temperature, she can assume that she has ovulated. Various rules determine a temperature shift for use in NFP; the most common is the rule of 3 over 6 (i.e., six low temperatures followed by at least a 0.2 of a degree rise, and then the next three temperatures remain at or above the 0.2 degree rise). Another approach is to average the temperatures from the previous menstrual cycle and use that average as the coverline. When there are three temperatures above that coverline, then the woman is in the infertile phase of her menstrual cycle.

Cervical mucus changes also serve as a marker for estimating the beginning, peak, and end of the fertile phase. These changes are a result of estrogen stimulation of the cells lining the endocervical canal.[18] Rising estrogen levels produce a mucus that is at first cloudy and thick, but becomes watery, slippery, and clear at the ovulatory stage, then changes back to cloudy and thick, and finally to dry. If a woman pays attention to her cervical mucus sensations at the vulva throughout the day and finger tests the mucus to observe the characteristics, she should have a fairly good marker for tracking her fertile window from cycle to cycle.

The cervix also changes during the fertile phase of the menstrual cycle. At first the cervix is hard, like the cartilage of the nose, and situated low in the vagina; but as estrogen stimulates the cervix, it becomes soft, like the lips. At the same time, the os of the cervix opens, mucus pours from the opening, and the position of the cervix rises as felt internally in the vagina.[19] Once ovulation takes place, the cervix again becomes hard and closed, and its position shifts lower in the vagina. A woman can feel internally for the position and characteristics of the cervix and make daily judgments on her fertile or infertile phase. However, there has been scant research on the accuracy of the cervical sign in estimating the fertile phase. There is also the concern that through self-examination the woman can introduce germs into the vagina and inadvertently damage the cervix.

The final markers used to estimate the fertile window are metabolites of reproductive hormones that can be detected in the urine.[20] Antibody assay technology has enabled researchers to develop simple test strips that can be dipped into urine, or held under the urine stream while voiding, to detect reproductive hormones. The most common test strip, of course, is the pregnancy test developed to detect levels of human chorionic gonadotropin (hCG), which is produced after an ovum is fertilized. Detectable levels can be found about fourteen days post-ovulation, at the first missed menstrual period. Another popular test is the ovulation detection kit and test strip used to help predict ovulation by detecting the LH surge in the urine, in order to

18. See Moghissi, "Cervical Mucus Changes and Ovulation Prediction and Detection," 748–53.

19. See E. Keefe, "Self-Examination of the Cervix as a Guide in Fertility Control," *International Review of Natural Family Planning* 10 (1986): 322–38.

20. See F. Batzer, "Test Kits for Ovulation and Pregnancy," *Technology 1987: Contemporary OB/GYN* 28 (1986): 7–16; G. Corson, D. Ghaz, and E. Kemmann, "Home Urinary Luteinizing Hormone Immunoassay: Clinical Applications," *Fertility and Sterility* 53 (1990): 591–601; P. G. Crosignani et al., "Optimal Use of Infertility Diagnostic Tests and Treatments," *Human Reproduction* 15 (2000): 723–32.

determine the best time for intercourse to achieve pregnancy.[21] These test strips can be used as markers for NFP by estimating the day of ovulation.

Recently, more sophisticated, hand-held electronic hormonal fertility monitors (the Persona and Clearblue Easy Fertility monitors) have been developed.[22] Both monitors detect metabolites of estrogen and LH on test strips which are inserted into the monitor for an automatic reading, similar to the glucose test strips and electronic readers used by diabetics. The Persona monitor, designed to help women avoid pregnancy, is sold in Europe but not in the United States; the Clearblue monitor was designed to help couples achieve pregnancy, even though it has a higher threshold of estrogen and thus a shorter estimated fertile phase than the Persona. The Clearblue's high fertility reading is triggered when the monitor detects a twofold increase of estrogen from baseline levels; its peak reading is triggered when the LH threshold is detected. This monitor thus provides a marker for the beginning, peak, and end of the fertile window.

Accuracy of Natural Markers of Fertility

All natural markers used to estimate fertility for NFP methods are imprecise, and each has its strengths and benefits. Researchers have investigated the accuracy of these markers in comparison with the "gold standard" in ovulation detection: serial ultrasound of the dominant ovarian follicle, with the follicle's visual collapse indicating the day of ovulation. Prior to the use of serial ultrasound, the urinary or serum surge in LH or a ratio of estrogen and progesterone was used as a marker for ovulation. These studies indicated a strong correlation between the peak in cervical mucus and the estimated day of ovulation; however, 98 percent of the time, the mucus peak varied from the day of ovulation plus or minus three days.[23] Thus, the peak in cervical mucus provides a seven-day estimate of the actual day of ovulation.

Since ultrasound technology came into use, serial ultrasound of the dominant follicle's growth and collapse have been compared in studies with the BBT shift, the peak in cervical mucus, and the LH surge as detected in the urine.[24] The studies show that the LH surge is the most precise indirect marker of ovulation, followed by the

21. See M. Seibel, "Luteinizing Hormone and Ovulation Timing," *Journal of Reproductive Medicine* 31 Supp. (1986): 754–59; Consumer Reports, "The Fertility Window," *Consumer Reports* 68 (2003): 48–50; J. B. Stanford, G. L. White, and H. Hataska, "Timing Intercourse to Achieve Pregnancy: Current Evidence," *Obstetrics and Gynecology* 100 (2002):1333–41.

22. See K. May, "Home Monitoring with the ClearPlan Easy Fertility Monitor for Fertility Awareness," *Journal of International Medical Research* 29 S1 (2002): 14A–20A; J. Bonnar et al., "Personal Hormone Monitoring for Contraception," *British Journal of Family Planning* 24 (1999): 128–34.

23. See Fehring, "Accuracy of the Peak Day of Cervical Mucus as a Biological Marker of Fertility," 231–35.

24. See M. Guida et al., "Efficacy of Methods for Determining Ovulation in a Natural Family Planning Program," *Fertility and Sterility* 72 (1999): 900–904; K. Tanabe et al., "Prediction of the Potentially Fertile Period by Urinary Hormone Measurements Using a New Home-Use Monitor: Comparison with Laboratory Hormone Analyses," *Human Reproduction* 16 (2001): 1619–24; R. Ecochard et al., "Chronological Aspects of Ultrasonic, Hormonal, and Other Indirect Indices of Ovulation," *British Journal of Obstetrics and Gynecology* 109 (2001): 822–29.

cervical mucus peak and the BBT shift. Another study showed that ovulation, as detected by ultrasound, occurred 97 percent of the time on the two days of peak readings on the electronic hormonal monitor and never occurred prior to the peak reading.[25] Thus far no studies have validated self-detected changes in the cervix with accurate markers of ovulation. NFP developers are still debating how best to detect, observe, and rate self-detected cervical changes.

Methods of NFP

Over the past eighty years, a number of NFP methods have been developed; these can be generally classified as calendar-based methods, single-indicator methods, and combination methods. There are also such low-tech methods as the fixed-day calendar-based system, and high-tech methods that use electronic hormonal monitoring of fertility and monoclonal assays.

The first methods of NFP were developed by two physician scientists, Hermann Knaus from Germany and Kyusako Ogino from Japan, in the mid to late 1920s.[26] The calendar-based systems they devised, sometimes called the Ogino-Knaus methods, involve taking the shortest menstrual cycle from the last twelve and subtracting twenty days (or nineteen to be less rigorous) from that length to determine the beginning of the infertile time. Similarly, subtracting ten days from the longest menstrual cycle of the previous twelve indicates the day on which the fertile time ends. For example, if the length of the shortest menstrual cycle over the previous twelve cycles was twenty-six days, and the longest was thirty days, the first day of fertility would be day 6 of the menstrual cycle and the last day of fertility would be day 20; thus, the estimated fertile phase is from days 6 to 20.

In the United States, the calendar-based NFP method was made popular by a young obstetrician-gynecologist from Loyola University School of Medicine, Dr. Leo Latz.[27] He traveled to Europe to study under Knaus and returned to the United States to write a book titled *The Rhythm of Sterility and Fertility in Women*, published in 1932. Over the next twenty years, his foundation sold more than six hundred thousand copies of the book, in which he declared that his simple method could be taught by physicians, professional nurses, or social workers in a twelve-minute office session. Latz's book gave us the term "rhythm method" for calendar-based methods, a term still commonly (and erroneously) used for NFP by health professionals and the lay public.

The rhythm method was one of the most popular methods of family planning among U.S. women, and Catholic women in particular, from the 1930s through the

25. See H. M. Behre et al., "Prediction of Ovulation by Urinary Hormone Measurements with the Home Use of the ClearPlan Fertility Monitor: Comparison with Transvaginal Ultrasound Scans and Serum Hormone Measurements," *Human Reproduction* 15 (2000): 2478–82.

26. See H. Knaus, *Periodic Fertility and Sterility in Woman: A Natural Method of Birth Control* (Vienna: Wilhelm Maudrich, Publisher, 1934); K. Ogino, *Conception Period of Women* (Harrisburg, Penn.: Medical Arts Publishing, 1934).

27. See L. Latz, *The Rhythm of Sterility and Fertility in Women* (Chicago: Latz Foundation, 1932).

1950s. Upward of 30 percent of women of reproductive age, and 55 percent of Catholic women, used calendar-based methods well into the 1950s.[28] With the advent of the hormonal birth control pill, that statistic dramatically changed.

The ease of use of birth control pills, coupled with anecdotal evidence of couples unintentionally becoming pregnant with the rhythm method, led to a decline in use of calendar-based methods. Interestingly, more women of reproductive age in the United States currently use "rhythm" than the so-called modern methods of NFP, which rely on cervical mucus and basal body temperature.[29] Furthermore, efforts have been renewed to investigate calendar-based methods using a careful scientific approach. Researchers at Georgetown University's Institute for Reproductive Health have developed a fixed-day calendar-based method of NFP. The days of fertility for this method are days 8 to 19 of the menstrual cycle for women who generally have menstrual cycle lengths between twenty-six and thirty-two days.[30] A bead system is used to help couples track fertility. The Institute for Reproductive Health researchers have found this method to be comparable in efficacy to barrier methods of contraception.

In the 1930s, a parish priest in Germany who was teaching couples in his parish the Knaus rhythm method found that they were getting pregnant with its use, even though they were attempting to avoid pregnancy.[31] At the advice of his physician brother, he added daily morning body temperature readings to detect the BBT shift, thus initiating the use of temperature readings for birth control. Since then, many physician scientists have developed and tested BBT methods, notably British physician John Marshall, who conducted the first large prospective-efficacy study of the BBT method of NFP.[32] The BBT shift is usually used with calendar-based calculations to determine the beginning of the fertile phase, but it is also used alone as a post-ovulatory-only method of NFP.

Since the mid-1800s, physicians have been aware of a vaginal mucus discharge that has some correlation with fertility. However, it was not until the early 1950s that a number of physician researchers combined calendar-based formulas, BBT, and the tracking of changes in the cervix and cervical mucus as a method of NFP.[33] This method was called the sympto-thermal method and is considered one of the "modern methods" of NFP. Women who use this method can also track secondary signs of fertility, such as ovulatory pain (mittleschmertz) and breast tenderness. A modern

---

28. See C. F. Westoff and N. R. Ryder, "Conception Control among American Catholics," in *Catholics/ U.S.A.: Perspectives on Social Change*, ed. W. T. Liu and N. J. Pallone (New York: John Wiley and Sons, 1970), 257–68.

29. See W. D. Mosher and J. Jones, "Use of Contraception in the United States: 1982–2008," *Vital and Health Statistics* 23.29 (2010): 1–77, see especially table 1, for example.

30. See M. Arevalo, V. Jennings, and I. Sinai, "Efficacy of a New Method of Family Planning: The Standard Days Method," *Contraception* 65 (2002): 333–38.

31. See R. Vollman, "Brief History of Natural Family Planning," in *Natural Family Planning: Introduction to the Methods*, ed. Clara R. Ross (Washington, D.C.: Human Life Foundation, 1977), 1–5.

32. See J. Marshall, "A Field Trial of the BBT Method of Regulating Births," *Lancet* 292 (1968): 8–10.

33. See Keefe, "Self-Examination of the Cervix as a Guide in Fertility Control"; J. Roetzer, "Further Evaluation of the Sympto-thermal Method," *International Review of Natural Family Planning* 1 (1977): 139–50.

form of this combination method, developed by a European NFP group, is called the European double-check method, referring to a double check for the beginning and end of the fertile phase.[34] Research has established efficacy rates comparable to the birth control pill among German women who use this method.

In the mid-1960s, several physicians working with various NFP methods deduced that changes in cervical mucus could be used alone as a natural marker for the beginning, peak, and end of the estimated fertile phase. The best-known of these ovulation methods, developed by Drs. John and Evelyn Billings from Australia, is known as the Billings Ovulation Method.[35] A large multicountry efficacy study of the generic ovulation methods was carried out by the World Health Organization in the late 1970s (the results will be discussed below).[36] A standardized variation of the ovulation methods, called the Creighton Model, was developed by Dr. Thomas Hilgers, along with his wife and two professional nurses.[37] The Creighton Model uses a standardized method of grading and charting cervical mucus observations.

Over the years, many devices have been tested and developed to help women observe and track natural indicators of fertility. However, it was not until the 1990s that micro-electronics, modern biochemistry, and immunoassay techniques allowed the consumer to measure hormones as they are excreted in the urine. In 1990, Carl Djerassi, one of the developers of the first hormonal contraceptive pill, predicted what he called "Jet-Age NFP," in which the woman herself would be able to measure her reproductive hormones with simple hand-held electronic devices.[38] Urine-based pregnancy tests and ovulation test kits have been around since the 1980s, but the late 1990s saw the introduction of the Persona and Clearblue monitors we have already discussed. The Clearblue device has been used as an aid for monitoring fertility and for either achieving or avoiding pregnancy in a model of NFP developed at Marquette University.[39] It has been used effectively as a second marker, along with cervical mucus monitoring, for determining the beginning and end of the fertile window, or as the primary marker along with a simple fertility algorithm.

34. See P. Frank-Herrmann et al., "Determination of the Fertile Window: Reproductive Competence of Women—European Cycle Databases," *Gynecology and Endocrinology* 20 (2005): 305–12.

35. See E. L. Billings, *The Billings Ovulation Method* (Melbourne, Australia: Ovulation Method Research and Reference Centre of Australia, 1995); E. L. Billings and J. J. Billings, *Teaching the Billings Ovulation Method* (Melbourne, Australia: Ovulation Method Research and Reference Centre of Australia, 1997); E. L. Billlings, J. J. Billings, and M. Caterinich, *Billings Atlas of the Ovulation Method* (Melbourne, Australia: Ovulation Method Research and Reference Centre of Australia, 1989).

36. See World Health Organization, "A Prospective Multicentre Trial of the Ovulation Method of Natural Family Planning. II. The Effectiveness Phase," *Fertility and Sterility* 36 (1981): 591–98.

37. See T. W. Hilgers, *The Medical Applications of Natural Family Planning* (Omaha, Neb.: Pope Paul VI Institute Press, 1991); T. W. Hilgers, *The Scientific Foundations of the Ovulation Method* (Omaha, Neb.: Pope Paul VI Institute Press, 1995); T. W. Hilgers, *The Creighton Model NaProEducation System* (Omaha, Neb.: Pope Paul VI Institute Press, 1996).

38. See C. Djerassi, "Fertility Awareness: Jet-Age Rhythm Method?" *Science* 248 (1990): 1061–62.

39. See R. Fehring, "New Low and High Tech Calendar Methods of Family Planning," *Journal of Nurse Midwifery and Women's Health* 50 (2005): 31–37.

Efficacy of NFP Methods

The understanding of efficacy and effectiveness of NFP methods has evolved during the last seventy years as family planning methods have evolved. When Leo Latz first reported on the efficacy of the rhythm method, he reported 15,924 cases of intercourse in the sterile time with no pregnancies.[40] Modern efficacy studies of family planning methods are the result of controlled prospective studies (usually cohort) of the given method.[41] Effectiveness studies are based on the unintended pregnancy rate of a population that uses a method of family planning; this rate is usually determined retrospectively through chart review or surveys. Most studies of NFP (like those of contraceptive methods) are of a prospective controlled study nature over time (usually 12 to 24 months of use) and are considered "efficacy" studies rather than "effectiveness" studies.

In the early days of determining the effectiveness of NFP methods or contraception, simple Pearl rates were calculated based on the number of unintended conceptions multiplied by 1300 and divided by the number of months of use. This provided a pregnancy rate based on 100 woman-years of use. However, Pearl pregnancy rates become inflated as people drop out of the study or become pregnant. Today, contraceptive efficacy is based on modern survival analysis statistical techniques, which take into account the varying lengths of use of a given method and are less affected by the drop-out of participants.

Generally, two statistics are used to describe the efficacy of a family planning method. These are the perfect, or "correct-use," pregnancy rate, which includes only those unintended pregnancies which occurred during proper use of the method in question (in other words, during what was determined to be the fertile phase of each cycle in the study, these couples did not have intercourse), and the "typical use" or total pregnancy rate, which includes pregnancies resulting from both correct use and imperfect (that is, inconsistent or incorrect) use. The perfect-use unintended pregnancy rates are based only on the months or, ideally, the menstrual cycles of correct use by couples in the study. The total or typical-use unintended pregnancy rate includes both correct-use and imperfect-use unintended pregnancies and the total months of use or the total number of menstrual cycles of use in the analysis.[42] Perfect-use efficacy rates can be obtained only in prospective clinical studies; retrospective survey studies of populations can provide only typical-use pregnancy rates.

Unintended pregnancy rates will be affected by the number of actions the couple must perform to use the method effectively. The "use and forget about it" aspect of such methods as sterilization, IUD, or implants results in very low unintended pregnancy rates. Methods that require more behaviors, such as daily use of the hormonal

---

40. J. Latz, and E. Reiner, "Further Studies on the Sterile and Fertile Periods in Women," *American Journal of Obstetrics and Gynecology* 43 (1942): 74–79.

41. J. Trussell, "Contraceptive Failure in the United States," *Contraception* 70 (2004): 89–96.

42. Ibid.; V. Lamprect and J. Trussell, "Natural Family Planning Effectiveness: Evaluating Published Reports," *Advances in Contraception* 13 (1997): 155–65.

birth control pill, usually result in higher unintended pregnancy rates. This is why the birth control pill has a typical-use rate of approximately 8 unintended pregnancies per 100 women over twelve months of use. Since NFP methods require not only daily monitoring of fertility but also periodic abstinence, more behaviors are involved. Therefore, the unintended pregnancy rates of NFP methods tend to be higher than the birth control pill and other nonbehavioral birth control methods. For example, the imperfect use rate of the ovulation method (mucus only) is about 86 unintended pregnancies per 100 users over twelve months of use. Imperfect-use rates are not the same as total pregnancy rate,[43] since they are based on the menstrual cycles in which the method was not used consistently and correctly. Total pregnancy rates are based on all menstrual cycles, whether the method was used correctly or not.

NFP methods, however, have a very low correct or perfect-use unintended pregnancy rate, usually between 1 and 3 pregnancies per 100 women users over thirteen menstrual cycles or twelve months of use. One reason for this low rate is that the methods tend to overestimate the fertile window (on average) by twofold or more. The longer the estimated fertile window, the less likely there will be perfect-use pregnancies. For example, if only the first and last days of the menstrual cycle were considered infertile, the method would be 100 percent perfect but would have a high imperfect use rate, unless the couples use near-total abstinence from intercourse. When the methods are used post-ovulation, there is a very low unintended pregnancy rate, especially with more objective markers of ovulation, like the BBT shift in addition to cervical mucus observations.

Table 5-1 provides the general perfect- and typical-use unintended pregnancy rates for contraceptive and select NFP methods. These figures are adapted from an article by James Trussell from the Population Institute at Princeton University;[44] the estimated pregnancy rates Trussell presents are frequently cited in journal articles and in medical and nursing textbooks and are believed to be authoritative and accurate. In Trussell's ranking, NFP methods are considered second-rung methods in efficacy and effectiveness, since their use involves a fair number of behaviors. They are rated about the same as male condoms, lower than the pill, IUD, and sterilization, but with lower pregnancy rates than spermicides and withdrawal.

A recent evidence-based review of NFP efficacy studies concluded that NFP methods were not very effective for use in avoiding pregnancy and intimated that they are not recommended for use in modern medicine.[45] The conclusion was based on only two randomized control trials, which were conducted in the late 1970s and were methodologically flawed.[46] Randomized control trials of NFP methods are dif-

43. J. Trussell and L. Grummer-Strawn, "Contraceptive Failure of the Ovulation Method of Periodic Abstinence," *Family Planning Perspectives* 22 (1990): 65–75, doi:10.2307/2135511.

44. Trussell, "Contraceptive Failure in the United States."

45. D. A. Grimes et al., "Fertility Awareness-Based Methods for Contraception: Systematic Review of Randomized Controlled Trials," *Contraception* 72 (2005): 85–90.

46. J. E. Medina et al., "Comparative Evaluation of Two Methods of Natural Family Planning in Columbia," *American Journal of Obstetrics and Gynecology* 138 (1980): 1142–47; M. E. Wade et al., "Randomized Prospective Study of the Use-Effectiveness of Two Methods of Natural Family Planning: An Interim Report,"

Table 5-1. **Unintended Pregnancy Rates per 100 Women over 12 Months of Use, by Family Planning Method**

	Perfect Use	*Typical Use*
Chance	85	85
Spermicides	18	29
Withdrawal	4	27
Condoms	2	15
Standard Days Method	5	12
Ovulation Method	3	22
Symptothermal	2	7
Pill	0.3	8
IUD	0.1	0.6

Note: Contraceptive pregnancy rates are based on the article J. Trussell, "Contraceptive Failure in the United States," *Contraception* 70 (2004): 89–96; NFP pregnancy rates are based on the following articles: M. Arevalo, V. Jennings, and I. Sinai, "Efficacy of a New Method of Family Planning: the Standard Days Method," *Contraception* 65 (2002): 333–38; World Health Organization, "A Prospective Multicentre Trial of the Ovulation Method of Natural Family Planning. II. The Effectiveness Phase," *Fertility and Sterility* 36 (1981): 591–98; P. Frank-Herrmann et al., "The Effectiveness of a Fertility Awareness Based Method to Avoid Pregnancy in Relation to a Couple's Sexual Behavior During the Fertile Time: A Prospective Longitudinal Study," *Human Reproduction* 22 (2007): 1310–19.

ficult to undertake: it would be morally wrong to randomize participants into a contraceptive group, such as a comparison group using condoms; and it is often difficult to randomize participants into NFP methods that they are not interested in using. There are, however, many good cohort studies of NFP methods. Table 5-2 lists studies that have been published in peer-reviewed journals over the past ten years, along with the large, classic, five-country study of the ovulation method conducted by the World Health Organization.[47]

As can been seen in table 5-2, the unintended pregnancy rates of natural family planning methods are variable. It is hard to compare them, because of the different interpretations of unintended pregnancies, along with such methodological variations as whether they were calculated based on months of use or cycles of use, or whether they only included perfect-use cycles in the correct-use rates. Efficacy studies conducted by developers or promoters of various NFP methods have built-in bias and tend to underreport unintended pregnancies or to explain them away. Furthermore,

---

American Journal of Obstetrics and Gynecology 134 (1979): 628–31; M. E. Wade et al., "A Randomized Prospective Study of the Use-Effectiveness of Two Methods of Natural Family Planning," *American Journal of Obstetrics and Gynecology* 141 (1981): 368–76.

47. World Health Organization, "The Effectiveness Phase."

Table 5-2. **Classic and Recent NFP Efficacy Studies: Correct Use and Total Survival Rates per 100 Women over 12 Months of Use**

Study	Indicators	Length**	Correct	Typical
World Health Organization[a]	Mucus	(25–32)	97	78
Howard et al.[b]	Mucus	(25–32)	100	86
Arevalo et al.[c]	Fixed Calendar	(26–32)	95	88
Arevalo et al.[d]	Mucus	(13–42)	96	86
Frank-Hermann et al.[e]	Mucus & Temp	(25–35)	99	92
Fehring et al.[f]	Mucus/E3G/LH	(21–42)	98	87
Fehring et al.[g]	Mucus/Temp/LH	(21–42)	99	89

Note: Survival rate = number of women per 100 who did not have an unintended pregnancy.

** Range of length of menstrual cycles in study.

a. World Health Organization, "A Prospective Multicentre Trial of the Ovulation Method of Natural Family Planning. II. The Effectiveness Phase," *Fertility and Sterility* 36 (1981): 591–98.

b. M. P. Howard and J. B. Stanford, "Pregnancy Probabilities During Use of the Creighton Model Fertility Care System," *Archives of Family Medicine* 8 (1999): 391–402.

c. M. Arevalo, V. Jennings, and I. Sinai, "Efficacy of a New Method of Family Planning: The Standard Days Method," *Contraception* 65 (2002): 333–38.

d. M. Arevalo et al., "Efficacy of the New TwoDay Method of Family Planning," *Fertility and Sterility* 82 (2004): 885–92.

e. P. Frank-Herrmann et al., "Determination of the Fertile Window: Reproductive Competence of Women—European Cycle Databases," *Gynecology and Endocrinology* 20 (2005): 305–12.

f. R. J. Fehring et al., "Efficacy of Cervical Mucus Observations Plus Electronic Hormonal Fertility Monitoring as a Method of Natural Family Planning," *Journal of Obstetric Gynecologic and Neonatal Nursing* 36 (2007): 152–60.

g. R. J. Fehring, M. Schneider, and M. L. Barron, "Efficacy of the Marquette Method of Natural Family Planning," *American Journal of Maternal Child Nursing* 54 (2008): 165–70.

the menstrual cycles included in these studies tend to be of regular length, that is, between twenty-six and thirty-five days long. Given these caveats, there still are some very good efficacy studies of NFP methods.

Table 5-2 summarizes the results of several such studies. These studies included only women with regular menstrual cycle lengths. The second study by M. Arevalo et al. and the two studies by Richard Fehring et al. have the most liberal menstrual cycle length of thirteen to forty-two days. The total unintended pregnancy rate of the World Health Organization study is the highest, at 22 percent. The P. Frank-Herrmann et al., European double-check method has the lowest total rate, similar to that found with oral hormonal contraceptives.

The unintended pregnancy rates increase considerably when irregular-length menstrual cycles (including post–birth control pill, postpartum, and perimenopause) are included in the efficacy calculations. For example, in the Howard and Stanford study, the total unintended pregnancy rate of a cervical-mucus-only method jumps to 17 percent,[48] and a database of the same method from Marquette University indicates

48. M. P. Howard and J. B. Stanford, "Pregnancy Probabilities during Use of the Creighton Model Fertility Care System," *Archives of Family Medicine* 8 (1999): 391–402.

a cervical-mucus-only method rate of approximately 22 percent (similar to the World Health Organization study rate) when all unintended pregnancies from all reproductive categories are included.[49]

In summary, NFP methods are fairly effective when used by women with menstrual cycles of fairly regular length who follow the method's rules consistently. Efficacy suffers when the methods are not used consistently and correctly, or when they are used by women with irregular menstrual cycle lengths, especially during postpartum and breastfeeding. It remains to be seen whether Clearblue Easy Fertility Monitor (CEFM)-enhanced methods of NFP are more effective than other traditional methods. The five-country World Health Organization ovulation method efficacy study has an unintended imperfect use pregnancy rate around 25 per 100 women over twelve months of use;[50] Most of these pregnancies were couples who had intercourse even though they knew they were in the fertile period. Trussell observed that, while the ovulation method can be very effective when used correctly, the method is "unforgiving"; if the couple has intercourse during the fertile phase of the menstrual cycle, they most likely will become pregnant.[51]

Two simplified NFP methods developed by the researchers at Georgetown's Institute for Reproductive Health were devised to integrate simple but effective NFP methods into family planning programs in developing countries.[52] The standard days method is a simple fixed-day calendar-based method (i.e., days 8 to 19 are always fertile) for women who have menstrual cycles between twenty-six and thirty-two days in length.[53] The TwoDay Method is based on asking whether the woman has observed mucus secretions that day and the day before; if she answers no to both questions, she can consider herself infertile on that day.[54] Both methods have respectable correct and imperfect use records among a variety of people in various developing countries: the standard days method has a perfect use pregnancy rate of 5 per 100 women and a typical use of 12 per 100 over 12 months of use; the TwoDay Method has a correct use pregnancy rate of 4 and a typical use of 14 per 100 women over 12 months of use.

Studies have also examined the European double-check method and the Marquette University method, which combines the use of the electronic hormonal fertility monitor with cervical mucus monitoring. Both these methods provide a double check for the beginning and end of the estimated fertile phase. The European method was found in a recent study to produce both perfect-use and typical-use efficacy pregnancy rates that rival the birth control pill. A prospective, retrospective, and cohort comparison study of the Marquette method's efficacy showed that a combination of

---

49. R. J. Fehring et al., "Cohort Comparison of Two Fertility Awareness Methods of Family Planning," *Journal of Reproductive Medicine* 54 (2007): 165–70.

50. See World Health Organization, "The Effectiveness Phase," 597.

51. See Trussell and Grummer-Strawn, "Contraceptive Failure of the Ovulation Method of Periodic Abstinence."

52. See Arevalo, Jennings, and Sinai, "Efficacy of a New Method of Family Planning"; M. Arevalo et al., "Efficacy of the New TwoDay Method of Family Planning," *Fertility and Sterility* 82 (2004): 885–92.

53. See Arevalo, Jennings, and Sinai, "Efficacy of a New Method of Family Planning."

54. See Arevalo et al., "Efficacy of the New TwoDay Method of Family Planning."

mucus with the fertility monitor as a double check yielded significantly fewer unintended pregnancies compared to the mucus-only method.[55] These results are similar to the earlier randomized study, which demonstrated that the addition of BBT to mucus observations enhanced efficacy.[56] Randomized control trials are needed for a more precise comparison of the efficacy of NFP methods. Of note is that the first randomized control trial comparing two methods of NFP (since 1980) has recently been published comparing use of CEFM with cervical mucus monitoring.[57]

Use of NFP with Special Circumstances

While most efficacy studies of NFP methods have been conducted with women who have fairly regular cycle lengths (some studies may even require regular cycle lengths for participation), providers of NFP services often work with women who do not fit the pattern. These women include those who are breastfeeding, who are discontinuing hormonal contraception, or who are in the perimenopausal transition.

The postpartum breastfeeding transition, in which the woman goes from a state of amenorrhea to one of irregular patterns of ovulation, cycle length, and cervical mucus, is particularly difficult for NFP users to navigate without an unintended pregnancy.[58] Earlier studies of breastfeeding women and the use of the sympto-thermal method indicated that using NFP might actually enhance the unintended pregnancy rate.[59] A more recent study of a mucus-only method provided a total pregnancy rate of 33 percent among the breastfeeding participants.[60] Studies also show a dissociation between the traditional signs of fertility (mucus and temperature), the actual days of fertility, and days with estrogen rises.[61] In fact, a recent study showed that during the breastfeeding transition, follicles continue to mature but not necessarily proceed to an ovulatory event.[62] This seems to indicate some type of disconnect in the

55. See Fehring et al., "Cohort Comparison of Two Fertility Awareness Methods of Family Planning."

56. See Wade et al., "A Randomized Prospective Study of the Use-effectiveness of Two Methods of Natural Family Planning."

57. See R. Fehring et al, "Randomized Comparison of Two Internet-Supported Fertility Awareness Based Methods of Family Planning," *Contraception* 88, no. 1 (2013): 24–30.

58. See M. Arevalo, V. Jennings, and I. Sinai, "Application of Simple Fertility Awareness-Based Methods of Family Planning to Breastfeeding Women," *Fertility and Sterility* 80 (2003): 1241–48.

59. See M. H. Labbok et al., "Ovulation Method Use during Breastfeeding: Is There Increased Risk of Unplanned Pregnancy?" *American Journal of Obstetrics and Gynecology* 165 Supp (1991): 2031–36.

60. See Howard and Stanford, "Pregnancy Probabilities during Use of the Creighton Model Fertility Care System."

61. See L. Hatherley, "Lactation and Postpartum Infertility: The Use-Effectiveness of Natural Family Planning (NFP) after Term Pregnancy," *Clinical Reproduction and Fertility* 3 (1985): 319–34; G. A. Tomaselli et al., "Using Complete Breast-Feeding and Lactational Amenorrhoea as Birth Spacing Methods," *Contraception* 61 (2000): 253–57; M. Zinaman, and W. Stevenson, "Efficacy of the Symptothermal Method of Natural Family Planning in Lactating Women after the Return of Menses," *American Journal of Obstetrics and Gynecology* 165 Supp (1991): 2037–39; K. I. Kennedy et al., "Breastfeeding and the Symptothermal Method," *Studies in Family Planning* 26 (1995): 107–15; W. Li and Y. Qiu, "Relation of Supplementary Feeding to Resumption of Menstruation and Ovulation in Lactating Postpartum Women," *Chinese Medical Journal* 120 (2007): 868–70.

62. See E. V. Velasquez et al., "Pituitary-Ovarian Axis during Lactational Amenorrhoea. I. Longitudinal Assessment of Follicular Growth, Gonadotrophins, Sex Steroid and Inhibin Levels before and after Recovery of Menstrual Cyclicity," *Human Reproduction* 4 (2006): 909–15.

pituitary-hypothalamic-ovarian access. However, researchers have been working on evidenced-based protocols to bolster the confidence of couples using NFP methods during the breastfeeding transition. One protocol involves using a hormonal fertility monitor to measure estrone-3-glucuronide (E3G) and LH patterns during the transition, and creating "artificial" twenty-one-day cycles until ovulatory menstrual cycles resume.[63]

The transition from use of hormonal contraception to NFP use can be difficult for some women. Studies show that there is often a delay in ovulation, longer menstrual cycle lengths, heavier menses, and variation and increase in the amount of cervical-vaginal secretions.[64] These changes can persist as long as nine menstrual cycles after discontinuation of oral hormonal contraception.[65] The type and length of changes with longer-acting hormonal contraception, such as injectables, is not known, but most likely is much longer. However, NFP use after hormonal contraception can be effective. This works best when the couple is patient, and when they use NFP conservatively (marking the beginning and end of the fertile phase with two markers of fertility, or reserving intercourse only for post-ovulation). Couples who discontinue hormonal contraception often have difficulty adjusting to the periodic abstinence required with NFP.

The perimenopausal time period is a much longer transition than breastfeeding or post-contraception. To complicate matters, women over age forty-two who have completed their families, resumed their careers, and are concerned about having a baby with defects can be fearful about another pregnancy and want to have secure methods of family planning. There is little current research on the use of NFP during perimenopause. Research indicates that the menstrual cycle length shortens somewhat as women progress through perimenopause, though it can remain very regular in length.[66] However, once the difference in menstrual cycle length varies by more than seven days, the woman is considered in an early perimenopause stage. It is generally thought that women at the age of forty-five have a very low chance of pregnancy, similar to a twenty-one-year-old woman on oral hormonal contraception. This fact, however, is not always comforting to the NFP user. Couples who use the post-ovulatory period as identified by cervical mucus peak, the BBT, or the urinary LH surge, or, preferably, some combination of these methods, are generally able to use NFP effectively.

The biological markers for the perimenopausal transition are modeled in the "Stages of Reproductive Aging Workshop" or STRAW.[67] According to this mod-

63. See R. Fehring, M. Schneider, and M. L. Barron, "Protocol for Determining Fertility while Breast-feeding," *Fertility and Sterility* 84 (2005): 805–7.

64. See C. Nassaralla et al., "Characteristics of the Menstrual Cycle after Discontinuation of Oral Contraceptives," *Journal of Women's Health* 20 (2011): 169–77.

65. See C. Gnoth et al., "Cycle Characteristics after Discontinuation of Oral Contraceptives," *Gynecology and Endocrinology* 16 (2002): 307–17.

66. See A. E. Treloar et al., "Variation of the Human Menstrual Cycle through Reproductive Life," *International Journal of Fertility* 12 (1967): 124.

67. See M. R. Soules et al., "Executive Summary: Stages of Reproductive Aging Workshop (STRAW)," *Fertility and Sterility* 76 (2001): 874–78.

el, when the differences in menstrual cycle length exceed seven days, and when on those days the follicle stimulating hormone (FSH) is high, fertility is unlikely and the woman can be considered in perimenopause. In addition, when there is a difference in the running lengths of the menstrual cycle of more than forty-two days, menopause most likely will take place within two years.[68] More research is needed to integrate this knowledge into the practice of NFP.

Use of NFP to Achieve Pregnancy

Although NFP can be used to achieve pregnancy, there have been very few prospective studies of pregnancy rates with couples using fertility-focused intercourse aided by NFP. Hilgers reported a study in which 49 of 50 couples of normal fertility achieved a pregnancy within five months by focusing intercourse on days of good-quality cervical mucus.[69] German researchers reported the largest prospective study to estimate the cumulative probability of conception among a cohort of 346 couples using the sympto-thermal method (cervical mucus and basal body temperature monitoring) from their first cycle onward.[70] This study found a total of 310 pregnancies among the 346 couples during a maximum of twenty-nine cycles of observation. The researchers labeled the couples who achieved a pregnancy "truly fertile." The cumulative pregnancy rates for cycles 1, 3, 6, and 12 for all couples (N = 340) were 0.38, 0.68, 0.81, and 0.92 respectively. For the truly fertile couples (N = 304) the pregnancy rates for the same cycles were 0.42, 0.75, 0.88, and 0.98. Therefore, close to 90 percent of the truly fertile couples and close to 80 percent of all couples in the study achieved a pregnancy within the first six cycles of fertility-focused intercourse. Based on these results, the researchers recommended that couples who do not achieve a pregnancy within a six-month period of fertility-focused intercourse seek a primary infertility workup. However, they also recommended that these couples continue fertility-focused intercourse for another twelve months. There was no comparison group in this study with couples who used random acts of intercourse, so we do not know if the truly fertile couples would have the same pregnancy rate with random intercourse.

Researchers from Unipath Diagnostics completed a study that randomized one thousand women volunteers into two groups of five hundred. The female volunteers were between the ages of twenty-one and forty years, and their partners were between twenty-one and fifty years of age. One group received the Clearblue Easy Fertility Monitor (CEFM), and the control group was asked to do what they wished to achieve a pregnancy, including the use of such devices as ovulation test kits and basal

68. See J. Taffe and L. Dennerstein, "Time to the Final Menstrual Period," *Fertility and Sterility* 78 (2002): 397–403.

69. See T. W. Hilgers et al., "Cumulative Pregnancy Rates in Patients with Apparently Normal Fertility and Fertility-Focused Intercourse," *Journal of Reproductive Medicine* 37 (1992): 864–66.

70. See C. Gnoth et al., "Time to Pregnancy: Results of the German Prospective Study and Impact on the Management of Infertility," *Human Reproduction* 18 (2003): 1959–66.

body temperature.[71] The pregnancy rate during the first cycle was 15.2 percent (or 46 of 302) for the CEFM group and 7.8 percent (27 of 347) for the control group. The two-cycle cumulative pregnancy rate was statistically higher for the CEFM at 22.7 percent, compared to the control group at 14.4 percent (p = 0.006). The researchers found that having a previous pregnancy and a young partner were significant factors in achieving a pregnancy. In addition, the researchers provided the users of the CEFM with a satisfaction tool, which determined that 90 percent of users found the device easy or very easy to use, and 80 percent found it convenient or very convenient. They concluded that the CEFM helped increase the likelihood of pregnancy during the first two cycles of use, compared to nonuse, among women who had been trying to conceive for up to two years. This study was limited, as its duration was only two months and it did not compare the CEFM with cheaper alternatives to tracking fertility, such as cervical mucus monitoring. A more recent study found that among 124 couples seeking pregnancy when they focused intercourse on the estimated fertile phase (by mucus or CEFM) the pregnancy rate was 87 per 100 women over 12 months of use compared to only 5 when they did not focus intercourse.[72]

There is growing evidence that focused intercourse during the fertile time (as estimated by self-monitoring of natural fertility markers) can increase the pregnancy rate and decrease the time to pregnancy. However, only one randomized trial exists that compares self-indicators of fertility to estimate the fertile phase and timed intercourse. In fact, claims have been made in the scientific literature that focused intercourse based on the estimation of fertility is no more effective than having intercourse two to three times a week.[73] The National Institute for Clinical Excellence (NICE) guidelines make this statement specifically, adding that focused intercourse is too stressful.[74] The policy committee of the American Society of Reproductive Medicine notes that electronic or other devices designed to aid in determining the optimal time of fertility may be useful for couples who have infrequent intercourse.[75] The usefulness of these devices needs to be determined through further research.

Integration of NFP into Women's Health Care

One of the benefits of NFP use is its great potential for enhancing women's health care. Subcommittees of both the American Academy of Pediatrics and the American College of Obstetricians and Gynecologists have recommended that adolescents

---

71. See J. E. Robinson, M. Waklin, and J. E. Ellis, "Increased Pregnancy Rate with Use of the Clearblue Easy Fertility Monitor," *Fertility and Sterility* 87 (2007): 329–34.

72. See Q. Mu and R. Fehring, "Efficacy of Achieving Pregnancy with Fertility Focused Intercourse," *MCN: The American Journal of Maternal Child Nursing* 39 (2014): 35–40.

73. See H. K. A. Snick, "Should Spontaneous or Timed Intercourse Guide Couples Trying to Conceive?" *Human Reproduction* 10 (2005): 2976–77.

74. See National Institute for Clinical Excellence (U.K.), *Fertility: Assessment and Treatment for People with Fertility Problems*, Clinical Guidelines 11 (London: NICE, 2004).

75. See American Society for Reproductive Medicine, Practice Committee, "Optimizing Natural Fertility," *Fertility and Sterility* 9, Supplement 3 (2008): S1–S6.

monitor their menstrual cycles, to provide information that can be used as another vital sign for adolescent health.[76] Cycle monitoring can reveal the presence of excessive bleeding, irregular menstrual cycles, and other pathological conditions.

NFP-only physicians have indicated many health benefits of menstrual cycle charting,[77] including early hints of such cycle pathologies as anovulation, dysmucorrhea, irregular bleeding patterns, and corpus luteum insufficiency. Charting the menstrual cycle certainly can be helpful for couples in preventing unintended pregnancies. Research has shown that couples with subfertility have a higher probability of conception with charting and focused intercourse during the fertile window. Women who chart are more knowledgeable about their fertility and can be alerted to potential problems when they occur. NFP charting can also be invaluable for the diagnosis, testing, treatment, and assessment of infertility. Time spent by the physician reviewing menstrual cycle charts with the woman patient can also be used to great advantage in providing health advice.

One simple example of the value of menstrual cycle charting is the treatment and management of polycystic ovarian disease (PCOS). The unmanaged PCOS menstrual cycle is fairly easy to pick up in menstrual cycle charts, with long cycle lengths, cervical mucus patches, multiple peak-type mucus, LH spikes, and undefined temperature patterns. As the woman with PCOS is treated, whether with medications (glucophage, Clomid, or both) or with lifestyle changes (weight loss, diet, and exercise), the efficacy of treatment will play out with a normalized menstrual cycle, a defined fertile window, a clear day of ovulation, normal cycle length, and normal luteal phase length.

Women who seek health care for various health problems, including painful menses, acne, unusual menstrual bleeding, PCOS, endometriosis, and other reproductive disorders, are often treated with hormonal birth control pills. Sometimes, "the Pill" might be the best treatment for a health problem. According to the papal encyclical *Humane Vitae*, the use of contraceptives as a form of treatment is morally valid if they are a standard treatment for that disorder.[78] The *Ethical and Religious Directives* of the USCCB state: "Procedures that induce sterility are permitted when their direct effect is the cure or alleviation of a present and serious pathology and a simpler treatment is not available."[79] Some argue, however, that since the pill can be abortifacient, its use as a therapeutic might be morally problematic. In any case, the pill is certainly overused in medical practice, and its use can mask the underlying problem.

One very notable means of integrating NFP into women's health care is the practice of NaProTech, or natural procreative technology.[80] NaProTech is the merging of the Creighton Model of NFP with medical protocols, to treat a comprehensive vari-

---

76. See American Academy of Pediatrics, "Menstruation in Girls and Adolescents: Using the Menstrual Cycle as a Vital Sign," *Pediatrics* 118 (2006): 2245–50.

77. See Frank-Herrmann et al., "Determination of the Fertile Window."

78. See Paul VI, *Humanae Vitae*, no. 15.

79. USCCB, *Ethical and Religious Directives*, dir. 34.

80. See Thomas W. Hilgers, *The Medical and Surgical Practice of NaProTechnology* (Omaha, Neb.: Pope Paul VI Institute Press, 2004).

ety of women's health problems in a way that respects Catholic moral principles and seeks to find and treat the underlying medical cause. While one example of the use of NaProTech in managing infertility and related problems was recently published,[81] some of the NaProTech protocols have not been vetted in research or through medical associations, and some NFP-only physicians have not integrated NaProTech into their practice in family medicine or in obstetrics and gynecology. Many morally sound standardized and evidence-based treatments exist for women's health problems. These include medical and surgical treatment of endometriosis, medical and lifestyle treatment of PCOS, medical and surgical treatment of infertility that does not involve in vitro fertilization, and surgical and medical treatments for dysfunctional uterine bleeding, among others. Dr. Raviele's chapter in this book illustrates how a physician is able to manage common women's health problems effectively without recourse to contraception and other possibly immoral treatments.

Spiritual and Psychological Dynamics

There is little research on the psychological and spiritual dynamics of the use of NFP in married life. In response to the introduction of the birth control pill and concerns about worldwide population growth, Pope Paul VI called for a commission to study these questions.[82] After several years of meetings, this commission recommended a change in the Church's teaching on contraception: that it could be justified for right reasons so long as couples were generally open to having children. However, the commission was influenced by a study conducted by the Catholic Family Life Movement, which was led by Patti and Patrick Crowley.[83] The Crowleys' study examined the rhythm method's effects on married life, concluding that its use was detrimental to marriage. However, this study was methodologically flawed, agenda-driven, and biased; and the results, by today's scientific standards, are essentially useless.

In response to the Crowley study, J. Marshall from England (who had been a member of the papal commission) and a physician and wife couple from France produced studies that exhibited the opposite results.[84] Qualitative and survey studies in the late 1970s and early 1980s indicated that couples who used NFP felt that it improved communication, gave them greater knowledge of human reproduction, enhanced intimacy, and helped to develop self-mastery.[85] Two cohort comparison

---

81. See J. B. Stanford, T. A. Parnell, and P. C. Boyle, "Outcomes from Treatment of Infertility with Natural Procreative Technology in an Irish General Practice," *Journal of the American Board of Family Medicine* 21 (2008): 375–84.

82. See R. McClory, *The Turning Point* (New York: Crossroad Publishing Company, 1995).

83. See P. Crowley and P. Crowley, "Report to the Papal Birth Control Commission," Patrick and Patricia Crowley Papers, 1965–1966, University of Notre Dame Archives.

84. See J. Marshall and B. Rowe, "Psychological Aspects of the Basal Body Temperature Methods of Regulating Births," *Fertility and Sterility* 21 (1970): 14–19.

85. See M. P. McCusker, "Natural Family Planning and the Marital Relationship: The Catholic University of America Study," *International Review of Natural Family Planning* 1 (1977): 331–40; J. Tortorici, "Conception Regulation, Self-Esteem, and Marital Satisfaction among Catholic Couples," *International Review of Natural Family Planning* 3 (1979): 191–205; T. Borkman and M. Shivanandan, "The Impact of Natural Family

studies, comparing couples who used NFP with those who used various method of contraception, demonstrated greater intimacy and spiritual well-being among the NFP couples.[86] A more recent qualitative study confirmed that the great majority of NFP users felt that it enhanced their marriage, improved knowledge of human fertility, enriched their spirituality, and was helpful with their desires to either avoid or achieve pregnancy.[87] Some couples did express problems with managing abstinence and the daily work of monitoring fertility. The dearth of physicians who promoted or provided NFP services was identified by some of these couples as a drawback of NFP.

Of particular interest was a study of satisfaction levels among a population sample of German women who used various methods of family planning.[88] The German researchers found that satisfaction with NFP use by both current and previous users was only 43 percent (N = 428) compared with 92 percent among those who were sterilized (N = 139) and 68 percent (1,303) among those who used hormonal oral contraception. However, when the authors looked at specific psychological characteristics related to the individual method of family planning, the findings were more subtle. For example, 71 percent of hormonal pill users and 37 percent of those who were sterilized felt that they had health risks, compared to 0 percent of NFP users. Thirteen percent of pill users and 7 percent of those sterilized felt more irritable with their method of family planning, compared to only 5 percent of those using NFP. Ten percent of pill users and 5 percent of those sterilized felt depressed, compared to only 3.8 percent of those using NFP. Finally, 8.4 percent of those using the pill felt they had a better sex drive, as did 19 percent of those who were sterilized, but 21.5 percent of NFP users felt an increased sex drive. So, in a sense, women on the hormonal pill have a greater sense of health risks, are more irritable and depressed, and have lower sex drives. Women using NFP, on the other hand, might be more anxious about an unintended pregnancy, but they have no health risk, are less irritable and less depressed, and have a higher sex drive.

Marital Dynamics of Using NFP

NFP is based on an integrated, holistic view of human sexuality, which recognizes its spiritual, physical, intellectual, communicative/creative, and emotional elements, not just intercourse or genital contact. Couples who use NFP are encouraged to express

---

Planning on Selected Aspects of the Couple Relationship," *International Review of Natural Family Planning* 8 (1984): 58–66; G. A. Boys, *Natural Family Planning Nationwide Survey. Final Report to the National Conference of Catholic Bishops* (Washington, D.C.: Diocesan Development Program for NFP, 1989).

86. See R. J. Fehring, D. M. Lawrence, and C. M. Sauvage, "Self-Esteem, Spiritual Well-Being, and Intimacy: A Comparison among Couples Using NFP and Oral Contraceptives," *International Review of Natural Family Planning* 13 (1989): 227–36; R. Fehring and D. Lawrence, "Spiritual Well-Being, Self-Esteem, and Intimacy among Couples Using Natural Family Planning," *Linacre Quarterly* 61 (1994): 18–29.

87. See L. VandeVusse, R. Fehring, and L. Hanson, "Marital Dynamics of Practicing Natural Family Planning," *Journal of Nursing Scholarship* 35 (2003): 171–76.

88. See B. J. Oddens, "Women's Satisfaction with Birth Control: A Population Survey of Physical and Psychological Effects of Oral Contraceptives, Intrauterine Devices, Condoms, Natural Family Planning, and Sterilization among 1466 Women," *Contraception* 59 (1999): 227–86.

their sexuality in a non-genital way during times of periodic abstinence. This provides the couple with an opportunity to develop a holistic expression of sexuality and a greater control over their sexual drives. As self-control is developed, the genital expression of sexuality becomes more an act of giving and less an act of merely satisfying physical drives. This makes it less likely that one or the other of the marital partners will become solely an object of sexual gratification. Abstinence also helps keep the physical expression of sexuality new and fresh, a result often referred to by couples as the "honeymoon effect." By being more creative in expressing a broader sexuality, the couple becomes more sexually mature and can experience a deeper closeness, understanding, and peace.

The fertility monitoring and periodic abstinence required by NFP can lead to frustrations for some couples, who may dislike daily monitoring, experience stress over the possibility of becoming pregnant, or perceive a lack of spontaneity. This is most likely to occur with couples or individual spouses who have not yet learned to integrate an awareness of their fertility into their daily lives. However, for most couples, the practice of NFP results in a greater understanding of fertility and in better communication, since couples need to discuss daily their intention of using their fertility to achieve or avoid pregnancy. This communication then leads to sharing information, to making mutual decisions and to mutual trust. NFP promotes greater understanding between husband and wife and enables a shared responsibility.

Learning to live with the rhythms of life is important for a married couple; this includes the times of fertility and infertility in a woman's menstrual cycle. Married couples who use NFP to monitor their cycles will be aware of those times of fertility and infertility. By sharing these times with each other, they can give of themselves and make shared decisions of their intentions. When the NFP couple experiences the fertile time, they realize the awesomeness of their potential to collaborate with God in creating new human life. This power is best exercised in the context of love between husband and wife in a co-creative relationship with God.

Future Perspectives on NFP

One perceived problem with many of the current methods of NFP is that they can be complex and time-consuming, both for couples to learn and use and for health professionals to provide.[89] Some of the user manuals for current methods of NFP are longer than two hundred pages, which might account for the drop in NFP use over the past ten years. Furthermore, many parts of the country lack NFP service providers, some of whom must cover large areas of counties or states.

NFP service providers and researchers over the past ten years have been trying to develop simple-to-use, easily taught methods of NFP. Good examples of this are the two simplified methods developed by the Georgetown Institute for Reproduc-

---

89. See M. Arevalo, "Expanding the Availability and Improving Delivery of Natural Family Planning Services and Fertility Awareness Education: Providers' Perspectives," *Advances in Contraception* 13 (1997): 275–81.

tive Health, the standard days method and the TwoDay Method; and the European double-check methods discussed earlier in this chapter.

The Internet has also proven to be a valuable tool in providing NFP instructions and guidance. A number of NFP systems have online instructions or some type of web-based support system. One such example is the Northwest Family Service, which features online instruction and an online course leading to teacher certification in the sympto-thermal method system of NFP.[90] Online charting systems, such as the Taking Charge of Your Fertility (TCYF) charting system developed by T. Weschler, include access to user support.[91]

Marquette University's Institute for Natural Family Planning has developed an online NFP education, charting, and support system, with information on NFP, special circumstances protocols, and instructions on how to observe and chart fertility indicators. It also features a downloadable user manual and charting system, a user forum, and consultation services with a bioethicist, professional nurses, and physicians. The charting system has an automatic algorithm to calculate and display the estimated fertile window, based on charted fertility indicators. The system's Quickstart instructions tab provides the user with a one-page guide to using NFP; this is simple enough to get the reader started in observing and charting fertility. In a two-year period more than three hundred topics, ranging from special reproductive circumstances to unusual menstrual bleeding, have been broached by its more than twelve hundred online users, yielding more than twenty-four hundred responses from the site's health professionals. The site's accessibility allows engaged couples to learn NFP, chart at least one menstrual cycle, take a simple fertility quiz, and receive a certificate of completion for marriage preparation, which is automatically sent electronically to the engaged couple upon completion of the requirements.[92] Future NFP websites likely will be more user friendly and interactive, and will feature tailored education programs and links to handheld devices and fertility monitoring apps.

Future advances in technology to estimate the fertile phase of the menstrual cycle will most likely make tests kits and devices easier to use and even more accurate. One such device already in the development and testing phase measures a metabolite of progesterone through a simple urine test kit, which could help the woman confirm that ovulation has taken place and that she is in the post-ovulatory infertile phase. The test would pick up the rise in progesterone that occurs after ovulation and the development of the corpus luteum. Another possible future development is the use of a hand-held ultrasound device to allow home monitoring of the developing and dominant follicle and its eventual collapse after ovulation. Small hand-held devices already exist and are being used by health professionals, so it seems logical that this

90. See R. J. Huneger and R. Fuller, *A Couple's Guide to Fertility* (Portland, Ore.: Northwest Family Services, 1997). See also Northwest Family Services, http://www.nwfs.org/natural-family-planning.

91. See T. Weschler, *Taking Charge of Your Fertility* (New York: Harpers Collins, 2002). See also her website, http://www.tcoyf.com/.

92. See Marquette University College of Nursing Institute for NFP, http://nfp.marquette.edu. The author of this chapter is the institute director.

technology might eventually be put into the hands of couples. There currently are more than two hundred fertility monitoring apps that women can download on their smart phones, tablets, or computers.

NFP teacher training programs for health professionals offer another field for future expansion. A variety of NFP teacher training programs exist today, with a wide range of content and actual classroom time. Most of these programs are in-person and involve three to four full days of content; other programs take place over a seven- to ten-day period and involve an extensive practicum.[93] Marquette has an online NFP teacher training program for health professionals, offered in two six-module courses, one in theory and one in a case-study-focused practicum, offered for continuing education. Future training programs will likely be shorter in duration, offered online, and targeted to help the health professional discern which NFP method or fertility indicators are best for the couple user. An example of a short online course in providing an NFP method is the one developed by the Georgetown Institute for Reproductive Health to help health professionals provide the standard days method.[94]

Other Bioethical Issues with the Practice of NFP

There are some common bioethical issues with the practice and teaching of NFP that are of concern to Catholic health professionals and bioethicists, namely, can a couple enter into marriage with the intent to practice NFP before having their first child, can a couple practice NFP with a contraceptive mentality, and are there limits to non-genital contact in avoiding pregnancy (e.g., should the couple avoid masturbation or mutual masturbation)? These issues are briefly addressed for this chapter; however, the answers provided here are not intended to be an in-depth bioethical and philosophical analysis (which is beyond the scope of this chapter).

The answer to whether a couple can practice NFP before having their first child is "yes." Catholic Church teaching is clear that it is up to the couple to discern when and how many children they are called to have. They are guided to be generous to life, to prayerfully discern serious reasons to avoid having a child, and to take into account their relation with God, their spouse, their children already born, and the good of society.[95] Although a couple is required to be open to life before marriage it is reasonable to imagine serious reasons for putting off having a first child. For example, a man or woman in a relationship could be on chemotherapy or radiation therapy for cancer. A pregnancy in this situation could result in severe birth defects and would be a serious reason for avoiding pregnancy. The key point is that it is up to the couple to discern whether they have serious reasons for avoiding pregnancy for a short time or an indeterminate time period. Furthermore, Pope John Paul II stated that all married

---

93. See R. Fehring, "The Future of Professional Education in Natural Family Planning," *Journal of Obstetric, Gynecological and Neonatal Nursing* 33 (2004): 34–43.

94. See Georgetown University Institute for Reproductive Health, http://www.irh.org.

95. See Paul VI, *Humanae Vitae*, no. 10.

couples should learn NFP.[96] NFP is not just for avoiding pregnancy but also for helping couples to become pregnant; that is one reason why NFP is not like contraception. A more in-depth analysis and discussion of this issue can be found in the chapter
"Co-Creating with the Creator: A Virtue-Based Approach" by Melanie Barrett in
the book *Science, Faith, and Human Fertility*.[97] The couple should keep in mind that,
from a medical and health perspective, it is better for them to become pregnant and
have children while they are young and at the peak of their fertility.

The answer to whether a couple can practice NFP with a contraceptive mentality
is no. Pope John Paul II was specific that a contraceptive mentality refers to the use
of contraception and being closed to having children, treating fertility like an enemy,
and rejecting pregnancy when contraception fails.[98] Paul VI said that the practice
of NFP (periodic abstinence) strengthens married relationships and confers on it a
higher human value, helps couples develop self-mastery, allows them to fully develop
their personalities, and be open to life.[99] A couple could use NFP for selfish reasons
(i.e., for not having children), but this is not likely, considering the challenges that
NFP presents: periodic abstinence, living with fertility, and daily discerning of their
fertility status. Using NFP and integrating fertility within a marital conjugal relationship is a good that matures and strengthens the relationship. A more in-depth
analysis of this question was developed by this author and professor Kevin Miller
from Franciscan University of Steubenville.[100]

The final bioethical concern is what moral sexual practices married couples can
use during the fertile phase of the menstrual cycle when they are using NFP to avoid
pregnancy. First of all, most NFP providers and NFP methods are not very prescriptive as to what sexual practices married couples can use in their marital relations,
other than to say that they should not use condoms, withdrawal, or genital to genital
contact during the fertile phase if they want to avoid pregnancy. The practice of masturbation (alone, or even in tandem) is considered an immoral sexual practice by the
Catholic Church. The other dictum is that sexual foreplay should lead to a completion of intercourse, that is, the act of intercourse should not be frustrated. *Catholic
Sexual Ethics* by William E. May, Ronald Lawler, and Joseph Boyle is recommended
for a more in-depth analysis and discussion of this topic.[101]

96. See Pope John Paul II, *Evangelium Vitae, The Gospel of Life* [Encyclical Letter, March 25, 1995] (St. Paul,
Minn.: The Leaflet Missal Company, 1995), no. 97.

97. See Melanie Barrett, "Co-Creating with the Creator: A Virtue-Based Approach," in *Science, Faith
and Human Fertility*, ed. R. Fehring and T. Notare (Milwaukee, Wisc.: Marquette University Press, 2012),
267–302.

98. See John Paul II, *Evangelium Vitae*, no. 13.

99. See Paul VI, *Humanae Vitae*, no. 21.

100. See R. Fehring and K. Miller, "Is It Possible for NFP to Be Used (Immorally) with Contraceptive
Intent?" *Linacre Quarterly* 78 (2011): 86–90.

101. See W. E. May, R. Lawler, and J. Boyle, *Catholic Sexual Ethics: A Summary, Explanation, and Defense*,
3rd ed. (Huntington, Ind.: Our Sunday Visitor, 2011).

Case Studies

Here are two case studies taken from the Marquette practice course in NFP for health professionals.

Case Study One

Susan is a thirty-five-year-old married Catholic woman with two children, ages five and three. She was diagnosed and treated for breast cancer, and underwent surgery to remove her right breast with follow-up chemotherapy. Her oncologist placed her on Tamoxifen for five years and told her that she should not get pregnant because of the deleterious effect the drug might have on a developing baby. He asked her to discuss birth control with her obstetrician-gynecologist, who recommended that either she or, preferably, her husband should seek sterilization. She refused for two reasons: she and her husband follow Church teaching on family planning, and she still wished to have another child.

The patient and her husband previously used the sympto-thermal method of NFP (i.e., basal body temperature plus cervical mucus observations). However, she was not comfortable continuing with that method since her small children routinely interrupted her sleep patterns and interfered with her temperature readings, making it difficult for her to establish a waking temperature baseline necessary for that method of NFP. She heard of a new method of NFP that used electronic hormonal monitoring and sought out that method at the Marquette University Institute for Natural Family Planning.

1. Must the patient rely only on NFP to avoid pregnancy while on Tamoxifen, or, based on the potential danger to her or to a developing fetus, could she or her husband be sterilized or encouraged to use condoms?

The answer to sterilization or condoms is no, the couple cannot be offered either sterilization or the use of condoms. The *Ethical and Religious Directives* are very specific on this matter. Directive 53 states:

Direct sterilization of either men or women, whether permanent or temporary, is not permitted in a Catholic health-care institution. Procedures that induce sterility are permitted when their direct effect is the cure or alleviation of a present and serious pathology and a simpler treatment is not available.[102]

Furthermore, no contraceptive can be used or recommended. According to the *Directives*,

The Church cannot approve contraceptive interventions that "either in anticipation of the marital act, or in its accomplishment or in the development of its natural consequences, have the purpose, whether as an end or a means, to render procreation impossible." Such interven

---

102. USCCB, *Ethical and Religious Directives*, dir. 54.

tions violate "the inseparable connection, willed by God . . . between the two meanings of the conjugal act: the unitive and procreative meanings."[103]

To put it simply, one cannot use an immoral act to achieve a good. This is not the same as the principle of double effect, whereby hormonal contraception or sterilization would be used for the intention and purpose of treating a disease process, such as a cancerous uterus. In this situation, the treatment of the cancer is the direct and intended effect, and the sterilization is indirect and unintended. Providing sterilization or condoms in the case of the woman on Tamoxifen would be a direct act for the purpose of contraception, not an indirect act of treating a valid medical problem, and therefore would be prohibited.

2. What type of family planning method could a Catholic physician recommend for such a case? Doesn't the use of Tamoxifen, an estrogen antagonist, rule out the use of NFP, since it interferes with ovulation, the development of the follicle, estrogen production, and the natural signs of fertility?

Yes, Tamoxifen does interfere with some of the natural markers of fertility, specifically the production of cervical mucus. Some speculate that the use of Tamoxifen prevents ovulation, but this has not been documented. However, other markers of fertility still can be used to track fertility with confidence. Basal body temperature and the LH surge are not affected by Tamoxifen. The couple could use the "heroic" approach and practice abstinence from intercourse for five years, but this would be both unnecessary and detrimental to marital intimacy.

3. If the woman and her husband must use a method of NFP, which method would be the most effective to prevent an unintended pregnancy?

The patient described in this case came to the Marquette Institute for NFP for help because of its use of the electronic hormonal fertility monitor with the NFP method they provide. It was decided, in discussion with the couple, that she should use three indicators for estimating her fertility: temperature, cervical mucus, and readings from the monitor. She had a follow-up at the institute after every menstrual cycle to assess both her progress and the effects of the drug on her natural fertility indicators.

As expected, during the first three menstrual cycles the mucus ratings and patterns were not discernable. Mucus levels and ratings were high, indicating high fertility for most of the menstrual cycle. However, clear temperature shifts were detected, and the monitor displayed a clear fertile window by detecting the baseline rise of estrogen and the LH surge in the urine. After the third menstrual cycle, the woman reported having trouble in consistently obtaining a temperature reading prior to rising in the morning because of her small children's needs. She said that she was comfortable using just the monitor with the Marquette algorithm.

Data downloaded from her monitor to the institute's computer showed the patient's first six menstrual cycles of hormonal fertility monitor use. The data charts

---

103. Ibid., pt. 4, intro., quoting Paul VI, *Humanae Vitae*, nos. 14 and 12 resp.

showed the length of each menstrual cycle, the day of the E3G rise from baseline , and the estimated day of ovulation The data indicated that the menstrual cycles varied in range from twenty-seven to forty-two days, and that the estimated day of ovulation (the second peak day shown on the monitor) varied from day 13 to day 27. The monitor was able to identify both the fertile phase and its variability from cycle to cycle, enabling this couple to successfully avoid pregnancy for the five years of therapy. However, when there is a severe reason for avoiding pregnancy, the institute recommends the use of two indicators for the beginning and two for the end of the fertile phase, along with a conservative approach that allows intercourse only in the post-ovulatory phase.

Case Study Two

This case involves a Catholic married couple in their early thirties; both are college graduates and serious about their faith, and they participate frequently in the sacraments. However, they now have five small children, the last two conceived unintentionally during the breastfeeding transition. They presented themselves to the NFP teacher with the problem of trying to be faithful to Church teaching but frustrated that NFP was not working for them. They were using a mucus-based method of NFP, but there was no mucus pattern that would help them to discern a fertile phase during the breastfeeding transition. They tried the traditional methods of distinguishing what is called a basic infertile pattern of cervical mucus but could not differentiate an infertile pattern from a fertile pattern. The wife visited her obstetrician, who checked her cervix and determined it to be normal, with no inversion of cervical tissue to cause a continuous mucus pattern. They pleaded for help.

We have already discussed how the breastfeeding transition, from amenorrhea to the first three menstrual cycles postpartum, can be one of the most difficult transitions for NFP users; it is in this transition that NFP often fails to help couples to avoid pregnancy. Unintended pregnancy and confusing natural signs of fertility encountered during this transition are reasons couples tend to give for discontinuing the use of NFP.

1. Since NFP was not working for this breastfeeding woman and there was no discernable fertile phase with typical signs of fertility, could she use contraception until she returned to fertility and was able at least to use basal body temperature as a marker?

The answer to this question is no, based both on Catholic morality and on good medical practice. It does not make sense to put her on hormonal contraception (the progestin-only pill), because a physician or health professional should not use evil to produce a good. While hormonal contraception might bring the couple psychological peace in avoiding pregnancy, for faithful Catholics it would not produce spiritual peace. Although the woman in question was currently amenorrheic, the intent for contraception would be not treating a disease but avoiding conception, and in so doing, separating intercourse from fertility. In addition, hormonal contraception would interfere with discerning when her menstrual cycles resume.

When the hormonal contraceptive pill was first introduced, it was proposed by Catholic physicians as an aid to establishing regular menstrual cycles in women, so they could use the calendar-rhythm method.[104] Use of the pill might be morally justified if it did somehow help regularize the menstrual cycle, especially if given post-ovulation, but not if it is prescribed to suppress ovulation. Morally approved protocols are available to help women normalize the menstrual cycle, especially for those women with polycystic ovarian disease or with short luteal phases. Use of the pill to suppress ovulation and normal menses only avoids helping the woman determine the probable underlying cause of her menstrual irregularity, such as low thyroid levels. Furthermore, if the hormonal pill (especially with the progestin-only pill) is used to suppress ovulation, it has the even more serious potential of acting as an abortifacient.

2. If the couple cannot use any contraceptive during the breastfeeding period, what NFP method could they use?

This is a more difficult question. The woman should be encouraged to continue to breastfeed at least for one year, as recommended by the American Pediatric Association. Breastfeeding has many health benefits for both mother and infant and is encouraged by the Catholic Church. The woman can be assured that during the first six months after childbirth, if she is breastfeeding exclusively and has not experienced menses, she has less than a 2 percent chance of conceiving a child. This is known as the lactational amenorrhea method or LAM, which has been extensively researched for its efficacy among a variety of populations.[105]

However, once the woman no longer meets the LAM criteria, what can she do to avoid pregnancy? This patient's cervical mucus sign was not useful, as she could not discern any infertile pattern. Studies have indicated that the mucus sign is very inaccurate in discerning fertility during the breastfeeding transition.[106] Other signs, such as the BBT shift in temperature, are also not very helpful and in fact might increase the possibility of an unintended pregnancy.

Researchers at Marquette's institute have developed a breastfeeding protocol using the electronic hormonal fertility monitor.[107] This protocol entails creating "arti-

104. See J. J. Lynch, "The Oral Contraceptives: A Review of Moral Appraisement," *Linacre Quarterly* 29 (1962): 168–75.

105. See M. H. Labbok et al., "Multicenter Study of the Lactational Amenorrhea Method (LAM): I. Efficacy, Duration, and Implications for Clinical Applications," *Contraception* 55 (1999): 327–36; V. Valdes et al., "The Efficacy of the Lactational Amenorrhea Method (LAM) among Working Women," *Contraception* 62 (2000): 217–19; World Health Organization Task Force, "The World Health Organization Multinational Study of Breast-Feeding and Lactational Amenorrhea. III. Pregnancy during Breast-Feeding," *Fertility and Sterility* 72 (1999): 431–39.

106. See Tommaselli et al., "Using Complete Breast-feeding and Lactational Amenorrhoea as Birth Spacing Methods."

107. See Richard J. Fehring, "Breastfeeding Protocol for the Clearblue Fertility Monitor," Marquette University, Natural Family Planning, March 2004, http://nfp.marquette.edu/sc_breastfeed_monitor.php.

ficial" twenty-day menstrual cycles and using the monitor to track fertility by testing for the E3G rise and the first LH surge before ovulation. This is done by re-triggering the monitor every twenty days. The monitor will test for twenty days in a row if it does not sense an LH surge. The efficacy of this protocol is now being tested through the Marquette website for NFP services and support. An efficacy study with 198 post-partum women who have used the protocol was recently published; with correct use there were 2 pregnancies per 100 women users, and the imperfect-use pregnancy rate was 8 per 100 women over twelve months of use.[108]

The woman in this case study was one of the first to use the protocol. Her fertility monitoring charts showed five artificial cycles by using the monitor settings; in the fifth cycle, the monitor detected the urinary LH surge with presumed subsequent ovulation and a short luteal phase, both typical for a breastfeeding woman. The first three "cycles" were twenty-eight days long, since she did not retrigger the monitor after the twenty days of testing. That left four days in which she was not apprised of her fertility status. For this reason, the current protocol was modified to twenty-one-day cycles. Canadian physicians have proposed some further modifications to this protocol.[109]

The Marquette researchers are also working to modify the protocol, especially for the first six menstrual cycles after ovulation resumes postpartum. The current protocol has a default onset of fertility on day 6 of the menstrual cycle. However, the first few menstrual cycles typically have a pattern of delayed ovulation. Because of this, one tentative protocol will mark the onset of fertility on day 10 (or earlier if indicated by a high reading on the monitor or a high cervical mucus level). If the menstrual cycle is very long and the twenty days of testing run out, users are asked to re-trigger the monitor for another twenty days of testing. Research showed the first menstrual cycle postpartum of a woman who followed the re-trigger instructions and successfully identified the delayed ovulation in her menstrual cycle. Further research is needed to help women more confidently progress through the breastfeeding transition.

3. Should the couple just abstain from intercourse until the woman has progressed through the breastfeeding transition?

Morally, this course of action presents no problem; sadly, some couples feel this is their only recourse to remain faithful to Catholic teaching. More research in this area of reproductive transition is needed, as well as in the transition through the peri-menopause. Catholic physicians and scientists should view this as a significant challenge, and, at the invitation of Pope Paul VI, bend their backs to solve such problems and to help Catholic couples live according to their faith.[110]

---

108. See T. Bouchard, M. Schneider, and R. Fehring, "Efficacy of a New Postpartum Transition Protocol for Avoiding Pregnancy," *Journal of the American Board of Family Medicine* 26 (2013): 35–44.

109. See S. J. Genius and T. P. Bouchard, "High-tech Family Planning: Reproductive Regulation through Computerized Fertility Monitoring," *European Journal of Obstetrics and Gynecology* 153 (2010): 124–30.

110. See Pope Paul VI, Address to Participants in the Twenty-Fifth General Assembly of Pharmacology, September 7, 1974, in Zimmerman, *Natural Family Planning*, 257.

Summary

Although the Catholic Church teaches that NFP is the only form of birth control that can be used by married Catholic couples to regulate the size of their family, in actual practice few Catholic couples do so.[111] In fact, in the United States there is little difference in contraceptive use between Catholic couples and other couples of reproductive age; in both groups, sterilization and hormonal oral contraception are the most frequently used methods. In fact, sterilization seems to be used more by Catholics than by the general U.S. population, and is the number one method used by Hispanic couples. Only about 0.2 percent of Catholic couples of reproductive age currently use NFP methods, and only about 2 to 3 percent of Catholic couples ever have used NFP.

One reason for these statistics is the reluctance of Catholic health-care providers, and of physicians in particular, to prescribe and promote the use of NFP. As the primary gatekeepers of health, physicians can do much to promote healthy behaviors, but in this matter they seldom take the initiative. Furthermore, Catholic educational institutions, especially Catholic medical and nursing schools, offer little to no education on NFP. Thus it is not surprising that NFP is not widely used in the United States by either Catholics or other women of reproductive age. Physicians, advanced practice nurses, and physician assistants are the gatekeepers of family planning methods. Without Catholic physicians and Catholic professional nurses learning about and promoting NFP, it is doubtful that NFP will spread. It often takes tremendous courage for physicians and other professionals to use, promote, and provide NFP services. NFP is largely ridiculed or ignored in medical schools, scientific journals, and medical societies as being ineffective, too complicated, and old fashioned.

However, the Catholic Church and in particular the popes from Pius XI through Benedict XVI and Francis have called on and pleaded with Catholic health-care providers and Catholic institutions of higher education to provide NFP services, education, and research in this area of family planning.[112] Pius XII, in a 1951 address to Catholic obstetric nurses, said that it is rightly expected that they be well informed about natural methods of family planning and that it is "your office, not that of the priest, to instruct married people" and that "your apostolate demands of you as women that you know and defend this theory."[113] Paul VI, in *Humanae Vitae*, implored physicians that "their proper professional duty is the task of acquiring all the knowledge necessary in this delicate sector, so as to be able to give to the married persons who consult them the wise counsels and sound directives."[114] John Paul II, in a 1981

---

111. See R. Fehring and A. Schlidt, "Trends in Contraceptive Use among Catholics in the United States: 1988–1995," *Linacre Quarterly* 68 (2001): 170–85; Ohlendorf and Fehring, "The Influence of Religiosity on Contraceptive Use among US Catholic Women."

112. See R. Fehring, "The Catholic Physician and Natural Family Planning: Helping to Build the Culture of Life," *National Catholic Bioethics Quarterly* 9 (2009): 305–23.

113. Pius XII, Address to Italian Catholic Union of Midwives, October 29, 1951, in Zimmerman, *Natural Family Planning*, 229–30.

114. Paul VI, *Humanae Vitae*, no. 27.

address to nurse midwives (echoing Pius XII), mentioned the important contribution of advice and practical guidance they can offer to individual couples, who wish to carry out responsible procreation, while respecting the order established by God.[115] He also encouraged all married Catholic couples to learn NFP, and declared that establishing centers for the study of natural birth regulation is one of the primary means of building a culture of life.[116] Furthermore he said that a unique responsibility belongs to health-care personnel, to be guardians and servants of human life, and that educating in the service of life involves the training of married couples in responsible procreation. It is hoped that this overview will help stimulate Catholic physicians and other Catholic health professionals to learn more about NFP and to integrate it into their practices.

In aid of this process, two simple NFP protocols are available on the website for the Marquette University Institute for Natural Family Planning;[117] these quick instructions can be handed to women or couples who wish to use NFP to avoid or achieve pregnancy. The first protocol uses the electronic hormonal monitor and the second uses cervical mucus; both protocols also involve a simple algorithm. If couples wish to use both mucus and monitor to avoid pregnancy, they need to wait to have intercourse until both the monitor and mucus indicate infertility. Fertility monitoring charts can be downloaded at the same website,[118] and a short Powerpoint slide program to support the protocols may be obtained by e-mail.[119] The introductory slide program lasts about twelve minutes and is accompanied by commentary for each slide. The protocols and the slide program are intended to make a simple NFP method available to couples on a computer, tablet, or cell phone during an office visit.

Bibliography

American Academy of Pediatrics. "Menstruation in Girls and Adolescents: Using the Menstrual Cycle as a Vital Sign." *Pediatrics* 118 (2006): 2245–50.

American Society for Reproductive Medicine, Practice Committee. "Optimizing Natural Fertility." *Fertility and Sterility* 9 S3 (2008): S1–S6.

Arevalo, M. "Expanding the Availability and Improving Delivery of Natural Family Planning Services and Fertility Awareness Education: Providers' Perspectives." *Advances in Contraception* 13 (1997): 275–81.

Arevalo, M., V. Jennings, M. Nikula, and I. Sinai. "Efficacy of the New TwoDay Method of Family Planning." *Fertility and Sterility* 82 (2004): 885–92.

Arevalo, M., V. Jennings, and I. Sinai. "Efficacy of a New Method of Family Planning: The Standard Days Method." *Contraception* 65 (2002): 333–38.

115. See John Paul II, Address to Midwives (January 26, 1980), in Zimmerman, *Natural Family Planning*, 259–60.

116. See John Paul II, *Evangelium Vitae*, no. 97.

117. See http://nfp.marquette.edu/nfp_quick_inst_intro.php

118. The fertility monitor chart can be found at http://nfp.marquette.edu/pdf/MonitorChart.pdf; the mucus recording chart, http://nfp.marquette.edu/pdf/MucusChart.pdf; and a chart to track both, http://nfp.marquette.edu/pdf/MonitorPlusMucus.pdf

119. E-mail address for the Marquette University Institute for Natural Family Planning is muinstnfp@marquette.edu.

Arevalo, M., V. Jennings, and I. Sinai. "Application of Simple Fertility Awareness-Based Methods of Family Planning to Breastfeeding Women." *Fertility and Sterility* 80 (2003): 1241–48.

Barrett, Melanie. "Co-Creating with the Creator: A Virtue-Based Approach." In *Science, Faith and Human Fertility*, ed. R. Fehring and T. Notare, 267–302. Milwaukee, Wisc.: Marquette University Press, 2012.

Barron, M. L., and R. J. Fehring. "Basal Body Temperature Assessment: Is It Useful to Couples Seeking Pregnancy?" *MCN American Journal of Maternal Child Nursing* 30 (2005): 290–96.

Batzer, F. "Test Kits for Ovulation and Pregnancy." *Technology 1987: Contemporary OB/GYN* 28 (1986): 7–16.

Behre, H. M., J. Kuhlage, C. Gassner, B. Sonntag, C. Schem, H. P. Schneider, and E. Nieschlag. "Prediction of Ovulation by Urinary Hormone Measurements with the Home Use of the ClearPlan Fertility Monitor: Comparison with Transvaginal Ultrasound Scans and Serum Hormone Measurements." *Human Reproduction* 15 (2000): 2478–82.

Billings, E. L. *The Billings Ovulation Method*. Melbourne, Australia: Ovulation Method Research and Reference Centre of Australia, 1995.

Billings, E. L., and J. J. Billings. *Teaching the Billings Ovulation Method*. Melbourne, Australia: Ovulation Method Research and Reference Centre of Australia, 1997.

Billlings, E. L., J. J. Billings, and M. Caterinich. *Billings Atlas of the Ovulation Method*. Melbourne, Australia: Ovulation Method Research and Reference Centre of Australia, 1989.

Bonnar, J., G. Freundl, and R. Kirkman. "Personal Hormone Monitoring for Contraception." *British Journal of Family Planning* 24 (1999): 128–34.

Borkman, T., and M. Shivanandan. "The Impact of Natural Family Planning on Selected Aspects of the Couple Relationship." *International Review of Natural Family Planning* 8 (1984): 58–66.

Bouchard, T., M. Schneider, and R. Fehring. "Efficacy of a New Postpartum Transition Protocol for Avoiding Pregnancy." *Journal of the American Board of Family Medicine* 26 (2013): 35–44.

Boys, G. A. *Natural Family Planning Nationwide Survey. Final Report to the National Conference of Catholic Bishops*. Washington, D.C.: Diocesan Development Program for NFP, 1989.

Clubb, E., and J. Knight. *Fertility*. Exeter, U.K.: David and Charles, 1999.

Consumer Reports. "The Fertility Window." *Consumer Reports* 68 (2003): 48–50.

Corson, G., D. Ghaz, and E. Kemmann. "Home Urinary Luteinizing Hormone Immunoassay: Clinical Applications." *Fertility and Sterility* 53 (1990): 591–601.

Crosignani, P. G., and B. L. Rubin. "Optimal Use of Infertility Diagnostic Tests and Treatments." *Human Reproduction* 15 (2000): 723–32.

Crowley, P., and P. Crowley. "Report to the Papal Birth Control Commission." Patrick and Patricia Crowley Papers, 1965–1966. University of Notre Dame Archives.

Djerassi, C. "Fertility Awareness: Jet-Age Rhythm Method?" *Science* 248 (1990): 1061–62.

Dunson, D. B., D. D. Baird, A. J. Wilcox, and C. R. Weinberg. "Day-Specific Probabilities of Clinical Pregnancy Based on Two Studies with Imperfect Measures of Ovulation." *Human Reproduction* 14 (1999): 1835–39.

Dunson, D. B., B. Columbo, and D. D. Baird. "Changes with Age in the Level and Duration of Fertility in the Menstrual Cycle." *Human Reproduction* 17 (2002): 1399–403.

Ecochard, R., H. Boehringer, M. Rabilloud, and H. Marret. "Chronological Aspects of Ultrasonic, Hormonal, and Other Indirect Indices of Ovulation." *British Journal of Obstetrics and Gynecology* 109 (2001): 822–29.

Fehring, Richard J. "Physician and Nurse's Knowledge and use of Natural Family Planning." *The Linacre Quarterly* 63 (1995): 22–28.

——. "Accuracy of the Peak Day of Cervical Mucus as a Biological Marker of Fertility." *Contraception* 66 (2002): 231–35.

——. "Breastfeeding Protocol for the Clearblue Fertility Monitor." Marquette University, Natural Family Planning. March 2004. http://nfp.marquette.edu/sc_breastfeed_monitor.php.

——. "The Future of Professional Education in Natural Family Planning." *Journal of Obstetric, Gynecological and Neonatal Nursing* 33 (2004): 34–43.

——. "New Low and High Tech Calendar Methods of Family Planning." *Journal of Nurse Midwifery and Women's Health* 50 (2005): 31–37.

———. "The Catholic Physician and Natural Family Planning: Helping to Build the Culture of Life." *National Catholic Bioethics Quarterly* 9 (2009): 305–23.

Fehring, R., L. Hanson, and J. Stanford. "Nurse-Midwives' Knowledge and Promotion of Lactational Amenorrhea and Other Natural Family Planning Methods for Child Spacing." *Journal of Nurse Midwifery and Women's Health* 46 (2001): 68–73.

Fehring, R., and D. Lawrence. "Spiritual Well-Being, Self-Esteem, and Intimacy among Couples Using Natural Family Planning." *Linacre Quarterly* 61 (1994): 18–29.

Fehring, R. J., D. M. Lawrence, and C. M. Sauvage. "Self-Esteem, Spiritual Well-Being, and Intimacy: A Comparison among Couples Using NFP and Oral Contraceptives." *International Review of Natural Family Planning* 13 (1989): 227–36.

Fehring, R., and K. Miller. "Is It Possible for NFP to Be Used (Immorally) with Contraceptive Intent?" *Linacre Quarterly* 78 (2011): 86–90.

Fehring, R., and A. Schlidt. "Trends in Contraceptive Use among Catholics in the United States: 1988–1995." *Linacre Quarterly* 68 (2001): 170–85.

Fehring, R., and M. Schneider. "Variability of the Fertile Phase of the Menstrual Cycle." *Fertility and Sterility* 90 (2008): 1232–35.

Fehring, R., M. Schneider, and M. L. Barron. "Protocol for Determining Fertility while Breast-feeding." *Fertility and Sterility* 84 (2005): 805–7.

Fehring, R. J., M Schneider, M. L. Barron, and K. Raviele. "Cohort Comparison of Two Fertility Awareness Methods of Family Planning." *Journal of Reproductive Medicine* 54, no. 3 (2009): 165–70.

Fehring, R., M. Schneider, K. Raviele, D. Rodriguez, and J. Pruszynski. "Randomized Comparison of Two Internet-Supported Fertility Awareness Based Methods of Family Planning." *Contraception* 88, no. 1 (2013): 24–30.

Frank-Herrmann, P., C. Gnoth, S. Baur, T. Strowitzki, and G. Freundl. "Determination of the Fertile Window: Reproductive Competence of Women—European Cycle Databases." *Gynecology and Endocrinology* 20 (2005): 305–12.

Genius, S. J., and T. P. Bouchard. "High-tech Family Planning: Reproductive Regulation through Computerized Fertility Monitoring." *European Journal of Obstetrics and Gynecology* 153, no. 2 (2010): 124–30.

Gnoth, C., P. Frank-Herrmann, A. Schmoll, E. Godehardt, and G. Freundl. "Cycle Characteristics after Discontinuation of Oral Contraceptives." *Gynecology and Endocrinology* 16 (2002): 307–17.

Gnoth, C., D. Godehardt, E. Godehardt, P. Frank-Herrmann, and G. Freundl. "Time to Pregnancy: Results of the German Prospective Study and Impact on the Management of Infertility." *Human Reproduction* 18 (2003): 1959–66.

Grimes, D. A., M. F. Gallo, V. Grigorieva, K. Nanda, and K. F. Schulz. "Fertility Awareness-Based Methods for Contraception: Systematic Review of Randomized Controlled Trials." *Contraception* 72, no. 2 (2005): 85–90.

Guida, M., G. A. Tommaselli, S. Palomba, M. Pellicano, G. Moccia, C. Di Carlo, and C. Nappi. "Efficacy of Methods for Determining Ovulation in a Natural Family Planning Program." *Fertility and Sterility* 72 (1999): 900–904.

Hatherley, L. "Lactation and Postpartum Infertility: The Use-effectiveness of Natural Family Planning (NFP) after Term Pregnancy." *Clinical Reproduction and Fertility* 3 (1985): 319–34.

Heffner, L. J., and D. J. Schust. *The Reproduction System at a Glance.* 4th edition. Malden, Mass.: Wiley Blackwell, 2014.

Hilgers, T. W. *The Medical Applications of Natural Family Planning.* Omaha, Neb.: Pope Paul VI Institute Press, 1991.

———. *The Scientific Foundations of the Ovulation Method.* Omaha, Neb.: Pope Paul VI Institute Press, 1995.

———. *The Creighton Model NaProEducation System.* Omaha, Neb.: Pope Paul VI Institute Press, 1996.

———. *The Medical and Surgical Practice of NaProTechnology.* Omaha, Neb.: Pope Paul VI Institute Press, 2004.

Hilgers, T. W., K. D. Daly, A. M. Prebil, and S. K. Hilgers. "Cumulative Pregnancy Rates in Patients with Apparently Normal Fertility and Fertility-Focused Intercourse." *Journal of Reproductive Medicine* 37, no. 10 (1992): 864–66.

Howard, M. P., and J. B. Stanford. "Pregnancy Probabilities during Use of the Creighton Model Fertility Care System." *Archives of Family Medicine* 8 (1999): 391–402.

Huneger, R. J., and R. Fuller, *A Couple's Guide to Fertility.* Portland, Ore.: Northwest Family Services, 1997.

John Paul II, Pope. *Familiaris Consortio, On the Role of the Christian Family in the Modern World* [Apostolic Exhortation. November 22, 1981]. Boston: Daughters of St. Paul, 1981.

——. *Evangelium Vitae, The Gospel of Life* [Encyclical Letter. March 25, 1995]. St. Paul, Minn.: The Leaflet Missal Company, 1995.

Keefe, E. "Self-Examination of the Cervix as a Guide in Fertility Control." *International Review of Natural Family Planning* 10 (1986): 322–38.

Kennedy, K. I., B. A. Gross, S. Parenteau-Carreau, A. M. Flynn, J. B. Brown, and C. M. Visness. "Breastfeeding and the Symptothermal Method." *Studies in Family Planning* 26, no. 2 (1995): 107–15.

Knaus, H. *Periodic Fertility and Sterility in Woman: A Natural Method of Birth Control.* Vienna: Wilhelm Maudrich, 1934.

Labbok, M. H., V. Hight-Laukaran, A. E. Peterson, V. Fletcher, H. von Hertzen, and P. F. Van Look. "Multicenter Study of the Lactational Amenorrhea Method (LAM): I. Efficacy, Duration, and Implications for Clinical Applications." *Contraception* 55, no. 6 (1999): 327–36.

Labbok, M. H., R. Y. Stallings, F. Shah, A. Pérez, H. Klaus, M. Jacobson, and T. Muruthi. "Ovulation Method Use during Breastfeeding: Is There Increased Risk of Unplanned Pregnancy?" *American Journal of Obstetrics and Gynecology* 165 Supp (1991): 2031–36.

Lamprect, V., and J. Trussell. "Natural Family Planning Effectiveness: Evaluating Published Reports." *Advances in Contraception* 13 (1997): 155–65.

Latz, J., and E. Reiner. "Further Studies on the Sterile and Fertile Periods in Women." *American Journal of Obstetrics and Gynecology* 43 (1942): 74–79.

Latz, L. *The Rhythm of Sterility and Fertility in Women.* Chicago: Latz Foundation, 1932.

Li, W., and Y. Qiu. "Relation of Supplementary Feeding to Resumption of Menstruation and Ovulation in Lactating Postpartum Women." *Chinese Medical Journal* 120 (2007): 868–70.

Lynch, J. J. "The Oral Contraceptives: A Review of Moral Appraisement." *Linacre Quarterly* 29 (1962): 168–75.

Marshall, J. "A Field Trial of the BBT Method of Regulating Births." *Lancet* 292 (July 6, 1968): 8–10.

Marshall, J., and B. Rowe. "Psychological Aspects of the Basal Body Temperature Methods of Regulating Births." *Fertility and Sterility* 21 (1970): 14–19.

May, K. "Home Monitoring with the ClearPlan Easy Fertility Monitor for Fertility Awareness." *Journal of International Medical Research* 29 S1 (2002): 14A–20A.

May, W. E., R. Lawler, and J. Boyle. *Catholic Sexual Ethics A Summary, Explanation, and Defense.* 3rd edition. Huntington, Ind.: Our Sunday Visitor, 2011.

McCarthy, J. J., and H. E. Rockette. "A Comparison of Methods to Interpret the Basal Body Temperature Graph." *Fertility and Sterility* 39 (1983): 640–46.

McClory, R. *The Turning Point.* New York: Crossroad, 1995.

McCusker, M. P. "Natural Family Planning and the Marital Relationship: The Catholic University of America Study." *International Review of Natural Family Planning* 1 (1977): 331–40.

Medina, J. E., A. Cifuentes, J. R. Abernathy, J. M. Spieler, and M. E. Wade. "Comparative Evaluation of Two Methods of Natural Family Planning in Columbia." *American Journal of Obstetrics and Gynecology* 138 (1980): 1142–47.

Menarguez, M., L. M. Pastor, and E. Odeblad. "Morphological Characterization of Different Human Cervical Mucus Types Using Light and Scanning Electron Microscopy." *Human Reproduction* 18 (2004): 1782–89.

Moghissi, K. S. "Cervical Mucus Changes and Ovulation Prediction and Detection." *Journal of Reproductive Medicine* 31 Supp. (1986): 748–53.

Mosher, W. D., and J. Jones. "Use of Contraception in the United States: 1982–2008." *Vital and Health Statistics* 23, no. 29 (2010): 1–77.

Mu, Q., and R. Fehring. "Efficacy of Achieving Pregnancy with Fertility Focused Intercourse." *MCN: The American Journal of Maternal Child Nursing* 39 (2014): 35–40.

Nassaralla, C., J. B. Stanford, K. D. Daly, M. Schneider, K. C. Schliep, and R. J. Fehring. "Characteristics of the Menstrual Cycle after Discontinuation of Oral Contraceptives." *Journal of Women's Health* 20, no. 2 (2011): 169–77.

National Institute for Clinical Excellence (U.K.). *Fertility: Assessment and Treatment for People with Fertility Problems*. Clinical Guidelines 11. London: NICE, 2004.

Oddens, B. J. "Women's Satisfaction with Birth Control: A Population Survey of Physical and Psychological Effects of Oral Contraceptives, Intrauterine Devices, Condoms, Natural Family Planning, and Sterilization among 1466 Women." *Contraception* 59 (1999): 227–86.

Odeblad, E. "Cervical Mucus and Their Functions." *Journal of the Irish Colleges of Physicians and Surgeons* 26 (1997): 27–32.

Ogino, K. *Conception Period of Women*. Harrisburg, Penn.: Medical Arts Publishing, 1934.

Ohlendorf, J., and R. Fehring. "The Influence of Religiosity on Contraceptive Use among US Catholic Women." *Linacre Quarterly* 74 (2007): 135–44.

Palter, S., and D. Olive. "Reproductive Physiology." In *Novak's Gynecology*, ed. S. J. Berek, 149–74. Philadelphia: Lippincott Williams and Wilkins, 2002.

Paul VI, Pope. *Humanae Vitae, Of Human Life* [Encyclical Letter. July 25, 1968]. Boston: Pauline Books, 1968.

Robinson, J. E., M. Waklin, and J. E. Ellis. "Increased Pregnancy Rate with Use of the Clearblue Easy Fertility Monitor." *Fertility and Sterility* 87 (2007): 329–34.

Roetzer, J. "Further Evaluation of the Sympto-thermal Method." *International Review of Natural Family Planning* 1 (1977): 139–50.

Seibel, M. "Luteinizing Hormone and Ovulation Timing." *Journal of Reproductive Medicine* 31 Supp. (1986): 754–59.

Snick, H. K. A. "Should Spontaneous or Timed Intercourse Guide Couples Trying to Conceive?" *Human Reproduction* 10 (2005): 2976–77.

Soules, M. R., S. Sherman, E. Parrott, R. Rebar, N. Santoro, W. Utian, and N. Woods. "Executive Summary: Stages of Reproductive Aging Workshop (STRAW)." *Fertility and Sterility* 76 (2001): 874–78.

Speroff, L., and M. Fritz. *Clinical Gynecologic Endocrinology and Infertility*. 7th edition. Philadelphia: Lippencott Williams and Wilkins, 2005.

Stanford, J. B., T. A. Parnell, and P. C. Boyle. "Outcomes from Treatment of Infertility with Natural Procreative Technology in an Irish General Practice." *Journal of the American Board of Family Medicine* 21 (2008): 375–84.

Stanford, J. B., P. B Thurman, and J. C. Lemaire. "Physicians' Knowledge and Practices Regarding Natural Family Planning." *Obstetrics and Gynecology* 94 (1999): 672–78.

Stanford, J. B., G. L. White, and H. Hataska. "Timing Intercourse to Achieve Pregnancy: Current Evidence." *Obstetrics and Gynecology* 100 (2002):1333–41.

Taffe, J., and L. Dennerstein. "Time to the Final Menstrual Period." *Fertility and Sterility* 78 (2002): 397–403.

Tanabe, K., N. Susumu, K. Hand, K. Nishii, I. Ishikawa, and S. Nozawa. "Prediction of the Potentially Fertile Period by Urinary Hormone Measurements Using a New Home-Use Monitor: Comparison with Laboratory Hormone Analyses." *Human Reproduction* 16 (2001): 1619–24.

Tomaselli, G. A., M. Guida, S. Palomba, M. Barbato, and C. Nappi. "Using Complete Breast-Feeding and Lactational Amenorrhoea as Birth Spacing Methods." *Contraception* 61 (2000): 253–57.

Tortorici, J. "Conception Regulation, Self-Esteem, and Marital Satisfaction among Catholic Couples." *International Review of Natural Family Planning* 3 (1979): 191–205.

Treloar, A. E., R. E. Boynton, B. G. Behn, and B. W. Brown. "Variation of the Human Menstrual Cycle through Reproductive Life," *International Journal of Fertility* 12 (1967): 77–126.

Trussell, J. "Contraceptive Failure in the United States." *Contraception* 70 (2004): 89–96.

Trussell, J., and L. Grummer-Strawn. "Contraceptive Failure of the Ovulation Method of Periodic Abstinence." *Family Planning Perspectives* 22 (1990): 65–75. doi:10.2307/2135511.

United States Conference of Catholic Bishops (USCCB), *Ethical and Religious Directives for Catholic Health Care Services*. 5th edition. Washington, D.C.: USCCB, 2009.

Valdés, V, M. H. Labbok, E. Pugin, and A. Pérez. "The Efficacy of the Lactational Amenorrhea Method (LAM) among Working Women." *Contraception* 62, no. 5 (2000): 217–19.

VandeVusse, L., R. Fehring, and L. Hanson. "Marital Dynamics of Practicing Natural Family Planning." *Journal of Nursing Scholarship* 35 (2003): 171–76.

Velasquez, E. V., R. V. Trigo, S. Creus, S. Campo, and H. B. Croxatto. "Pituitary-Ovarian Axis during Lactational Amenorrhoea. I. Longitudinal Assessment of Follicular Growth, Gonadotrophins, Sex Steroid and Inhibin Levels before and after Recovery of Menstrual Cyclicity." *Human Reproduction* 4 (2006): 909–15.

Vollman, R. "Brief History of Natural Family Planning." In *Natural Family Planning: Introduction to the Methods*, ed. Clara R. Ross, 1–5. Washington, D.C.: Human Life Foundation, 1977.

Wade, M. E., P. McCarthy, J. R. Abernathy, G. S. Harris, H. C. Danzer, and W. A. Uricchio. "Randomized Prospective Study of the Use-effectiveness of Two Methods of Natural Family Planning: An Interim Report." *American Journal of Obstetrics and Gynecology* 134 (1979): 628–31.

Wade, M. E., P. McCarthy, G. D. Braunstein, J. R. Abernathy, C. M. Suchindran, G. S. Harris, H. C. Danzer, and W. A. Uricchio. "A Randomized Prospective Study of the Use-Effectiveness of Two Methods of Natural Family Planning." *American Journal of Obstetrics and Gynecology* 141 (1981): 368–76.

Weschler, T. *Taking Charge of Your Fertility*. New York: Harpers Collins, 2002.

Westoff, C. F., and N. R. Ryder. "Conception Control among American Catholics." In *Catholics/U.S.A.: Perspectives on Social Change*, ed. W. T. Liu and N. J. Pallone, 257–68. New York: John Wiley and Sons, 1970.

Wilcox, A. J., D. B. Dunson, and D. D. Baird. "The Timing of the 'Fertile Window' in the Menstrual Cycle: Day Specific Estimates from a Prospective Study." *British Medical Journal* 321 (2000): 1259–62.

Wilcox, A. J., C. R. Weinberg, and D. D. Baird. "Timing of Sexual Intercourse in Relation to Ovulation: Effects on the Probability of Conception, Survival of the Pregnancy, and Sex of the Baby." *New England Journal of Medicine* 333 (1995): 1517–21.

World Health Organization Task Force. "The World Health Organization Multinational Study of Breast-Feeding and Lactational Amenorrhea. III. Pregnancy during Breast-Feeding." *Fertility and Sterility* 72 (1999): 431–39.

World Health Organization. "A Prospective Multicentre Trial of the Ovulation Method of Natural Family Planning. II. The Effectiveness Phase." *Fertility and Sterility* 36 (1981): 591–98.

Zimmerman, Anthony, ed. *Natural Family Planning: Nature's Way—God's Way*. Milwaukee, Wisc.: DeRance, 1980.

Zinaman, M., and W. Stevenson. "Efficacy of the Symptothermal Method of Natural Family Planning in Lactating Women after the Return of Menses." *American Journal of Obstetrics and Gynecology* 165 Supp (1991): 2037–39.

Christopher O'Hara

6. CATHOLIC WITNESS IN PEDIATRICS

The field of pediatrics affords perhaps the widest scope of clinical opportunity for a practitioner seeking to align his or her practice with authentically Catholic medical care. The issues are varied over childhood development, and the advice and influence that the pediatrician has on his or her patients' parents, as well as on the patient, is great. Coupled with these relationships among parents, child, and pediatrician, often the cumulative time spent by the children and parents with the pediatrician over years is also significant. The respected pediatrician, perhaps more than physicians practicing in other medical disciplines, may in a major way help the formation of the child. In this chapter, Dr. O'Hara outlines an approach to advising parents, children, and teenagers about what is good, true, and beautiful in a culture that too often obscures the view of these transcendental realities. O'Hara makes no apology for presenting a form of practice that accords with authentic Catholic witness. He also provides specifics about how to practice in this way.—*Editors*

Introduction

It is not enough for a Catholic pediatrician to be an excellent clinician; even the most hardcore atheist can be excellent clinically. The Catholic difference pediatrics should be founded in a Catholic worldview of man's origin, nature, and destiny,[1] and should be expressed in our love, our compassion rooted in love,[2] and our virtue. The reason for this difference is found in our formation. As Catholics, we are called to be faithful to the Gospel, so our outlook and our work should be different from that of general society. But our culture, like many cultures before it, claims we are mistaken, and is

---

1. See P. Kreeft, "Why a Christian Anthropology Makes a Difference," paper presented at Catholic Medical Association 79th Educational Conference, Seattle, Wash., October 2010.

2. See P. Guinan, "Hippocrates and Christian Medicine," *Ethics and Medics* 34, no. 11 (November 2009): 3–4.

determined to destroy Judeo-Christian principles by excising them from the social landscape. This approach will leave society with nothing but totalitarian materialism, and materialism has never led to happiness.

Virtue

The *Catechism* defines virtue as "habitual and firm disposition to do the good. It allows the person not only to perform good acts, but to give the best of himself. The virtuous person tends toward the good with all his sensory and spiritual powers; he pursues the good and chooses it in concrete actions."[3] Secular humanism, by contrast, relies on everyone treating each other with respect for respect's sake, enforcing this rule with the law of the jungle. Like the house built on sand, it will not weather the storm.

Of the four cardinal virtues (prudence, justice, fortitude, and temperance), the most important is prudence, the virtue that "disposes our reason" to discern what is good and to choose the proper way of achieving it.[4] Catholic physicians, like all Catholics, should "grasp the beauty and attraction of right dispositions towards goodness."[5] Sadly, many Catholics are lacking in formation and role models of virtue; what lessons they learned were like seeds scattered among thorns or on rocky soil (Mt 13:5–7).

Catholic physicians must possess the virtue of fortitude to practice virtuously. Much of today's medical literature reveals the researchers' materialist and secular leanings, and our pluralistic society values individual autonomy above all else, even to the exclusion of human dignity. However, Catholic principles have stood the test of time over the centuries, and have proven to be effective in protecting individuals from behaviors that are ultimately harmful to themselves and to society.

Infancy

The birth of a child should bring joy to a home, but frequent late-night awakenings, diaper changes, doctor visits, and fears of the unknown can make new parenthood an unnerving experience. New parents need words of encouragement, sympathetic listening, and patient responses to their questions to help them cope with the first months of their child's life. Physician visits in the newborn nursery should focus on key points, to avoid information overload. The initial office visit for first-time parents, or for families whose child carries a serious diagnosis, should be done at one week (regardless of the feeding method or payment schedule) and should allow additional time for questions, to allay fears and provide reassurance.

Unfortunately, the blessings a new baby brings are not always obvious. Some mothers who are no longer in a relationship with the child's father will transfer their

---

3. *Catechism of the Catholic Church* (Fort Wayne, Ind: The Faith Database, 2008), no. 1803, https://www.faithdatabase.com/.
4. Ibid., no. 1806.
5. Ibid., no. 1697.

negative feelings for the father to the child; this is especially common with single, teenage mothers. Other parents may view the child as a threat to a career, a relationship or a lifestyle; they may display negative feelings toward the child or toward his or her normal behaviors. When this becomes evident, it is important to delve into these issues, so as to raise the parent's awareness and provide the child with a healthier environment. Questions like "What kind of home life do you want for your child?" and "How do you plan to provide that?" create a starting point. It may be important to explore why an absent parent is no longer involved with the family. Some parents may lack the insight to perceive the importance of these questions, but those who do will have made the first necessary step toward correcting the problem.

Many secular physicians ignore parents' negative feelings or behaviors, ascribing them to societal ills instead of personal problems. While this may remove the "blame," it does nothing to protect the child. Developing rapport with these parents may be difficult, but it is essential. The Catholic pediatrician should strive to imitate St. Philip Neri, who befriended the struggling souls he encountered before trying to lead them back to the fold.

For the affected parent, it may help to remember that forgiveness is healthier for the forgiver than resentment. A fine book titled *The Process of Forgiveness*, by Fr. William Meninger, is an excellent starting point for physicians who are interested in this dynamic. For parents who struggle with these wounds, a number of websites can be helpful, including Marital Healing, its YouTube channel, and Child Healing.[6]

For those parents with insight who try but struggle with change, the lessons of love and forgiveness are paramount. Love atones for a myriad of sins. Repeating this phrase often in the presence of families with difficulties is more effective than the blame-free attitude of modern medicine. Obviously, while the gift of forgiveness should never be withheld, abusive or neglectful parental behaviors must always be reported to the appropriate authorities.

Parental Mental Health and Attachment

Infancy is a time to build a strong parent-child relationship. When an infant experiences warmth and affection, a secure attachment is created. As the infant grows, he or she mimics the emotional reactions of the parents. In emotionally and mentally healthy parents, this sets the stage for early discipline, since older infants and toddlers will learn to stop behaviors that upset their parents.[7] If a parent does not respond warmly to the infant (if, for example, the parent ignores the infant's crying), the foundation for insecure attachment is laid. This can occur in mothers who have postpartum depression or another mental illness.[8]

---

6. http://www.maritalhealting.com; http://www.YouTube.com/Marital Healing; http://www.child healing.com.

7. See L. Bissonnette-Pitre and the Most Reverend R. F. Vasa, *Healthy Families: Safe Children; The Power of Relationships* (Bend, Ore.: Ardor, Inc., 2007), DVD.

8. See M. W. Wan and J. Green, "The Impact of Maternal Psychopathology on Child–Mother Attachment," *Archives of Women's Mental Health* 12 (2009): 123–34.

Postpartum depression affects more than 500,000 women in the United States annually.[9] This is a rather staggering statistic, given the effects of the mother's illness on the infant. Insecure attachment is just one of these effects; it occurs 5.4 times more often in infants whose mothers suffered from postpartum depression, and 9.8 times more often in infants whose mothers suffered with postpartum depression and a previous history of depression.[10] Mothers who are depressed tend to be either disengaged or authoritarian in their interactions; their infants are generally less attentive and have higher levels of arousal.[11] If the mother's depression persists beyond six months, the infant will be more likely to exhibit delays of growth and development by 1 year of age;[12] the child's long-term intellectual functioning may also suffer.[13] Positive interventions, such as music and massage therapy, can help improve the mother-child bond in such cases.[14]

Since Catholics understand that the body and the soul interact and are interdependent, Catholic pediatricians understand that the mother's mental and spiritual health are directly linked to the health of the child (an approach now commonly referred to as "holistic"). Because the pediatrician sees the mother more frequently in the postpartum period than does the ob-gyn, evaluating all mothers with a depression screening tool can facilitate referral to a mental health provider and can spare their children from adverse effects. A number of validated tools for this screening are available, including the Edinburgh Postnatal Depression Scale.[15]

Parents who have anger issues, or those who experienced emotional rejection as children, may also have difficulty forming a secure attachment with their infant. This is problematic, since children with insecure attachment will have trouble with relationships in adulthood as well.[16] The Catholic pediatrician should maintain a list of mental health resources to which to refer parents who need help in establishing positive emotional bonds with a new baby.

9. See R. E. Blackmore and L. H. Chaudron, "Postpartum Depression: Recognition and Intervention," *Journal of Clinical Outcomes Management* 19 (2012): 133–42.

10. See L. Murray, "The Impact of Postnatal Depression on Infant Development," *Journal of Child Psychology and Psychiatry* 33 (1992): 543–61.

11. See T. Field, M. Diego, and M. Hernandez-Reif, "Infants of Depressed Mothers Are Less Responsive To Faces and Voices: A Review," *Infant Behavior and Development* 32 (2009): 239–44.

12. See T. Field, "Maternal Depression Effects on Infants and Early Interventions," *Preventive Medicine* 27 (1998): 200–203.

13. See D. F. Hay et al., "Intellectual Problems Shown by 11-Year-Old Children Whose Mothers Had Postnatal Depression," *Journal of Child Psychology Psychiatry and Allied Disciplines* 42 (2001): 871–89; D. Sharp, D. F. Hay, S. Pawlby et al., "The Impact of Postnatal Depression on Boys' Intellectual Development," *Journal of Child Psychology and Psychiatry* 36 (1995): 1315–36; S. L. Sohr-Preston and L. V. Scaramella, "Implications of Timing of Maternal Depressive Symptoms for Early Cognitive and Language Development," *Clinical Child and Family Psychology Review* 9 (2006): 65–83.

14. See Field, "Maternal Depression Effects on Infants and Early Interventions"; Field, Diego, and Hernandez-Reif, "Infants of Depressed Mothers Are Less Responsive to Faces and Voices."

15. J. L. Cox, J. M. Holden, and R. Sagovsky, "Detection of Postnatal Depression: Development of the 10-Item Edinburgh Postnatal Depression Scale," *British Journal of Psychiatry* 150 (1987): 782–86.

16. See Bissonnette-Pitre and Vasa, "Program III: Authoritative Parenting," in *Healthy Families: Safe Children*, DVD.

Selfless Parenting

Parenting requires selflessness, but this virtue does not come easily to some parents. Like many things, it is best learned when modeled by a loving caregiver; thus, adults who grew up lacking in loving parental attention can find it difficult to provide such attention to their own children. This does not mean it is impossible for such a parent to learn how to form a loving parent-child relationship; such training can be had through parenting classes offered by a local charity or other agency. The pediatrician can help new parents discern their need to develop selflessness through sensitive questioning: "Did you feel loved by your parents?" "Do you want to raise your children differently from the way you were raised? In what way?" "What relationships did you have with adults in your childhood that you would like to emulate?" If the parent is interested in this kind of dialogue, it is worth discussing specific actions and behaviors that can build a positive relationship, since long-term goals and concrete objectives require habit formation. Guiding the parent to establish habits, goals, and objectives can help create positive changes.

It is never too early to ask parents what kind of person they want the infant to be when he or she is grown. This does not mean finding out their career aspirations for the child (although that may prove illuminating), but rather is a jumping-off point for parents to begin making their child's moral, ethical, and spiritual growth a priority. Everyone is born with some capacity to use reason, even if it is impossible to measure; thus, moral training is possible in (nearly) everyone. "Is it your goal to raise a moral child?" "What does that mean to you?" "How can you help your child learn to behave morally?" are some of the questions physicians can use to begin this dialogue and encourage parental discernment. Parents should be helped to understand that the foundation for a healthy relationship with their child in adolescence is rooted in early attachment. A securely attached child will be more personally satisfied, suffer less stress in the face of major life events, and more willingly seek support when feeling lonely, anxious, angry, or depressed in the future.[17]

Making the Infant a Priority

Ideally, both parents should attend the well-child checkup in infancy. When both parents are present, the pediatrician can encourage them to foster cooperation or suggest that they switch off with scheduled naps to prevent sleep deprivation. Despite the popular misconception that babies can be spoiled, pediatricians should make it a point to encourage parents to hold their infant as much as they want, especially to comfort the child who is crying. This approach nurtures parent-child attachment and enhances the infant's cognitive and social development; moreover, babies who are held and comforted cry less at 12 months than those who are not.[18]

---

17. See G. C. Armsden and M. T. Greenburg, "The Inventory of Parent and Peer Attachment: Individual Differences and Their Relationship to Psychological Well-Being in Adolescence," *Journal of Youth and Adolescence* 16 (1987): 427–54.

18. See Bissonnette-Pitre and Vasa, "Authoritative Parenting," in *Healthy Families: Safe Children*, DVD.

The security felt by the infant has long-range effects: it assists in the development of self-control, allows for effective discipline, plays a role in moral development in early childhood, and protects adolescents against a variety of unhealthy behaviors.

Making the Parents a Priority

Parents of all infants, not just those with colicky babies, should be reminded that when they are frustrated, it is okay to let the baby cry for a while. This is the only real exception to the "comfort your infant" rule, but it is significant, since frustration can drive even loving parents to hurt their infants. For non-intact families, even more caution is required, as non-biological partners commit a disproportionately large amount of physical abuse.[19]

Parents should also be encouraged to nurture their marriage. Sometimes new parents are so enamored of their infant that they need to be reminded of how much they love each other. An intact family stemming from a healthy marriage will allow the growing child to avoid much of the self-destructive behavior of adolescence and to develop healthy relationships into adulthood.[20] Family meals, leisure time together, and exercise can and should be planned in advance, so that they take precedence and are less likely to be squeezed out of the schedule. A parent who can schedule a haircut should rank family time as an even higher priority that is worthy of its own designated time slot. Exercise is especially useful, since it helps to alleviate the effects of stress and has anxiolytic and anti-depressant effects.[21]

These ideas can help couples nurture their marriage through the challenges of parenthood:

- Sit down, and talk every day for at least ten minutes. Do not use this time to go over schedules; instead, listen to and talk about each other's goals and dreams. For families with a traveling parent, schedule time for a phone call every day.
- Eat meals together as often as possible and never with the distraction of television and other electronic devices.
- Remind your spouse that you love him or her, every day, in front of the children.
- Set aside thirty minutes of family time every day for parents and children to spend time together playing. This should be uninterrupted time—no phone calls, television, Internet, or distractions. A family walk is one way to combine this with exercise.
- For families with a traveling parent, set aside one day each week that is for family only.

19. See L. Margolin, "Child Abuse by Mother's Boyfriends: Why the Overrepresentation?" *Child Abuse and Neglect* 16 (1992): 541–51; P. G. Schnitzer and Barnard G. Ewigman, "Child Deaths Resulting from Inflicted Injuries: Household Risk Factors and Perpetrator Characteristics," *Pediatrics* 116 (2005): e687–e693.

20. See R. A. Barry and G. Kochanska, "A Longitudinal Investigation of the Affective Environment in Families with Young Children: From Infancy to Early School Age," *Emotion* 10 (2010): 237–49.

21. See Peter Salmon, "Effects of Physical Exercise on Anxiety, Depression and Sensitivity to Stress: A Unifying Theory," *Clinical Psychology Review* 21 (2001): 33–61.

- Intimacy can be as simple as holding hands. It is necessary for a healthy marriage.

Late Infancy and Toddlerhood

Unhealthy Adjustments

If parents have established a secure attachment with their child in infancy, the "terrible twos" will not be so terrible. Once infants gain mobility by crawling or walking, the world is open to them, but this time of discovery is also marked by stranger anxiety and the child's struggle to develop independence. It is hard for some parents to adjust to the toddler's need to use mommy or daddy as home base while exploring the environment. It is equally hard for some parents who view the infant as no longer "needing" them. It's important to challenge this assumption, turning it into a teachable moment. A child will always need his or her parent, but the nature of the needs changes as the child develops. Parents who "need to be needed" to an excessive degree may have other issues bubbling under the surface, such as poor self-esteem or fear of abandonment, and are at risk for depression.[22] It may help the parent to provide a calm but stimulating home environment, with the parent doing things the child cannot do for him- or herself, such as reading books, telling stories, playing beautiful music, or singing songs. Further, more focused dialogue with the parent will determine whether therapy is needed.

Dangers in the Home

For the infant and young toddler, everything is new. A safe environment is essential, since young children learn by exploring. It is hard for children at this age to avoid touching everything they see, and expecting them to exercise caution is unrealistic, as children's brains do not develop the capacity for self-control until about 18 months of age. While close supervision is vital and the word "no" helps to set limits, too many "no's" make the child feel uncertain of him- or herself.[23] This is why it is absolutely crucial that homes with toddlers have childproof covers over outlets and locked cabinets for storing medications, cleaning agents, and alcohol. This includes homes of grandparents, relatives, or other frequent caregivers, and should begin at 6 months of age in preparation for the infant becoming mobile.[24] Even if parents or grandparents protest that poisons are "up high" or that the child "doesn't get into things," there is no good reason for neglecting to protect a child from such dangers.

22. See A. Cogswell, L. B. Alloy, and J. Spasojevic, "Neediness and Interpersonal Life Stress: Does Congruency Predict Depression," *Cognitive Therapy and Research* 30 (2006): 427–43.
23. See Bissonnette-Pitre and Vasa, "Authoritative Parenting," in *Healthy Families: Safe Children*, DVD.
24. See ibid.

Discipline's Foundation

While the child has no true capacity for self-control prior to 18 months, the foundation for this virtue is already being laid through the relationship with his or her parent. A warm relationship and attachment built in infancy sets the stage for later interactions, in which the child's behavior can be modified in a nonthreatening way. If a parent smiles and shows joy over the child's actions, the child's behavior is rewarded and may persist. Parents can set a positive stage for later discipline by hugging their child often, telling the child they love him or her, and holding him or her whenever the opportunity presents itself.

Early Childhood: Ages 2 through 5

One of the great joys of early childhood for parents is the ability to communicate verbally with their young person. This stage of development is a time of wonder and excitement over the little things in life that many adults take for granted. Parents should be encouraged to take the time to revel in these moments with their child, so that the small discoveries of the day are not dismissed as mundane.

Innocence in Early Childhood

Too many parents and caregivers treat young children in their care as if they were adults, and the harm that results can be difficult to repair. The most offensive of these mistakes is to damage a child's innocence, a term we use here in its most general sense. Damage to innocence can take many forms: inappropriate physical contact, emotional neglect (including verbal abuse), exposure to pornographic or violent images or behaviors, and unrealistic expectations that set up the child for failure. While sexual contact does occur with unnerving frequency, exposure to inappropriate words, images, or behaviors is almost universal. Parents will expose children to all sorts of inappropriate details in the interest of "honesty," particularly in materials meant to teach about human sexuality that read more like how-to manuals. The pediatrician can take the lead here, recommending more appropriate sex education materials like *The Miracle of Me from Conception to Birth* by Amy Pedersen and *Angel in the Waters* by Regina Doman, both of which are excellent for this age group.[25] The physician can also model the kind of language that preserves the child's innocence, even instituting a policy that bans use of vulgar language in the medical practice. Parents should be urged to remove objectionable materials from the child's home, including blocking television and Internet access to such material. Affronts to children's innocence must be taken seriously.

Parents may ask about children seeing their own naked bodies or those of siblings

---

25. Amy Pedersen, *The Miracle of Me from Conception to Birth* (Stockbridge, Mass.: Marian Press, 2007); and Regina Doman, *Angel in the Waters* (Manchester, N H.: Sophia Institute Press, 2004).

at home. While adults in the home should try to remain covered, they should not indicate that the natural state is cause for shame. As children become older, their modesty will develop naturally. Shaming children for nudity at this age sends the wrong message about the beauty of the body. There is a profound and obvious difference between nakedness without shame in young children or in classic art and the nudity of pornography; Michelangelo's *David* is a case in point. His nude body is a creation of God, but he is not on display for erotic pleasure. Pornography objectifies a person's body for the sensual pleasure of another; this "use" was described by Pope John Paul II, in his *Theology of the Body*, as the opposite of love.[26]

Unrealistic Expectations

The damage to a child's innocence from the overbearing parent or caregiver is under-recognized and harder to define; much depends on the individual child's temperament, developmental level, and intelligence. This is where open-ended questions and sound judgment are important. The physician can begin this conversation by asking parents what they want to change about life at home, or perhaps what annoys the parent most about the child's behavior. Simply asking the latter question, acknowledging that annoying behaviors exist, can be validating for parents. It is important to remember that adults who are perfectionists were raised by perfectionists. They especially need to hear the message that no one is perfect, that we all need mercy, compassion, and forgiveness. Does expecting perfection teach mercy or compassion? The two websites Marital Healing, and Child Healing: Strengthening Families have excellent resources for interested parents on this topic as well.[27]

Discipline in Early Childhood

The adage "don't cry over spilt milk" is a valuable lesson for parents and children alike. For parents, it might be amended to "don't get angry over spilled milk." The biggest mistakes of parental discipline are made when parents act in a state of anger; corporal punishment is a good example of this. Corporal punishment teaches children that the "law of the jungle applies"—the bigger, stronger person wins, and the weaker must be reduced to fear and helplessness. It teaches children to act on their anger in a nonconstructive way, and it is not as effective a form of discipline as praise for good behavior.

Discipline and punishment must be done without emotions.[28] "Time-out" is not meant to serve as a punishment itself, but provides time for both child and parent to cool down after an infraction. Parents should be reassured that young children may cry as a result of proper disciplinary actions; this is part of the pain of growing up and

---

26. See Pope John Paul II, *Man and Woman He Created Them: A Theology of the Body*, trans. Michael Waldstein (Boston: Pauline Books and Media, 2006).

27. http://www.maritalhealing.com and http://www.childhealing.com.

28. Bissonnette-Pitre and Vasa, "Authoritative Parenting," in *Healthy Families: Safe Children*, DVD.

learning, and is a signal for a parent to express compassion and love while remaining firm. Changing the rules because a child cries is not helpful and sets a bad precedent for future manipulation by the child. Parents should acknowledge those hurt feelings and follow up redirection and time-out with a hug and reassurance of the parent's love. Besides large helpings of praise for good behaviors, along with modeling good examples, stories can help children learn about good behaviors. The *Let's Talk About* series by Joy Berry is a source of stories about subjects such as selfishness, fighting, and disobedience, using examples and language that children easily understand.[29]

Some guidelines for effective early childhood discipline:

- Praise and rewards for good behaviors are the most effective discipline.
- In young children, redirection rather than punishment works well, but time-outs will be needed as a way to calm a child who is resistant.
- Redirection involves suggesting some better behaviors, allowing the child to choose.
- The child should get at least one warning to change a bad behavior before parents resort to time-out. In some cases, such as hitting, however, time-out can be immediate to cool down a volatile emotional state.
- The reason for a time-out or redirection must always be explained in the simplest way possible; one good gauge is to use the number of words of the child's age in years ("No biting" or "we don't hit").

For the parent who punishes too harshly, by yelling or spanking, admitting the mistake and asking for forgiveness benefits both parent and child. Both parties learn the lesson of humility, and more importantly, the child's doubts about parental love may be erased. In cases where parents repeatedly struggle to maintain their composure, anger management counseling may be necessary. From a medical perspective, anger is like a cancerous growth. Unless it is dealt with, it will continue to grow and consume the individual.

St. John Bosco wrote, "Discipline yourself first, and then you'll be fit to discipline the children."[30] Modeling good behavior is the most important part of instilling discipline, since children learn best by example. Bad behavior, as well, has a trickle-down effect: parents who act unjustly will raise unjust children, and those who are unfair will raise disrespectful children. Three distinct parenting styles can be identified: the authoritarian ("do as I say"), the permissive ("do whatever you want"), and the authoritative style, in which clear limits are set and the child is given limited choices (both good and bad). Authoritative parenting is the most challenging of these styles in practice, but research has shown it to be the most effective.[31] St. John Bosco com-

---

29. Joy Berry, *Let's Talk About* series (New York: Scholastic, 1982–2008).

30. St. John Bosco, "Youth Ministry and Parenting: Guiding Principles," in *Epistolario*, vol. 4 (Turin, 1959), 201–3, quoted from the Roman Missal, January 31, https://www.crossroadsinitiative.com/media/articles/youth-ministry-john-bosco.

31. See E. R. DeVore and K. R. Ginsburg, "The Protective Effects of Good Parenting on Adolescents," *Current Opinion in Pediatrics* 17 (2005): 460–65.

mented on this approach in an instruction to his fellow priests, who helped him to care for homeless boys: "It is easier to become angry than to restrain oneself, and to threaten a boy than persuade him."[32]

While Catholics and non-Catholics alike can agree on authoritative parenting, the Catholic worldview offers a specific rationale for following this parenting style. Catholic parents raise their children to be virtuous and to eventually go to heaven. To achieve this goal, children need guidance, rules (morals), and structure; this framework allows the child to feel secure and thus to thrive within clear and known boundaries. Structure also allows children to learn about nature and its consequences.[33] In a sense, they learn the natural law as they learn to control their own behavior over time.

Authoritative Parenting

When parents propose choices to a child, they should give a virtue as the reason behind the good choice. When a child has committed a transgression, the parent should give immediate feedback, and any punishment should be commensurate with the crime. The ideal punishment must teach a lesson, which ought to be less superficial than "be nice." It should identify the sin behind the crime, invoke the virtue that was not followed, and assist the child in discerning how to do better in the future, all in a developmentally appropriate way. Likewise, when a parent praises a job well done, identifying the virtue will teach the child that acting virtuously is deserving of praise. Parents can give immediate praise to a child when a good decision is made. Besides helping to condition the child's behavior, using moments of praise to identify the virtue will instill its meaning and associate it with praise and choosing well. This approach to discipline goes back to the book of Genesis, where God gave Adam and Eve a directive, allowed them choices, and warned them of the consequences of a bad choice (Gn 2:16–17). In Exodus, God gave his chosen people the Ten Commandments as guides for behavior (Ex 20:1–17; Dt 5:6–21); in Deuteronomy, he offered his people a choice between life and death and noted the consequence, urging them to "choose life, that you and your descendants may live" (Dt 30:19). While secular culture may disdain the Commandments, most reasonable people will admit that following these rules helps to maintain tranquility in the home and in the community.

In imagining their children's future, many parents harbor hopes of raising an Ivy League graduate, a Broadway star, or a professional athlete. But a child's virtue is infinitely more important than his or her GPA or batting average. The goal of a parent should be to raise a saint. This is a tough sell even to some Catholics, but it is important to encourage even secular parents to focus on raising a virtuous child who can be trusted with all things. The goal of raising a "nice" person is nebulous; permissive parenting that raises a child to do "whatever makes him happy" leads to an endless, fruitless search for meaning. The idea can be better understood if we speak

---

32. St. John Bosco, "Youth Ministry and Parenting: Guiding Principles."
33. See Bissonnette-Pitre and Vasa, "Authoritative Parenting," in *Healthy Families: Safe Children*, DVD.

of every child having a calling (we may even call it a vocation); the parent's job is to equip the child with the tools (education) and wisdom (discernment) to follow his or her calling. Education provides the tools—reading, writing, and arithmetic—with which children interact with the world, but it is not equivalent to wisdom. Instead, wisdom is a way of observing and processing, both intellectually and spiritually, what the world shows us.

Today's relativists see morality as evidence of rigid, restrictive thinking, instead of as a framework of principles and structure; this is where authoritative parenting diverges into the secular and Catholic worlds. Catholics recognize that it is good both to teach morals to a child and to attempt to live by them oneself. Wise parents teach the difference between right and wrong, allowing children to make increasingly complex decisions as they grow older and develop their ability to use reason.

Modeling Good Behaviors

Parents can and should model good behaviors, like problem solving, and virtues such as patience. Parents who set a good example will foster virtue in their children, and the best way to teach children is by example. An observant parent will notice his or her bad habits in the children as they grow; children will mimic bad habits regardless of where they are or who they are with.

Patience is a virtue that parents are wise to cultivate, despite the sacrifice it entails. When children misbehave, a patient parent can acknowledge the frustration they feel but still accept the sacrifice involved in not acting on those feelings. Such a parent can acknowledge and affirm a child's feelings better than a parent who is controlling or one who lacks self-control and acts on his or her emotions.[34]

Responding to a child's anger with anger will only frighten the child or feed the cycle of hostility. Confronting anger calmly but firmly defuses the negative emotion and teaches self-control. Love is rooted in sacrifice and self-denial, and thus it requires self-discipline. Any advice on discipline for parents with children of preschool age or older should include the importance of modeling how to work through differences in a civilized manner. Parents should make an effort to do the following:

- Work out differences in front of children. This will help teach them to compromise and to respect differences of opinion.
- Never raise their voices, especially when working out differences.
- Reassure the child that he or she is loved and that the argument was not about him or her.

---

34. See ibid.

Innocence and Unrealistic Expectations

In early childhood, the parent who pushes a child to perform is potentially harming the child's innocence with unrealistic expectations. Few parents do this purposely; they are simply living what they know. This kind of overbearing parenting can lead to psychological and emotional problems in both childhood and adolescence, which in turn can lead to such physical symptoms as fibromyalgia, irritable bowel syndrome, reflex neuropathic dystrophy, and pseudo-seizures. Treating these maladies requires a fuller understand of what it means to be loved unconditionally. It is helpful for the pediatrician to introduce the mind-body interaction and its role in child development as early as possible, while engaging in a medical work-up that is as limited as possible.

Diet in Early Childhood and Beyond

Good dietary habits are taught most easily in early childhood. Parents should be instructed to place a healthy meal in front of their child and, ideally, eat the healthy meal with him or her. Expecting a child to "clean the plate" is not the goal of a meal; it will eventually teach a child to eat whether or not he or she is hungry. It is good to leave the table hungry now and then; such a practice fights off gluttony. God created the senses of taste and smell so that we could enjoy food. Having too much food can cause health problems.

Like other issues of early childhood, healthy eating is best achieved in young children through the parents' example. Providing healthy meals can be difficult for parents who never learned the skill; for them, the USDA has a very useful website with recipes and information on healthy food choices.[35] Classes aimed at changing the diet and exercise habits of mothers have been shown to be effective in changing the eating habits of their families.[36] Linking diet and exercise with integrity of the body and mind is one way of getting some families to buy into healthy eating.

While sweets and unhealthy foods are fine in moderation, good foods should predominate in the home, so that they predominate in the diet. A house that is full of potato chips is likely to be full of potato chip eaters, whereas a house with plentiful fruit will be full of fruit eaters. Arming parents with knowledge involves teaching about healthy and balanced meals, and teaching that modeling healthy eating is more effective than trying to limit intake.[37]

In our endeavors to care for children's health, we need to introduce the concept of spiritual elements in addition to the physical. A Catholic worldview understands the importance of integrity of the physical (body), and the spiritual (soul). A disruption

---

35. See http://www.choosemyplate.gov.

36. See D. M. Klohe-Lehman et al., "Low-Income, Overweight and Obese Mothers as Agents of Change to Improve Food Choices, Fat Habits, and Physical Activity in their 1-to-3-Year-Old Children," *Journal of the American College of Nutrition* 26 (2007): 196–208.

37. See R. Brown and J. Ogden, "Children's Eating Attitudes and Behaviour: A Study of the Modeling and Control Theories of Parental Influence," *Health Education Research* 19 (2004): 261–71.

of either of these is an affront to both, as demonstrated by failure to thrive in children who are emotionally neglected or physically abused, as well as by the binging and purging seen in older children who suffer from bulimia.

There is a growing body of evidence in the medical literature that family meals are pivotal in children's lives. The frequency of family meals is inversely related to behavioral problems in adolescents and correlates positively with vegetable, fruit, grain, and calcium-rich food consumption in adolescents.[38] When families sit down together, they have an opportunity to share news and conversation, model good behavior, and encourage healthy food choices.

Books and Electronic Media in Early Child Development

Because the first five years are vital in the development of discipline and socialization, it makes sense for children to avoid the television and computer as much as possible, spending time instead in creative play or in some activity with a loving adult. Creative play need not be artistic in nature; even outdoor activities where a child uses his or her imagination can be considered creative play. The "let's pretend" years should be taken advantage of and relished. Simple and inexpensive items that can be found around the house are all a child this age needs to create a make-believe world.

Research has determined that electronic media in the first years of life has a negative effect on development,[39] and that watching violent programming is linked to aggressive behavior in boys as well as girls.[40] This is true despite marketing claims that some media products enhance the brain development of infants.[41] By contrast, reading to a child helps to foster language and social development, as it establishes a dialogue between reader and listener.

Pediatricians should encourage parents to make reading or storytelling time a priority and an everyday event, not just a bedtime activity. The child should be allowed to ask lots of questions, and the parents should be encouraged to ask open-ended

38. On the correlation to behavior, see J. A. Fulkerson et al., "Family Dinner Meal Frequency and Adolescent Development: Relationships with Developmental Assets and High-Risk Behaviors," *Journal of Adolescent Health* 39 (2006): 337–45. On the correlation to diet, see D. Neumark-Sztainer et al., "Family Meal Patterns: Associations with Sociodemographic Characteristics and Improved Dietary Intake among Adolescents," *Journal of the American Dietetic Association* 103 (2003): 317–22.

39. See F. J. Zimmerman and D. A. Christakis, "Children's Television Viewing and Cognitive Outcomes: A Longitudinal Analysis of National Data," *Archives of Pediatrics and Adolescent Medicine* 159 (2005): 619–25; F. J. Zimmerman, D. A. Christakis, and A. N. Meltzoff, "Associations between Media Viewing and Language Development in Children under Age 2 Years," *Journal of Pediatrics* 151 (2007): 364–68.

40. See D. A. Christakis and F. J. Zimmerman, "Violent Television Viewing during Preschool Is Associated with Antisocial Behavior during School Age," *Pediatrics* 120 (2007): 993–99; J. R. Milavsky et al., "Television and Aggression: Results of a Panel Study," in *Television and Behavior: Ten Years of Scientific Progress and Implications for the Eighties*, vol. 2, *Technical Reviews*, eds. D. Pearl, L. Bouthilet, and J. Lazar, DHHS Publication no. ADM 82-1196 (Washington, D.C.: U.S. Government Printing Office, 1982), 138–57, as cited in C. A. Anderson et al., "The Influence of Media Violence on Youth," *Psychological Science in the Public Interest* 4 (2003): 81–110.

41. See Zimmerman, Christakis, Meltzoff, "Association between Media Viewing and Language Development in Children under Age 2 Years."

questions. Parents can begin reading books with a message early as well, although the primary goal is language and intellectual development. Children's books need not always have a moral message, but children deserve great books since "we become the books we read."[42] The goal is to provide a treasured memory of physical closeness, along with a learning experience.

Electronic Media

Discouraging the use of "educational media" at this age is crucial. Passive viewing of electronic media, or its use as "background noise," throws up barriers to real conversational exchange. Would parents expect their pediatrician to talk to them with a television in the background? This is the age at which habits are formed, and these are the most vital years for the foundation of relationships and discipline. Pediatricians can foster a love of reading by providing a free book at each office visit or by keeping at the desk a supply of applications for library cards. Reading lists of recommended books can be available as office handouts or posted online at the office's website. An excellent list that is comprehensive for all age groups is *A Mother's List of Books*, by Theresa Fagan.[43]

One special situation of note is the military parent who is deployed far from home. The USO sponsors a United Through Reading program with books provided by First Books, which allows a parent to read a book and record it on DVD so that it can be played to the child or children at home.[44]

Play in Early Childhood: Parallel Play

What escapes many and is explained by few pediatricians is the phenomenon of parallel play in toddlers and preschool children. During these early years, children are engaged in play that is both imitative and creative. Children should be given the tools to explore their environment and the opportunity to play outdoors, an activity that is sadly in decline.[45] Early childhood toys should be simple; while electronic gadgets may be fun and stimulating in the short term, a child's imagination can turn a box into anything. Many parents are tempted to seek out daycare in an effort to provide playmates for their young children, but except in cases where a parent is unable to care for the child because of health reasons, the home environment is usually more than adequate.

---

42. M. Kelly, *The Seven Levels of Intimacy* (Sycamore, Ill.: Lighthouse Catholic Media, NFP, 2011).

43. Theresa Fagan, *A Mother's List of Books* (Chevy Chase, Md.: Theresa Fagan, 2009).

44. http://www.unitedthroughreading.org.

45. See R. Clements, "An Investigation of the Status of Outdoor Play," *Contemporary Issues in Early Childhood* 5 (2004): 68–80.

Middle Childhood: Ages 6 through 11

Starting at age 7, when children are able to discern right from wrong, the lessons of self-care that were started in early childhood can be solidified. Much can be accomplished in the child's character formation. The child of this age is reading and learning on his or her own. Once the child can use reason, parents may take a more Socratic approach, asking leading questions to help the child reach conclusions about his or her behavior. This method facilitates learning how to make good choices and fosters moral development.[46] Parents should be urged to expect great things of their children. This does not mean parents should expect their child to throw a 100 mph fastball, or be at the top of the class; this kind of excellence means always doing one's best, making every day count, and avoiding experiences that do not elevate the soul. The pediatrician can serve as a resource by posting in the office a list of educational venues or events that offer free activities for families. Middle childhood is an important stage for parents to spend a lot of time with their child, applying love in generous portions; time invested in the relationship now will go a long way to protecting the child in adolescence.

Sports, Organized and Otherwise

In a perfect world, team sports allow children in middle childhood to have fun, interact with friends or classmates, exercise, and experience the influence of a role model—the coach. Our culture, however, has allowed organized sports for children to become an obsession for parents and coaches, and this mindset has filtered down to the young players. The rising incidence of sports injuries in younger children today is evidence of this: young children stop when something hurts, unless pushed on by an overbearing coach or parent. Some parents, even at this stage in their child's life, are looking forward to a possible college athletic scholarship. The pediatrician should confront these inflated expectations directly, asking parents to identify the purpose of their child's participation in organized sport. The bottom line question is "how will participation in these activities make your child a better person?" The primary goals of organized athletics should be exercise and fun. If the sports league's primary focus is skill acquisition, parents should think twice about enrolling their child. Though playing a team sport may teach the value of hard work, dedication, self-sacrifice, and teamwork, such virtues may also be taught in the home, especially where chores are often part of a child's daily routine.

Team sports in middle childhood do provide some benefits:

- The habit of frequent exercise teaches one how to stay in shape.
- Making mistakes and losing teach one how to cope with setbacks, both personally and communally.

46. See M. Kelly, *Building Better Families: 5 Practical Ways to Build Family Spirituality* (Sycamore, Ill.: Lighthouse Catholic Media, 2009), audiobook.

- Teamwork helps people of varying talents work together toward a common goal.
- Sports have rules, and athletes who follow them learn to control impulses.
- Learning to be a good sport means competing without bearing grudges or ill will.
- Winning is not everything.
- Having fun and doing one's best are the most important lessons of playing a sport.

Young prepubescent athletes are at higher risk for repetitive motion injuries; those who compete in the same sport throughout the year face a greater chance for these injuries than those who change activities from season to season. Participation in team sports can be fun for a child, but it can also be a distraction from the more important aspects of life, such as school, family, faith, and friends. For some families, the sport becomes the center of family life, and children are caught in an identity trap: they are defined by what they do and not by who they are.

The Challenges of Electronic Media

The impact of television on children's everyday lives was vividly demonstrated in a 1973 study by T. M. Williams, which examined the population of a remote British Columbia town before and after the introduction of television. Her findings showed that exposure to television led to decreased creativity, impaired acquisition of reading skills, and decreased participation in nontelevision leisure activities.[47] The Center for Screen Time Awareness, recognizing the difficulties families face in giving up television, promotes Game Nights and Turn Off weeks in an effort to promote social engagement within families and communities.[48] Families are encouraged to pick a specific night every week or month on which electronics are turned off and the family spends time together playing board games, taking a walk, or engaging in another enriching activity. Parents who decide to allow television in their homes should take advantage of content screening tools such as the Parents Television Council website and books such as *Raising Kids in the Media Age*, by Jay Dunlap.[49]

Watching television is a passive activity that discourages social interaction between the viewers and does little to build healthy relationships. Healthier choices include visiting the local library or park, making a craft, looking at books, or talking about hopes and dreams.[50]

Parents who restrict their child's access to electronic media may face pressure from the child or from other parents to allow viewing of content they deem inappropriate.

47. See *The Impact of Television: A Natural Experiment in Three Communities*, ed. T. M. Williams (New York: Academic Press, 1986).

48. http://unplugyourkids.com.

49. http://www.parentstv.org/welcome.asp; Jay Dunlap, *Raising Kids in the Media Age* (Hamden, Conn.: Circle Press, 2008).

50. See Kelly, *The Seven Levels of Intimacy*.

Catholic pediatricians must support those parents who protect their children from this content. Violent images on television or computer games show the child that the world is a scary place and, in effect, rob the child of his or her childhood innocence. A large body of evidence points to the negative effects of media violence. Aggressive behavior has been linked to the absorption of violent media even in low-risk individuals.[51] One disturbing finding is that violence often occurs in content that is not obviously labeled "violent," such as in movies classified as comedies.[52]

Guarding young eyes from inappropriate content in movies is more challenging in the age of DVD home delivery and streaming online content. Parents who wish to eliminate exposure to indecency in films have many resources at their disposal; these include the free websites of the Dove Foundation and Movie Guide, as well as the movie review site sponsored by movie critic Michael Medved and the fee-based website screenit.[53]

The Importance of Play

Creative play is vital for children; they need time for activities that are interesting and require imagination. Leisure and play can serve as a time for bonding between the child and parent or other important adult, and will shape the child as much as, if not more than, school work. The author Eric Hoffer has observed:

Art is older than production for use, and play older than work. Man was shaped less by what he had to do than by what he did in playful moments. It is the child in man that is the source of his uniqueness and creativeness, and the playground is the optimal milieu for the unfolding of his capacities.[54]

Creative, child-centered activities such as hobbies can provide an ideal environment for this kind of growth. Because of electronic media's influence, along with over-filling children's schedules with adult-structured activities, participation in hobbies has been on a downswing in recent years.[55] Hobbies do not need to be expensive or equipment-intensive: a child who likes to draw does not need an easel and watercolors, but can have a creative outlet with crayons and scrap paper. The focus of leisure should be re-creation, activities that give our bodies and souls the rest they need and deserve. This kind of recreation shifts the focus away from activities aimed at placing the child ahead of his or her peers.

In families in postindustrial America, many children live with one parent, or both parents work outside of the home; as a result, some children spend a considerable

51. See P. Boxer et al., "The Role of Violent Media Preference in Cumulative Developmental Risk for Violence and General Aggression," *Journal of Youth and Adolescence* 38 (2009): 417–28.

52. See W. D. McIntosh et al., "What's So Funny about a Poke in the Eye? The Prevalence of Violence in Comedy Films and Its Relation to Social and Economic Threat in the United States, 1951–2000," *Mass Communication and Society* 6 (2003): 345–60.

53. http://www.dove.org, http://www.movieguide.org, http://www.michaelmedved.com, http://www.screenit.com.

54. Eric Hoffer, *Reflections on the Human Condition* (New York: Harper and Row, 1973), 20.

55. See Clements, "An Investigation of the Status of Outdoor Play." 73–75.

chunk of each day unsupervised. For these children, the Internet and television often provide companionship and escape, albeit not of the best kind, given the content of programs and websites that children can access. This is where a hobby, especially one that requires little adult supervision, can fill otherwise idle hours and provide a far greater sense of accomplishment and satisfaction, while keeping both mind and body busy and out of mischief. Adults can give children room to stretch creatively on their own, yet still be involved by sharing the fruits of the child's efforts and offering insight into the child's progress. A final word about hobbies and all the activities of childhood: they should be reflective of great things, not just good things. The words of St. Paul echo this: "whatsoever things are true, whatsoever modest, whatsoever just, whatsoever holy, whatsoever lovely, whatsoever of good fame, if there be any virtue, if any praise of discipline, think on these things" (Phil 4:8).[56]

Preparing for Adolescence

One of the more difficult decisions for parents is when to discuss human sexuality with their child. Children in early or middle childhood can learn about simple anatomy and function, but the push for early graphic sex education is both an assault to the child's innocence and an "easy out" for the adults in the child's life. The body often matures earlier than the psyche, and, once the maturation process starts, graphic sex education serves as little more than titillation. Such lessons should not start with anatomy and end with lessons in sexual technique, all in the same conversation. A parent should arm the child with information about the parts of the body, not just the genitals, and how they work. Children can also learn about the beauty of the body in art, and the beauty of marital love, without graphic descriptions of intercourse.

Books about sexual development should never be offered to children in a vacuum: parents need to be proactive, talking beforehand about what the child will read and then following up with discussion afterward. This is a conversation that deserves to be scheduled ahead of time so it is not given short shrift. A helpful guide for Catholic parents is "The Truth and Meaning of Human Sexuality: Guidelines for Education within the Family" by the Pontifical Council for the Family.[57] It is not a curriculum to explain sexual development, but offers a roadmap for structuring this discussion in a developmentally appropriate way. Since not all books on sexual development written for children are acceptable and appropriate, parents should be cautioned to be selective. These are among the books that help explain the maturation process of puberty without damaging the child's innocence:

Beyond the Birds and the Bees by Gregory Popcak;
Before I Was Born by Carol Nystrom (may be too verbally graphic for the recommended age range of 5 to 8 years);

---

56. Douay Rheims translation.
57. http://www.vatican.va/roman_curia/pontifical_councils/family/documents/rc_pc_family_doc_08121995_human-sexuality_en.html.

Parents, Children and the Facts of Life by Rev. Harry V. Sattler;
The Joyful Mysteries of Life by Catherine Scherrer and Bernard Scherrer.[58]

Adolescence

Character Formation and Discipline

During the adolescent years, character formation is challenged by expanding freedoms and growing social pressures. Good listening, though often difficult, is a key skill for the parent to cultivate in these years. When parents make space in the family schedule for one-on-one time and family time, especially at mealtime, they are creating a favorable environment for listening. While it is true that teenagers become incrementally more autonomous in making choices for themselves, they need guidance from caring adults more than ever. True freedom involves responsibility and is not merely carte blanche to "do what you want." Parents or physicians who adopt the latter approach abdicate their responsibility for the young person. The need for guidance does not end at the age of 18; as recent research indicates, brain development is not complete until sometime between ages 23 and 25.[59] The author Matthew Kelly has explained how behaviors affect an individual's character:

If you can tell me what your habits are, I can tell you what sort of person you are. If you can tell me what your habits are, I can tell you what your future looks like. Because habits create character, and your character is your destiny. Good habits create good character, and create a wonderful destiny. Bad habits create bad character and create misery in our future.[60]

Parents of adolescents, just like parents with elementary school–aged children, may be conflicted about cultural exposure to media, saying they want their children to be "normal." Whether or not media influences adolescents is still debatable, since most of today's parents were raised with television images and musical lyrics that do not reflect their deeply held beliefs, and they seem immune to it. Even so, it is important to recommend exposing adolescents to art and music forms that are classical and thus counter-cultural. They need a counterpoint to the pop culture message that having more—more things, more food, more sex—will lead to happiness. True happiness cannot be found in food or sex, and those who seek it there are destined to misuse these sensual pleasures.

For secular families who understand the dangers of the culture, one figure to hold up as an example is Mohandas Gandhi, who is still an influential figure many years after his assassination. Gandhi considered these traits the most spiritually perilous to humanity:

---

58. Gregory Popcak, *Beyond the Birds and the Bees* (West Chester, Penn: Ascension Press, 2012); Carol Nystrom, *Before I Was Born* (Colorado Springs, Colo.: NavPress, 2007); Rev. Harry V. Sattler, *Parents, Children and the Facts of Life* (Patterson, N.J.: Saint Anthony's Guild, 1952); Catherine Scherrer and Bernard Scherrer, *The Joyful Mysteries of Life* (San Francisco: Ignatius Press, 1997).

59. See American College of Pediatricians, "The Teenage Brain: Under Construction," American College of Pediatricians Best for Children, 2016, http://www.acpeds.org/The-Teenage-Brain-Under-Construction.html.

60. Kelly, *Building Better Families.*

Wealth without Work
Pleasure without Conscience
Science without Humanity
Knowledge without Character
Politics without Principle
Commerce without Morality
Worship without Sacrifice[61]

Though he was not Christian, Gandhi's words echo the seven deadly sins familiar to Catholics. For adolescents, reading works of great literature is one way to learn these truths. Since public schools use the "great books" less and less, pediatricians should arm parents with a list of these so that they can encourage children to read them at home. William Shakespeare, C. S. Lewis and J. R. R. Tolkien are just a few examples of great Christian writers. Other excellent books for this age level can be found in "A Mother's List of Books."[62]

Even more important than great books to the adolescent's character formation is the virtuous behavior of parents. Virtues are expressed through actions, and they have a broad appeal to non-Christian or anti-Christian parents. Fr. Robert Barron has compiled a contrasting list of "lively virtues" as antidotes for the seven deadly sins:

Humility vs. Pride
Admiration vs. Envy
Forgiveness vs. Anger
Zeal vs. Sloth
Generosity vs. Greed
Asceticism vs. Gluttony
Chastity vs. Lust[63]

Character formation and discipline go hand-in-hand; self-discipline goes a step further. A young person's self-discipline has a powerful impact on his or her academic achievement. Research has shown that self-discipline has more of an effect than IQ on an adolescent's grades, time spent on homework, school attendance, and the time of day when the student begins to do homework.[64]

Character Formation and Sexuality

It is imperative that pediatricians encourage parents to discuss sexual development with preteens and sexuality with teens, to counter the prevailing cultural attitudes. In the Catholic view, sex is far from dirty: it is a gift to be saved for marriage and used responsibly. Waiting to have sex until one is married makes it special rather than

61. M. K. Gandhi, http://www.deadlysins.com/features/gandhi.htm.

62. Fagan, *A Mother's List of Books*.

63. R. Barron, *Seven Deadly Sins, Seven Lively Virtues* (Sycamore, Ill.: Lighthouse Catholic Media, NFP, 2011), audiobook.

64. See A. L. Duckworth and M. E. P. Seligman, "Self Discipline Outdoes IQ in Predicting Academic Performance of Adolescents," *Psychological Science* 16 (2005): 939–44.

dirty, and represents "a proper ordering of the sexual passions and sensuality."[65] These conversations between parent and child should be an ongoing dialogue, starting out with the basics and progressing to more detail of what God's plan entails. For atheist or agnostic parents who are open to the message of chastity, the concept of giving the self as a gift is still relevant. Risk mitigation should not be the message's main point, but rather respect for one's self and for the other. The argument against using another individual is one that can be universally understood, like all lessons about virtue. Living chastely allows one to see the true beauty in all persons and frees one from slavery to passions. The primary goal of chastity is purity in thoughts and deeds; the additional goals, if the person marries, include lifelong fidelity to one's spouse and a wonderful, fulfilling sex life. Young people can reach these goals if they learn about the beauty of marital love and understand that delaying gratification is worth the wait.

Parents can and should talk to their adolescents about remaining pure even if they did not themselves. Adolescents do not need to have a parent who was pure, only one who believes purity is right. A parent who lives a life of good moral choices is helping to foster morality in an adolescent. When parents say they are uncomfortable discussing chastity because of their own youthful indiscretions, the pediatrician should remind them that they need not disclose this. The more important aspect is not what they did but what they expect. In addition, these parents may feel some relief to know that their own experience may give them a good perspective on what leads adolescents to be unchaste.

Case: The Birds and the Bees

The mother of a 15-year-old boy asks the pediatrician to "have the talk with him." She explains in front of him that she knows he is having sex, because "as his mother I can tell." She also says that she has asked him, but he denies being sexually active. The boy lives with his mother and his maternal grandmother; his mother reports that he sees his father only at church on Sundays. After the mother leaves the room, the boy reveals that he is sexually active with a girl the same age whom he met at church.

Discussion: A mother who makes a request like this is not generally asking the physician to convince her child to be chaste. Parents who are permissive about sex may want a physician to hand out condoms for protection against STDs and birth control pills to help prevent pregnancy. Faced with this request, a secular pediatrician will ask a parent to leave the room and go on to discuss moral-free sexuality with the adolescent. Permissive parents and pediatricians usually have the viewpoint that teens will have sex no matter what, so they might as well be safe. Before the Catholic pediatrician tackles this subject, he or she should ask parents what they expect to be discussed and determine their frame of reference. If parents are permissive about sex, a message centered on chastity will not be supported at home. The realities are that premarital sex is more common today than it was prior to the widespread use

---

65. Barron, *Seven Deadly Sins, Seven Lively Virtues.*

and availability of contraceptives; that adolescents have a bad track record with the use of condoms and birth control pills; and that the increase in premarital sex may be due to risk compensation—taking greater risks when one perceives the risks as lower because of technology. However, condoms are far from perfect protection, and adolescents who engage in sex at an early age are at extremely high risk (in part due to cumulative risk) for pregnancy, STDs, marital dissolution later in life, and having children who grow up in poverty.[66] In addition, the safer-sex message shows an intellectual disconnect between prevention and risk. We would not tell a teen he can carry a gun if he wears a bulletproof vest, or that she can smoke as long as she only smokes filtered cigarettes. Why then does secular medicine regard adolescent premarital sex as fine so long as the participants use protection?

This young man can be educated about the world around him, and the Socratic method can allow him to reach his own conclusions about chastity in ways he can understand. The questions might include: What do you want to do with your life? Do you want to attend college or trade school, to travel and see the world? Do you see yourself married to this girl? Can you pursue your dreams if you father a child? Do you love this girl? Do you want what's best for her? Will it be easy to spend time with her and not engage in intercourse? Would it be best to stop seeing her, since it will be much more difficult to avoid having intercourse with her now? When you do have a date, what are some better ways to spend time with a girl so that it does not lead to intercourse?

Human Papilloma Virus Vaccine

Perhaps no other immunization since Jenner's smallpox injection has raised the public's ire as much as the recently introduced human papilloma virus vaccine. Proponents claim that it will prevent cervical cancer in women by preventing infection with the HPV strains linked to the development of cancer. A study showing a reduction in cancer per se has not been done; efficacy trials of the vaccine actually utilized sex workers and measured HPV acquisition. It is presumed, probably rightly so, that preventing infection with the virus will prevent the latent stage which later leads to cancer. But an efficacy trial with this endpoint would require many years, since the latency period can be quite long. Still, it may be disingenuous to make cancer prevention the thrust of its use and the promise behind promotional campaigns.

The number of people who are infected with these viruses is astronomical, dwarfing the number of HIV infections. While a recent study showed that condoms provide some protection from HPV,[67] recommending condom use to reduce risk again reveals an intellectual disconnect with other medical advice. The advice is akin to accepting this patient's bad choices. Despite the evidence from many studies about

66. See S. E. Wills, "Condoms and AIDS: Is the Pope Right or Just 'Horrifically Ignorant'?" *Linacre Quarterly* 77 (2010): 17–29.

67. See C. M. Nielson et al., "Consistent Condom Use Is Associated with Lower Prevalence of Human Papillomavirus Infection in Men," *Journal of Infectious Diseases* 202 (2010):445–51.

the ineffectiveness of condoms at preventing many STDs, the current advice of most physicians and the party line of most professional bodies is to advise the use of condoms.[68] Apart from the ineffectiveness of this barrier, areas of skin not covered by a condom can pass the virus to a sexual partner.

Since the introduction of the vaccine, a number of school districts have added HPV to their list of mandated vaccines, and in 2007 an executive order from the governor of Texas briefly mandated it statewide until the legislature quickly rescinded it. The Catholic Church has always recognized that we are a fallen people subject to temptations of the flesh; in addition, the *Catechism* exhorts us to preserve our health. Based primarily on this latter argument, the Catholic Medical Association has made a statement approving the vaccine's use in late adolescence, as opposed to the age of eleven originally recommended by the Centers for Disease Control's Advisory Committee on Immunization Practices.[69]

Administering this vaccine provokes some questions about the child's readiness to discuss sexual development. The best judges of the child's readiness are the parents, and even they may be unsure of the exact right time.

Case: HPV Vaccination

A mother is concerned about her 9-year-old daughter and asks the pediatrician about the new HPV vaccine. She is hesitant to use this vaccine because she wants to teach her daughter to save sex until marriage, and is afraid of talking to her about the vaccine because her daughter shows no interest in boys.

Discussion: Some pediatricians insist on giving the vaccine at the youngest age possible and will discuss "safe sex" with the patient. This is a one-size-fits-all approach, but not all 10- or 11-year-olds are ready to have that discussion. The mother in this case is taking a thoughtful approach. Parents are the child's first teachers, and in most cases they know better than the physician when the child is ready to learn more about sex. The best time to delve into details about sex is different for every child, but it should wait until the child has started to show signs of pubertal development. Since emotional and psychological maturation lag behind physical maturation, the discussions should take place over time, starting with basic information and gradually expanding into details.

One concern that has been dismissed by the vaccine's proponents is the problem of risk compensation: individuals will take greater risks when they perceive they are being protected by technology. This has been demonstrated in the sexual risk-taking behavior of homosexual men and IV drug users in light of the availability of highly active retroviral therapy.[70] In this case, allowing the parent, or the parent and the

---

68. See J. R. Mann, C. C. Stine, and J. Vessey, "The Role of Disease-Specific Infectivity and Number of Disease Exposures on Long-Term Effectiveness of the Latex Condom," *Sexually Transmitted Diseases* 29 (2002): 344–49; V. Kataja et al., "Risk Factors Associated with Cervical Human Papillomavirus Infections: A Case-Control Study," *American Journal of Epidemiology* 138 (1993): 735–45.

69. See Catholic Medical Association, "Position Paper on HPV Immunization" (2007), http://www.cathmed.org/assets/files/Position%20Paper%20on%20HPV%20Immunization.pdf.

70. See Wills, "Condoms and AIDS."

adolescent, to decide about the vaccine once she has reached her eighteenth birthday is optimal.

Chastity

Chastity falls under the cardinal virtue of temperance, the use of reason to control the passions.[71] Mastering the passions is a lifelong process, one that requires more work during the process of formation in childhood and adolescence.[72] The chaste person has fully integrated the physical and spiritual aspects of sexuality and has learned to balance freedom with responsibility.[73] The human heart cannot be at peace when mastered by passions; such a path is self-destructive. Consciously choosing the good and freely following reason rather than passion imparts dignity upon the person through developing power over base human tendencies.[74] The chaste person's achievement of this dignity may be personal, but it also has a positive impact on society.[75]

Chastity and Friendship

Chastity blossoms within friendship, so it is wise to encourage adolescents and parents to forge friendships with people who share their beliefs and views;[76] such friendships offer moral encouragement and social support that makes choosing the good an easier task.[77] Love is about acceptance.[78] A child who does not feel accepted by the parent will seek acceptance elsewhere, possibly with a group of "friends" who expose the child to alcohol, cigarettes, drugs, sex, or some form of victimization. The message of chastity starts with this message of love established by parental acceptance.

Parents must provide ample monitoring of their children's friendships, as friends can have a profound effect on children. While having friends with a similar moral outlook can have a positive effect, the opposite is also true. Studies indicate that children or adolescents who engage in risky behaviors are a risk factor for such behaviors in their close friends.[79] This is particularly true for sexual activity, and it still applies if an adolescent *perceives* that peers are sexually active, even if they are not.[80]

71. See *Catechism of the Catholic Church*, no. 2341.

72. Ibid., no. 2342.

73. Ibid., no. 2337.

74. Ibid., no. 2339.

75. Ibid, no. 2344.

76. Ibid., no. 2347.

77. See A. Adamczyk and J. Felson, "Friends' Religiosity and First Sex," *Social Science Research* 35 (2006): 924–47.

78. See Kelly, *Building Better Families*.

79. See S. B. Kinsman et al., "Early Sexual Initiation: The Role of Peer Norms," *Pediatrics* 102 (1998):1185–92.

80. See U. Upadhyay and M. Hindin, "Do Perceptions of Friends' Behaviors Affect Age at First Sex? Evidence from Cebu, Philippines," *Journal of Adolescent Health* 39 (2006): 570–77.

Helping Parents Teach the Message of Chastity

Today, children experience sex visually on television, and in magazines, movies, and the Internet; and they hear music with demeaning or sexually suggestive lyrics. As adolescents spend less time with family, limiting their exposure requires repeated discussion about why certain lyrics or images are wrong and how to walk away from them, turn them off, or avoid them. This requires young people to develop self-discipline; yet the delayed gratification of chastity is not just about sex, but about self-control in general.

Teaching a teen to be chaste involves spending time growing together in Christ through the everyday activities of playing, praying, eating, talking, and above all listening. Communication is crucial in setting clear rules, discussing what is right and wrong, and teaching the adolescent how to refuse sexual temptation.[81] This does not involve a simple, one-time talk. When parents repeatedly express expectations, stay on message, and listen carefully, an adolescent will feel closer to parents and be better able to talk with them.[82]

Adolescents who perceive parental communication as good are less likely to become sexually active.[83] Studies also indicate that a healthy parental marriage relationship helps prevent the teen from engaging in premarital sex.[84] The Catholic pediatrician should remind mothers and fathers that time spent keeping the marriage healthy is a good investment in the child. Many simple, everyday actions can promote marital intimacy: holding hands, talking every day, telling each other "I love you" often and in front of the children, and never going to bed angry—as St. Paul said to the Church in Ephesus, "do not let the sun go down on your anger" (Eph 4:26).

Guidance for parents can be found in a number of books and websites. *Raising Pure Teens*, by Jason Evert and Chris Stefanick, takes a direct approach and includes a practical resource section with advice on technology for monitoring an adolescent's computer activity, including unsolicited messages.[85] Parents or parishes interested in a sex education curriculum will find the Respect, Inc., website to be a good resource.[86]

A number of books can help parents who want to promote a chaste life for their adolescent, although the same caveat mentioned above applies here: such books should not be presented without before-and-after discussion between parent and child. Some of these books are

---

81. See C. B. Aspy et al., "Parental Communication and Youth Sexual Behavior," *Journal of Adolescence* 30 (2007): 449–66.

82. See S. C. Martino et al., "Beyond the 'Big Talk': The Roles of Breadth and Repetition in Parent-Adolescent Communication about Sexual Topics," *Pediatrics* 121 (2008): e612–e618.

83. See P. S. Karofsky, L. Zeng, and M. R. Kosorok, "Relationship between Adolescent–Parental Communication and Initiation of First Intercourse by Adolescents," *Journal of Adolescent Health* 28 (2000): 41–45.

84. See M. Cunningham and A. Thorton, "The Influence of Parents' Marital Quality on Adult Children's Attitudes toward Marriage and Its Alternatives: Main and Moderating Effects," *Demography* 43 (2006): 659–72.

85. See Jason Evert and Chris Stefanick, *Raising Pure Teens* (El Cajon, Calif.: Catholic Answers, 2010).

86. http://www.sexrespect.com.

If You Really Loved Me, by Jason Evert (written in a question-and-answer format
    with a distinctly Catholic viewpoint. It is too graphic for preteens.)
Sex and the New You, by Richard Bimler (for early adolescence)
Sex and the New You: For Young Men 13–15, by Richard Bimler
How to Find Your Soulmate without Losing Your Soul, by Jason Evert and Crys-
    talina Evert (aimed at young women)
Theology of His Body/Theology of Her Body, by Jason Evert (two books in one;
    distinctly Catholic and frank without being explicit. Useful throughout ado-
    lescence but not a beginner's book.)[87]

Chastity of the Senses

Our culture values heroism, but it overlooks the daily grind of self-sacrifice required
by love. Young people need to hear, over and over, that love is about sacrifice, not
about getting what they want from others. Secular sex education teaches about sex
and contraceptives, isolated from any message about the adolescent's value as an individual. Even the American Psychological Association recognizes the trend; it recently
published a paper warning that the mass media's portrayal of women has a negative
impact on young women's self-image.[88]

The Catholic view rejects neither the beauty of the body nor the reality of desire, but it does demand that sexual desire be disciplined. Jesus taught that looking at
someone with lust was committing adultery in one's heart (Mt 5:27–28). Our Lord
read the human heart and understood what it meant to be human; even so, his statement did not sit well with his listeners, and today it is rejected outright. The women
of Christ's time were dressed modestly by any standards; if their male contemporaries
had difficulty fighting off impure thoughts about women in such modest clothing,
does it make sense to flaunt the human body in revealing garments? Current evidence
bears out Jesus' counsel: adolescents exposed to high levels of sex on television had
twice the likelihood of initiating sexual activity over a one-year period,[89] and twice
the likelihood of experiencing a pregnancy in a three-year period.[90] It only follows,
then, that other forms of media with sexual content increase the likelihood of intercourse as well.[91]

---

87. Jason Evert, *If You Really Loved Me* (El Cajon, Calif.: Catholic Answers, 2009); Richard Bimler, *Sex and the New You* (St. Louis, Mo.: Concordia Publishing House, 1998); Richard Bimler, *Sex and the New You: For Young Men 13–15* (St. Louis, Mo.: Concordia Publishing House, 2008); Jason Evert and Crystalina Evert, *How to Find Your Soulmate without Losing Your Soul* (San Diego: Totus Tuus Press, 2011); Jason Evert, *Theology of His Body/Theology of Her Body* (West Chester, Penn.: Ascension Press, 2009).

88. American Psychological Association, Task Force on the Sexualization of Girls, *Report of the APA Task Force on the Sexualization of Girls* (Washington, D.C.: American Psychological Association, 2007), http://www.apa.org/pi/wpo/sexualization.html.

89. See R. L. Collins et al., "Watching Sex on Television Predicts Adolescent Initiation of Sexual Behavior," *Pediatrics* 114 (2004): e280–e289.

90. See A. Chandra et al., "Does Watching Sex on Television Predict Teen Pregnancy? Findings from a National Longitudinal Survey of Youth," *Pediatrics* 112 (2008): 1047–54.

91. See J. D. Brown et al., "Sexy Media Matter: Exposure to Sexual Content in Music, Movies, Television, and Magazines Predicts Black and White Adolescents' Sexual Behavior," *Pediatrics* 117 (2006): 1018–27.

The sexual content of television has been on the increase in recent years, and the content has become more explicit.[92] Although the entertainment industry denies any link between its portrayals of certain behaviors and subsequent behaviors in children, the results of numerous studies refute this claim.[93] Statistics associated with sexual content should especially concern the Catholic pediatrician. Children ages 12 to 14 who experience high levels of exposure to sexual media content are more than twice as likely to have sexual intercourse by the time they are 16 than children who are exposed to the lowest levels of these media.[94] If parents doubt this link, the pediatrician should point out that corporations pay millions of dollars to advertise because they understand television's effect on people's behaviors.

Parents who want to fight the culture can create a home environment that nurtures respect for the body; limits on television viewing are a necessary step in this process. A 2008 study showed that adolescents who reported screen time limits and higher levels of parental disapproval of watching television did not initiate oral or vaginal sex as frequently as the group with more lenient attitudes or limits. In addition, co-viewing was found to be protective against the initiation of sexual activity, perhaps because parents can express disapproval of the images or messages they watch with their teens.[95]

Chastity of the Senses: Speech and Music

A person's character is judged by his or her words, and the use of profanity or immodest speech is a sign of indiscretion. If someone is unable to show restraint in speech, what other behaviors might he or she have trouble restraining? Parents have the right to insist on decent use of language from their son or daughter's dates, as an indicator that the young person can be trusted. They should also teach their own children that using profanity will not help a person get or keep a job, and it causes listeners to lose the message of one's words. One study showed that individuals were less likely to acquire the content or follow the instructions of a videotaped instructor who used profanity.[96] Another study found that students were less willing to go to a counselor for help after listening to an audiotape of that counselor using profanity in a counseling session, and that counselors who used profanity were rated as less effective by their clients.[97]

92. See J. D. Brown, K. Walsh Childers, and C. Waszak, "Television and Adolescent Sexuality," *Journal of Adolescent Health Care* 11 (1990): 62–70.

93. See S. Villani, "Impact of Media on Children and Adolescents: A 10-Year Review of the Research," *Journal of the American Academy of Child and Adolescent Psychiatry* 40 (2001): 392–401; K. L. L'Engle, J. D. Brown, and K. Kenneavy, "The Mass Media Are an Important Context for Adolescents' Sexual Behavior," *Journal of Adolescent Health* 38 (2006): 186–92; Collins, Elliott, Berry, Kanouse, Kunkel, Hunter, and Miu, "Watching Sex on Television Predicts Adolescent Initiation of Sexual Behavior."

94. See Brown, L'Engle, Pardun, et al., "Sexy Media Matter."

95. See M. Bersamin et al., "Parenting Practices and Adolescent Sexual Behavior: A Longitudinal Study," *Journal of Marriage and the Family* 70 (2008): 97–112.

96. See L. Sazer and H. Kassinove, "Effects of Counselor's Profanity and Subject's Religiosity on Content Acquisition of a Counseling Lecture and Behavioral Compliance," *Psychological Reports* 69 (1991): 1059–70.

97. See J. L. Kottke and C. D. MacLeod, "Use of Profanity in the Counseling Interview," *Psychological Reports* 65 (1989): 627–34.

If speech has such an effect on listeners, music's effect is exponentially greater. The lyrics of popular music often portray the culture's distorted view of sexuality, and research has confirmed that adolescents who listened to more music with sexually degrading lyrics advanced more quickly into coital and non-coital sexual activity.[98] In a study of college-aged adolescents, listening to music with lyrics deemed misogynous was shown to cause increased aggression in males toward females.[99] While some parents might contend that they listened to sexually charged music and "turned out okay," Catholic pediatricians need to arm parents with these statistics and help them recognize that the slope is indeed slippery.

Chastity of the Senses: Pornography

No discussion of chastity of the senses would be complete without some discussion of pornography. The goal of pornography is to display the model as an object of sexual pleasure. The effect is to dehumanize the person and reduce him or her to an object of sexual pleasure. This corrupts the true meaning of sexuality into a selfish relationship, where a sexual "partner" is appreciated only for the ability to provide physical pleasure. Does an attitude like this send a positive loving message? A study by C. Y. Senn and H. L. Radtke showed mood disturbance effects on women who were shown both sexist and violent pornography.[100]

If viewing violent video games increases a child's aggressive behavior, it only makes sense that a similar effect—a devaluation of the true meaning of human sexuality—can occur as a result of viewing pornographic material. It would seem to be difficult to prevent this kind of objectification from spreading to other facets of one's life. Perhaps the Holy Father Pope Benedict XVI has recognized this objectification seeping into society; during his 2008 visit to the United States, he described and lamented a general "coarsening of social relations."[101] Does pornography depict human sexuality as selfless concern for the well-being of another individual, or does it portray fantasies of power and desirability? Perhaps these fantasy portrayals are linked with recent theories about pornography addiction—that pornography is an escape from the effects of childhood humiliation.

The widespread media depiction of women as sexual objects and of sex as nothing more than a spectator sport transcends pornography. Society is becoming increasingly desensitized to images of sex; the use of increasingly younger girls in advertising and entertainment media with overtly sexual themes has been recognized by the American Psychological Association.[102] Catholic pediatricians must ask parents

98. See S. C. Martino et al., "Exposure to Degrading versus Nondegrading Music Lyrics and Sexual Behavior among Youth," *Pediatrics* 118 (2006): e430–e441.

99. See P. Fischer and T. Greitemeyer, "Music and Aggression: The Impact of Sexual-Aggressive Song Lyrics on Aggression-Related Thoughts, Emotions, and Behavior toward the Same and the Opposite Sex," *Personality and Social Psychology Bulletin* 32 (2006): 1165–76.

100. C. Y. Senn and H. L. Radtke, "Women's Evaluations of and Affective Reactions to Mainstream Violent Pornography, Non-Violent Pornography and Erotica," *Violence and Victims* 5 (1990): 143–55.

101. Pope Benedict XVI, "I Have Come to America to Confirm You in the Faith of the Apostles," Homily at Nationals Stadium, Washington, D.C., April 17, 2008, http://www.michaeljournal.org/benedictusa.asp.

102. See American Psychological Association, Task Force on the Sexualization of Girls, *Report of the APA Task Force on the Sexualization of Girls*.

whether they want their daughters to be treated as objects with nothing more to offer than their bodies, or if they want their sons to believe that they are incapable of controlling their sexual urges.

A picture of mom, or of the family, near the computer can help fortify the adolescent who struggles with Internet pornography. For Catholic youth, small prayer cards with images of our Lord, the Blessed Mother, or a saint can be attached to a corner of the computer. Images in wall or locker posters should be positive rather than titillating (mountain vistas or sports figures, rather than a model in a bikini); even blank walls are better than soft pornography. This will help the adolescent work on fostering other interests and friendships that are supportive of the chaste life. A Catholic perspective can help fight off the temptation to indulge in pornographic imagery: a parent might suggest, "Send those images in your mind up to God and he will take them from you." Even nonreligious youth can be advised to visualize placing such images into a bottomless pit, where they will fall away forever. These steps by families can help their young people avoid the temptations of pornography:

- Use a filter on the computer to screen out pornography.
- Keep the computer out of the child's room and in high-traffic areas with the screen fully visible.
- Block access to pornographic channels, HBO, or Cinemax; better yet, eliminate cable entirely.
- Remove any pornographic books, DVDs, or magazines from the home.
- Discard magazines or catalogues that feature pictures of models in suggestive poses or scanty clothing.

Modesty in Dress

It has become harder for young people to dress modestly in recent years, because the clothing being sold in stores limits choices. Young women should be helped to understand that a man who is attracted to her body or clothes may not be the kind of man who will care for her through good times and bad. Equally, young men need to learn that a woman who feels the need to show off her body may not feel good about herself and might have other issues that could derail a relationship. Modesty guidelines for parents can be found at Pure Style Fashion Show Clothing Guidelines.[103]

Chastity of the Body

Recognizing that his life of sensual pleasures had left him empty, St. Augustine of Hippo wrote "our hearts are restless till they find rest in Thee."[104] Augustine saw that only God can satisfy the deepest longing of our hearts and lead us to true happiness. The longing he experienced is the same longing of people today who use the physical closeness of intercourse to compensate for the emptiness of their own hearts. In using

---

103. http://affiliate.purefashion.com/modesty.
104. St. Augustine of Hippo, *Confessions*, bk. I, ch. 1 (New York: The Collier Press, 1909).

erotic or sensual love to try to satisfy the need for an unselfish and unconditional love, they are misusing another person, their partner. John Paul II described it as "treating another human not as an end but merely as a means for the satisfaction of sexual desires."[105] Fr. Robert Barron writes that chastity is the "refusal in … sexual practice to turn the other [individual] into an object or a means"; thus, chastity is an action rather than a passive state.[106] The Church, like Augustine, recognizes that sex loses the fullness of its meaning when it is focused on the sensual or when it is experienced out of the context of marriage. Parents have the life experience to recognize the sacrifice and commitment necessary for a marriage to succeed. A Catholic pediatrician must help parents acknowledge that the way they view their vocation as spouses will affect how their adolescent children respond to the call of sensual self-discipline.

Many authors attempt to cover the topic of adolescent sexuality by answering the question "how far is too far?" Going "too far" implies that the road being traveled has dangers; and adolescents need to understand that if they take this road, they are likely to get burned. Intimacy has many levels; the deepest form of intimacy involves sharing one's weaknesses and one's dreams.[107] Teens can learn good relationship habits from parents who are willing to be vulnerable and to model the closeness that vulnerability brings. Parents can help young people understand the intimacy involved in simply holding hands or sharing conversation, building the selflessness and maturity that will bode well for a marriage relationship in the future.

Secular medicine thinks this view of sex is old-fashioned. D. E. Greydanus and E. R. MacAnarney wrote that, while physicians are not obliged to provide birth control for their adolescent patients, they should at least provide information and advice to sexually active teens who want some form of contraception. They also warn against "judgmental views" and "quasi-parental power struggles."[108] This stance is both relativistic and permissive and stands in contrast to most pediatric advice. If an adolescent asked for advice on what cigarettes he should smoke, would the pediatrician offer suggestions or take a stand against the behavior? Would we assist this same adolescent if he or she asked for advice on purchasing drugs? From a health standpoint, the pediatrician is bound to recommend against any behavior, sexual or otherwise, that threatens the young person's health, safety, and future happiness.

Dating

Parents should be advised of the dangers of allowing teens to date or be involved in serious romantic relationships in early adolescence. Studies indicate that a male who is involved in a serious relationship in seventh grade has twice the average risk of becoming sexually active by ninth grade; for a girl, that risk is close to three times the average, with early menarche being an additional risk factor.[109] Dating should be

---

105. Quoted in Barron, *Seven Deadly Sins, Seven Lively Virtues.*
106. Ibid.
107. See Kelly, *The Seven Levels of Intimacy.*
108. D. E. Graydanus and E. R. McAnarney, "Letter to the Editor," *Pediatrics* 66 (1980): 475.
109. See B. VanOss Marín et al., "Boyfriends, Girlfriends and Teenagers' Risk of Sexual Involvement," *Perspectives on Sexual and Reproductive Health* 38 (2006): 76–83.

reserved for late adolescence—age 16 and older. It is true that few pediatricians make such a recommendation at well checkups in an office setting, and school-sponsored dances for seventh graders do not help matters. But knowledge is power, and parents deserve to be informed of the dangers of early dating and unsupervised time. Parents who are receptive to this message may need "permission" to be counter-cultural, to teach proper dating behaviors, to set expectations and to stick to them despite pressure from friends, family, children, and neighbors. A pediatrician is able to provide moral support about dating and limit-setting. Besides the age-16 rule, limits can include dating in the home as a start, and any potential date being subject to parental approval.

Chastity and Sex Education in the Home

The safest sex occurs with one and only one married partner; all other forms offer a declining safety profile. Chastity is thus the safest route. The virtue of chastity is an expression of integration; this requires training, just like any other worthwhile goal, but it offers profound rewards. As Francis Cardinal Arinze wrote, "The discipline and self-mastery which it entails bring much peace and self-respect to the individual."[110]

Parents may be uncomfortable discussing sexuality with their teen. The pediatrician can help parents clarify what they want their young person to know about sexuality, and possibly bring to light the obstacles they face in having this discussion. Often parents who themselves were unable to remain chaste as teens feel that their conversation with their teen may seem hypocritical. But our faith tells us that the evil one wants us to feel unworthy and powerless because of our sins. If only perfect people were allowed to speak, the world would be a very quiet place. C. S. Lewis describes how fear can paralyze good intentions in his book *The Screwtape Letters*, a book that can be recommended to parents who are even marginal Christians.[111]

Some articles in the literature declare that abstinence education does not work. As one article from 2000 claims, "no credible published studies have suggested that programs promoting abstinence only, without addressing risk reduction, do any better."[112] If they are no better, they are presumably at least equivalent to other programs in risk reduction. Another article describes abstinence-only programs as morally problematic, claiming they promote "questionable and inaccurate opinions" and even threaten fundamental human rights to health, information, and life.[113] An editorial in the *Journal of the American Medical Association* lamented the government's funding of abstinence programs.

---

110. Francis Cardinal Arinze, "Chastity Elevates and Builds Up," *Linacre Quarterly* 77 (2010): 143.

111. C. S. Lewis, *The Screwtape Letters* (New York: HarperCollins, 2001).

112. L. D. Lieberman et al., "Long-Term Outcomes of an Abstinence-Based, Small-Group Pregnancy Prevention Program in New York City Schools," *Family Planning Perspectives* 32 (2000): 237

113. J. Santelli et al., "Abstinence and Abstinence-Only Education: A Review of U.S. Policies and Programs," *Journal of Adolescent Health* 38 (2006): 72–81.

It is difficult to understand the logic behind the decision to earmark funds specifically for abstinence programs. Unfortunately, much of the public health policy debate appears to have been ideologically motivated rather than empirically driven. However, no matter how widespread, politically viable, or popular a program may be, efficacy in preventing and modifying behaviors associated with STI/HIV must remain the primary criterion by which programs are judged.[114]

The Society for Adolescent Medicine recommended doing away with these programs altogether.[115] Secular medicine is taking a harm-reduction approach to the problem of adolescent sexuality, choosing to focus on prevention of pregnancy and sexually transmitted diseases. The rationale is that adolescents are going to have sex anyway. But there would still be a failure rate even if all sex were practiced with a condom. While we all want to prevent harm, the medical establishment, in this case, is turning a blind eye to the evidence. The rate of STDs has grown apace with the increase in the number of sexually experienced adolescents. Since adolescents have a much higher user-failure rate with all forms of contraception, including condoms, secular medicine is taking a risk-reduction strategy rather than a harm-elimination approach to sexual activity.

The most promising of the abstinence-based education programs is Teen STAR. One of its interventions in Chile was shown to reduce pregnancy rates from 18.9 percent to 3.3 percent.[116] Additionally it has been shown to delay sexual initiation and actually lessen the sexual activity of sexually experienced adolescents.[117] The curriculum does mention birth control, but it does not recommend it. Program participants are asked to research the topic and bring this information to the class, where it is shared and discussed (but again, not recommended). It includes a fertility awareness component, in which young women monitor their cervical mucus changes and learn to appreciate their body cycles, increasing their self-respect.[118] Since the sexually experienced population is typically the most difficult to reach, this reversal of sexual activity is encouraging. Catholic pediatricians should strive to learn this program and promote it in the local Catholic schools, since at present it is not being offered in many U.S. cities.

Risks of Adolescent Premarital Sexual Activity

Physical and verbal abuse are nearly twice as common in adolescent heterosexual relationships that involve sexual intercourse.[119] Studies have also found a link between

114. R. J. DiClemente, "Preventing Sexually Transmitted Infections among Adolescents: A Clash of Ideology and Science," *Journal of the American Medical Association* 279 (1998): 1575.

115. See Society for Adolescent Medicine, "Abstinence-Only Education Policies and Programs: A Position Paper of the Society for Adolescent Medicine," *Journal of Adolescent Health* 38 (2006): 83–87.

116. See C. Cabezón et al., "Adolescent Pregnancy Prevention: An Abstinence-Centered Randomized Controlled Intervention in a Chilean Public High School," *Journal of Adolescent Health* 36 (2005): 64–69.

117. See P. Vigil et al., "Effects of TeenSTAR, an Abstinence-Only Sexual Education Program, on Adolescent Sexual Behavior, *Revista médica de Chile* 113 (2005): 1173–82.

118. See H. Klaus, "Valuing the Procreative Capacity: A New Approach to Teens," *International Review of Natural Family Planning* 8 (1984): 206–13.

119. See C. E. Kaestle and C. T. Halpern, "Sexual Intercourse Precedes Partner Violence in Adolescent Romantic Relationships," *Journal of Adolescent Health* 36 (2005): 386–92.

adolescent sexual activity and depression,[120] especially in female adolescents with multiple partners.[121]

The literature also supports the notion of increased suicidal ideation and attempts in sexually active versus abstinent youth. In addition, adolescents bear a disproportionate burden of the sexually transmitted diseases reported in the United States (50 percent of new cases), even though they are a minority of the sexually active population (25 percent).[122] The number of lifetime sexual partners is inversely related to a person's age at first intercourse,[123] and early sexual intercourse is understood to be a risk factor for having more sex partners over time, as well as for STD acquisition.

Case: Premarital Sex and STDs

A 16-year-old girl comes to the emergency department complaining of abdominal pain and vomiting. She admits to being sexually active with only one partner. She is found to have cervical motion tenderness on a bimanual exam and she is admitted with pelvic inflammatory disease. No parent is at the bedside during a visit on rounds the following day. A more thorough social history finds that she lives with her mother, who she claims does not care about her, and that her father is uninvolved in her life.

Discussion: Trying to scare adolescents away from having intercourse is ineffective, especially since so many of them use it as a means of finding love or a connection with someone. Since adolescents put so much emphasis on feeling, this is a good place to start, and the Socratic approach of posing questions allows the adolescent to solve the problem herself and to realize that someone cares. The pediatrician can ask, "Does intercourse make you feel loved? If this boy loved you, would he have been having intercourse with someone else? If sex makes you feel close and bonded to your boyfriend, but you break up, are you going to have sex with the next boyfriend, or the next after that? When you find the man you want to marry, will sex mean anything if you've had it with every one of your boyfriends? Which one of your boyfriend's other partners gave him an STD to pass on to you?" These arguments hit home, and help the young woman hear the truth: if she does not have more than one sexual partner, her boyfriend either has one now or had one in the past. She has been attempting to fill the void of affection at home, and she lacks a father who could understand the boy's motives and could try to protect her from him. Will searching for love by having

---

120. See A. M. Meier, "Adolescent First Sex and Subsequent Mental Health," *American Journal of Sociology* 112 (2007): 1811–47; D. D. Hallfors et al., "Which Comes First in Adolescence—Sex and Drugs or Depression?" *American Journal of Preventive Medicine* 29 (2005): 163–70; A. L. Spriggs and C. T. Halpern, "Sexual Debut Timing and Depressive Symptoms in Emerging Adulthood," *Journal of Youth and Adolescence* 37 (2008): 1085–96; D. D. Hallfors et al., "Adolescent Depression and Suicide Risk Association with Sex and Drug Behavior," *American Journal of Preventive Medicine* 27 (2004): 224–30.

121. See Meier, "Adolescent First Sex and Subsequent Mental Health."

122. See Centers for Disease Control, "Announcement: STD Awareness Month – April 2012," *Morbidity and Mortality Weekly* 61 (2012): 223.

123. See E. J. McGuire III et al., "Sexual Behavior, Knowledge, and Attitudes about AIDS among College Freshmen," *American Journal of Preventive Medicine* 8 (1992): 226–34.

sex with multiple partners until she finds the "right one" make her feel loved for her unique qualities as an individual?

Family Influence and Premarital Sexual Activity: Creating a Culture at Home

Parents often say that their teens will make their own decisions no matter what they tell them, but study after study has demonstrated the link between parents' messages and adolescent behavior. According to a paper by J. Jaccard and P. J. Dittus, the message of birth control approval from the mother increases the likelihood that a virgin will engage in premarital sexual activity by an odds ratio of 1.2. The odds ratio increased to 2.1 if the adolescent also perceived the mother's approval level of premarital sexual activity to be high.[124] In a similar way, a lack of parental disapproval is associated with a rate of sexual initiation that is double that of peers.[125] Maternal "demandingness" (setting rules for conduct, discussion and explanation of these rules, and enforcement of expected behavior) and parental responsiveness (warmth, affection, emotional support, and an atmosphere of self-regulation for teens) were also shown to be associated with a decreased risk of sexual activity.[126]

The teen's perception of a parent's attitudes and behaviors influences the behaviors of the adolescent more strongly than the parent's stated beliefs. In another survey, young people who communicated with their parents about delaying sexual activity were less likely to have had intercourse than those who did not report such discussions. Despite evidence that sex education does not promote sexual activity, communication with parents about birth control and STD prevention was associated here with youth having had sexual intercourse.[127]

Despite the persistent pull of extracurricular activities, sports, and other drains on family time, parents must work on their relationship with their children just as they would work on the relationship with their spouse. High satisfaction levels with the parent-child relationship have been linked to delaying sex.[128] Family "connectedness"—an inviting, nurturing environment where teens can find positive activities—also serves to protect youth from early sexual activity.[129] Healthy relationships between parents and children of all ages are warm, caring, and consistent in limit-setting and expecta-

---

124. See J. Jaccard and P. J. Dittus, "Adolescent Perceptions of Maternal Approval of Birth Control and Sexual Risk Behavior," *American Journal of Public Health* 90 (2000): 1426–30.

125. See S. L. Ashby, C. M. Arcari, and M. B. Edmonson, "Television Viewing and Risk of Sexual Initiation by Young Adolescents," *Archives of Pediatrics and Adolescent Medicine* 160 (2006): 375–80; H. Hahm et al., "Longitudinal Effects of Perceived Maternal Approval on Sexual Behaviors of Asian and Pacific Islander (API) Young Adults," *Journal of Youth and Adolescence* 37 (2008): 74–84.

126. See M. Cox, "Maternal Demandingness and Responsiveness as Predictors of Adolescent Abstinence," *Journal of Pediatric Nursing* 22 (2007): 197–205.

127. See Aspy et al., "Parental Communication and Youth Sexual Behavior."

128. See C. McNealy et al., "Mother's Influence on the Timing of First Sex Among 14- and 15-year-olds," *Journal of Adolescent Health* 31 (2002): 256–65.

129. See N. Parera and J. C. Surís, "Having a Good Relationship with Their Mother: A Protective Factor against Sexual Risk Behavior among Adolescent Females?" *Pediatric and Adolescent Gynecology* 17 (2004): 267–71; M. D. Resnick, L. J. Harris, and R. W. Blum, "The Impact of Caring and Connectedness on Adolescent Health and Well-Being," *Journal of Paediatric and Child Health* 29, supplement 1 (1993): S3.

tions. One can draw analogies to the workplace: a boss who is cold and uncaring will find the employees disgruntled, uncooperative, and searching for a job elsewhere. By the same token, a boss who is no-nonsense but fair will earn the respect of employees

Substance Abuse Issues

Tobacco

Tobacco use is a risk factor for cancer, heart disease, and stroke, but cigarettes in adolescence act as a gateway drug and are even linked with early sexual intercourse.[130] Like drinking, adolescent smoking is a social activity, though it begins much earlier, on average around age 12. Many children see their parents smoke, but others view it as a kind of initiation into a peer group. While adolescent smoking is often linked to slick marketing, teens who feel accepted at home and have a strong sense of attachment are less likely to seek out acceptance within a group that practices deviant behaviors.

Getting a child to quit smoking will be far more successful if the adult in his or her life quits as well. As the author Matthew Kelly describes it, decisions create habits, habits create character, and character controls destiny.[131] The facts alone will not be effective; most smokers know the dangers. More likely than not, the smoking parent knows someone who has died of lung cancer, and does not want this painful fate for his or her son or daughter. Parents and teens who attempt to quit may need counseling, along with activities that involve using their hands to offset the motor component of smoking. Since the appetite suppression of cigarettes will be gone and the oral motor habit will need to be replaced, specific information about how to prevent weight gain through healthy foods should be stressed. A pediatrician can provide support through referral to a smoking cessation program, suggestions on diet and oral stimulation, and even by offering free serial weight measurements using the office scale.

Alcohol

The abuse of and addiction to alcohol has caused a staggering amount of harm to children. Separate estimates say that between 11 million and 17.5 million children grow up with an alcoholic parent.[132] At least half of these children suffer long-term effects of one kind or another. Alcohol has been shown to be a gateway drug;[133] its use at an early age is a factor in alcohol dependence that cannot be explained by familial or environmental factors alone.[134] This alone supports encouraging young people to wait

---

130. On tobacco as a gateway drug, see S. A. Everett et al., "Other Substance Use among High School Students Who Use Tobacco," *Journal of Adolescent Health* 23 (1998): 289–96. On the link between tobacco use and sexual activity, see A. L. Coker et al., "Correlates and Consequences of Early Initiation of Sexual Intercourse," *Journal of School Health* 64 (1994): 372–77.

131. See Kelly, *Building Better Families*, audiobook.

132. See N. Ronel and R. Haimoff-Ayali, "Risk and Resilience: The Family Experience of Adolescents with an Addicted Parent," *International Journal of Offender Therapy and Comparative Criminology* 54 (2010): 448–72.

133. See J. W. Welte and G. M. Barnes, "Alcohol: The Gateway to Other Drug Use among Secondary-School Students," *Journal of Youth and Adolescence* 14 (1985): 487–98.

134. See J. D. Grant et al., "Adolescent Alcohol Use Is a Risk Factor for Adult Alcohol and Drug Dependence: Evidence from a Twin Design," *Psychological Medicine* 36 (2006): 109–18.

until age 21 to try alcohol. It has been shown that increased availability leads to an increase in drinking prevalence and an increase in the amount of alcohol consumed.[135] Fortunately, the most recent statistics show its use among adolescents is declining.[136]

Alcohol use is connected with an array of adolescent problem behaviors ranging from the foolish to the deadly. Apart from the obvious risks involved in drunk driving, alcohol is linked to early sexual initiation, and in females, receiving unwanted sexual advances and passively consenting to these advances.[137] In college students, drinking is associated with having multiple sexual partners, and with engaging in casual sex.[138] More worrisome, however, is the association of alcohol use with the increased risk of nonconsensual sexual activity.[139]

Since most parents think adolescents are already uninhibited enough when they are sober, alcohol's effect of reducing inhibitions should be pointed out to parents who may see alcohol use in adolescents as a mere rite of passage. While parents may insist that their adolescent would never ride with a drunk driver or drive drunk themselves, they need to understand the other dangers as well. Disapproval from parents and close parental monitoring has been shown to help prevent teen alcohol use.[140] For both males and females, having friends with similar views supports their healthy choices, while friends with antagonistic views may lead to risk-taking behaviors.[141]

Drugs

Drug abuse has destroyed families all over the world. While the drugs of choice and the number of abusers change like the tide, the underlying problem is one of spiritual destitution. This topic is rarely discussed by the medical community, because the culture of medicine is atheistic and spiritual emptiness defies scientific explanation or treatment. But from a Catholic perspective, drug use, much like acts of lust or glut-

---

135. See J. D. Hawkins, R. F. Catalano, and J. Y. Miller, "Risk and Protective Factors for Alcohol and Other Drug Problems in Adolescence and Early Adulthood: Implications for Substance Abuse Prevention," *Psychological Bulletin* 112 (1992): 64–105.

136. See B. M. Kuehn, "Marijuana Use on the Rise," *Journal of the American Medical Association* 305 (2011): 242.

137. For links to sexual initiation, see Coker et al., "Correlates and Consequences of Early Initiation of Sexual Intercourse". For links to unwanted sexual advances, see M. Testa and K. H. Dermen, "The Differential Correlates of Sexual Coercion and Rape," *Journal of Interpersonal Violence* 14 (1999): 548–61; S. Small and D. Kerns, "Unwanted Sexual Activity among Peers during Early and Middle Adolescence: Incidence and Risk Factors," *Journal of Marriage and the Family* 55 (1993): 941–52. For links to passive consent, see K. Cue Davis, W. H. George, and J. Norris, "Women's Responses to Unwanted Sexual Advances: The Role of Alcohol and Inhibition Conflict," *Psychology of Women Quarterly* 28 (2004): 333–43.

138. For links to multiple sexual partners, see K. M. Caldeira et al., "Prospective Associations between Alcohol and Drug Consumption and Risky Sex among Female College Students," *Journal of Alcohol and Drug Education* 53 (2009): 1–14. For links to casual sex, see C. M. Grello, D. P. Welsh, and M. S. Harper, "No Strings Attached: The Nature of Casual Sex in College Students," *Journal of Sex Research* 43 (2006): 255–67.

139. See A. Abbey, "Alcohol-Related Sexual Assault: A Common Problem among College Students," *Journal of Studies on Alcohol* Supplement No. 14 (2002): 118–28.

140. See K. Bogenschneider et al., "Parent Influences on Adolescent Peer Orientation and Substance Use: The Interface of Parenting Practices and Values," *Child Development* 69 (1998): 1672–88.

141. See K. Maxwell, "Friends: The Role of Peer Influence across Adolescent Risk Behaviors," *Journal of Youth and Adolescence* 31 (2002): 267–77.

tony, can be seen as an effort to gain temporary respite from spiritual emptiness. Perhaps this accounts for the strong association between adolescent drug use and early sexual activity; a study by C. Lammers et al. demonstrated a relative risk of 7.7 of early sexual activity in moderate to heavy drug users.[142] This point is also illustrated by the increase in suicidal behaviors in adolescents who use marijuana and, in particular, cocaine.[143]

Addiction is a spiritual, or existential, problem. It has a physical component, particularly evident when the addict abstains from the addictive substance, but, at its root, the addiction is a sign that something is missing. Typically, addicts do not cope with problems in the same way as do non-addicts; instead of processing their problems, they use substances to drown out the pain they feel. The drugs or drink produce more than the sensation of being high; for the addict, they provide temporary relief from pain. The addict's behavior when high or drunk frequently exacerbates the initial problems—family relationships become fractured, or the addict loses a job. The cycle will repeat itself again and again until the addict reaches a point of no escape—rock bottom—and seeks help. Even with rehabilitation and therapy, many addicts suffer multiple relapses over their lifetime.

Not all adolescent drug use will lead to addiction; the danger lies in the fact that no one can predict who will become an addict. Certainly, anyone with a family history of addiction who uses drugs or alcohol is playing with fire, yet 50 percent of those admitted to a hospital for addiction have no family history of it. Here again, parental influence is more powerful than is commonly held; drug use by parents has a direct correlation with drug use by their adolescent children.[144] In a paper by D. McDermott, parental attitudes toward adolescent drug use are also related to use in the adolescent.[145] As with many other adolescent behaviors, parental monitoring and family closeness play a role in prevention; and family disruption, lack of parental involvement, and low academic aspirations are risk factors.[146]

Safe Driving

Permissive parenting in the case of adolescent drivers can be deadly. Motor vehicle accidents are the leading cause of death for teenagers in the United States; in 2009, fifty-five hundred children under age 18 were killed in traffic accidents.[147] While the

142. See C. Lammers et al., "Influences on Adolescents' Decision to Postpone Onset of Sexual Intercourse: A Survival Analysis of Virginity among Youths Aged 13–18 Years," *Journal of Adolescent Health* 26 (2000): 42–48.

143. See V. Burge et al., "Drug Use, Sexual Activity and Suicidal Behavior in U.S. High School Students," *Journal of School Health* 65 (1995): 222–27.

144. See J. A. Andrews et al., "Parental Influence on Early Adolescent Substance Use: Specific and Nonspecific Effects," *Journal of Early Adolescence* 13 (1993): 285–310.

145. See D. McDermott, "The Relationship of Parental Drug Use and Parent's Attitude concerning Adolescent Drug Use to Adolescent Drug Use," *Adolescence* 19 (1984): 89–97.

146. See D. R. Simkin, "Adolescent Substance Use Disorders and Comorbidity," *Pediatric Clinics of North America* 49 (2002): 463–77.

147. See Julie Gilchrist, Michael F. Ballesteros, Erin M. Parker, "Vital Signs: Unintentional Deaths among Persons Aged 0–19 Years—United States, 2000–2009," *Morbidity and Mortality Weekly Report* 61 (2012): 270–76.

media raises the specter of the dangers of drunk driving every year at prom time, in reality 21.2 percent of all adolescent driver accidents leading to a child passenger death actually involved alcohol. The everyday risks of adolescent driving reveal even deeper concerns; accidents in cars driven by teens under age 16 as compared to older drivers result in the highest risk of death to their young passengers; and the passenger fatality rate is double with drivers aged 16 to 17 versus drivers aged 25 and above.[148] Of all adolescent drivers involved in fatal crashes, 65 percent were males, and one third of them were speeding at the time of the accident.[149] How is this addressed from the Catholic perspective? Secular pediatricians encourage parents to "pick your battles"; the Catholic message endorses limit-setting to protect adolescents. Parents should be encouraged not to cave in to the age-old argument that "everyone else is doing it" as they consider their teen's level of maturity and fitness to drive.

The idea that age alone qualifies a person to perform a task is flawed, as can be seen when considered in light of the reality of psychosocial maturity. While an adolescent may not be ready to drive, a parent's judgment may be clouded by the desire for an extra driver to free the parent from chauffeuring duties. Judging a teen's fitness to take the wheel requires much objectivity from parents, and the picture is complicated when the time comes to determine if a teenager should drive at night, on high-speed roads (45 mph or greater), or with younger passengers. These situations represent some of the highest risk situations for accidents. A good place to start is limiting night driving with the use of a curfew.[150] Pediatricians can use open-ended questions to help parents assess their adolescent's maturity, but such questions, and the parents' answers, are just one measure of an adolescent's readiness. One study points to "adopting adult roles, attitudes and behaviors and completing developmental tasks associated with becoming an adult" as signs of psychosocial maturity. Such "mature" individuals demonstrated lower levels of high-risk driving behaviors.[151] A useful system would initially limit teens to less risky situations, gradually allowing the young person to drive in more risky situations as he or she demonstrates mature behavior behind the wheel. More and more states are using this kind of system, whereby young drivers must prove their worthiness before moving on to the next level of driving. These laws set requirements that an adolescent driver must meet before advancing, including minimum numbers of hours of supervised driving, road skills tests, written tests, and driver's education classes. Any pediatrician whose state does not have laws like this should advise parents to institute their own comparable system.[152]

148. See F. Koplin Winston et al., "Risk Factors for Death among Older Child and Teenaged Motor Vehicle Passengers," *Archives of Pediatrics and Adolescent Medicine* 162 (2008): 253–60.

149. See Centers for Disease Control, "Drivers Aged 16 or 17 Years Involved in Fatal Crashes—United States, 2004–2008," *Morbidity and Mortality Weekly Report* 59 (2010): 1329–1330.

150. See D. F. Pruesser, A. F. Williams, and A. K. Lund, "Parental Role in Teenage Driving," *Journal of Youth and Adolescence* 14 (1985): 73–84.

151. See C. Raymond Bingham et al., "Problem Driving Behavior and Psychosocial Maturation in Young Adulthood," *Accident Analysis and Prevention* 40 (2008): 1758–64.

152. See J. T. Shope et al., "Graduated Driving Licensing in Michigan: Early Impact on Motor Vehicle Crashes among 16-Year-Old Drivers," *Journal of the American Medical Association* 286 (2001): 1593–98;

Given the danger associated with alcohol use and driving, parents must set a standard of zero tolerance. Driving after drinking, or riding with an individual who has been drinking, must result in suspension of the adolescent's license. The Centers for Disease Control (CDC) website has resources for parents, which include a parent-teen driving agreement.[153]

Specific Medical Issues

Attention Deficit Disorders

Much has been written about ADD and ADHD in the last few decades, and blame for its recent upsurge has been placed on everything from sugar to preservatives and food coloring in the diet. While attention problems have a biological link, television has also been implicated. A study looking specifically for attention-issue links with television content type revealed no connection with such problems with educational programming, but a marked association with non-educational programming shown to children aged 0 to 36 months. The strongest association was linked to violent programming, with an odds ratio of 2.2 of subsequent attention problems (1.19–4.08).[154] A recent prospective study demonstrated a link with video games as well; the amount of time spent playing games was a predictor of impulse and attention problems. The study showed bidirectional influences, leading to the conclusion that impulsive children tend to play more video games, which compounds their existing attention problems.[155]

While many children (mostly boys) have been successfully medicated for this condition, a number of children carry this diagnosis mistakenly; other children carry it as a sole diagnosis when much more is lurking beneath the surface. Individuals with ADHD are more likely than the general population to be affected by other mental health conditions, including depression, anxiety, oppositional defiant disorder, obsessive compulsive disorder, drug abuse, and bipolar disorder. The frequency of these other conditions and the challenge of parenting these children raise the likelihood of future failures unless appropriate action is taken. These children deserve closer scrutiny from their health-care providers for mental health problems related to the common comorbidities.

In addition, parents must understand that the issue transcends hyperactivity, so that they develop realistic expectations for their children. Attention problems can be confusing to parents, especially when the child seems to zone out instructions yet can

---

R. D. Foss, J. R. Feaganes, and E. A. Rodgman, "Initial Effects of Graduated Driver Licensing on 16-Year-Old Driver Crashes in North Carolina," *Journal of the American Medical Association* 286 (2001): 1588–92.

153. Centers for Disease Control, "Parents Are the Key," https://www.cdc.gov/parentsarethekey/index.html.

154. See F. J. Zimmerman and D. A. Christakis, "Associations between Content Types of Early Media Exposure and Subsequent Attentional Problems," *Pediatrics* 120 (2007): 986–92.

155. See Douglas A. Gentile et al., "Video Game Playing, Attention Problems and Impulsiveness: Evidence of Bidirectional Causality," *Psychology of Popular Media Culture* 1 (2012): 62–70.

focus attention on things he or she likes. Helping parents to reduce this tension may lessen the risk of frustration that might escalate into abuse. Quite often, the stress of childhood ADHD leads to maladaptive parenting strategies.[156] Many resources are available to parents. Some advice that has a refreshing and positive approach is "10 Tips for Parenting a Child with ADHD."[157] Another excellent source of information for parents is the website for the Texas Partners Resource Network, which goes beyond the usual advocacy to offer practical advice.[158] The site includes many handouts for parents to help them understand their child's needs, and suggestions for ways to help ensure the child's success at home and at school.

Children with attention deficits need patient caregivers, since dealing with them is often frustrating. They are typically scolded frequently and receive far more negative than positive feedback. One way to counteract this tension is to help parents focus on the child's talents and positive attributes. Doing so benefits both parent and child psychologically and emotionally. While most children will not grow up to be Nobel Prize winners or Olympic medalists, everyone has at least one talent or one strong point, even if they do not truly "excel." Our cultural preference for winners should never get in the way of a parent's acceptance, since this is a profound expression of parental love.

Children who carry the diagnosis of ADD or ADHD are overwhelmingly boys, and their successful education in a standard classroom is less likely. The odds improve considerably with one-on-one teaching and multimodal education that encourages hands-on learning. ADD/ADHD children process information differently from the general population; since it is hard for them to remain attentive to one stimulus, the information they receive does not register. Despite appearances, they are not trying to ignore the information or its source. Registration is the first action required for information to get into short-term memory (whence it can be transferred into long-term memory). Parents may come to recognize the kinds of sensory input that work for their child, and use them to their advantage.

Parents with ADD/ADHD children may want to consider homeschooling, since it provides the kind of individualized attention that works best for these children. It behooves Catholic pediatricians to learn more about the homeschooling movement; it includes a large Catholic contingent, and since it is countercultural, the Catholic pediatrician may be the only person willing to advise it. A home environment can be ideal for these children in many ways: it provides the child with individual attention and sensory stimuli specific to the child's needs; scheduling can be flexible, with study breaks and extended lessons where they seem necessary; and classmate bullying is absent. Everyday tasks and items can be used to engage children in a home setting. A parent who is cooking can turn the project into a math lesson, using measuring cups and a kitchen scale; cash register receipts can teach addition and subtraction.

---

156. See V. Modesto-Lowe, J. S. Danforth, and D. Brooks, "ADHD: Does Parenting Style Matter?" *Clinical Pediatrics* 47 (2008): 865–72.

157. http://www.emedicinehealth.com/10_tips_for_parenting_a_child_with_adhd/article_em.htm.

158. http://www.partnerstx.org.

Daily chores and, indeed, almost any household event can be part of the lesson plan if the parent can find the teachable moment. The homeschooled child learns alongside his parents, the people who love him the most.

If homeschooling is not an option, parents may need encouragement to act as advocates for their children in the traditional school system. While medication may prove helpful for children with ADD/ADHD, it is not the sole solution and certainly is not a substitute for the use of appropriate teaching methods. Educators today have access to volumes of research on effective teaching strategies for children with attention deficits; they simply need to provide such strategies in the classroom.

Vaccinations

Vaccinations from Morally Illicit Sources

The antigens for a number of vaccines are grown in human cell cultures that were harvested from aborted infants. The first of these cell lines was developed decades ago. The cells originate from an infant aborted in Sweden because the woman did not want any more children.[159] The concern of physicians over the morality of giving and of parents of consenting to these vaccines is mostly limited to Catholic circles. Some parents may take solace in that the Vatican has already examined the issue and determined that the use of these vaccines was "a passive material cooperation . . . morally justified as an extreme ratio due to the necessity to provide for the good of one's children." The Vatican's statement went so far as to describe "the duty to avoid passive material cooperation" as "not obligatory if there is grave inconvenience." However, the same letter urged pharmaceutical companies to make alternatives, that is, morally acceptable vaccines, and described the situation wherein parents had to make such a decision as "moral coercion" and "unjust."[160] Since the letter's publication, Merck has stopped making morally acceptable measles and mumps vaccines while continuing to make its morally tainted measles, mumps, and rubella combination vaccine.

Vaccines obtained from morally illicit sources for which there are no morally licit alternatives:[161]

- Varicella: Varivax, Varilrix
- Hepatitis A: Vaqta, Havrix Avaxim, Epaxal
- Measles, Mumps and Rubella: MMR, Priorix
- MMRV: ProQuad/MMR-V Priorix Tetra
- Shingles: Zostavax
- Typhoid: Vivaxim

159. See M Wadman, "Medical Research: Cell Division," Nature 498 (June 27, 2013): 422–26.
160. Elio Sgreccia, President of the Pontifical Academy of Life, to Debra Vinnedge, Executive Director, Children of God for Life, June 9, 2005, http://www.immunize.org/concerns/vaticandocument.htm.
161. Children of God for Life, "USA and Canada—Aborted Fetal Cell Line Products and Ethical Alternatives (November 2015)," https://cogforlife.org/wp-content/uploads/vaccineListOrigFormat.pdf.

Vaccines obtained from morally illicit sources for which
morally licit alternatives exist:[162]

- Polio: Poliovax, DT PolAds Polio Sabin (oral)
- Polio combination: Pentacel, Quadracel
- Rabies: Imovax
- Smallpox: Acambis 1000

Vaccines and Vaccine Refusal

Most parents who refuse vaccination today are generally not doing so over concerns about the cell lines used. For the majority, the concerns are vaccine safety and the proposed link with autism. Vaccine refusal is not a new phenomenon. The smallpox vaccine caused a great deal of public apprehension, and the arm-to-arm transfer used to inoculate against cowpox transmitted other viruses and bacteria (e.g., syphilis) as well.[163] The anti-vaccine movement in the United States reportedly began in 1982 after a television documentary implicated the DTP vaccine in untoward reactions.[164] Much of the fear over vaccines today may be related to the now-retracted 1998 article from the *Lancet* in which Wakefield et al. presumably identified colitis in children with neuropsychiatric dysfunction.[165] Wakefield even held a press conference at which he suggested that alternatives to a combined MMR vaccine might be preferable. He stated, "There is sufficient anxiety in my own mind for the long term safety of the polyvalent vaccine—that is, the MMR vaccination in combination—that I think it should be suspended in favour of the single vaccines."[166] At the time of the announcement, Wakefield had entered a patent application for a new vaccine (he had failed to disclose this),[167] and his patients were not randomly selected but included children recruited by a lawyer acting for an anti-vaccine group in the United Kingdom. The same lawyer used Child 2 from Wakefield's paper as the lead case in a lawsuit against vaccine manufacturers.[168] It does not help when well-intentioned scientists draw conclusions about vaccine safety that their research does not support.[169] Fortunately, other scientists are happy to refute those conclusions in the medical literature,[170] and still others are able to scientifi-

---

162. Ibid. Morally licit alternatives: *Polio*—IPOL, IMOVAX Polio; *Polio combination*—Pediacel, Pediarix, any HiB, DTap, IPOL, InfanrixHexa; *Rabies*—RabAvert; *Smallpox*—ACAM2000, MVA3000.

163. See J. Blake, E. Hoyme, and P. L. Crotwell, "A Brief History of Autism, the Autism/Vaccine Hypothesis and a Review of the Genetic Basis of Autism Spectrum Disorders," *South Dakota Medicine* 15 (2013): 58–65.

164. See ibid.

165. See ibid.

166. B. Deer, "How the Vaccine Crisis Was Meant to Make Money," *British Medical Journal* 342 (2011): c5258.

167. See C. Dyer, "*Lancet* Retracts Wakefield's MMR Paper," *British Medical Journal* 340 (2010): c696; Deer, "How the Vaccine Crisis Was Meant to Make Money."

168. See Deer, "How the Vaccine Crisis Was Meant to Make Money"; B. Deer, "The *Lancet*'s Two Days to Bury Bad News," *British Medical Journal* 342 (2011): c7001.

169. See L. E. Taylor, A. L. Swerdfeger, and G. D. Eslick, "Vaccines Are Not Associated with Autism: An Evidence-Based Meta-Analysis of Case-Control and Cohort Studies," *Vaccine* 32 (2014): 3623–29.

170. See C. Turville, "Autism and Vaccination: The Value of the Evidence Base of a Recent Meta-Analysis," *Vaccine* 33 (2015): 5495–96.

cally demonstrate vaccine safety and a lack of association with MMR and autism.[171]

The number of children diagnosed with autism spectrum disorders and the medical community's inability to explain all of the risk factors no doubt fuels the creation of alternative theories. The disease has a genetic component: The relative risk for siblings is greater than 20,[172] and the concordance rate in identical twins is around 80 percent.[173] But the fact that the number is less than 100 percent implies other risk factors as well, and these have yet to be identified. As with many situations, the thing that is feared the most is often the unknown.

For parents, the perceived risk (whether or not it is scientifically valid) is quite real, and Catholic pediatricians should avoid vilifying vaccine-fearful parents, as sometimes occurs in the pages of secular medical media.[174] The perceived risks of vaccines may seem to outweigh the benefits of avoiding a disease, particularly when the disease has faded from society's collective memory. Both the risks and the benefits have emotional components. Vaccines for Haemophilus influenza type B and pneumococcus protect against meningitis (among other things). The devastation of a central nervous system infection is easily understood. The word "meningitis" strikes fear in families. A decision to not vaccinate against these bacteria is a calculated risk. In contrast, recent measles outbreaks have not caused any deaths in the United States. People fail to remember, however, the 123 deaths that occurred during the previous outbreak between 1989 and 1991.[175] The perception of the benign nature of vaccine-preventable illnesses feeds into the push back against immunizations. The long-term devastating complication of measles, subacute sclerosing panencephalitis, is rare, and it occurs in a time frame that precludes association in the average person's mind.[176] Another example of perceived risk-benefit imbalance is hepatitis A. It is rarely symptomatic in children under age 4. It carries a risk of acute liver failure, but this is uncommon in the United States.[177] Given that the immediate risk of serious illness is low in children and the complications uncommon, some parents may decline the vaccine. Since it is important to meet people where they are, it may help to advise parents that while children in daycare are often asymptomatic, adults who acquire hepatitis A miss, on average, thirty days of work.[178]

---

171. See H. Honda, Y. Shimizu, and M. Rutter, "No Effect of MMR Withdrawal on the Incidence of Autism: A Total Population Study," *Journal of Child Psychology and Psychiatry* 46 (2005): 572–79; T. Uno et al., "Early Exposure to the Combined Measles–Mumps–Rubella Vaccine and Thimerosal-Containing Vaccines and Risk of Autism Spectrum Disorder," *Vaccine* 33 (2015): 2511–16.

172. See Y. Uno et al., "The Combined Measles, Mumps, and Rubella Vaccines and the Total Number of Vaccines Are Not Associated with Development of Autism Spectrum Disorder: The First Case-Control Study in Asia," *Vaccine* 30 (2012): 4292–98.

173. See Blake, Hoyme, and Crotwell, "A Brief History of Autism."

174. See W. T. Gerson, "'On Narrow Minds Rests the Future of Children … ,'" *Infectious Diseases in Children Newsletter*, July 2015: 18.

175. See Centers for Disease Control, "Epidemiology and Prevention of Vaccine-Preventable Diseases," http://www.cdc.gov/vaccines/pubs/pinkbook/meas.html.

176. See ibid.

177. See M. Rook and P. Rosenthal, "Hepatitis A in Children," in *Viral Hepatitis in Children: Unique Features and Opportunities*, ed. Maureen M. Jonas (New York: Humana Press, 2010), 1–11.

178. See ibid.

Proportionate and Disproportionate Means in Medically Complex Children

Given the medical advances of recent decades, many children who would have died in infancy now survive much longer. These children may have survived extreme prematurity, have a congenital heart defect, or suffer from a neurological disorder that is associated with dysphagia. In 1980, the Church addressed individual judgments as to the proportionality of medical treatments in the *Declaration on Euthanasia*. The teaching states that judgment must be based on the type of treatment, its complexity or risk, and its cost in comparison to the expected results. The "state" of the patient and "his or her physical and moral resources" must also be considered. The document also addresses situations in which no remedies exist; many parents of children with special medical needs find themselves in such a situation on a daily basis.[179] Genetic disorders are an example of this. Parents may be faced with difficult decisions about medical treatments that will allow the child to survive but will never cure the underlying disorder. In these situations, a goals-oriented discussion needs to take place with the family in order to help determine the best course of action for that child.

Conclusion

The effect of the artificial separation of faith and reason in modern science during the Enlightenment has led to many of the problems we see in medicine today. With the moral decline in our culture, the sanctity of life is no longer valued. With the government's help, medicine has turned into a corporate establishment where physicians are "providers" and patient throughput is of the utmost importance. In the trenches, where medicine is practiced, however, we are faced with constant suffering; and suffering, even when it is caused by physical pain, is a spiritual matter. By focusing on the spiritual aspect of patient care, Catholic pediatricians care for the whole patient. By using the parents'—and in some cases the patient's—understanding of self, we may set them on a journey that leads to healing of the body and soul.

We have to remember that we are responsible for our little corner of the world, beginning with ourselves and our families. It appears that this is God's plan. For while the evil one works night and day, and has lots of help, we toil nearly alone. This is our suffering. If we embrace it, we may well be redeemed. If we run from it, we may be asked why we did not use our talents to build up the Kingdom. For in the end, it is not just our patients' lives that we save, it is our own.

179. Congregation for the Doctrine of the Faith, *Declaration on Euthanasia,* May 5, 1980, sec. 4, http://www.vatican.va/roman_curia/congregations/cfaith/documents/rc_con_cfaith_doc_19800505_euthanasia_en.html.

Bibliography

Abbey, A. "Alcohol-Related Sexual Assault: A Common Problem among College Students." *Journal of Studies on Alcohol,* Supplement 14 (2002): 118–28.

Adamczyk, A., and J. Felson. "Friends' Religiosity and First Sex." *Social Science Research* 35 (2006): 924–47.

American College of Pediatricians. "The Teenage Brain: Under Construction." American College of Pediatricians Best for Children. 2016. http://www.acpeds.org/The-Teenage-Brain-Under-Construction.html.

American Psychological Association. Task Force on the Sexualization of Girls. *Report of the APA Task Force on the Sexualization of Girls.* Washington, D.C.: American Psychological Association, 2007. http://www.apa.org/pi/wpo/sexualization.html.

Anderson, C. A., L. Berkowitz, E. Donnerstein, R. L. Huesmann, J. Johnson, and D. Linz, N. M. Malamuth, and E. Wartella. "The Influence of Media Violence on Youth." *Psychological Science in the Public Interest* 4 (2003): 81–110.

Andrews, J. A., H. Hops, D. Ary, E. Tildesley, and J. Harris. "Parental Influence on Early Adolescent Substance Use: Specific and Nonspecific Effects." *Journal of Early Adolescence* 13 (1993): 285–310.

Arinze, Francis. "Chastity Elevates and Builds Up." *Linacre Quarterly* 77 (2010): 139–46.

Armsden, G. C., and M. T. Greenburg. "The Inventory of Parent and Peer Attachment: Individual Differences and Their Relationship to Psychological Well-Being in Adolescence." *Journal of Youth and Adolescence* 16 (1987): 427–54.

Ashby, S. L., C. M. Arcari, and M. B. Edmonson. "Television Viewing and Risk of Sexual Initiation by Young Adolescents." *Archives of Pediatrics and Adolescent Medicine* 160 (2006): 375–80.

Aspy, C. B., S. K. Vesely, R. F. Oman, S. Rodine, L. Marshall, and K. McLeroy. "Parental Communication and Youth Sexual Behavior." *Journal of Adolescence* 30 (2007): 449–66.

Augustine of Hippo. *Confessions.* New York: Collier Press, 1909.

Barron, R. *Seven Deadly Sins, Seven Lively Virtues.* Sycamore, Ill.: Lighthouse Catholic Media, NFP, 2011. Audiobook.

Barry, R. A., and G. Kochanska. "A Longitudinal Investigation of the Affective Environment in Families with Young Children: From Infancy to Early School Age." *Emotion* 10 (2010): 237–49.

Berry, Joy. *Let's Talk About* series. New York: Scholastic, 1982–2008.

Benedict XVI, Pope. "I Have Come to America to Confirm You in the Faith of the Apostles." Homily at Nationals Stadium, Washington, D.C. April 17, 2008. http://www.michaeljournal.org/benedictusa.asp.

Bersamin, M., M. Todd, D. A. Fisher, D. L. Hill, J. W. Grube, and S. Walker. "Parenting Practices and Adolescent Sexual Behavior: A Longitudinal Study." *Journal of Marriage and the Family* 70 (2008): 97–112.

Bimler, Richard. *Sex and the New You.* St. Louis, Mo.: Concordia Publishing House, 1998.

———. *Sex and the New You: For Young Men 13–15.* St. Louis, Mo.: Concordia Publishing House, 2008.

Bingham, C. Raymond, Jean T. Shope, Jennifer Zakrajsek, and Trivellore E. Raghunathan. "Problem Driving Behavior and Psychosocial Maturation in Young Adulthood." *Accident Analysis and Prevention* 40 (2008): 1758–64.

Bissonnette-Pitre, L., and the Most Reverend R. F. Vasa. *Healthy Families: Safe Children; The Power of Relationships.* Bend, Ore.: Ardor, 2007. DVD.

Blackmore, R. E., and L. H. Chaudron. "Postpartum Depression: Recognition and Intervention." *Journal of Clinical Outcomes Management* 19 (2012): 133–42.

Blake, J., E. Hoyme, and P. L. Crotwell. "A Brief History of Autism, the Autism/Vaccine Hypothesis and a Review of the Genetic Basis of Autism Spectrum Disorders." *South Dakota Medicine* 15 (2013): 58–65.

Bogenschneider, K., M. Y. Wu, M. Raffaelli, and I. C. Tsay. "Parent Influences on Adolescent Peer Orientation and Substance Use: The Interface of Parenting Practices and Values." *Child Development* 69 (1998): 1672–88.

Bosco, John. "Youth Ministry and Parenting: Guiding Principles." In *Epistolario*, vol. 4, 201–3. Turin,

1959. Quoted from the Roman Missal, January 31. https://www.crossroadsinitiative.com/media/articles/youth-ministry-john-bosco/.

Boxer, P., L. R. Huesmann, B. J. Bushman, M. O'Brien, and D. Moceri. "The Role of Violent Media Preference in Cumulative Developmental Risk for Violence and General Aggression." *Journal of Youth and Adolescence* 38 (2009): 417–28.

Brown, J. D., K. L. L'Engle, C. J. Pardun, G. Guo, K. Kenneavy, and C. Jackson. "Sexy Media Matter: Exposure to Sexual Content in Music, Movies, Television, and Magazines Predicts Black and White Adolescents' Sexual Behavior." *Pediatrics* 117 (2006): 1018–27.

Brown, J. D., K. Walsh Childers, and C. Waszak. "Television and Adolescent Sexuality." *Journal of Adolescent Health Care* 11 (1990): 62–70.

Brown, R., and J. Ogden. "Children's Eating Attitudes and Behaviour: A Study of the Modeling and Control Theories of Parental Influence." *Health Education Research* 19 (2004): 261–71.

Burge, V., M. Felts, T. Chenier, and V. Parrillo. "Drug Use, Sexual Activity and Suicidal Behavior in U.S. High School Students." *Journal of School Health* 65 (1995): 222–27.

Cabezón, C., P. Vigil, I. Rojasc, M. E. Leivad, R. Riquelme, W. Arandaf, and C. García. "Adolescent Pregnancy Prevention: An Abstinence-Centered Randomized Controlled Intervention in a Chilean Public High School." *Journal of Adolescent Health* 36 (2005): 64–69.

Caldeira, K. M., A. M. Arria, K. E. O'Grady, E. M. Zarate, K. B. Vincent, and E. D. Wish. "Prospective Associations between Alcohol and Drug Consumption and Risky Sex among Female College Students." *Journal of Alcohol and Drug Education* 53 (2009): 1–14.

Catechism of the Catholic Church. Fort Wayne, Ind: The Faith Database, 2008. https://www.faithdatabase.com/.

Catholic Medical Association. "Position Paper on HPV Immunization." Bala Cynwyd, Penn.: Catholic Medical Association, 2007. http://www.cathmed.org/assets/files/Position%20Paper%20on%20HPV%20Immunization.pdf.

Centers for Disease Control. "Drivers Aged 16 or 17 Years Involved in Fatal Crashes—United States, 2004–2008." *Morbidity and Mortality Weekly Report* 59 (2010): 1329–30.

———. "Announcement: STD Awareness Month—April 2012." *Morbidity and Mortality Weekly* 61 (2012): 223.

———. "Epidemiology and Prevention of Vaccine-Preventable Diseases." http://www.cdc.gov/vaccines/pubs/pinkbook/meas.html. Accessed March 2, 2016.

Chandra, A., S. C. Martino, R. L. Collins, M. N. Elliott, S. H. Berry, D. E. Kanouse, and A. Miu. "Does Watching Sex on Television Predict Teen Pregnancy? Findings from a National Longitudinal Survey of Youth." *Pediatrics* 112 (2008): 1047–54.

Children of God for Life. "USA and Canada—Aborted Fetal Cell Line Products and Ethical Alternatives." November 2015. https://cogforlife.org/wp-content/uploads/vaccineListOrigFormat.pdf.

Christakis, D. A., and F. J. Zimmerman. "Violent Television Viewing during Preschool Is Associated with Antisocial Behavior during School Age." *Pediatrics* 120 (2007): 993–99.

Clements, R. "An Investigation of the Status of Outdoor Play." *Contemporary Issues in Early Childhood* 5 (2004): 68–80.

Cogswell, A., L. B. Alloy, and J. Spasojevic. "Neediness and Interpersonal Life Stress: Does Congruency Predict Depression." *Cognitive Therapy and Research* 30 (2006): 427–43.

Coker, A. L., D. L. Richter, R. F. Valois, R. E. McKeown, C. Z. Garrison, and M. L. Vincent. "Correlates and Consequences of Early Initiation of Sexual Intercourse." *Journal of School Health* 64 (1994): 372–77.

Collins, R. L., M. N. Elliott, S. H. Berry, D. E. Kanouse, D. Kunkel, S. B. Hunter, and A. Miu. "Watching Sex on Television Predicts Adolescent Initiation of Sexual Behavior." *Pediatrics* 114 (2004): e280–e289.

Congregation for the Doctrine of the Faith. *Declaration on Euthanasia.* May 5, 1980. http://www.vatican.va/roman_curia/congregations/cfaith/documents/rc_con_cfaith_doc_19800505_euthanasia_en.html.

Cox, J. L., J. M. Holden, and R. Sagovsky. "Detection of Postnatal Depression: Development of the 10-Item Edinburgh Postnatal Depression Scale." *British Journal of Psychiatry* 150 (1987): 782–86.

Cox, M. "Maternal Demandingness and Responsiveness as Predictors of Adolescent Abstinence." *Journal of Pediatric Nursing* 22 (2007): 197–205.

Cue Davis, K., W. H. George, and J. Norris. "Women's Responses to Unwanted Sexual Advances: The Role of Alcohol and Inhibition Conflict." *Psychology of Women Quarterly* 28 (2004): 333–43.

Cunningham, M., and A. Thorton. "The Influence of Parents' Marital Quality on Adult Children's Attitudes toward Marriage and Its Alternatives: Main and Moderating Effects." *Demography* 43 (2006): 659–72.

Deer, B. "How the Vaccine Crisis Was Meant to Make Money." *British Medical Journal* 342 (2011): c5258.

———. "The *Lancet*'s Two Days to Bury Bad News." *British Medical Journal* 342 (2011): c7001.

DeVore, E. R., and K. R. Ginsburg. "The Protective Effects of Good Parenting on Adolescents." *Current Opinion in Pediatrics* 17 (2005): 460–65.

DiClemente, R. J. "Preventing Sexually Transmitted Infections among Adolescents: A Clash of Ideology and Science." *Journal of the American Medical Association* 279 (1998): 1574–75.

Doman, Regina. *Angel in the Waters.* Manchester, N.H.: Sophia Institute Press, 2004.

Duckworth, A. L., and M. E. P. Seligman. "Self-Discipline Outdoes IQ in Predicting Academic Performance of Adolescents." *Psychological Science* 16 (2005): 939–44.

Dunlap, Jay. *Raising Kids in the Media Age.* Hamden, Conn.: Circle Press, 2008.

Dyer, C. "*Lancet* Retracts Wakefield's MMR Paper." *British Medical Journal* 340 (2010): c696.

Everett, S. A., G. A. Giovino, C. W. Warren, L. Crossett, and L. Kann. "Other Substance Use among High School Students Who Use Tobacco." *Journal of Adolescent Health* 23 (1998): 289–96.

Evert, Jason. *If You Really Loved Me.* El Cajon, Calif.: Catholic Answers, 2009.

———. *Theology of His Body/Theology of Her Body.* West Chester, Penn.: Ascension Press, 2009.

Evert, Jason, and Crystalina Evert. *How to Find Your Soulmate without Losing Your Soul.* San Diego: Totus Tuus Press, 2011.

Evert, Jason, and Chris Stefanick. *Raising Pure Teens.* El Cajon, Calif.: Catholic Answers, 2010.

Fagan, Theresa. *A Mother's List of Books.* Chevy Chase, Md.: Teresa Fagan, 2009.

Field, T. "Maternal Depression Effects on Infants and Early Interventions." *Preventive Medicine* 27 (1998): 200–203.

Field, T., M. Diego, and M. Hernandez-Reif. "Infants of Depressed Mothers Are Less Responsive to Faces and Voices: A Review." *Infant Behavior and Development* 32 (2009): 239–44.

Fischer, P., and T. Greitemeyer. "Music and Aggression: The Impact of Sexual-Aggressive Song Lyrics on Aggression-Related Thoughts, Emotions, and Behavior toward the Same and the Opposite Sex." *Personality and Social Psychology Bulletin* 32 (2006): 1165–76.

Foss, R. D., J. R. Feaganes, and E. A. Rodgman. "Initial Effects of Graduated Driver Licensing on 16-Year-Old Driver Crashes in North Carolina." *Journal of the American Medical Association* 286 (2001): 1588–92.

Fulkerson, J. A., M. Story, A. Mellin, N. Leffert, D. Neumark-Sztainer, and S. A. French. "Family Dinner Meal Frequency and Adolescent Development: Relationships with Developmental Assets and High-Risk Behaviors." *Journal of Adolescent Health* 39 (2006): 337–45.

Gentile, Douglas A., Edward L. Swing, Angeline Khoo, and Choon Guan Lim. "Video Game Playing, Attention Problems and Impulsiveness: Evidence of Bidirectional Causality." *Psychology of Popular Media Culture* 1 (2012): 62–70.

Gerson, W. T. " 'On Narrow Minds Rests the Future of Children ….' " *Infectious Diseases in Children Newsletter*, July 2015: 18.

Gilchrist, Julie, Michael F. Ballesteros, Erin M. Parker. "Vital Signs: Unintentional Deaths among Persons Aged 0–19 Years—United States, 2000–2009." *Morbidity and Mortality Weekly Report* 61 (2012): 270–76.

Grant, J. D., J. F. Scherrer, M. T. Lynskey, M. J. Lyons, S. A. Eisen, M. T. Tsuang, W. R. True, and K. K. Bucholz. "Adolescent Alcohol Use Is a Risk Factor for Adult Alcohol and Drug Dependence: Evidence from a Twin Design." *Psychological Medicine* 36 (2006): 109–18.

Graydanus, D. E., and E. R. McAnarney. "Letter to the Editor." *Pediatrics* 66 (1980): 475.

Grello, C. M., D. P. Welsh, and M. S. Harper. "No Strings Attached: The Nature of Casual Sex in College Students." *Journal of Sex Research* 43 (2006): 255–67.

Guinan, P. "Hippocrates and Christian Medicine." *Ethics and Medics* 34, no. 11 (November 2009): 3–4.

Hahm, H., J. Lee, L. Zerden, A. Ozonoff, M. Amodeo, and C. Adkins. "Longitudinal Effects of Perceived Maternal Approval on Sexual Behaviors of Asian and Pacific Islander (API) Young Adults." *Journal of Youth and Adolescence* 37 (2008): 74–84.

Hallfors, D. D., M. W. Waller, D. Bauer, C. A. Ford, and C. T. Halpern. "Which Comes First in Adolescence—Sex and Drugs or Depression?" *American Journal of Preventive Medicine* 29 (2005): 163–70.

Hallfors, D. D., M. W. Waller, C. A. Ford, C. T. Halpern, P. H. Brodish, and B. Iritani. "Adolescent Depression and Suicide Risk Association with Sex and Drug Behavior." *American Journal of Preventive Medicine* 27 (2004): 224–30.

Hawkins, J. D., R. F. Catalano, and J. Y. Miller. "Risk and Protective Factors for Alcohol and Other Drug Problems in Adolescence and Early Adulthood: Implications for Substance Abuse Prevention." *Psychological Bulletin* 112 (1992): 64–105.

Hay, D. F., S. Pawlby, D. Sharp, P. Asten, A. Mills, and R. Kumar. "Intellectual Problems Shown by 11-Year-Old Children Whose Mothers Had Postnatal Depression." *Journal of Child Psychology Psychiatry and Allied Disciplines* 42 (2001): 871–89.

Honda, H., Y. Shimizu, and M. Rutter. "No Effect of MMR Withdrawal on the Incidence of Autism: A Total Population Study." *Journal of Child Psychology and Psychiatry* 46 (2005): 572–79.

Jaccard, J., and P. J. Dittus. "Adolescent Perceptions of Maternal Approval of Birth Control and Sexual Risk Behavior." *American Journal of Public Health* 90 (2000): 1426–30.

John Paul II, Pope. *Man and Woman He Created Them: A Theology of the Body.* Translated by Michael Waldstein. Boston: Pauline Books and Media, 2006.

Kaestle, C. E., and C. T. Halpern. "Sexual Intercourse Precedes Partner Violence in Adolescent Romantic Relationships." *Journal of Adolescent Health* 36 (2005): 386–92.

Karofsky, P. S., L. Zeng, and M. R. Kosorok. "Relationship between Adolescent–Parental Communication and Initiation of First Intercourse by Adolescents." *Journal of Adolescent Health* 28 (2000): 41–45.

Kataja, V., S. Syrjänen, M. Yliskoski, M. Hippeläinen, M. Väyrynen, S. Saarikoski, R. Mäntyjärvi, V. Jokela, J. T. Salonen, and K. Syrjänen. "Risk Factors Associated with Cervical Human Papillomavirus Infections: A Case-Control Study." *American Journal of Epidemiology* 138 (1993): 735–45.

Kelly, M. *Building Better Families: 5 Practical Ways to Build Family Spirituality.* Sycamore, Ill.: Lighthouse Catholic Media, 2009. Audiobook.

———. *The Seven Levels of Intimacy.* Sycamore, Ill.: Lighthouse Catholic Media, NFP, 2011. Audiobook.

Kinsman, S. B., D. Romer, F. F. Furstenberg, and D. F. Schwarz. "Early Sexual Initiation: The Role of Peer Norms." *Pediatrics* 102 (1998):1185–92.

Klaus, H. "Valuing the Procreative Capacity: A New Approach to Teens." *International Review of Natural Family Planning* 8 (1984): 206–13.

Klohe-Lehman, D. M., J. Freeland-Graves, K. K. Clarke, C. Guowen, S. Voruganti, T. J. Milani, H. J. Nuss, J. M. Proffitt, and T. M. Bohman. "Low-Income, Overweight and Obese Mothers as Agents of Change to Improve Food Choices, Fat Habits, and Physical Activity in Their 1-to-3-Year-Old Children." *Journal of the American College of Nutrition* 26 (2007): 196–208.

Koplin Winston, F., M. J. Kallan, T. M. Senserrick, and M. R. Elliott. "Risk Factors for Death among Older Child and Teenaged Motor Vehicle Passengers." *Archives of Pediatrics and Adolescent Medicine* 162 (2008): 253–60.

Kottke, J. L., and C. D. MacLeod. "Use of Profanity in the Counseling Interview." *Psychological Reports* 65 (1989): 627–34.

Kreeft, P. "Why a Christian Anthropology Makes a Difference." Paper presented at the Catholic Medical Association 79th Educational Conference, Seattle, Wash., October 2010.

Kuehn, B. M. "Marijuana Use on the Rise." *Journal of the American Medical Association* 305 (2011): 242.

Lammers, C., M. Ireland, M. Resnick, and R. Blum. "Influences on Adolescents' Decision to Postpone Onset of Sexual Intercourse: A Survival Analysis of Virginity among Youths Aged 13–18 Years." *Journal of Adolescent Health* 26 (2000): 42–48.

L'Engle, K. L., J. D. Brown, and K. Kenneavy. "The Mass Media Are an Important Context for Adolescents' Sexual Behavior." *Journal of Adolescent Health* 38 (2006): 186–92.

Lewis, C. S. *The Screwtape Letters*. New York: HarperCollins, 2001.

Lieberman, L. D., H. Gray, M. Wier, R. Fiorentino, and P. Maloney. "Long-Term Outcomes of an Abstinence-Based, Small-Group Pregnancy Prevention Program in New York City Schools." *Family Planning Perspectives* 32 (2000): 237–45.

Mann, J. R., C. C. Stine, and J. Vessey. "The Role of Disease-Specific Infectivity and Number of Disease Exposures on Long-Term Effectiveness of the Latex Condom." *Sexually Transmitted Diseases* 29 (2002): 344–49.

Margolin, L. "Child Abuse by Mother's Boyfriends: Why the Overrepresentation?" *Child Abuse and Neglect* 16 (1992): 541–51.

Martino, S. C., R. L. Collins, M. N. Elliott, A. Strachman, D. E. Kanouse, and S. H. Berry. "Exposure to Degrading versus Nondegrading Music Lyrics and Sexual Behavior among Youth." *Pediatrics* 118 (2006): e430–e441.

Martino, S. C., M. N. Elliott, R. Corona, D. E. Kanouse, and M. A. Schuster. "Beyond the 'Big Talk': The Roles of Breadth and Repetition in Parent-Adolescent Communication about Sexual Topics." *Pediatrics* 121 (2008): e612–e618.

Maxwell, K. "Friends: The Role of Peer Influence across Adolescent Risk Behaviors." *Journal of Youth and Adolescence* 31 (2002): 267–77.

McDermott, D. "The Relationship of Parental Drug Use and Parent's Attitude concerning Adolescent Drug Use to Adolescent Drug Use." *Adolescence* 19 (1984): 89–97.

McGuire, E. J., III, S. G. Nicholls, P. Deese, and C. S. Landefeld. "Sexual Behavior, Knowledge, and Attitudes about AIDS among College Freshmen." *American Journal of Preventive Medicine* 8 (1992): 226–34.

McIntosh, W. D., J. D. Murray, R. M. Murray, and S. Manian. "What's So Funny about a Poke in the Eye? The Prevalence of Violence in Comedy Films and Its Relation to Social and Economic Threat in the United States, 1951–2000." *Mass Communication and Society* 6 (2003): 345–60.

McNealy, C., M. L. Shew, T. Beuhring, R. Sieving, B. Miller, and R. W. Blum. "Mother's Influence on the Timing of First Sex among 14- and 15-Year-Olds." *Journal of Adolescent Health* 31 (2002): 256–65.

Meier, A. M. "Adolescent First Sex and Subsequent Mental Health." *American Journal of Sociology* 112 (2007): 1811–47.

Modesto-Lowe, V., J. S. Danforth, and D. Brooks. "ADHD: Does Parenting Style Matter?" *Clinical Pediatrics* 47 (2008): 865–72.

Murray, L. "The Impact of Postnatal Depression on Infant Development." *Journal of Child Psychology and Psychiatry* 33 (1992): 543–61.

Neumark-Sztainer, D., P. J. Hannan, M. Story, J. Croll, and C. Perry. "Family Meal Patterns: Associations with Sociodemographic Characteristics and Improved Dietary Intake among Adolescents." *Journal of the American Dietetic Association* 103 (2003): 317–22.

Nielson, C. M., R. B. Harris, A. G. Nyitray, E. F. Dunne, K. M. Stone, and A. R. Giuliano. "Consistent Condom Use Is Associated with Lower Prevalence of Human Papillomavirus Infection in Men." *Journal of Infectious Diseases* 202 (2010): 445–51.

Nystrom, Carol. *Before I Was Born*. Colorado Springs, Colo.: NavPress, 2007.

Parera, N., and J. C. Surís. "Having a Good Relationship with Their Mother: A Protective Factor against Sexual Risk Behavior among Adolescent Females?" *Pediatric and Adolescent Gynecology* 17 (2004): 267–71.

Pedersen, Amy. *The Miracle of Me from Conception to Birth*. Stockbridge, Mass.: Marian Press, 2007.

Pontifical Council for the Family. "The Truth and Meaning of Human Sexuality: Guidelines for Education Within the Family." http://www.vatican.va/roman_curia/pontifical_councils/family/documents/rc_pc_family_doc_08121995_human-sexuality_en.html.

Popcak, Gregory. *Beyond the Birds and the Bees*. West Chester, Penn.: Ascension Press, 2012.

Pruesser, D. F., A. F. Williams, and A. K. Lund. "Parental Role in Teenage Driving." *Journal of Youth and Adolescence* 14 (1985): 73–84.

Resnick, M. D., L. J. Harris, and R. W. Blum. "The Impact of Caring and Connectedness on Adolescent Health and Well-Being." *Journal of Paediatric and Child Health* 29, Supplement 1 (1993): S3.

Ronel, N., and R. Haimoff-Ayali. "Risk and Resilience: The Family Experience of Adolescents with an Addicted Parent." *International Journal of Offender Therapy and Comparative Criminology* 54 (2010): 448–72.

Rook, M., and P. Rosenthal. "Hepatitis A in Children." In *Viral Hepatitis in Children: Unique Features and Opportunities*, ed. Maureen M. Jonas, 1–11. New York: Humana Press, 2010.

Salmon, Peter. "Effects of Physical Exercise on Anxiety, Depression and Sensitivity to Stress: A Unifying Theory." *Clinical Psychology Review* 21 (2001): 33–61.

Santelli, J., M. A. Ott, M. Lyon, J. Rogers, D. Summers, and R. Schleifer. "Abstinence and Abstinence-Only Education: A Review of U.S. Policies and Programs." *Journal of Adolescent Health* 38 (2006): 72–81.

Sattler, Harry V. *Parents, Children and the Facts of Life*, Patterson, N.J.: Saint Anthony's Guild, 1952.

Sazer, L., and H. Kassinove. "Effects of Counselor's Profanity and Subject's Religiosity on Content Acquisition of a Counseling Lecture and Behavioral Compliance." *Psychological Reports* 69 (1991): 1059–70.

Scherrer, Catherine, and Bernard Scherrer. *The Joyful Mysteries of Life*. San Francisco: Ignatius Press, 1997.

Schnitzer, P. G., and Barnard G. Ewigman. "Child Deaths Resulting from Inflicted Injuries: Household Risk Factors and Perpetrator Characteristics." *Pediatrics* 116 (2005): e687–e693.

Senn, C. Y., and H. L. Radtke. "Women's Evaluations of and Affective Reactions to Mainstream Violent Pornography, Non-Violent Pornography and Erotica." *Violence and Victims* 5 (1990): 143–55.

Sharp, D., D. F. Hay, S. Pawlby, G. Schmücker, H. Allen, and R. Kumar. "The Impact of Postnatal Depression on Boys' Intellectual Development." *Journal of Child Psychology and Psychiatry* 36 (1995): 1315–36.

Shope, J. T., L. J. Molnar, M. R. Elliott, and P. F. Walker. "Graduated Driving Licensing in Michigan: Early Impact on Motor Vehicle Crashes among 16-Year-Old Drivers." *Journal of the American Medical Association* 286 (2001): 1593–98.

Simkin, D. R. "Adolescent Substance Use Disorders and Comorbidity." *Pediatric Clinics of North America* 49 (2002): 463–77.

Small, S., and D. Kerns. "Unwanted Sexual Activity among Peers During Early and Middle Adolescence: Incidence and Risk Factors." *Journal of Marriage and the Family* 55 (1993): 941–52.

Society for Adolescent Medicine. "Abstinence-Only Education Policies and Programs: A Position Paper of the Society for Adolescent Medicine." *Journal of Adolescent Health* 38 (2006): 83–87.

Sohr-Preston, S. L., and L. V. Scaramella. "Implications of Timing of Maternal Depressive Symptoms for Early Cognitive and Language Development." *Clinical Child and Family Psychology Review* 9 (2006): 65–83.

Spriggs, A. L., and C. T. Halpern. "Sexual Debut Timing and Depressive Symptoms in Emerging Adulthood." *Journal of Youth and Adolescence* 37 (2008): 1085–96.

Taylor, L. E., A. L. Swerdfeger, and G. D. Eslick. "Vaccines Are Not Associated with Autism: An Evidence-Based Meta-Analysis of Case-Control and Cohort Studies." *Vaccine* 32 (2014): 3623–29.

Testa, M., and K. H. Dermen. "The Differential Correlates of Sexual Coercion and Rape." *Journal of interpersonal Violence* 14 (1999): 548–61.

Turville, C. "Autism and Vaccination: The Value of the Evidence Base of a Recent Meta-Analysis." *Vaccine* 33 (2015): 5495–96.

Upadhyay, U., and M. Hindin. "Do Perceptions of Friends' Behaviors Affect Age at First Sex? Evidence from Cebu, Philippines." *Journal of Adolescent Health* 39 (2006): 570–77.

Uno, Y., T. Uchiyama, M. Kurosawa, B. Aleksic, and N. Ozaki. "The Combined Measles, Mumps, and Rubella Vaccines and the Total Number of Vaccines Are Not Associated with Development of Autism Spectrum Disorder: The First Case-Control Study in Asia." *Vaccine* 30 (2012): 4292–98.

——. "Early Exposure to the Combined Measles–Mumps–Rubella Vaccine and Thimerosal-Containing Vaccines and Risk of Autism Spectrum Disorder." *Vaccine* 33 (2015): 2511–16.

VanOss Marín, B., D. B. Kirby, E. S. Hudes, K. K. Coyle, and C. A. Gómez. "Boyfriends, Girlfriends and

Teenagers' Risk of Sexual Involvement." *Perspectives on Sexual and Reproductive Health* 38 (2006): 76–83.

Vigil, P., R. Riquelme, R. Rivadeneira, and W. Aranda. "Effects of TeenSTAR, an Abstinence-Only Sexual Education Program, on Adolescent Sexual Behavior." *Revista médica de Chile* 113 (2005): 1173–82.

Villani, S. "Impact of Media on Children and Adolescents: A 10-Year Review of the Research." *Journal of the American Academy of Child and Adolescent Psychiatry* 40 (2001): 392–401.

Wadman, M. "Medical Research: Cell Division." *Nature* 498 (June 27, 2013): 422–26.

Wan, M. W., and J. Green. "The Impact of Maternal Psychopathology on Child–Mother Attachment." *Archives of Women's Mental Health* 12 (2009): 123–34.

Welte, J. W., and G. M. Barnes. "Alcohol: The Gateway to Other Drug Use among Secondary-School Students." *Journal of Youth and Adolescence* 14 (1985): 487–98.

Williams, T. M., ed. *The Impact of Television: A Natural Experiment in Three Communities*. New York: Academic Press, 1986.

Wills, S. E. "Condoms and AIDS: Is the Pope Right or Just 'Horrifically Ignorant'?" *Linacre Quarterly* 77 (2010): 17–29.

Zimmerman, F. J., and D. A. Christakis. "Children's Television Viewing and Cognitive Outcomes: A Longitudinal Analysis of National Data." *Archives of Pediatrics and Adolescent Medicine* 159 (2005): 619–25.

———. "Associations between Content Types of Early Media Exposure and Subsequent Attentional Problems." *Pediatrics* 120 (2007): 986–92.

Zimmerman, F. J., D. A. Christakis, and A. N. Meltzoff. "Associations between Media Viewing and Language Development in Children under Age 2 Years." *Journal of Pediatrics* 151 (2007): 364–68.

Sister Mary Diana Dreger and James S. Powers

7. CARING FOR OLDER ADULTS

Human dignity is not time sensitive. There is no expiration date for the dignity of the person. This reality sets the stage for Drs. Dreger and Powers to share specifically Catholic principles of geriatric care in this chapter. Through the use of clinical vignettes from their experience, they illustrate how physicians and health-care providers in general may successfully navigate through sometimes difficult medical-ethical dilemmas that arise in the course of caring for elderly patients. Simultaneously, the authors hold out in relief the preeminence of the dignity of every person. As in chapters 6, 8, 10, and 11, expressions of authentic Catholic care and witness are presented in specific, concrete ways. The accounts offered by Dreger and Powers invite—and perhaps challenge—the reader to reflect upon what the practice of Catholic health care may look like.—*Editors*

The care of older patients follows the long tradition of Christian caring for the needy, the poor, and the sick. Following a more than one-thousand-year tradition, caring religious and lay persons have opened their homes, monasteries, and hostels to care for those in need. The origin of hospitals and hospices dates back to the Middle Ages of Europe and to such champions as Sts. Francis and Clare of Assisi, who founded, in the thirteenth century, the first orders of religious to care for the poor and sick. In the seventeenth century, St. Vincent de Paul's communities founded hospitals and hospices to provide nursing care; in the nineteenth century, St. Jeanne Jugan of France began an order dedicated to serving the indigent sick and later developed nursing homes. Cicely Saunders, a twentieth-century nurse, social worker, and physician, founded the modern hospice movement; Marjory Warren, a surgeon, initiated the field of geriatrics when she was asked to run the poor houses of 1930s London. In more recent times, St. Teresa of Calcutta was famed for her community's care for India's dispossessed and dying people. And in the new millennium, St. John Paul II, in his words and by his personal example, taught the world to love the elderly, to embrace redemptive suffering, and to approach death from the perspective of eternity.

There is a worldwide need to care for an increasing number of elderly people. By

2030, developing countries will experience a doubling of their elderly populations, and in the United States more than 25 percent of the population will be over age 65. An ever-increasing portion of the world's population is achieving the human potential to reach extreme old age. While many are living healthier older lives than ever before, many also experience chronic illness and increasing levels of disability as they age. This burden of illness places demands on health-care systems, providers, and family caregivers. As Catholic health-care professionals, it is incumbent on us to educate ourselves in sensitivity to the special needs of our older patients, to engage in appropriate goal-setting, and to appreciate the special place of old age in creation and the cycle of life.

This sensitivity to the needs of the elderly is rooted in Catholic moral teaching, which holds at its foundation the human person's inherent dignity. The life of the human person is fundamentally sacred because it involves God's special creative action in the infusion of the soul. This rational being can enter into a relationship with the Holy Trinity in a way that occurs with no other creature on earth.[1] Circumstances of aging or of illness do not diminish human dignity, even if they limit the patient's physical or rational functions. Rather, these changes call us as caregivers to be more sensitive to a person who may no longer be able to claim this respect by his or her own means. Catholic health-care professionals should recognize the critical role they play in serving and safeguarding the life of the elderly person, and truly become witnesses to all of society concerning the value of old age. "There must be a growing conviction that a fully human civilization shows respect and love for the elderly," advised Pope John Paul II.[2]

Physicians are sometimes guilty of displaying ageism when older patients are categorically considered more complex and difficult to care for; when illness symptoms are attributed to age itself; when histories and exams are rushed and important patient concerns neglected; and when specific treatment consideration is based solely on age rather than patient-specific characteristics, wishes, and goals.[3]

The physician faces a continuing challenge in differentiating among aging, chronic illness, and frailty. Aging is not the same as bad health, and is a very individual experience. In general terms, comorbidity refers to the simultaneous presence of multiple diseases; disability represents loss of function; and frailty represents a state of decreased reserve with a high risk for developing adverse health outcomes. A person's increased lifespan brings with it a higher potential for disability. The goal of care for older patients is to understand the patient's wishes and to maximize personal well-being. Optimizing care and focusing on the prevention and relief of disability, which accompanies the burden of illness, is a noble calling that will continue to challenge physicians.

1. See Congregation for the Doctrine of the Faith, *Donum Vitae, Instruction on Respect for Human Life in Its Origin and on the Dignity of Procreation*, February 22, 1987, intro., no. 5, http://www.vatican.va/roman_curia/congregations/cfaith/documents/rc_con_cfaith_doc_19870222_respect-for-human-life_en.html.

2. Pope John Paul II, *Letter to the Elderly*, October 1, 1999, no. 12, http://www.vatican.va/holy_father/john_paul_ii/letters/documents/hf_jpii_let_01101999_elderly_en.html.

3. See Ronald D. Adelman, Michele G. Greene, and Marcia G. Ory, "Communication between Older Patients and Their Physicians," *Clinics in Geriatric Medicine* 16 (2000): 1–24.

Using authentic case examples, we hope to explore ways the health-care professional can enhance professionalism, communication skills, and ethical competencies in caring for elderly individuals. The discussions that follow each case will illustrate specific Catholic and geriatric principles of care.

Case 1

Mrs. Bonnie Stewart was a 64-year-old woman who appeared much older than her stated age. She had advanced, steroid-dependent rheumatoid arthritis as well as oxygen-dependent chronic obstructive pulmonary disease (COPD). She had two caregivers at home: her husband, who required a walker, and an overburdened daughter. Over a two-year period, Mrs. Stewart had developed numerous skin wounds, and she had suffered through several episodes of osteomyelitis, which were treated with long-term IV antibiotics. Her weight was down to 90 pounds, her albumin hovered around 2.5 g/dl (normal is 3.6 to 5.1), and she became bedfast. Essentially she was a total-care patient. Her daughter was distressed over the situation, and she became very demanding of the medical staff. While health-care professionals tried to encourage a different care setting, no amount of discussion could convince the family to consider a skilled nursing facility. Most of this resistance came from the daughter, who felt the need to participate in her mother's care. Mrs. Stewart's level of pain required the use of transdermal narcotics, as well as oral hydromorphone for breakthrough pain. Her goal was to be free from her burden of pain. While she was still in the hospital, hospice was consulted, but she remained hospitalized for an extended time because of a line infection. Eventually she was able to be discharged to her home with hospice care, for her bedfast state, chronic pain, osteomyelitis, and decubiti. At home she received the Sacrament of the Sick during a visit from the hospice chaplain. She died on Christmas Day, surrounded by her family members. Her funeral was a celebration of her life, and the family later expressed great satisfaction with the care she had received. This case demonstrates respect for the elderly and individual goals of care.

Respect for the Elderly

Long life can be seen as a sign of God's favor, and it marks the final stage of human maturity. The wisdom of experience gained over a long life can be a precious gift.[4] However, respect for the elderly as human persons endowed with a rational nature by divine design can test our skills as caregivers. Rheumatoid arthritis as in the example above is a disease that disfigures the human body. Long-term steroid use further adds to physical impairment; its effects on the body are described in such non-human terms as "buffalo hump" and "moon faces." The oxygen-dependent patient is attached

---

4. See John Paul II, *To the Elderly*.

to a mechanical device, which tends to encourage more attention to numbers like oxygen saturation levels than to the person they describe. Yet the Catholic physician should always be attentive to the human person.

It is not uncommon for us to approach our patients assuming we may start the relationship on a first-name basis. Particularly with our elderly patients, it is best not to make this assumption. Some will invite us to address them more informally, but studies show that the elderly are more likely to prefer a level of professionalism in which both patient and physician address each other by surnames.[5] Our first encounter with the elderly patient and the way we use his or her name will say much about our respect for that person. John Paul II, in his *Letter to the Elderly*, encourages us to "continue to give the elderly the respect which the sound traditions of many cultures on every continent have prized so highly."[6]

How we communicate with the elderly patient frames the picture of our respect for that person. Often a third party, such as a spouse, child, or other caregiver, is involved in the physician-patient interaction with a geriatric patient. The older person may be limited in communication due to sensory (vision, hearing) problems or cognitive deficits. These may slow down the interview portion of the clinical visit, and the physician may be tempted to interact with the younger caregiver, who can respond to questions more quickly and perhaps more reliably. Certainly it is appropriate to involve caregivers, but the Catholic physician will first of all be attentive to the patient.

The content of this communication is just as important. Caring for any person requires knowing the person, not just the medical history. Our first meetings with a new elderly patient should include time simply to "get to know" the person. Understanding the older patient's personal history—the patient's home town and educational experience, marriage, employment, children, hobbies—helps the physician to understand both the patient's past accomplishments and future goals.

Ronald D. Adelman, Michele G. Greene, and Marcia G. Ory, in their article "Communication between Older Patients and Their Physicians," explain:

Accessing this narrative history may be time consuming initially, but it is worth the time extended because it gives a formidable jump-start to the development of trust, which is unfortunately missing so often in the medical encounter. The simple act of listening to the patient's story can be poignant for the patient as well as to the physician. Indeed, the very act of listening to an older patient's overall history acknowledges the unique personhood of the patient; the older patient sees that the physician is interested in him or her as more than a disease entity. Through discussions of the patient's life history, the physician comes to understand the patient's present life, value system, achievements, and failures; and this knowledge assists in diagnosis and treatment of current problems.[7]

5. See Joyce Allman et al., "Elderly Women Speak about Their Interactions with Health Care Providers," in *Language and Communication in Old Age: Multidisciplinary Perspectives*, ed. Heidi E. Hamilton (New York: Garland Publishing, 1999), 332–33.

6. John Paul II, *To The Elderly*, no. 11.

7. Adelman, Green, and Ory, "Communication between Older Patients and Their Physicians," 14.

The physician has a great opportunity to validate the importance of the elderly person's life, but this can happen only if the physician *knows* the history behind the patient. John Paul II quoted Cicero in saying "the burden of age is lighter for those who feel respected and loved by the young."[8] The physician has this same occasion to lighten the burden of old age and learn who the patient is. By doing so, the physician can help the patient recognize the value of the patient's life and what this means for his or her future care.

Part of this respect for the elderly patient includes sensitivity to the family. Mrs. Stewart's identity is not to be seen in isolation: Mr. Stewart is part of Mrs. Stewart's self. His own limitations may leave him on the sidelines of her care, but the sidelines are no less important. His own health-care goals may be influenced by what he sees happening with his wife, and Mrs. Stewart herself will have in her mind how her choices of care will affect her lifelong spouse. Grief reactions may play a role long before physical death is declared at the bedside.[9]

This case history also implies the grief of the quiet spouse in the background and the grief of the demanding daughter, but also the grief of the patient herself. The physician who sees the elderly patient not as an isolated "case" but as part of her domestic community is demonstrating great respect for that person.

Pain Management/Palliative Care

Palliative care refers to medical care that focuses on comfort measures rather than on the treatment of specific disease processes. The word "palliative" comes from the Latin "palliare" which means "to cloak"; this might imply that we are cloaking or hiding the symptoms from the patient. Health-care professionals may mistakenly think that palliative care is a distinct or final level of care. Rather, we would do better to understand that all through the life process, we provide palliative care, treating disease entities while simultaneously incorporating symptom management. While a physician prescribes antibiotics to cure a bacterial pneumonia, antipyretics, analgesics, and cough suppressants may also be offered to palliate the patient's symptoms. Similarly at the end of life, we should see palliative care measures as within the scope of medical care, and not simply a different stage of care.[10]

Sometimes palliative care is considered the type of care used when "there is nothing more to do." If symptom management is always part of medical care, palliative care is very much something that we *are* doing to care for the patient. While it is true that palliative care is not associated with cure, it certainly is a form of treatment. An ancient proverb reminds physicians that we "cure sometimes, treat often, and comfort always"; another version of this saying substitutes "heal" for "treat." In fact, treatment

8. John Paul II, *To The Elderly*, no. 12.

9. See Randy S. Hebert et al., "Preparing Family Caregivers for Death and Bereavement: Insights from Caregivers of Terminally Ill Patients," *Journal of Pain and Symptom Management* 37 (2009): 3–12.

10. See R. Sean Morrison, and Diane E. Meier, "Palliative Care," *New England Journal of Medicine* 350 (2004): 2582–90.

of pain, nausea, and other distressing symptoms does bring a level of healing to suffering patients. Physicians should not belittle their own ability to provide this kind of care, nor mislead patients into thinking that nothing more can be done for them. Even the language we use around the issue of palliative care is important for the comfort of the patient and the family.[11] And should there really be no other procedures or interventions to perform, or medications to prescribe, we still cannot say there is "nothing more," for there is always room for greater love for the one who suffers.

Treatment of pain, in particular, can be a challenge to the physician and is of concern to patients and caregivers alike. Pain has many components. While inflammation and neuropathy can explain particular types of symptoms, and have associated specific pharmacologic treatment, other aspects of pain must be considered as well. Individuals may have differences in pain perception and particularly in pain thresholds. Anxiety and fear can heighten perceived pain.[12] In considering treatment, an astute practitioner will likely need to address pharmacologic treatment in a variety of ways. For example, while benzodiazepines are not analgesics, their anxiolytic effect can contribute to pain control. In treating depressive symptoms, selective serotonin re-uptake inhibitors (SSRIs) may assist in the treatment of pain as well. Formal cognitive-behavior therapy can lessen pain. Even reassuring words from physician and caregiver that a patient's symptoms will not be ignored can contribute to pain management.

Narcotics are the core pharmacologic treatment for pain that does not respond to other means. Patients may have underlying fears about this class of medications, with preconceived notions of the nature of morphine and other opioids. Physicians may have their own concerns related to abuse of these medications by patients or family members, or even about legal actions that may result if they are judged to be overprescribing controlled substances. Some may have ethical concerns related to hastening death by respiratory suppression if narcotics are used inappropriately. Church teaching on this is clear.

The use of painkillers to alleviate the sufferings of the dying, even at the risk of shortening their days, can be morally in conformity with human dignity if death is not willed as either an end or a means, but only foreseen and tolerated as inevitable. Palliative care is a special form of disinterested charity. As such it should be encouraged.[13]

In the *Ethical and Religious Directives*, we are advised, "Patients should be kept as free of pain as possible.... Medicines capable of alleviating or suppressing pain may be given to a dying person, even if this therapy may indirectly shorten the person's life, so long as the intent is not to hasten death."[14] Catholic physicians owe it to the proper

11. See Steven Z. Pantilat, "Communicating with Seriously Ill Patients: Better Words to Say," *Journal of the American Medical Association* 301 (2009): 1279–81.

12. See Adam T. Hirsh et al., "Fear of Pain, Pain Catastrophizing, and Acute Pain Perception: Relative Prediction and Timing of Assessment," *Journal of Pain* 9 (2008): 806–12.

13. *Catechism of the Catholic Church for the United States of America*, trans. United States Catholic Conference (Boston, Mass.: St. Paul Books and Media, 1994), no. 2279.

14. United States Conference of Catholic Bishops, *Ethical and Religious Directives for Catholic Health Care Services*, 5th ed. (Washington, D.C.: USCCB, 2009), dir. 61.

care of their suffering patients to understand the use of pain-relieving medications and to apply this knowledge appropriately to them.

Physicians can refer to published evidence-based guidelines for help in understanding the scope of palliative care and for encouragement to address these issues with patients.[15] Specific recommendations are given for pharmacologic agents to be used for pain. Symptoms such as dyspnea and depression are addressed in these guidelines. Other distressing symptoms, including, but not limited to, fatigue, nausea, vomiting, diarrhea, constipation, cough, and respiratory secretions, are treated with appropriate medications and other interventions. At times, the care team may need to explain to the patient and family the etiology of various symptoms, the types of treatment and expected outcomes, as well as to assure them that addiction to medications at this stage is not a concern. Many hospice organizations publish resources which offer physicians suggested methods for managing symptoms. These are useful, even if not strictly evidence based.[16]

Medical professionals also must recognize that, just as they cannot cure every illness, sometimes patients reach a level of suffering that cannot be alleviated. The Church calls us to address these situations with great consideration for the patient in full personhood, both body and soul. We read in the *Ethical and Religious Directives*: "Patients experiencing suffering that cannot be alleviated should be helped to appreciate the Christian understanding of redemptive suffering."[17]

With St. Paul, each of us has an opportunity to participate in the redemptive act of Jesus: "Now I rejoice in my sufferings for your sake, and in my flesh I complete what is lacking in Christ's afflictions for the sake of his body, that is, the church" (Col 1:24).[18] The Catholic physician may assist a Christian patient in understanding Christ's passion more deeply and personally, and how we are individually called to unite ourselves with him in our own sufferings. In the Old Testament, too, Isaiah describes the Suffering Servant of the Lord, and, as the *Catechism* says, "intuits that suffering can also have a redemptive meaning for others."[19] Based on this understanding, the *Ethical and Religious Directives* explain, "Since a person has the right to prepare for his or her death while fully conscious, he or she should not be deprived of consciousness without a compelling reason."[20] It is for this reason that palliative sedation is ethically and morally improper.

No less than a surgeon navigating a delicate procedure in the operating room, the physician caring for a dying patient should recognize the treasure in the experience of caring for the elderly patient at the end of life.

---

15. See Amir Qaseem et al., "Evidence-Based Interventions to Improve the Palliative Care of Pain, Dyspnea, and Depression at the End of Life: A Clinical Practice Guideline from the American College of Physicians," *Annals of Internal Medicine* 148 (2008): 141–46.

16. See Daniel C. Johnson, Cordt T. Kassner, and Jean S. Kutner, "Current Use of Guidelines, Protocols, and Care Pathways for Symptom Management in Hospice." *American Journal of Hospice and Palliative Care* 21 (2004): 51–57.

17. USCCB, *Ethical and Religious Directives*, dir. 61.

18. All quotations from Scripture are taken from the Revised Standard Version.

19. *Catechism of the Catholic Church*, no. 1502.

20. USCCB, *Ethical and Religious Directives*, dir. 61.

Sacramental Care

Health-care professionals are becoming more attuned to the importance of taking a "spiritual history" of the patient.[21] At a minimum, this includes inquiring about the patient's faith background. It is important that this question be asked in relationship to the patient, not simply the family. In the Hispanic community, for example, many elderly members will refer to themselves as Catholic, even if they have had little or no opportunity to participate in Mass and the sacraments. Often this is because their children are attending other faith communities, and their parents have no way to get to a Catholic church.

When the patient's faith has been established, the physician might inquire as to how his or her faith can be of assistance in times of illness or at the end of life. Patients and their families can differ in their understanding of the seriousness of the illness. Sometimes introducing the idea of help from their faith community is best done by the team attending to them, so that this important aspect of their care is not missed. Of course, this need not be left to the patient's hour of impending death. A spiritual history of the patient is recommended as part of the initial visit with any patient.

For Catholic patients, the Catholic physician has a unique opportunity to share the life of the Church with one who is suffering. Again, this kind of intervention should not be missed at any point in the path of the physician-patient relationship. Preventive care visits can provide a unique moment to delve into issues of spiritual well-being, and to suggest ways to maintain spiritual health. Indeed, good Catholic friends should do this for each other always! Yet for the elderly, and especially for those who are dying, the offerings are even greater.

Our love for our patients must be, above all, a love that hopes for their greatest good, which is their eternal happiness with the Father in heaven. Patients may fear their last days, and may sense a kind of hopelessness if we suggest calling in the priest. The *Catechism* expresses well the various emotions experienced in sickness:

Illness can lead to anguish, self-absorption, sometimes even despair and revolt against God. It can also make a person more mature, helping him discern in his life what is not essential so that he can turn toward that which is. Very often illness provokes a search for God and a return to him.[22]

The Catholic physician should be attentive to the call to be an intercessor for others, not only in prayer, but also in advocating for the Catholic patient by recommending the sacraments of healing.[23] The sacrament of Reconciliation and the sacrament of the Anointing of the Sick are not limited to those with terminal illness, but they do take on a distinctive role in the Catholic patient's last days. As physicians, we re-

---

21. Daniel P. Sulmasy, "Spiritual Issues in the Care of Dying Patients: '… It's Okay between Me and God,'" *Journal of the American Medical Association* 296 (2006): 1385–92.

22. *Catechism of the Catholic Church*, no. 1501.

23. See James Francis Stafford, Address on the Occasion of the Annual General Conference of the Society for Catholic Liturgy, September 9, 2006, http://www.vatican.va/roman_curia/tribunals/apost_penit/documents/rc_trib_appen_doc_20060921_stafford-reconciliation_en.html.

call Jesus as the Divine Physician of both bodies and souls. He used material means to effect healing in others. The *Catechism* elaborates: "He makes use of signs to heal: spittle and the laying on of hands, mud and washing. The sick try to touch him, 'for power came forth from him and healed them all.' And so in the sacraments Christ continues to 'touch' us in order to heal us."[24] So the Church recognizes, among the seven sacraments, one specifically for the sick. The Anointing, said Pope Paul IV,

is not a sacrament for those only who are at the point of death. Hence, as soon as anyone of the faithful begins to be in danger of death from sickness or old age, the fitting time for him to receive this sacrament has certainly already arrived.[25]

The *Catechism* also directs that "the faithful should encourage the sick to call for a priest to receive this sacrament."[26] A Catholic physician should take this call seriously, as his vocation is so closely associated to the healing mission of Jesus himself.

Case 2

Mrs. Doris Blakely was an 80-year old-woman who had recently been widowed. Her husband had expired soon after being diagnosed with a glioblastoma. In the years before her husband's death, he had helped her through treatment for breast cancer, as well as surgery for a perforated diverticulum, which had left her with a colostomy. Mrs. Blakely suffered from dementia, scoring 15 out of 30 on the Mini-Mental Status Exam. Without her husband for support, she became anxious, ruminating, and more dependent on her three daughters who lived nearby. She began to refuse to eat. A month following her husband's death, she presented weakened and delirious to the physician's office, requiring admission to the hospital with a urinary tract infection and profound volume depletion. The interdisciplinary team developed a care plan involving intravenous hydration and antibiotics, as well as physical, occupational, and speech therapy. She received supportive counseling, and was able to improve to the point that she could return to her home with her daughters taking turns providing care. Her physician and other health-care personnel had discussed with Mrs. Blakely and her daughters the option of an assisted-living facility. However, the daughters felt a duty to provide for their mother in her old age. This case highlights the burdens of caregiving and the support required for this important role.

---

24. *Catechism of the Catholic Church*, no. 1504.

25. Vatican Council II, *Sacrosanctum Concilium, Constitution on the Sacred Liturgy*, December 4, 1963, no. 73, http://www.vatican.va/archive/hist_councils/ii_vatican_council/documents/vat-ii_const_19631204_sacrosanctum-concilium_en.html.

26. *Catechism of the Catholic Church*, no. 1516.

Duty to Parents

My son, take care of your father when he is old; grieve him not as long as he lives. . . . For kindness to a father will not be forgotten, it will serve as a sin offering—it will take lasting root. In time of tribulation it will be recalled to your advantage, like warmth upon frost it will melt away your sins. (Sir 3:12–15)

Our duty to our parents is specified in the fourth commandment, which begins the second tablet of the Decalogue. The *Catechism* notes that it is placed after the first three commandments, which guide our relationship with God, and at the head of the next seven, which govern our relationships with others; thus, it shows us "the order of charity." "God has willed that, after him, we should honor our parents to whom we owe life and who have handed on to us the knowledge of God."[27]

This commandment is not without foundations, as the *Catechism* explains:

Respect for parents (*filial piety*) derives from *gratitude* toward those who, by the gift of life, their love and their work, have brought their children into the world and enabled them to grow in stature, wisdom, and grace. "With all your heart honor your father, and do not forget the birth pangs of your mother. Remember that through your parents you were born; what can you give back to them that equals their gift to you?"[28]

Nor is the commandment limited to youth. The *Catechism* points out that even as adults, we do not outgrow our duty to our parents. "The fourth commandment reminds grown children of their *responsibilities toward their parents*. As much as they can, they must give them material and moral support in old age and in times of illness, loneliness, or distress."[29]

Cultures across the world have this sense of obligation to our elders and in particular to our parents. This is not unique to Christianity. Studies show that family caregivers find unique rewards in their generous work. Their personal sense of self-worth is increased as they recognize the reality of the good they are providing for their loved ones. This perspective is important for patients themselves to realize, as they are often led to believe that they are simply a heavy physical, emotional, or financial "burden" on their family members; and this perception may unnecessarily color end-of-life decisions.[30]

However, in Western society, as individuality, self-determination, and independence become the hallmarks of successful adulthood, this awareness of duty to our parents has been eroded. Instead, phrases such as "I have my own life to live" are not uncommon, and the elderly themselves express a desire not to interfere with the lives of their children. John Paul II noted this change in society. "Elsewhere, and especially in the more economically advanced nations, there needs to be a reversal of the current trend, to ensure that elderly people can grow old with dignity, without having to fear that they will end up no longer counting for anything."[31]

---

27. Ibid., no. 2179, quoting Sir 7:27–28.

28. *Catechism of the Catholic Church*, no. 2215.

29. Ibid., no. 2218.

30. See Jennifer L. Wolff et al., "End-of-Life Care: Findings from a National Survey of Informal Caregivers," *Archives of Internal Medicine* 167 (2007): 40–46.

31. John Paul II, *To The Elderly*, no. 12.

Some would have faulted Mrs. Blakely's daughters for their selfless attention to their mother. In fact, they were responding to their inherent understanding of the natural relationship to her, and thus could be assured of the supernatural graces needed to fulfill this call. A Catholic physician must be supportive of family caregivers, acknowledging their struggles and sufferings as well as their generosity. This support should extend to conversations that seek to understand the difficulties faced by these most loyal of caregivers, and to incorporate their needs in the patient's care plan.[32]

Nutrition and Hydration

Elderly patients commonly face issues related to nutritional needs and dietary insufficiencies; these can occur in either the primary care setting or the hospital setting.[33] Changes in the gastrointestinal system result in the elderly being more susceptible to vitamin B12 deficiency, and to its concomitant hematologic and neurologic manifestations. Perceptions of taste are altered, and osmoreceptors in the brain appear to function differently in the older patient. Changes in activity levels will modify caloric requirements. Certain biomarkers of inflammation can be mistaken for those of nutritional status. The astute clinician of the elderly will be attentive to the patients' nutritional care, and will view evidence of change in nutritional status as a possible sign that some disease process needs to be addressed.

Volume depletion associated with infection in the elderly is not uncommon. Replacing and maintaining intravascular volume is important for fever control, maintaining circulation, and continuing renal function. Delirium and cognitive dysfunction in a patient may originate in dehydration; thus, replacing fluids may be crucial not only for maintaining physical processes, but for terminally ill patients to retain cognitive ability at the end of life.[34] Loss of appetite may indicate an underlying pathology, but is also associated with anxiety and depression. Caring for the physical and psychological needs of our older patients includes their need for food and water.

The right to food and water is accepted universally, and a number of nations actually specify this right in their constitutions.[35] Yet this right is sometimes represented as a medical treatment for those who are chronically ill, or even for the elderly who present with an acute illness. The Church continues to maintain that nutrition and hydration are to be considered as elements of usual care for a patient, not as components of a medical treatment plan. Catholic bioethical teachings always bring us back to respect for the human person, calling us to consider all types of care, first and foremost, in light of its benefit or burden to the patient him- or herself.

32. See Michael W. Rabow, Joshua M. Hauser, and Jocelia Adams, "Supporting Family Caregivers at the End of Life: 'They Don't Know What They Don't Know,'" *Journal of the American Medical Association* 291 (2004): 483–91.

33. See Sonya Brownie, "Why Are Elderly Individuals at Risk of Nutritional Deficiency?" *International Journal of Nursing Practice* 12 (2006): 110–18.

34. See Peter G. Lawlor, "Delirium and Dehydration: Some Fluid for Thought?" *Supportive Care in Cancer* 10 (2002): 445–54.

35. See United Nations, Food and Agricultural Organization, *The Right to Food in National Constitutions*, http://www.fao.org/docrep/w9990e/w9990e12.htm.

In the fifth edition of the *Ethical and Religious Directives*, issues related to hydration and nutrition are delineated. "In principle, there is an obligation to provide patients with food and water, including medically assisted nutrition and hydration for those who cannot take food orally."[36] First, the general principle is set forth: no less than to the poor and hungry of the world, we have an obligation to the patient to provide food and water; at times, this must take place through medical assistance. Depending on the situation of the particular patient, and the means available, this may include intravenous fluid repletion including necessary electrolytes, enteral feedings via nasal or gastric tubes, epidermal clysis, or even total parenteral nutrition. The clinician's first priority must be the patient's needs and the benefit to that individual human person.

The directive continues, pointing out that chronic illness itself is not a contraindication to providing nutrition. "This obligation extends to patients in chronic and presumably irreversible conditions (e.g., the 'persistent vegetative state') who can reasonably be expected to live indefinitely if given such care."[37] Again, it is made clear that food and water as such fall into the category of care, not that of medical treatment, even if they are provided in a way that requires a medical intervention. The medical means (for example, an intravenous catheter or a gastrostomy tube) does not transform a human right into a negotiable option.

This does not mean, however, that the Church does not recognize that at some stage in life, disease processes can render medical intervention to provide food and water unreasonable or disproportionate, given the understanding of the illness at hand. The *Ethical and Religious Directives* continue:

Medically assisted nutrition and hydration become morally optional when they cannot reasonably be expected to prolong life or when they would be "excessively burdensome for the patient or [would] cause significant physical discomfort, for example, resulting from complications in the use of the means employed." For instance, as a patient draws close to inevitable death from an underlying progressive and fatal condition, certain measures to provide nutrition and hydration may become excessively burdensome and therefore not obligatory in light of their very limited ability to prolong life or provide comfort.[38]

A patient with an obstructing gastrointestinal tumor has a medical contraindication to placement of a gastrostomy tube to provide nutrition. The burden to the patient clearly outweighs the benefit. In each case, for the good of each individual person, we are called to consider not simply the nature of the intervention, but the benefit and burden to the patient.

The Catholic physician faces a particular challenge in the current medical ethics climate in the United States on this matter. Frequently, medical science is asked to defer to criteria other than evidence-based, patient-centered care. At times, the "bur-

---

36. USCCB, *Ethical and Religious Directives*, dir. 58.

37. Ibid.

38. Ibid., quoting Congregation for the Doctrine of the Faith, "Responses to Certain Questions of the United States Conference of Catholic Bishops concerning Artificial Nutrition and Hydration," August 1, 2007.

den" identified is a burden to the health-care system, and the patient is judged to be a drain on limited resources. In another schema, the issue is not that the intervention is deemed a burden to the patient, but that *life itself* is identified as the burden. Financial hardships or the challenges of sickness may prompt some to view providing medically assisted nutrition and hydration as a morally optional treatment. The Church asks the Catholic health-care professional to defend those who are ill and cannot speak for themselves against this kind of thinking.

But what of the case where the patient him- or herself signs an advance directive with a categorical refusal of medically assisted intervention to provide food and water? Is the Catholic physician to defer to this "higher good," designated as the absolute autonomy of the patient? In fact, the physician is not. The *Directives* explain that what is true on the corporate level for Catholic health-care institutions is likewise true to the individual health-care provider: "a Catholic health-care institution . . . will not honor an advance directive that is contrary to Catholic teaching. If the advance directive conflicts with Catholic teaching, an explanation should be provided as to why the directive cannot be honored."[39] Ideally, a Catholic physician should be able to explain to a patient why refusal of a particular type of care or treatment may not be in the best interests of that person's dignity. If disagreement continues between the patient and caregivers, then to avoid cooperation in evil and its associated scandal, it may be necessary for a Catholic hospital or a Catholic health-care professional to transfer the care of the patient to another institution or provider.

Case 3

Mr. Theodore Baxter was a 90-year-old man who had been widowed for many years. He was a retired business executive who had always been, and still was, intensely independent. His daughter was a nurse, and she recognized a change in her father as he became progressively more forgetful and exhibited deterioration in his housekeeping skills. She became distressed as he became more frustrated and argumentative. He became lost while driving one day, frightening both his daughter and himself. At that point, he reluctantly agreed to an office consultation. His physical exam was unremarkable, but he scored 25 out of 30 on the Mini-Mental Status Exam. He was started on a cholinesterase inhibitor, but over a period of months, his dementia continued to progress. He agreed to a personal care service, a model of support for him that was consistent with his previous position as an executive. A resourceful care manager assisted him with his errands, accompanied him to his appointments, and eventually encouraged him to relinquish driving. Mr. Baxter also came to accept designating his daughter as his power of attorney. After a year, he moved to an assisted-living residence, which improved his living conditions still more. At times his dementia was associated with episodes of agitation, requiring psy-

---

39. USCCB, *Ethical and Religious Directives*, dir. 24.

chiatric consultation and ongoing adjustment of his medication appropriate to his condition. This case highlights the many losses associated with aging, especially independence and the need for special living arrangements.

Location of Care

Respect for the elderly includes an appreciation for the unique features of their lives that continue to be important to them. Independence is acquired when we reach adulthood; and for most of us, it is only with difficulty that we agree to relinquish this. Those caring for the elderly must be attentive to this ongoing inclination to self-sufficiency, as it is closely tied to decisions related to location of care.

Almost universally, as in the case presented, older patients want to continue to live in their own homes, which in many ways is a great benefit to them. On a personal level, they can maintain a sense of self-reliance. They can continue to be part of their community, where they know their neighbors and can participate in their local church. Familiarity with their surroundings and with their personal possessions brings consolation. Their personal history exists in their long-standing place of residence.

Yet difficulties can arise. Rather than remaining part of community, the elderly person can become isolated in this situation. Life can be lonely after the death of a spouse and after children are no longer part of the household. Familiar neighbors themselves may have died or moved, and relationships with new ones are harder to develop. The size and required upkeep of the house and surrounding property may strain the elderly person's resources. Physical limitations can interfere with the person's ability to care for him- or herself properly.

Both family members and health-care professionals must be sensitive to these conflicting realities. Decisions about location of care must be considered with great respect for the individual patient. The Pontifical Council for Pastoral Assistance to Health Care Workers, elaborates: "This requires love: availability, attention, understanding, sharing, benevolence, patience, dialogue. 'Scientific and professional expertise' is not enough; what is required is 'personal empathy with the concrete situations of each patient.' "[40] John Paul II reminded us of the family's importance in all stages of life, making special note of the needs of the elderly.

[T]he most natural place to spend one's old age continues to be the environment in which one feels most "at home," among family members, acquaintances, and friends, where one can still make oneself useful.... The ideal is still for the elderly to remain within the family, with the guarantee of effective social assistance for the greater needs which age or illness entail.[41]

40. Pontifical Council for Pastoral Assistance to Health Care Workers, *Charter for Health Care Workers* (Boston, Mass.: Pauline Books and Media, 1995), no. 2, quoting John Paul II, Address to the Congress of Italian Catholic Doctors, *L'Osservatore Romano*, October 18, 1988.
41. John Paul II, *To The Elderly*, no. 13.

Health-care professionals and families are encouraged to find ways to make it possible for the elderly to be cared for in their homes.

The home care setting is faced with some limitations. These may include the patient's physical limitations, dementia and its related safety issues, distance from supportive family and friends, and financial considerations. The patient may ultimately benefit from moving to a smaller independent living arrangement specialized for the elderly, to an assisted-living facility, or even to a home that provides nursing care.

[T]here are situations where circumstances suggest or demand that they be admitted to "homes for the elderly" where they can enjoy the company of others and receive specialized care. Such institutions are indeed praiseworthy, and experience shows that they can provide a valuable service when they are inspired not only by organizational efficiency but also by loving concern. Everything becomes easier when each elderly resident is helped by family, friends, and parish communities to feel loved and still useful to society.[42]

Besides providing for physical needs, special living arrangements for the elderly can have many social benefits as well.

Dementia

The wisdom from the Book of Sirach encourages care for our elderly parents, and makes special note of dementia. "My son, take care of your father when he is old.... Even if his mind fail, be considerate with him; revile him not in the fullness of your strength" (Sir 3:12–13). Our rational nature, the ability to reason, is a unique part of our human nature. The *Catechism* tells us: "Being in the image of God, the human individual possesses the dignity of a person, who is not just something, but someone. He is capable of self-knowledge, of self-possession, and of freely giving himself and entering into communion with other persons."[43]

When the elderly patient begins to lose the capability of reasoning, it is a difficult time for both patient and family, as it represents, in some sense, a loss of the human person's identity. As the patient loses connection with his or her surroundings, relationships with others, history, and even self, it may seem as if this diminution of reason lessens the patient's value as a person. But this is not true. In the words of the *Directives*, "The inherent dignity of the human person must be respected and protected regardless of the nature of the person's health problem or social status."[44]

Dementia is defined as memory loss along with a decline in function of at least one other cognitive domain. This may be impairment in handling complex tasks, reasoning ability, spatial ability and orientation, or language. For the diagnosis of dementia, the symptoms must be significant enough to interfere with work and social relationships, must mark a decline from previous function, and must be noted as both insidious in onset and progressive.[45]

---

42. Ibid.
43. *Catechism of the Catholic Church*, no. 357.
44. USCCB, *Ethical and Religious Directives*, dir. 23.
45. See American Psychiatric Association, *Diagnostic and Statistical Manual of Mental Disorders* (Washington, D.C.: American Psychiatric Association, 1994).

Those who care for persons with dementia face many challenges. It may be appropriate to conduct, for all patients as they age, a formal Mini-Mental Status Exam or other cognitive evaluation as part of a yearly preventive care visit.[46] Initially this provides a baseline for the patient, or it may pick up a subtle cognitive defect that is not obvious to the physician in the normal course of conversation with the patient. Appropriate medications may help, particularly in early stages of cognitive loss; thus, physicians should be vigilant in identifying the initial phases of dementia. It is also crucial to diagnose pseudo-dementia, in which the patient is really manifesting clinical depression. Proper treatment requires correct diagnosis.

The safety and well-being of the patient will necessitate involvement of the family or other caregivers. Relatives may have their own emotional responses to a parent's or sibling's decline in mental function. The health-care team should be sensitive to the family's reactions and should guide them to deeper understanding of dementia as an illness. This may include offering family members resources to help them recognize the common features of dementia. Children can become angry with parents, whom they judge to be not listening or not paying attention or not remembering, as if the elderly are at fault and able to choose appropriate behavior. They may fear that the parent's illness is going to impose itself on the adult children's lives and limit their freedom.

The wise health-care provider will know that patient care often involves care of family members as well. Just as would be the case if the elderly parent were dying of cancer or heart disease, the family of the patient with dementia needs support. In particular, the Catholic health-care professional may be a unique witness for the dignity of the human person, even in the face of the demeaning consequences of dementia. Fr. Tad Pacholczyk writes in "Defending the Dignity of Those with Dementia":

The medical profession in particular faces a unique responsibility towards each individual with dementia, a duty to approach each life, especially in its most fragile (and uncooperative) moments, with compassion, patience, and attention. When our ability to think rationally or choose freely becomes clouded or even eliminated by dementia, we still remain at root the kind of creature who is rational and free, and the bearer of inalienable human dignity.[47]

Advance Care Planning

The Patient Self-Determination Act (PSDA) of 1990 is a federal law enacted to ensure that competent adults admitted to health-care facilities are provided with information regarding their legal rights during treatment. Specifically the PSDA directs that patients be given information about their right to prepare an advance directive for their health care. Patients are not obliged to complete such a document, but doing so may facilitate care when critical medical situations arise.

---

46. See Malaz Boustani et al., "Screening for Dementia in Primary Care: A Summary of the Evidence for the U.S. Preventive Services Task Force," *Annals of Internal Medicine* 138 (2003): 927–37.

47. Tad Pacholczyk, "Defending the Dignity of Those with Dementia," Making Sense of Bioethics, October 2010. http://www.ncbcenter.org/files/1114/6982/1083/MSOB064_Defending_the_Dignity_of_Those_with_Dementia.pdf.

There are two types of advance care planning documents. If a patient has either one or both of these documents, the delineated plan goes into effect only if the patient is not able to communicate his or her wishes to the health-care team at the time of decision making. This is an important point: as long as the patient is able to engage in decision making with the physician on his or her own, neither document has any weight.

The first such document is one that designates a health-care proxy. This is a person identified as one who may make health-care decisions for the patient if the patient is unable to do so. The document presumes that the patient has discussed his or her health-care preferences, especially those related to the patient's medical history and moral values, with the proxy beforehand. One or more alternates may be designated on the document, in case of an emergency in which the first-named proxy cannot be contacted. The document appointing a health-care proxy may be called the "Durable Power of Attorney for Heath Care," the "Medical Power of Attorney," or the "Appointment of Health Care Agent."

The second document is one that specifies the patient's particular choices regarding health care at the end of life, or in a critical situation. Again, this document applies only when the patient cannot, at that time, engage in meaningful dialogue with the health-care team. Most of these documents currently address five treatment strategies that are considered "extraordinary" interventions in a situation in which prolonging life may be inappropriate. These treatments are: cardiopulmonary resuscitation (chest compressions); external defibrillation; intubation and artificial ventilation; artificial hydration and nutrition; and the use of antibiotics. The document may include whether the patient wants comfort measures alone, limited interventions, or full treatment. Some documents include subtleties related to particular "quality of life" indices. They may also state preferences related to organ donation. This document may be called a "Living Will," a "Medical Directive," an "Advance Directive," or simply an "Advance Care Plan." Another form that incorporates the designation of a health-care proxy as well as particular treatment guidelines is called the "Five Wishes."[48] These include: (1) the person I want to make care decisions for me when I can't; (2) the kind of medical treatment I want or don't want; (3) how comfortable I want to be; (4) how I want people to treat me; and (5) what I want my loved ones to know. A Catholic living will should also address the following five principles: (1) the desire for pain relief; (2) assessing treatments as either ordinary or extraordinary; (3) providing nutrition and hydration; (4) prohibiting euthanasia; and (5) providing for spiritual care.[49]

Additional directives have now been developed which require a physician's order. One such document is the "POST" form, an acronym which stands for Physician Order for Scope of Treatment, or in some states, "MOLST" or POLST" referring

48. Aging with Dignity, "Five Wishes," http://www.agingwithdignity.org/five-wishes.php.

49. P. T. Morrow, "The Catholic Living Will and Health Care Surrogate: A Teaching Document for Evangelization, and a Means of Ensuring Spirituality Throughout Life," *Linacre Quarterly* 80, no. 4 (2013): 317–22.

to Medical or Physician/authorized Healthcare Provider Order for Life Sustaining Therapy. This is a physician's order, binding whether the patient is at home, in a care facility, or being transported from one level of care to another, generated by the patient and physician. It gives guidance to emergency transport personnel and does not require that a separate DNR order be written for a patient in the hospital; emergency medical personnel are required to abide by the orders without requiring additional or alternate forms. The form is to be completed based on the physician's understanding of what the patient would want. This can occur through the physician's conversation with the patient, through discussion with family or other people close to the patient, or because the physician believes that he or she knows what is in the patient's best interests.

The Patient Self-Determination Act and advance care planning documents were developed out of respect for the dignity of the human person. In some circumstances, however, the physician can become preoccupied with treatment plans and lose sight of the suffering patient and family. This situation is described in the *Charter for Health Care Workers*:

Contemporary medicine, in fact, has at its disposal methods which artificially delay death, without any real benefit to the patient. It is merely keeping one alive or prolonging life for a time, at the cost of further, severe suffering. This is the so-called "therapeutic tyranny," which consists "in the use of methods which are particularly exhausting and painful for the patient, condemning him in fact to an artificially prolonged agony." This is contrary to the dignity of the dying person and to the moral obligation of accepting death and allowing it at last to take its course. "Death is an inevitable fact of human life": it cannot be uselessly delayed, fleeing from it by every means.[50]

The Catholic physician, who has a sense of eternity as the ultimate end of human life, will always strive to see patients in this light.

It is most appropriate, therefore, for the Catholic physician to discuss care preferences with patients before it is time to make critical decisions. A physician who has a long-term relationship with a patient should already know who the family members are. It should not be difficult, when the patient is well, to inquire about whom the patient would want involved in treatment decisions, should he or she be unable to make decisions alone. At the same time, a Catholic physician can use these conversations to assess that a patient or family would not request interventions that would constitute a kind of passive or active euthanasia. Respect for patient autonomy does not oblige a physician to acquiesce to treatment plans contrary to Catholic teaching. At times, a Catholic physician may need to explain to a patient why a particular advance directive cannot be honored. If a course of action cannot be agreed upon, the physician may need to help the patient find another caregiver.[51]

---

50. Pontifical Council for Pastoral Assistance to Health Care Workers, *Charter for Health Care Workers*, no. 119.

51. See USCCB, *Ethical and Religious Directives*, dir. 24. See also Lesley S. Castillo et al., "Lost in Translation: The Unintended Consequences of Advance Directive Law on Clinical Care," *Annals of Internal Medicine* 154 (2011): 121–28. Of interest, in appendix table 3: "However, nearly all states grant clinicians the right of

It must also be understood that there are limitations to the use of advance directives. Patients may neglect to discuss with their health-care proxies the criteria they wish to be used when the patient cannot make a health-care decision alone. Cultural norms may not be fully incorporated in directives that are more suited to a Western way of thinking about medical decisions. Directives may need to be updated, depending on the patient's change in relationships or modified views on health-care decisions. Finally, no advance directive can adequately address the complexities of medical, personal, and family interactions that take place in the health-care arena. In an increasingly protocol-driven medical world, physicians may put false hopes in an advance directive that appears to be well formulated yet does not fit the reality of the patient's situation in the clinical scene. The Catholic physician will never rely simply on preplanned arrangements, but will honor the dignity of the patient and family in difficult situations. Henry S. Perkins writes:

> Physicians surely have the duty to fight disease in most circumstances, but physicians always have the still greater duty to see patients and survivors through their suffering and thereby to bear witness to it. Perhaps that greater duty lifts medicine from a mere occupation to a true profession.[52]

Case 4

Sister Mary Joseph was an 87-year-old woman with end-stage congestive heart failure. At the age of 85, she had contracted a protracted and severe febrile diarrheal illness temporally related to a course of oral clindamycin. Initially she declined medical evaluation, fearing an admission to the hospital. Her stated goal was "to live to be 100," so her caregivers in her community suggested that reaching that goal would require inpatient evaluation and treatment. She acquiesced, recovered after an extended course of metronidazole, and returned to her usual independence. At the age of 86, severe chest pain and shortness of breath one morning prompted a limited cardiac evaluation in the infirmary of her convent. Changes in EKG and lab abnormalities suggested an acute cardiac event, and again, Sister Mary Joseph feared a hospital admission. Her primary care physician visited her that evening and suggested a brief hospitalization for consultation with a cardiologist, who might suggest a conservative course of action. Sister Mary Joseph acquiesced again, and with this new specialist, her cardiac symptoms were managed medically at home and well-controlled over the ensuing months. Occasional appointments at the cardiac clinic were supplemented with telephone and email follow-up, and

---

refusal based on conscience or other objections," and "Most states acknowledge that providers are not required to act contrary to the standard of care, whereas other states variously permit noncompliance on the basis of one's conscience and personal, moral, religious, and philosophical beliefs. If a provider invokes a conscience objection, states require the provider or institution to notify the patient and permit his or her transfer to another provider."

52. Henry S. Perkins, "Controlling Death: The False Promise of Advance Directives," *Annals of Internal Medicine* 147 (2007): 51–57.

Sister Mary Joseph was able to continue with nearly all of her normal daily routine including her community activities. In her last two weeks of life, she developed dyspnea that was increasingly resistant to diuretics, nitrates, and supplemental oxygen. She was convinced to try morphine; and while she was reluctant, because of negative connotations, she recognized the palliative effects and was pleased to continue with PRN doses. Neither the patient nor her caregivers at this point could see any benefit in hospitalization. Sister Mary Joseph asked her fellow religious to pray that she would have a peaceful death. Her condition improved one Sunday morning, she set new activity goals for herself and enjoyed a good lunch. That afternoon, her condition declined precipitously, and she died quietly, with several sisters at her bedside. This case demonstrates the difference between proportionate and disproportionate care, as well as symptom management in advanced disease processes.

Proportionate and Disproportionate Care

The Church recognizes that medicine is not simply about treating diseases but is about caring for the suffering patient. Medical interventions are not merely reflexive answers to a scientifically derived diagnosis. The human person is a complex being with physical, psychological, spiritual, and community needs, as can be seen in Sister Mary Joseph's case. Treatment plans should properly include consideration of all of these dimensions.

As early as 1957, Pope Pius XII distinguished between ordinary and extraordinary means of medical treatments. He made clear that one is held to use ordinary means, whereas extraordinary means are not obligatory. He identified ordinary means as those "that do not involve any grave burden for oneself or another."[53] They do, on the other hand, offer a reasonable hope of benefitting the patient. Later, the Vatican *Declaration on Euthanasia* (1980) commented that the terms "ordinary" and "extraordinary" are sometimes imprecise terms, and it recognized the use of the words "proportionate" and "disproportionate."

In any case, it will be possible to make a correct judgment as to the means by studying the type of treatment to be used, its degree of complexity or risk, its cost, and the possibilities of using it, and comparing these elements with the result that can be expected, taking into account the state of the sick person and his or her physical and moral resources.[54]

The Church has continued this important teaching, reiterating it in various publications, such as the *Ethical and Religious Directives*:

---

53. Pope Pius XII, "The Prolongation of Life: Address to an International Congress of Anesthesiologists, November 24, 1957," *The Pope Speaks* 4 (1958): 393–98.
54. Congregation for the Doctrine of the Faith, "Declaration on Euthanasia," May 5, 1980, http://www.vatican.va/roman_curia/congregations/cfaith/documents/rc_con_cfaith_doc_19800505_euthanasia_en.html.

While every person is obliged to use ordinary means to preserve his or her health, no person should be obliged to submit to a health-care procedure that the person has judged, with a free and informed conscience, not to provide a reasonable hope of benefit without imposing excessive risks and burdens on the patient or excessive expense to family or community.[55]

It is notable that the determining factor in whether a particular treatment is "proportionate" depends primarily on whether it is of benefit to the patient. This means that the treatment in and of itself is not deemed obligatory or optional. Rather there must be an understanding of the circumstances as they pertain to the particular patient at the actual time of the proposed intervention. According to the *Charter for Heath Care Workers*,

The health-care worker who cannot effect a cure must never cease to treat. He is bound to apply all "proportionate" remedies. But there is no obligation to apply "disproportionate" ones. In relation to the conditions of a patient, those remedies must be considered ordinary where there is due proportion between the means used and the end intended. Where this proportion does not exist, the remedies are to be considered extraordinary.[56]

Again, the proposed treatments must be examined based on whether they, as a means used, will promote the end intended: that is, the appropriate treatment of the patient's malady. The illness is not to be considered apart from the patient who is suffering it.

At times, the balance between the benefit of a treatment and its burden is misapplied. For example, a course of intravenous antibiotics administered in a hospital setting is a proportionate treatment, as a means to achieve the intended end, namely the eradication of a bacterial infection. This is not a particularly burdensome intervention. However, some will argue that the patient, in old age and chronic illnesses, is "burdened" by life, and therefore intravenous antibiotics are "disproportionate." This is not an accurate reading of the Church's teaching. The question is about the burden of the treatment, not about the burden of the medical condition. Again, this does not mean that intravenous antibiotics are always and in every case an obligatory treatment. It may be that the burden of hospitalization is too great for a patient who is nearing his or her last days. In this case, it is certainly reasonable to try less aggressive means of treatment at home (such as oral antibiotics), while being sure to care for the patient's real needs. The *Directives* tell us:

The task of medicine is to care even when it cannot cure. Physicians and their patients must evaluate the use of the technology at their disposal. Reflection on the innate dignity of human life in all its dimensions and on the purpose of medical care is indispensable for formulating a true moral judgment about the use of technology to maintain life. The use of life-sustaining technology is judged in light of the Christian meaning of life, suffering, and death. In this way two extremes are avoided: on the one hand, an insistence on useless or burdensome technology even when a patient may legitimately wish to forgo it and, on the other hand, the withdrawal of technology with the intention of causing death.[57]

---

55. USCCB, *Ethical and Religious Directives*, dir. 32.

56. Pontifical Council for Pastoral Assistance to Health Care Workers, *Charter for Health Care Workers*, no. 64.

57. USCCB, *Ethical and Religious Directives*, intro. to part 5.

At times, it is reasonable to allow some time to see how a patient's condition might progress, rather than insisting that interventions must be immediate or not at all. Families of patients are sometimes given unreasonable parameters in which to make decisions for their loved ones. A caring and astute clinician knows how to offer options in ways that allow for alternate decisions to be made, if changing circumstances warrant this. As we read in the *Catechism*,

Discontinuing medical procedures that are burdensome, dangerous, extraordinary, or disproportionate to the expected outcome can be legitimate; it is the refusal of "over-zealous" treatment. Here one does not will to cause death; one's inability to impede it is merely accepted. The decisions should be made by the patient if he is competent and able or, if not, by those legally entitled to act for the patient, whose reasonable will and legitimate interests must always be respected.[58]

Clinicians, patients, and their family members are all called upon to recognize humbly their limitations in the face of life and of death. We are all asked to participate with God as the creator of human life, who holds us all in existence. The *Directives* explain this further: "The truth that life is a precious gift from God has profound implications for the question of stewardship over human life. We are not the owners of our lives and, hence, do not have absolute power over life."[59]

Care for the Dying

The way a person understands life has much to do with how he or she thinks about death. For the Catholic, physical death marks the end of life on earth, but it also marks the passage into eternity. Although death is, in and of itself, an evil—insofar as the separation of body and soul disrupts that substantial unity that is the human person—our care for the dying can be a grace-filled time for patient, family, and caregivers alike.

Though it may seem obvious, it is important to recall that the dying person is the focus of care in the dying process. The patient's physical, intellectual, emotional, and spiritual needs are to remain central to all decisions related to the plan of care. There is no more important time to recognize the human person's dignity. The *Catechism of the Catholic Church* reminds us that "the dying should be given attention and care to help them live their last moments in dignity and peace."[60]

Physical care includes providing for the patient's comfort, and especially addressing pain, dyspnea, and other sufferings such as nausea or pruritus. Attention to temperature, cleanliness, food, and drink are all aspects of usual care. Caregivers must take care not to exclude the use of certain medications that have been a long-standing part of the patient's regimen simply because we are "allowing her to die," as rebound effects of withdrawal of medications may precipitate other discomfort.

---

58. *Catechism of the Catholic Church*, no. 2278.
59. USCCB, *Ethical and Religious Directives*, intro. to part 5.
60. *Catechism of the Catholic Church*, no. 2279.

Intellectual care means that the care team makes the patient aware as much as possible of diagnosis, prognosis, and anticipated course of care. The *Directives* advise:

Persons in danger of death should be provided with whatever information is necessary to help them understand their condition and have the opportunity to discuss their condition with their family members and care providers. They should also be offered the appropriate medical information that would make it possible to address the morally legitimate choices available to them.[61]

The reasoning ability of the human person is one of the unique capacities that image our creator; recognizing this ability in our dying patients as we care for them is central to acknowledging their dignity. For this reason, we should not, presuming that awareness of their condition will itself be a suffering, unnecessarily sedate patients. Again, the *Directives* tell us, "Since a person has the right to prepare for his or her death while fully conscious, he or she should not be deprived of consciousness without a compelling reason."[62] For example, intractable pain may require doses of sedating pain medication that interfere with consciousness. But the astute clinician will look for other factors (anxiety about family members, or unmet spiritual needs, for instance) that may be contributing to suffering but which call for treatment other than sedation.

Emotional care can be time consuming, but it is nonetheless essential to good medical care. A patient may fear dying alone or may harbor sadness over unresolved family conflicts. There may be anger over diagnosis and lack of cure. There may be hope that the patient can yet live to attend an important future event. The patient may even approach death with great courage, with a desire to give this final gift of example to loved ones. Love for our patients allows us to affirm feelings, offer help if needed, but especially to be present and accompany the patient on this final journey.

Finally, spiritual care is not outside the realm of the health-care team.[63] The Catholic physician recognizes the spiritual nature of every dying patient, whether or not the patient realizes it him- or herself. Talking with the patient and family members about death may encourage them to engage their religious community in appropriate ways. Even if the patient and family are not Catholic, the physician can suggest to them that they involve a chaplain or their pastor, rabbi, imam, or other religious leader in their care. Even when we are explicit in talking with patients and their loved ones about death, they may still need definite suggestions for spiritual preparation. This need not signal that we are "giving up" on the patient; it should, rather, indicate that we care about all that is important to him or her.

Care of the dying includes care for the patient's family and loved ones.[64] The physician and care team can recommend ways to the patient and relatives to "get things

---

61. USCCB, *Ethical and Religious Directives*, dir. 55.

62. Ibid., dir. 61.

63. See Martha Meraviglia et al., "Providing Spiritual Care to Terminally Ill Older Adults," *Journal of Gerontological Nursing* 34 (2008): 8–14.

64. See Debra Parker-Oliver, "Redefining Hope for the Terminally Ill," *American Journal of Hospice and Palliative Care* 19 (2002): 115–20.

in order" in their relationships. We hear of the "last five words"—thank you, I love you, forgive me, I forgive you, good bye—as a guideline to promote emotional healing and reaffirm family bonds. The family also needs the guidance of the health-care team to understand how the patient's death might manifest itself. For physicians who have seen death many times over, we may forget that this may be the first time that a wife, husband, child, or parent has ever seen someone die. Each experience of death will be unique because of the distinctive nature of each family member's relationship to the dying patient.

Respect for the dead should grace the aftercare and bereavement process. The Christian, giving up his spirit, dies with the belief in the resurrection of the body and its reuniting with the soul in glory. The body of the deceased is provided a reverent burial in anticipation of the resurrection. The Church permits cremation as long as it does not represent any lack of faith in the resurrection of the body. Also, the place of burial is sacred, for it receives the body which has been a temple of the Holy Spirit. The grave or tomb in burial is the final resting place destined for resurrection on the Last Day.

The physician and other health-care members should not be overlooked in the death of the patient. Each death, like each life, is unique. But we as health-care providers run the risk of moving on, without being mindful of the sacred moments in which we have been privileged to participate. The attending physician should be sensitive to the medical student who has never had a patient die, to the nurse who developed a close, if brief, relationship to the family, to the respiratory therapist who worked hard to assure the patient's comfort.[65] The Catholic physician should at least be grateful to all who collaborated in the patient's care. It would be worthwhile for the physician to speak to each team member, or even gather them as a group to recognize their contributions, to remember the patient, and to address any as yet unspoken concerns. This can be a grace-filled moment for all involved.

Concluding Remarks

The stages of human development through infancy, latency, adolescence, and adulthood are well recognized, but elderly persons have a number of developmental tasks to complete as well. These include preparing for retirement, establishing new living arrangements appropriate to one's health, adjusting to decreased physical and emotional reserves, confronting mortality, and loss of parents, spouses, siblings, and friends. The vulnerable elderly patient continues to progress through life's cycle, striking a new balance between dependency needs and the continual need for independence. The patient may also face challenges such as adapting to living alone, preventing social isolation, adjusting to possible institutional living, making sense of one's life, and accepting one's own approaching death.

65. Katharine Treadway and Neal Chatterjee, "Into the Water: The Clinical Clerkships," *New England Journal of Medicine* 364 (2011): 1190–93.

Annotated References of Key Geriatrics Resources

American Geriatrics Society. "Measuring Medical Care Provided to Vulnerable Elders: The Assessing Care of Vulnerable Elders-3 (ACOVE-3) Quality Indicators." *Journal of the American Geriatrics Society* 55 (2007): S247–S487.
Evidence-based guidelines for geriatric clinical care.

Boyd, C. M., J. Darer, C. Boult, L. P. Fried, L. Boult, and A. W. Wu. "Clinical Practice Guidelines and Quality of Care for Older Patients with Multiple Co-morbid Diseases." *Journal of the American Medical Association* 294 (2005): 716–24.
Provocative discussion of balancing clinical treatment decisions in the presence of multiple comorbidities.

Fried, L. P., Q. L. Xue, A. R. Cappola, et al. "Nonlinear Multisystem Physiological Dysregulation Associated with Frailty in Older Women: Implications for Etiology and Treatment." *Journals of Gerontology Series A: Biological Sciences and Medical Sciences* 64A (2009): 1049–57.
Comprehensive discussion of the concept of frailty.

Fries, J. F., and L. M. Crapo. *Vitality and Aging*. San Francisco: W. H. Freeman, 1981.
Detailed description of aging population dynamics and ways to differentiate age from disease.

Karasik, D., S. Demissie, L. A. Cupples, and D. P. Kiel. "Disentangling the Genetic Determinants of Human Aging: Biological Age as an Alternative to the Use of Survival Measures." *Journals of Gerontology Series A: Biological Sciences and Medical Sciences* 60A (2005): 574–87.
A comprehensive review of the concept of biological age and its measurement.

Lesser, C. S., C. R. Lucey, B. Egener, C. H. Braddock III, S. L. Linas, and W. Levinson. "A Behavioral and Systems View of Professionalism." *Journal of the American Medical Association* 304 (2010): 2732–37.
The American Board of Internal Medicine operationalizes the concept of professionalism according to learned habitual behaviors of physicians relative to health care delivery.

Medina-Walpole, A., J. T. Pacala, and J. F. Potter, eds. *Geriatrics Review Syllabus: A Core Curriculum in Geriatric Medicine*. 9th edition. New York: American Geriatrics Society, 2016.
An evidence-based syllabus of clinical geriatrics organized by syndromes and physiologic systems.

Morrison, R. S., and D. E. Meier. "Clinical Practice. Palliative Care." *New England Journal of Medicine* 350 (2004): 2582–90.
A comprehensive review of the philosophy, structure, and application of palliative care.

Powers, J. S., S. White, L. Varnell, C. Turvy, K. Kidd, D. Harrell, B. Knight, K. Floyd, and K. Zupko. "An Autonomy Supportive Model of Geriatric Team Function." *Tennessee Medicine* 93 (2000): 295–97.
Presents a model of team function which maximized individual team member skills to achieve optimum patient care.

Williams, B. C., G. Warshaw, A. R Fabiny, N. Lundebjerg Mpa, A. Medina-Walpole, K. Sauvigne, J. G. Schwartzberg, and R. M. Leipzig. "Medicine in the 21st Century: Recommended Essential Geriatrics Competencies for Internal Medicine and Family Medicine Residents." *Journal of Graduate Medical Education* 1 (2010): 373–83.
Consensus guidelines for geriatric competencies for completion of Internal Medicine and Family Medicine training.

Bibliography

Adelman, Ronald D., Michele G. Greene, and Marcia G. Ory. "Communication between Older Patients and Their Physicians." *Clinics in Geriatric Medicine* 16 (2000): 1–24.
Allman, Joyce, Sandra L. Ragan, Chevelle Newsome, Lucretia Scoufos, and Jon Nussbaum. "Elderly Women Speak about Their Interactions with Health Care Providers." In *Language and Communi-*

cation in Old Age: Multidisciplinary Perspectives, ed. Heidi E. Hamilton, 332–33. New York: Garland Publishing, 1999.

American Psychiatric Association. *Diagnostic and Statistical Manual of Mental Disorders.* Washington, D.C.: American Psychiatric Association, 1994.

Boustani, M., B. Peterson, L. Hanson, R. Harris, and K. N. Lohr. U.S. Preventive Services Task Force. "Screening for Dementia in Primary Care: A Summary of the Evidence for the U.S. Preventive Services Task Force." *Annals of Internal Medicine* 138 (2003): 927–37.

Brownie, Sonya. "Why Are Elderly Individuals at Risk of Nutritional Deficiency?" *International Journal of Nursing Practice* 12 (2006): 110–18.

Catechism of the Catholic Church for the United States of America. Translated by the United States Catholic Conference. Boston, Mass.: St. Paul Books and Media, 1994.

Congregation for the Doctrine of the Faith. *Declaration on Euthanasia.* May 5, 1980. http://www .vatican.va/roman_curia/congregations/cfaith/documents/rc_con_cfaith_doc_19800505_ euthanasia_en.html.

———. *Donum Vitae, Instruction on Respect for Human Life in Its Origin and on the Dignity of Procreation.* February 22, 1987. http://www.vatican.va/roman_curia/congregations/cfaith/documents/rc_con_ cfaith_doc_19870222_respect-for-human-life_en.html.

Hebert, Randy S., R. Schulz, V. C. Copeland, and R. M. Arnold. "Preparing Family Caregivers for Death and Bereavement: Insights from Caregivers of Terminally Ill Patients." *Journal of Pain and Symptom Management* 37 (2009): 3–12.

Hirsh, Adam T., S. Z. George, J. E. Bialosky, and M. E. Robinson. "Fear of Pain, Pain Catastrophizing, and Acute Pain Perception: Relative Prediction and Timing of Assessment." *Journal of Pain* 9 (2008): 806–12.

John Paul II, Pope. *Letter to the Elderly.* October 1, 1999. http://www.vatican.va/holy_father/john_ paul_ii/letters/documents/hf_jpii_let_01101999_elderly_en.html.

Johnson, Daniel C., Cordt T. Kassner, and Jean S. Kutner. "Current Use of Guidelines, Protocols, and Care Pathways for Symptom Management in Hospice." *American Journal of Hospice and Palliative Care* 21 (2004): 51–57.

Lawlor, Peter G. "Delirium and Dehydration: Some Fluid for Thought?" *Supportive Care in Cancer* 10 (2002): 445–54.

Meraviglia, Martha, R. Sutter, and C. D. Gaskamp. "Providing Spiritual Care to Terminally Ill Older Adults." *Journal of Gerontological Nursing* 34 (2008): 8–14.

Morrison, R. Sean, and Diane E. Meier. "Palliative Care." *New England Journal of Medicine* 350 (2004): 2582–90.

Morrow, P. T. "The Catholic Living Will and Health Care Surrogate: A Teaching Document for Evangelization, and a Means of Ensuring Spirituality Throughout Life." *Linacre Quarterly* 80, no. 4 (2013): 317–22.

Pantilat, Steven Z. "Communicating with Seriously Ill Patients: Better Words to Say." *Journal of the American Medical Association* 301 (2009): 1279–81.

Parker-Oliver, Debra. "Redefining Hope for the Terminally Ill." *American Journal of Hospice and Palliative Care* 19 (2002): 115–20.

Perkins, Henry S. "Controlling Death: The False Promise of Advance Directives." *Annals of Internal Medicine* 147 (2007): 51–57.

Pius XII, Pope. "The Prolongation of Life: Address to an International Congress of Anesthesiologists, November 24, 1957." *The Pope Speaks* 4 (1958): 393–98.

Pontifical Council for Pastoral Assistance to Health Care Workers. *Charter for Health Care Workers.* Boston, Mass.: Pauline Books and Media, 1995.

Qaseem, Amir, V. Snow, P. Shekelle, D. E. Casey Jr., J. T. Cross Jr., D. K. Owens. Clinical Efficacy Assessment Subcommittee of the American College of Physicians. "Evidence-Based Interventions to Improve the Palliative Care of Pain, Dyspnea, and Depression at the End of Life: A Clinical Practice Guideline from the American College of Physicians." *Annals of Internal Medicine* 148 (2008): 141–46.

Rabow, Michael W., Joshua M. Hauser, and Jocelia Adams. "Supporting Family Caregivers at the End of Life: 'They Don't Know What They Don't Know.'" *Journal of the American Medical Association* 291 (2004): 483–91.

Stafford, James Francis. Address on the Occasion of the Annual Conference of the Society for Catholic Liturgy. September 9, 2006. http://www.vatican.va/roman_curia/tribunals/apost_penit/documents/rc_trib_appen_doc_20060921_stafford-reconciliation_en.html.

Sulmasy, Daniel P. "Spiritual Issues in the Care of Dying Patients: '. . . It's Okay between Me and God.'" *Journal of the American Medical Association* 296 (2006): 1385–92.

Treadway, Katharine, and Neal Chatterjee. "Into the Water: The Clinical Clerkships." *New England Journal of Medicine* 364 (2011): 1190–93.

United States Conference of Catholic Bishops. *Ethical and Religious Directives for Catholic Health Care Services.* 5th edition. Washington, D.C.: USCCB, 2009.

Vatican Council II. *Sacrosanctum Concilium, Constitution on the Sacred Liturgy.* December 4, 1963.

Wolff, Jennifer L., S. M. Dy, K. D. Frick, and J. D. Kasper. "End-of-Life Care: Findings from a National Survey of Informal Caregivers." *Archives of Internal Medicine* 167 (2007): 40–46.

Stephen E. Hannan, Peter A. Rosario,
Dennis M. Manning, E. Wesley Ely, and
Deacon John M. Travaline

---

8. CATHOLIC PERSPECTIVES ON CARING
FOR THE CRITICALLY ILL

In this chapter, five physicians with many years' combined experience in caring for critically ill patients reflect upon the more commonly encountered ethical dilemmas presenting in the intensive care units of modern day acute care hospitals. The authors discuss important principles and guidelines for successfully navigating through ethically challenging circumstances, and propose ways of maintaining faithful witness to practicing as a Catholic physician. Beyond their spelling out of principles and guidelines, the authors also bring to the fore the spiritual dimension of the patient and provide commentary on the celebration of sacraments with patients in the critical care setting. This chapter, especially along with chapters 6, 7, 10, 11, and 12, clearly portrays a Catholic ethos for the practice of medicine in truth and love; it does so through relating some of the first-hand experience of clinicians in their respective fields.—*Editors*

Physicians have opportunities that a priest does not have, and our mission does not end when medicine is no longer of help. There still remains the soul that must be brought to God. Jesus says, "Whoever visits the sick is helping me." This is a priestly mission.

St. Gianna Beretta Molla

Introduction

In most hospitals, the intensive care unit (ICU) is the point of care for the sickest of all patients. In the ICU, patients face some of the most significant physical, psychological, and spiritual challenges of their lives. As a result, questions of a transcendent nature emerge on a daily basis as they seldom do elsewhere. Because care of the critically ill often involves therapies and interventions to postpone death and sustain life, the issues faced here are particularly crucial, and they offer an opportunity for

Catholic health-care providers, their patients, and the patients' family and friends to witness to their faith. There are many chapters in countless books on how to manage patients with all manner of critical illness. This chapter is designed to integrate some of the same life-threatening clinical scenarios with a faith-based approach to decision making that is in keeping with authentic Catholic witness.

Physicians and other health-care providers, irrespective of their faith tradition, must acknowledge that caring for ICU patients is never a time to proselytize. Rather, health-care professionals, like everyone in general, are called to live out their moral obligation to serve our patients of all faiths and no faith in light of the truth of the Gospel message to "love your neighbor as yourself." From this vantage point, physicians and other health-care professionals are then attuned to entering a covenantal relationship with their patients.

When disposed to this covenantal way of practice, imagining the ICU as a "holy" place can be instructive in caring for critically ill patients. Many patients at the end of life will pass through the ICU on their way to hospice or some other non-intensive care setting, and the situations that occur in the ICU provide good opportunities to reflect on the holy and where it can be found. Patients who are believers facing a serious illness often talk about God; if they sense that they may be dying, the situation calls to mind things that are holy. Even our behaviors as doctors in an ICU should be, on many levels, performed with reverence. We may not tend to think of reverential acts occurring in an ICU, especially since highly technologically sophisticated medical equipment used in the ICU setting can sometimes depersonalize patient interactions. But if we hold the idea of holiness in our mind and the notion of the ICU as sacred space, our behaviors and actions may be delivered with the intent toward "golden rule" service of a human in need; and with a focus on that person's ever-present dignity and immeasurable self-worth, we may better maintain a strong sense of the primacy of the patient as a person.[1]

In this chapter, some of the commonly encountered ethical issues—namely, withdrawing or withholding life-sustaining therapy, and the use of medically assisted nutrition and hydration—are discussed. As an added bonus to this chapter, reflections on true-life stories of the administration of sacraments to patients in the ICU are provided to bring to life the idea of the ICU as a holy environment.

Issues Concerning Withholding and Withdrawing Life-Sustaining Therapy

Well before cardiopulmonary resuscitation, advanced cardiopulmonary life support, sophisticated mechanical ventilators, and pacemaker-defibrillators were adopted and became commonplace, the Catholic Church was anticipating and advising us in matters of life-support technology. When mechanical ventilation was in its infancy, Pope

---

1. Adapted from Russell B. Connors Jr., "The ICU as Holy Ground," in *Ethics in Critical Care Medicine*, ed. James P. Orlowski (Hagerstown, Md.: University Publishing Group, 1999), 235–52.

Pius XII responded to physicians' questions about resuscitation in a 1957 address to the International Congress of Anesthesiologists.[2] Doctors had asked the Holy Father for guidance on using a mechanical ventilator if the patient's situation was "hopeless," and in establishing the fact of death in a brain-injured patient who is still supported by a ventilator and has evidence of blood circulation. In this address, Pius articulated the foundation of Catholic teaching about end-of-life care. That teaching is based on the dignity of the human person, the obligation that one has in cases of serious illness to use ordinary means for preserving life and health. Many of the ethical dilemmas in the practice of critical care involve analyses of ordinary, proportionate, or morally obligatory means of treatment, and those that are extraordinary, disproportionate, or morally optional. We refer the reader to the first two chapters of this book for more in-depth treatment of fundamental principles applicable to many of the clinical issues that arise in the ICU.

Do-not-resuscitate (DNR) orders disallow the use of efforts to reverse a cardiac or pulmonary arrest. In general, a DNR order should be considered when a disease is irreversible (no known therapy will be effective in reversing its course) and irreparable (medical care cannot significantly slow its process).[3]

Hospitalized patients often request a DNR order when the deteriorating trajectory of their disease is fairly obvious. But in many situations, like chronic obstructive pulmonary disease (COPD) or congestive heart failure (CHF), the timing of death is difficult to predict, and patients with such nonmalignant but severe chronic illnesses are typically very late to enter into end-of-life discussions.

The request for a DNR order should come from a competent and informed patient, or, if the patient cannot achieve this level of decision making, from a surrogate. The decision on the futility of cardiopulmonary resuscitation (CPR), however, should not be made unilaterally. The physician should advise on the effectiveness of such treatments, so that the patient or surrogate can make an informed judgment on benefits and burdens. The weight of each treatment should be carefully considered by the patient before a decision is made.

It is important to determine accurately the patient's capacity to make a DNR decision. An ethical analysis of pacemaker-ICD withdrawals described a criterion for decision-making capacity, which requires the patient's ability to communicate, to comprehend the nature and consequences of the request (the patient's death), and to persist in the request. The request should be consistent with the patient's previously expressed goals and values.[4]

In order for patients to reach an informed decision on whether or not to use CPR, it is important that they understand the effectiveness of these interventions. The Na-

2. Pope Pius XII, "The Prolongation of Life," in *Catholic Health Care Ethics : A Manual for Practitioners*, 2nd ed., ed. Edward J. Furton, Peter J. Cataldo, and Albert S. Moraczewski, OP (Philadelphia: National Catholic Bioethics Center, 2009), 299–301.

3. See Eugene F. Diamond, *A Catholic Guide to Medical Ethics* (Palos Park, Ill.: Linacre Institute, 2001).

4. See P. S. Mueller, C. C. Hook, and D. L. Hayes, "Ethical Analysis of Withdrawal of Pacemaker or Implantable Cardioverter-Defibrillator Support at the End of Life," *Mayo Clinic Proceedings* 78 (2003): 959–63.

tional Registry of Cardiopulmonary Resuscitation and others have produced several large studies that address the outcomes for CPR and advanced cardiopulmonary life support in hospitalized patients.[5] Although this information is not widely known to physicians except perhaps in general terms,[6] it becomes crucial in light of statistics that suggest that if patients knew the outcome data, they might be less inclined to undergo CPR.[7] In fact, this is the focus of the educational patient-care videos and research of Angelo Volandes, MD, and his popular book called *The Conversation*.[8] These clinical scenarios are provided to illustrate some key points about how to navigate this tough area of clinical decision making.

Case 1: Chronic Ventilatory Failure and Long-Term Mechanical Ventilation: Continuation or Withdrawal of Ventilatory Support

A 67-year-old woman presented to the clinic solely for the intention of meeting the pulmonologist. She wanted to be sure she would like her lung doctor. She related a brief history of asthma, which included a fifty-plus-pack-per-year history of smoking, yet her described symptoms could better be ascribed to irreversible chronic obstructive pulmonary disease (COPD), such as long-standing emphysema. Indeed, her pulmonary function tests (PFTs) showed severe COPD with an FEV_1 of only 1.8 liters and little reversibility with bronchodilation. She was started on appropriate medications, and within two weeks the physician received a call from the emergency room stating that she was in the ED in severe respiratory distress, demonstrating mild hypersomnolence and rapid, shallow respirations. A trial of noninvasive ventilation was begun. Serial arterial blood gases showed progressive CO_2 retention and continued hypoxemia, despite supplemental oxygen.

She was seen by the physician soon after admission into the ICU, where she was found to be less responsive, diaphoretic, and slightly cyanotic, with markedly diminished breath sounds, tachycardia, and distant heart sounds on auscultation. She was at that point intubated and mechanically ventilated. Within two days, she met criteria for extubation by passing a spontaneous breathing trial. She remained off of mechanical ventilation for two days, but on the third day she again developed respiratory failure and had to be reintu-

5. See, for example, M. A. Peberdy et al., "Cardiopulmonary Resuscitation of Adults in the Hospital: A Report of 14720 Cardiac Arrests from the National Registry of Cardiopulmonary Resuscitation," *Resuscitation* 58 (2003): 297–308; William J. Ehlenbach et al., "Epidemiologic Study of In-Hospital Cardiopulmonary Resuscitation in the Elderly," *New England Journal of Medicine* 361 (2009): 22–31.

6. See Mark H. Ebell et al., "The Inability of Physicians to Predict the Outcome of in-Hospital Resuscitation," *Journal of General Internal Medicine* 11 (1996): 16–22.

7. See D. J. Murphy et al., "The Influence of the Probability of Survival on Patients' Preferences Regarding Cardiopulmonary Resuscitation," *New England Journal of Medicine* 330 (1994): 545–49; Peberdy et al., "Cardiopulmonary Resuscitation of Adults in the Hospital."

8. Angelo Volandes, *The Conversation: A Revolutionary Plan for End-of-Life Care* (New York: Bloomsbury USA, 2015), https://lisa-wang-p49c.squarespace.com/the-conversation. See also Advanced Care Planning (ACP) Decisions, "Patient Resources," http://www.acpdecisions.org/patients/.

bated. This cycle repeated itself shortly afterwards. In addition to her severe COPD, she had a history of chronic anxiety disorder, which only added to the difficulty of keeping her out of respiratory failure and off mechanical ventilation.

After she failed yet a third time to remain off mechanical ventilation (this time she was off the ventilator less than forty-eight hours), the physician questioned the patient and her family about whether she should be reintubated, given the previous failures and mounting evidence that she was going to require long-term ventilatory support. He suggested the ventilator might even become permanent. It was decided through talking to her and the family that she would want a tracheostomy and then to continue treatment.

During the next thirty days, the second half of which was spent in a long-term acute care (LTAC) hospital, the patient received continuous mechanical ventilation, and a percutaneous endoscopic gastrostomy (PEG) tube was placed for nutritional feedings; in addition, she was treated aggressively with bronchodilators, corticosteroids, antibiotics, anti-anxiolytics. In time she was weaned from mechanical ventilation, and the tracheostomy tube was downsized and eventually removed, along with the feeding tube. Her emphysema remained stable for the next four years without re-hospitalization before she succumbed to her disease.

This patient's story brings up several points that are worthy of discussion:

- How can physicians establish a solid patient/physician relationship? What are our patients looking for?
- What are the needs of chronic ventilator patients and their families?
- Should mechanical ventilation be initiated on a patient with a poor prognosis?
- Should the unweanable patient remain on, or be withdrawn from, mechanical ventilation?
- Which approach—noninitiation or withdrawal of therapy—is the better approach for the patient with a terminal illness?
- How should we approach the patient with a good prognosis who wishes to withdraw life-sustaining therapy prematurely?

Often the introduction of a physician to a new patient is through a consultation. Such an encounter in the office or clinic setting is frequently easier to manage than the hospital consultation, especially a consultation in the ICU. The person is usually less ill, more able to communicate, and more comfortable discussing end-of-life issues in the office setting. In the hospital, a patient's ability to communicate might be seriously limited. Family members who would otherwise be present with the patient in the clinic may be unavailable in the hospital. Permission and understanding is essential to determination of matters such as the use of mechanical ventilation, dialysis, nutritional support and how it is to be administered, and a cardiopulmonary resuscitation status, among other things. As a result, when the patient is unable to communicate his or her wishes effectively, therapeutic decisions fall to family members or a surrogate who may mean well but may not truly or fully know the desires of the person they represent.

All too often we end up having to ask patients their wishes toward life-sustaining therapy when they are *in extremis*, which is very difficult and fraught with many confounding issues. Rather than feel frustrated about it, which is commonly expressed ("Why wasn't this dealt with in an outpatient clinic setting?"), anyone in this position should view it as a privilege to have such personal and important conversations with a patient and his or her family. It is never a burden and always a gift, and one might make a point of remembering the quote of St. Gianna Beretta Molla placed at the beginning of this chapter. Having said this, the reality, however, is that in urgent and life-threatening situations, it is often difficult to determine how well patients understand their situation as they attempt to make informed decisions.

As noted above, many physicians, whether in clinic or in hospital, shy away from discussions involving end-of-life issues, or else they treat them in a very desultory way. They may lack certainty in their treatment suggestions, fearing to give inadequate or wrong advice. Perhaps such discussions evoke emotional distress in physicians, or they simply do not know how to communicate in a way that promotes compassion, understanding, and empathy. Racial and cultural differences with patients may add to their hesitancy; language and pronunciation problems may hinder understanding. In addition, such discussions are time-consuming; the issues they involve cannot be easily resolved in a few minutes.

However, the patient-physician relationship is important enough, and of enough therapeutic value, to compel physicians to work on effective communication skills. Doctors should endeavor to develop empathy, simplicity of speech, truthfulness, hopefulness, and an understanding demeanor, and strive to be more than "a passive conduit of medical information."[9]

The challenge of forming a patient-physician relationship can be considerably more complicated in the ICU than within the clinic setting. Apart from the issues noted above, information can be inconsistent or even contradictory, especially when multiple health-care providers are involved. Ultimately, poor communication will adversely affect clinical therapies and family satisfaction. Physicians are urged to consider including all family members in discussions, provided the patient or surrogate gives permission, so every family member has an opportunity to understand the treatment plan. This may mean numerous meetings, or patiently going over the same information several times, to help family members comprehend the gravity of their loved one's illness.[10] It is also wise to consider having family members on rounds so that they can hear the entire medical presentation. Many ICUs have modeled this approach and find it actually saves time, because, through experiencing the presenta-

9. John Travaline, Robert Ruchinskas, and Gilbert D'Alonzo, "Patient-Physician Communication: Why and How," *Journal of the American Osteopathic Association* 105 (2005): 15.

10. See Gordon Wood, Elizabeth Chaitin, and Robert Arnold, "Communication in the ICU: Holding a Family Meeting," *UpToDate*, last updated June 24, 2016, http://www.uptodate.com/contents/communication-in-the-icu-holding-a-family-meeting.

tion on rounds, the family feels fully informed; the need for time-consuming and difficult-to-organize family meetings is greatly diminished or eliminated altogether. In circumstances where "family rounds" (having family on routine rounds) is not practiced or possible, early and frequent family conferences are ultimately more help-ful and less time-consuming than multiple individual discussions.

It is important to take a spiritual history. Patients must be respected regardless of religious belief or nonbelief, and so a way of asking this is "Do you have any spiritual values that you want your medical team to know that might affect your medical deci-sions?" This is nonjudgmental and can help them feel comfortable to express whatever it is that they need us to know about this intensely personal area of their "mind/body/spirit" triad.

Many Christians get confused about important differences between euthanasia and the withholding or withdrawal of life support. (Withholding support and with-drawing it are ethically equivalent acts; they will be discussed in depth later in the chapter.) It is true that the Church teaches that all life is sacred, but the Church also teaches that overly burdensome or extraordinary care is not warranted when in the eyes of the patient those burdens outweigh the potential benefits. It is key that the Church emphasizes that this risk/benefit ratio is to be ultimately determined by the patient himself or herself. Archbishop Cronin's thesis that emphasized this patient-centered decision-making process (published in 1958 and again as a fiftieth anniversary edition) was a major guiding light to bioethicists and to St. John Paul II in his writing of *Evan-gelium Vitae*.[11] In fact, what Cronin wrote, now sixty years ago, has remained essen-tially intact in all of its major opinions on these topics in the eyes of the Church.

The physician must attempt to gauge the true reality of the patient's condition and relay it to the patient, surrogate, and family directly, yet as compassionately as possible. He or she must try to convey the truth that use of extraordinary means for survival, particularly when such means can be construed as futile or excessively bur-densome to the patient, is not a mandatory requirement of the Church. In such cases, the patient does not die of failure to initiate therapy, but from the underlying disease process. The same can be said of withdrawing futile treatment from the dying patient, and as stated above, withdrawal of life support is ethically the same as withholding life support (that is, there is no ethical distinction between the two).

As stated earlier, the best opportunity to discuss issues of care, particularly those involving life-threatening illnesses, is in the doctor's office or clinic. Discussions of CPR, with or without airway intubation, should be commonplace. Recently, debate has arisen concerning Physician Orders for Life-Sustaining Treatment (POLST, also known as MOLST, for "medical orders for life-sustaining therapy") and whether such orders contain hidden dangers that might conflict with Catholic moral teach-ing and the *Ethical and Religious Directives for Catholic Health Care Services*.[12] With

11. D. A. Cronin, *The Moral Law in Regard to Ordinary and Extraordinary Means of Conserving Life* (Rome: Gregorian University, 1958).

12. United States Conference of Catholic Bishops (USCCB), *Ethical and Religious Directives for Catho-lic Health Care Services*, 5th ed. (Washington, D.C.: USCCB, 2009).

POLST and MOLST, the patient can exercise more autonomy, such as determining the use of antibiotics or dialysis for example. Restriction of treatments that are futile, excessively burdensome, or create excessive expense for the family or community is endorsed by Church teaching, and it is precisely this area of care that ought to be the goal of any such POLST or MOLST orders.

John Paul II, in *Evangelium Vitae,* and the U.S. Conference of Catholic Bishops have issued statements that help with the faithful application of Church teaching along the lines of balancing aggressive care with appropriate judgment regarding excessively burdensome care. For example, the bishops say the following: "We have a duty to preserve life, but the duty to preserve life is not absolute, for we may reject life-prolonging procedures that are insufficiently beneficial or excessively burdensome [disproportionate to expected results or excessively burdensome to patient and family]."[13] Further, we are taught this: "To forego extraordinary or disproportionate means is not the equivalent of suicide or euthanasia; it rather expresses acceptance of the human condition in the face of death."[14]

Some might fear that the patient's wishes might oblige the Catholic doctor to do something illicit. However, since POLST/MOLST orders also apply to entities outside of the hospital, they can augment the *Ethical and Religious Directives* by ensuring that interventions are reasonable and not excessively burdensome.[15] The Catholic Medical Association has taken a rather hardline stance (to protect the sanctity of life) against the use of "doctor signed" order forms about end-of-life decisions, stating that the forms do not take into account unanticipated changes in the person's clinical course.[16] On the other hand, it might be possible that the orders, carefully used, could be a form of communication between the patient and, for example, an ICU physician, who often does not know a person prior to caring for them in an incapacitated state with no available surrogate, though a simple check-box form does not lend itself to this.

In theory, the idea of having conversations with patients well in advance of the ICU, in an outpatient setting with a caring physician and medical team, is an ideal to achieve; and there are some positive aspects about POLST/MOLST orders. Further, they essentially are not contrary to Church teachings. However, there are some important caveats to point out. Although these orders are "signed" only by physicians and not by physician assistants or nurse practitioners, many states have adopted a more technical approach to having these filled out, meaning that people other than the physician will actually go through the POLST/MOLST form with the patient, and have it completed and signed later by the physician. Herein lies the rub. It is possible that the nuances of the most appropriate decisions for the particular patient might be poorly understood by nonmedical personnel or even someone

13. Ibid., dir. 29.

14. Pope John Paul II, *Evangelium Vitae, On the Value and Inviolability of Human Life*, Encyclical Letter, March 25, 1995, no. 65.

15. See John Tuoley, "POLST Orders Are Not Dangerous," *Ethics and Medics* 35, no. 10 (October 2010): 3–4; Lisa Gasbarre Black, "The Danger of POLST Orders," *Ethics and Medics* 35, no. 6 (June 2010): 1–2.

16. See Catholic Medical Association, "Physician Orders for Life-Sustaining Treatment" resources, http://www.cathmed.org/resources/polst/.

who is medical but not the patient's actual physician. Lastly, there are states in which physician-assisted suicide and euthanasia (PAS/E) are legal, and in such states a more aggressive approach is taken to having patients choose to not have, for example, fluids and nutrition. This has caused the Catholic Medical Association to create a white paper warning that "the benefits will be grossly outweighed by the harms and abuses that will result from use of the POLST form and the campaign to promote it."[17] An example of a good partnership between health care and the Church is to be found in the state of Illinois, which approached the POLST/MOLST conversation through the eyes of Catholic teaching.[18]

Moving on to other elements of this particular patient's story: a decision not to intubate and restart mechanical ventilation after the first or second extubation would most likely have resulted in the patient's demise. In such a situation, withholding mechanical ventilation could have been reasonable and morally justifiable if the patient and/or surrogate thought, after serious consideration of the details as they related to him or her, thought that this therapy was overly burdensome with little hope of ongoing benefit. In this particular situation, the family chose to continue therapies, which resulted in gradual improvement back to the patient's functional baseline for several years.

Individuals with COPD who also have poor nutritional status, impaired quality of life, older age, comorbid diseases (especially heart disease and depression), and a severe form of COPD obviously have a poor long-term prognosis. Though it is difficult to determine how long he or she might live, just as it is for CHF patients, the preferred approach to determining when to address end-of-life planning is triggered by the "surprise" question: "Would you be surprised if this patient was dead in one year?" If the answer to this question is "no, I would not be surprised if this patient was dead in one year," then an end-of-life conversation is warranted to determine the patient's preferences. A thorough approach to this is outlined nicely for hospitalized patients; it is similar to the approach found in the case presented above.[19] Using this "surprise" question will help one avoid waiting until the threat of death is imminent. Up until that time, even severe COPD may be perceived as just a "way of life."[20] Both physician and patient may be lulled into a false sense of security. The question then—when a crisis arrives—becomes, how aggressively should one treat exacerbated COPD that has resulted in acute respiratory failure. Even more uncertainty arises when the patient cannot be liberated from mechanical ventilation after a prolonged period or,

17. C. Brugger et al., "The POLST Paradigm and Form: Facts and Analysis," *Linacre Quarterly* 80, no. 2 (2013): 105, http://www.cathmed.org/assets/files/LNQ59%20FINAL.pdf.

18. See Catholic Conference of Illinois, "CCI Provides Answers on POLST," September 8, 2014, http://www.ilcatholic.org/cci-provides-answers-on-polst; and Catholic Conference of Illinois, POLST faq, http://www.ilcatholic.org/wp-content/uploads/POLST_FAQs_2014.pdf.

19. See John J. You, Robert A. Fowler, and Daren K. Heyland, on behalf of the Canadian Researchers at the End of Life Network (CARENET), "Just Ask: Discussing Goals of Care with Patients in Hospital with Serious Illness," *Canadian Medical Association Journal* 186, no. 6 (April 1, 2014): 425–32.

20. See Hilary Pinnock et al., "Living and Dying with Severe Chronic Obstructive Pulmonary Disease: Multi-perspective Longitudinal Qualitative Study," *BMJ* 342, January 24, 2011: d142.

as in the previous case, multiple episodes of respiratory failure develop, with the need for frequently reinstituting mechanical ventilation with progressive physical decline and absence of recovery to previous baseline.

Case 2: When a Patient with a Pacemaker-Defibrillator Is Nearing Death

A 75-year-old man with a severe ischemic cardiomyopathy (ejection fraction 15 percent), with an automated implantable cardioverter defibrillator, and with diabetes and very limited physical abilities (NYHA class IV) is found unresponsive by his family. Emergency personnel find him in a paced rhythm at 80 with a weak pulse, a low blood pressure of 80/40, and agonal respirations. He is intubated, given IV fluids, started on dopamine, and brought to the emergency department, where he is seen by his cardiologist, an intensivist, and his primary care physician. Interrogation of the defibrillator revealed episodes of ventricular tachycardia and ventricular fibrillation on the day of admission, with appropriate firings of the defibrillator. His serial cardiac enzymes were consistent with a myocardial infarction the day of admission. Noninvasive medical management was advised by his cardiologist.

Despite optimization of his fluids and cardiac medications and continuing mechanical ventilatory support, by day 3 he remained in a low cardiac output state, evidenced by physical exam and echocardiogram. Urine output was marginal, and his creatinine level was rising. When sedation was discontinued, he was able to open his eyes to voice stimulation, but he did not follow simple commands, and appeared to have anoxic encephalopathy.

His wife requested and received a written DNR order. By day 4, without having been given any psychoactive medications that would otherwise cloud his sensorium, the patient was deeper into a comatose state, unable to respond to commands, and with ongoing heart failure and pulmonary edema despite aggressive medical management. Based on his previously stated wishes, the wife requested both withdrawal of the ventilator and termination of the pacemaker and defibrillator functions. He died within twenty-four hours, peacefully and with his family at the bedside.

This patient's clinical course raises a number of issues: *Does a DNR order mean the implantable cardioverter-defibrillator should be deactivated?* In some patients the answer is yes, but not in all. Some patients request DNR status because they meet the previously discussed criteria for poor survival statistics and choose to avoid CPR as a treatment option. But if death is not imminent, ongoing implantable cardioverter-defibrillator (ICD) activity is a proportionate treatment. Patients with an ICD and a DNR order based on noncardiac problems (malignancy, sepsis, acute renal failure), may still benefit from continuing ICD, if the arrhythmia is caused by a cardiac condition rather than by their other underlying medical conditions. This presupposes that the patient has judged the benefits and burdens favorably. In this patient's clinical circumstance, death did appear imminent; and it was in keeping with the patient's previously stated wishes to discontinue the devices.

Can low-burden interventions, such as pacemakers and defibrillators, be deactivated? The short answer is yes; however, care must be taken to ensure that all involved are doing this for an appropriate patient and for the right reasons. This question has been analyzed and really is the same issue faced in withdrawing or withholding other, more burdensome treatments.[21]

The clinical course of heart failure is not a linear downhill trajectory, as is the clinical course of late-stage cancer; it is, rather, a saw-toothed or stuttering series of declines and rallies, with an overall decline.[22] This patient's most recent heart attack caused cardiogenic shock as well as anoxic encephalopathy. After the patient's prognosis was accurately understood by the patient's wife, it was her estimation that her husband would not want ongoing life support, because he had expressed to her (conversation not documented above but was recounted to the medical team) that this would be overly burdensome to him unless it was clear that there was a high likelihood of recovery (which there was not at this point). Thus, she chose on his behalf to heed his wishes, and he died naturally without ongoing life support and with the pacemaker disabled. She commented to the team that this peaceful dying process was exactly what he had hoped for when they had discussed things the month earlier.

Withdrawing Therapy versus Physician-Assisted Suicide (PAS) versus Euthanasia

The distinction between these terms was succinctly stated by Mueller, Hook, and Hayes in their analysis of pacemaker-defibrillator support at the end of life:

> In PAS, the patient personally terminates his or her life by using an external means provided by a clinician (e.g., lethal prescription). In euthanasia, the clinician directly terminates the patient's life (e.g., lethal injection). In PAS and euthanasia, a new intervention is introduced (e.g., drug), the sole intent of which is the patient's death. In contrast, when a patient dies after an intervention is refused or withdrawn, the underlying disease is the cause of death.[23]

Viewed by these standards, the physician in the above case legitimately could have had the pacemaker function of the device deactivated.

Many questions surrounding pacemaker deactivation remain. For example:

---

21. See Mueller, Hook, and Hayes, "Ethical Analysis of Withdrawal of Pacemaker or Implantable Cardioverter-Defibrillator Support at the End of Life"; W. R. Lewis et al., "Withdrawing Implantable Defibrillator Shock Therapy in Terminally Ill Patients," *American Journal of Medicine* 119 (2006): 892–96; J. T. Berger, "The Ethics of Deactivating Implanted Cardioverter Defibrillators," *Annals of Internal Medicine* 142, no. 8 (2005): 631–34; R. Lampert et al., "HRS Expert Consensus Statement on the Management of Cardiovascular Implantable Electronic Devices (Ceids) in Patients Nearing the End of Life or Requesting Withdrawal of Therapy," *Heart Rhythm* 7 (2010): 1008–26.

22. See S. J. Goodlin, "Palliative Care in Congestive Heart Failure," *Journal of the American College of Cardiology* 54 (2009): 386–96.

23. Mueller, Hook, and Hayes, "Ethical Analysis of Withdrawal of Pacemaker or Implantable Cardioverter-Defibrillator Support at the End of Life," 962.

- If the patient is pacemaker-dependent (such as in severe bradycardia syndromes), isn't the pacemaker having its intended effect and wouldn't turning it off amount to euthanasia?
- Is there a moral difference between withholding therapy and withdrawing it once it is in place? Certainly most of the burden of a pacemaker would seem to be related to its insertion and the immediate postoperative period.
- Are there other burdens (perhaps indirect) to be considered?
- Does it matter whether a device is internal or external?
- Is there a difference between an intermittent treatment, such as a defibrillator, and a continuous therapy, such as a pacemaker?
- What if a patient wanted the device surgically removed, or decided to just let the batteries wear out and not replace them?
- To extend the debate further, what if a transplant patient, or one with a prosthetic organ, asked to have the transplant or prosthesis removed?[24]

In 2000, Dr. Edmund Pellegrino commented on a case of pacemaker deactivation.[25] Assuming that a competent, informed patient or surrogate has made the request to deactivate the device, the central question is whether this action is morally defensible; Pellegrino affirmed that it is defensible if the pacemaker function is futile. Based on the standards of effectiveness, benefits, and burdens of a treatment, the cited patient's refractory low cardiac output state was not being helped by the pacemaker and thus the device was ineffective. Pellegrino cites indirect burdens that should also be considered. In this patient's case, these include interfering with a death that would occur naturally in the pacemaker's absence; the expense or use of resources of ongoing care; and the emotional burdens on the patient's wife and family of prolonging an irreversible and irreparable illness.

More on Withholding and Withdrawing
Life-Sustaining Therapy

We have already made points about withholding and withdrawing life-sustaining therapy, but the topic warrants a more in-depth discussion. Dr. Daniel Sulmasy provides a helpful reflection on questions of withholding or withdrawing treatment, as well as on other questions related to these issues.[26] Although many physicians and patients feel that there is a moral difference between starting a therapy and stopping it, most commentaries, including Sulmasy's, seem to indicate that there is no philosophical or ethical difference. Sulmasy recognizes this gap between the clinician and the ethicist/philosopher, and he advises doctors to be sensitive to these differences as they consider specific situations. In Sulmasy's view, the distinction between intermit-

24. See Daniel P. Sulmasy, "Within You/Without You: Biotechnology, Ontology, and Ethics," *Journal of General Internal Medicine* 23, Supplement 1 (2008): 69–72.

25. Edmund D. Pellegrino, "Decisions to Withdraw Life-Sustaining Treatment: A Moral Algorithm," *Journal of the American Medical Association* 283 (2000): 1065–67.

26. Sulmasy, "Within You/Without You: Biotechnology, Ontology, and Ethics."

tent and continuous therapy is not morally decisive; the general principles of withholding and withdrawing treatment still apply.

Internalized devices raise the question of whether they have in effect become part of the patient, or at least part of their physiology. To help frame these questions, Sulmasy describes therapies as either regulative or constitutive. Regulative treatments—for example, antidysrhythmic drugs, antipyretics, or defibrillators—coax the body back toward normal. Even if internal to the body, such treatments do not become part of the patient's "self," and thus they could be withheld or withdrawn should their use be deemed futile or if the burden-benefit analysis is disproportionate.

Constitutive therapy—examples of such therapies are pacemakers, mechanical ventilators, dialysis machines, or insulin—takes over a function that the body can no longer perform. Organ transplants and heart valve replacements also fall under this category. Here the decision to withhold or withdraw requires further thought, for deactivating a pacemaker, which may result in the immediate death of the person, is certainly different from removing a transplanted kidney.

To help sort through this, Sulmasy proposes the further division of constitutive therapy into replacement and substitutive categories. Replacement therapy participates in the organic unity of the patient as an organism and thus becomes part of the patient. Substitutive therapy, by contrast, literally substitutes for a pathologically disordered function. A kidney transplant would be considered replacement, but intermittent dialysis would be considered substitutive. Since the distinction between these types of treatment is not always clear, the physician should consider whether a therapy is responsive to changing physiology in an organism (as in the case of a kidney transplant); whether it can grow and repair itself and is independent of external energy sources; whether it is immunologically compatible; and whether it is integrated into the patient's body. Sulmasy proposes that, under the proper circumstances, most substitutive therapies can be withdrawn. The more a therapy can be understood as a replacement therapy, however, the less it seems morally appropriate to withdraw it.[27] Getting back to the patient in this case study, the pacemaker-defibrillator would be considered substitutive, so the decision to deactivate would have been appropriate for conditions of withdrawal.

The Heart Rhythm Society's consensus statement regarding withdrawal of these devices at the end of life also offers helpful guidance.[28] A committee of cardiologists/ electrophysiologists, geriatricians, hospice and palliative medicine specialists, bioethicists, nurses, pediatricians, legal experts, psychiatrists, and divinity scholars collaborated on this statement, which considers the issues from the many perspectives. The statement discusses Pellegrino's concepts from ten years earlier,[29] as well as the killing versus allowing to die issue, conscience issues, and means of communicating with patients and family members. Except for a single reference to withdrawing artificial nutrition and hydration, which does not specify the limited circumstances in

27. Ibid.
28. Lampert et al., "HRS Expert Consensus Statement."
29. See Pellegrino, "Decisions to Withdraw Life-Sustaining Treatment."

which this might be permissible for Catholics and other, like-minded persons, this document appears to be in line with Church teachings as well as with the previous writings of Pellegrino and Sulmasy.

Withdrawal of devices in instances such as this one need not be an admission of defeat, nor laden with guilt, even when viewed from a Catholic perspective. Rather it may be time for patient, physician, and family to listen to what the body is telling them and accept, indeed affirm, that God is calling this patient home. Such well-reasoned, rational (as opposed to *rationed*) care, which sees scientific reason as the companion, rather than the enemy, of faith, is the essence of what Pope John Paul II described in his encyclical *Fides et Ratio*.[30] Sadly, in many cases of terminal illness, rational care is yielding to its opposite, "desperation care."[31]

This prayer speaks to end-of-life circumstances and offers a faith-filled perspective on the origin and destiny of human life:

Lord, teach me not to hold on to life too tightly. Teach me to take it as a gift; to enjoy it, to cherish it while I have it, but to let go gracefully and thankfully when the time comes. The gift is great, but the Giver is greater still. You are the Giver and in You is a life that never ends.[32]

States of Unconsciousness: Permanent versus Unsure

Brain Death

Very often in the practice of critical care medicine, particularly when caring for patients with impaired consciousness, it is important to describe accurately the patient's condition. The physician must differentiate between death, brain death, coma, persistent vegetative state (PVS), and minimally conscious state.

John Paul II, in his address to the Eighteenth International Congress of the Transplantation Society, defined "death" as "a single event, consisting in the total disintegration of that unitary and integrated whole that is the personal self. It results from the separation of the life-principle (or soul) from the corporal reality of the person."[33] The patient in case 2 above, with his spontaneous eye opening, was alive, not dead.

Brain death is one of the two sets of criteria a clinician can use to determine that a patient has died; the cardiopulmonary criteria compose the other set. According to those criteria, death is recognized when there is irreversible cessation of both circulatory and respiratory functions.[34]

---

30. Pope John Paul II, *Fides et Ratio, On the Relationship between Faith and Reason*, Encyclical Letter, September 14, 1998, esp. no. 106.

31. M. J. DelVecchio Good et al., "Narrative Nuances on Good and Bad Deaths: Internists' Tales from High-Technology Work Places," *Social Science and Medicine* 58 (2004): 939–53.

32. Evening Prayers, Retreat Manual, Manresa-on-the-Mississippi Jesuit Retreat House, Convent, Louisiana.

33. Pope John Paul II, "Address to the Eighteenth Congress of the Transplantation Society" [August 29, 2000], in *Catholic Health Care Ethics*, ed. Furton, Cataldo, and Moraczewski, no. 4.

34. See National Conference of Commissioners on Uniform State Laws, *Uniform Determination of*

John Paul II leaves the standards for ascertaining the fact of death, including criteria for brain death, to medical experts.[35] The American Academy of Neurology's recent report reiterates the guidelines of the 1981 President's Commission report for the determination of death, which led to the Uniform Determination of Death Act (UDDA). This report states: "An individual who has sustained either 1) irreversible cessation of circulatory and respiratory functions, or 2) irreversible cessation of all functions of the entire brain, including the brainstem, is dead."[36] The prevailing consensus and current standard is that the brain death determination is legitimate, and guidelines help clinicians make this determination.[37] Despite the acceptance and use of guidelines, however, variability in the practice of using neurologic criteria for the determination of death is significant.[38] Catholic thought on brain death that emerged from a multidisciplinary symposium on the topic has tried to bring some clarity to the issue.[39]

Coma

The term "coma" describes a pathologic state of unconsciousness in which a patient is both unconscious and unarousable,[40] neither awake nor aware. Because this patient initially had spontaneous eye opening, he was considered arousable, and therefore he was not diagnosed as comatose. However, as his clinical circumstances progressed, he descended into a coma despite aggressive attempts to treat his cardiac dysfunction. This was a very telling and ultimately helpful clinically defining course that allowed the family to know how to apply his previously stated wishes in the specific clinical circumstance. This serves as an excellent example of avoiding a "one shoe fits all" or "cookie-cutter" approach to a situation.

Persistent Vegetative State

The term "persistent vegetative state" (PVS) has been in use since 1972 to describe a subgroup of patients who have had an anoxic injury to the brain and who progress to a state of being awake (eyes open) but not aware (not interacting with their

Death Act (Chicago: National Conference of Commissioners on Uniform State Laws, 1980), http://www .uniformlaws.org/shared/docs/determination%20of%20death/udda80.pdf.

35. John Paul II, "Address to the Eighteenth Congress of the Transplantation Society," no. 4.

36. E. F. Wijdicks et al., "Evidence-Based Guideline Update: Determining Brain Death in Adults: Report of the Quality Standards Subcommittee of the American Academy of Neurology," *Neurology* 74 (2010): 1911–18.

37. See E. F. M. Wijdicks, "The Diagnosis of Brain Death," *New England Journal of Medicine* 344 (2001): 1215–21.

38. See S. Ghoshal and D. M. Greer, "Why Is Diagnosing Brain Death So Confusing?" *Current Opinion in Critical Care* 21 (2015):107–12; S. Wahlster et al., "Brain Death Declaration: Practices and Perceptions Worldwide," *Neurology* 84 (2015):1870–79; D. M. Greer et al., "Variability of Brain Death Determination Guidelines in Leading US Neurologic Institutions," *Neurology* 70 (2008): 284–89.

39. M. Moschella and M. L. Condic, "Symposium on the Definition of Death: Summary Statement," *Journal of Medicine and Philosophy* 41 (2016): 351–61.

40. See F. Plum and J. Posner, *The Diagnosis of Stupor and Coma*, 3rd ed. (Philadelphia: F. A. Davis, 1996).

environment).[41] It is a somewhat controversial term to begin with, and many health-care professionals now prefer to avoid "vegetative" when referring to humans and thus turn toward terms such as "unresponsive wakefulness syndrome." For this chapter, we will continue with the term PVS but will acknowledge that even the authors are not particularly comfortable with this language. Such a clinical state may be a transition phase between coma and recovery, or between coma and death.[42] Specifically, such patients are unaware of self or environment and unable to interact with others. There are data, however, which suggest that some severely brain damaged individuals may be capable of conscious awareness of the outside world.[43] In general though, this term should be considered only when the patient has no evidence of sustained, reproducible, purposeful, or voluntary behavioral responses to visual, auditory, tactile, or noxious stimuli, as well as when there is no evidence of language comprehension or expression. Such patients have sleep-wake cycles and bowel and bladder incontinence. They have sufficiently preserved hypothalamic and brainstem autonomic function to permit survival with medical and nursing care, but they have variably preserved cranial nerve reflexes and spinal reflexes.

The prognosis for PVS is variable. Although there are long-term survivors, the average life expectancy is two to five years.[44] Most die from infection, most commonly in the lungs (pneumonia) or the urinary tract. Other causes of death include respiratory failure and other underlying diseases.

The term "permanent" vegetative state would be considered if a patient continued to fulfill the PVS criteria for more than three months, the standard for patients who have survived an anoxic injury. In patients whose PVS results from traumatic brain injury, the prognosis is somewhat better, a period of one year of PVS without improvement is required before their condition can accurately be called "permanent vegetative state."

Minimally Conscious State

It can be a challenge to distinguish between PVS and minimally conscious state. The patient in a minimally conscious state can intermittently demonstrate interaction with the environment, for example, by visually tracking, following simple commands, signaling yes or no (even if incorrectly), having restricted intelligible verbalization, or displaying restricted purposeful behavior. The prognosis in these patients is better than in those with PVS, especially if the etiology was from a traumatic insult.

A fully conscious person is both awake and fully aware of self and environment.

---

41. See B. Jennett and F. Plum, "Persistent Vegetative State after Brain Damage. A Syndrome in Search of a Name," *Lancet* 1 (1972): 734–37.

42. See Gerald L. Weinhouse "Hypoxic-Ischemic Brain Injury," *UpToDate* (2010), http://www.uptodate.com/contents/hypoxic-ischemic-brain-injury-evaluation-and-prognosis.

43. See Steve Connor, "Vegetative Patients May Be More Conscious of the World Than We Think," *Independent* (U.K.), October 16, 2014, http://www.independent.co.uk/news/science/vegetative-patients-may-be-more-conscious-of-the-world-than-we-think-9799650.html.

44. See ibid.

The minimally conscious person can awaken and demonstrate minimal interaction with the environment. The PVS person is awake, but not aware of self or environment. The comatose person is alive, but neither awake nor aware of self or environment. Awareness requires wakefulness, but wakefulness can be present without awareness.

Prognosis after Cardiac Arrest and Hypoxic-Ischemic Brain Injury

In a person who has undergone cardiac arrest, the pre–hospital admission factors associated with poor outcome include: lack of vital signs, presence of sepsis, stroke with severe deficit, cancer, Alzheimer's disease, two or more chronic illnesses, or CPR for more than five minutes.[45]

If a patient survives to be admitted to the hospital, he or she may face a poor prognosis based on several other indicators, including persistent coma, hypotension, need for intubation and mechanical ventilation, need for vasopressors to maintain perfusion, severe congestive heart failure, and older age.[46] The clinical, radiographic, and biochemical test examinations during the first few days of hospitalization after hypoxic-ischemic brain injury cannot provide any absolute prognostic conclusions as to whether a patient will or will not recover. However, data from the medical literature can allow prudent decisions in many cases such as this. Such information is crucial in helping families or surrogates to assess burden and benefit in order to be able to judge what treatments are proportionate or disproportionate in the case at hand.

A fairly antiquated method that is not routinely used any more (it is included here because it still helps us to understand the evolution of the medical approach to brain death) is the "fourteen-day series" of physical findings which, if considered together and in the context of anoxic brain injury, predict virtually no chance of regaining independence.[47] The criteria are given in table 8-1.

For a more practical assessment, two specific clinical criteria can be used: an absent or extensor motor response (extending the arms or legs to noxious stimuli) at day 3, or an absent pupillary or corneal response at day 3.[48] These criteria have been found in two systematic reviews to be 100-percent specific for poor outcome. The tests for the two criteria are highly specific and give very few false positive results.

Patients with myoclonic status epilepticus have sudden bilateral, synchronous, sometimes profound, movements of the face and limbs. Although this finding is strongly associated with poor outcomes (either death or persistent coma), the medical literature indicates that it has insufficient negative prognostic power in and of itself.

45. See Philip J. Podrid, Morton F. Arnsdorf, and Jie Cheng, "Outcome of Sudden Cardiac Arrest," *UpToDate,* 2010.

46. See Ibid.

47. Weinhouse, "Hypoxic-Ischemic Brain Injury."

48. See E. F. Wijdicks, A. Hijdra, and G. B. Young, "Practice Parameter: Prediction of Outcome in Comatose Survivors after Cardiopulmonary Resuscitation (an Evidenced-Based Review): Report of the Quality Standards Subcommittee of the American Academy of Neurology," *Neurology* 67 (2006): 203–10; D. G. Zandbergen et al., "Systematic Review of Early Prediction of Poor Outcome in Anoxic-Ischemic Coma," *Lancet* 352 (1998): 1808–12.

Table 8-1. **Fourteen-Day Series**

Initial Exam	No Pupillary Response
Day 1	Motor response is no better than flexor (flexing the arm or leg to noxious stimuli) Spontaneous eye movements neither orienting nor roving conjugate
Day 3	Motor response no better than flexor No spontaneous eye opening
Day 7	Motor response not obeying commands Spontaneous eye movements neither orienting nor roving conjugate (eyes move together, back and forth but are not fixating on anything)
Day 14	Oculocephalic response not normal (the doll's eye maneuver) Not obeying commands No spontaneous eye opening Eye movements not improved at least two grades from the initial exam

In particular, there have been patients with good recovery when this finding was associated with circulatory arrest from respiratory failure.

Electrical Tests and Lab Tests

An electroencephalogram (EEG) may help with prognostication in many cases of unresponsiveness; status epilepticus, for instance, can be diagnosed by EEG and is potentially treatable. Another example is an EEG finding of generalized and sustained suppression of the brain's electrical activity. In the absence of medications as the cause or of other metabolic derangements, this finding indicates a likelihood of poor outcome.

A somatosensory evoked potential (SSEP) test detects and records an electrical signal in the nervous system after the patient has been stimulated. This test may be especially useful in early prognostication. In a multicenter cohort study, patients without brain response to bilateral median nerve stimulation during the first week after injury had a 100-percent predictive value of a dismal outcome, namely, no better than persistent coma.[49]

Biochemical markers such as the neuron specific enolase (NSE) or the glial S-100 protein have no diagnostic utility in this area (or really in any major clinical area) and should not be used to help predict outcome after anoxic brain injury.[50]

49. See D. G. Zandbergen et al., "SSEPs and Prognosis in Postanoxic Coma: Only Short or Also Long Latency Responses?" *Neurology* 67 (2006): 583–86.

50. See D. G. Zandbergen, R. J. de Haan, and A. Hijdra, "Systematic Review of Prediction of Poor Outcome in Anoxic-Ischemic Coma with Biochemical Markers of Brain Damage," *Intensive Care Medicine* 27 (2001): 1661–67.

Use of Assisted Nutrition and Hydration

John Paul II, in a 2004 allocution, has provided guidance for cases in which patients fail to progress beyond the PVS: "I should like particularly to underline how the administration of water and food, even when provided by artificial means, always represents a natural means of preserving life, not a medical act. Its use, furthermore, should be considered, in principle, ordinary and proportionate, and as such morally obligatory insofar as and until it is seen to have attained its proper finality, which in the present case consists in providing nourishment to the patient and alleviation of his suffering."[51] One must apply this knowledge while keeping in mind that the patient (or the patient's qualified surrogate) is ultimately the one to judge what treatment is proportionate and what is disproportionate.

A very personal touch in weak patients is to attempt spoon-feeding, but this process requires a patient with enough cognitive abilities to cooperate and some semblance of a swallowing mechanism and cough reflex. It also implies that the caregiver has ample time and patience to keep up with the patient's nutritional needs. In the hospital, nurses can and do perform spoon-feeding, but the time this takes is potentially compromised by competing duties. The National Catholic Bioethics Center's bulletin *Ethics and Medics* has published helpful reflections on the value of spoon-feeding. Dr. Greg Burke, in an article about dementia and the downside of tube feedings, writes, "One cannot help but think of the isolation that tube feeding may cause in some patients."[52] Br. Ignatius Perkins, RN, describes some added implications and benefits of spoon-feeding:

The act of hand-feeding the sick then, requires that the clinician, family member, friend or volunteer engage the whole person, regardless of the person's station in life or the reason for the illness. What might seem to be a simple act of feeding the sick is really a profound affirmation of the intrinsic dignity of the human person, witnessing to the personhood of the one who is sick, and a commitment to remain physically present and to nourish the patient even though there may be little or no cognitive awareness of others or the environment.[53]

This harkens back to Pellegrino's advice that physicians be "present" to their patients.[54]

The Second Vatican Council, in *Gaudium et Spes*, described the conscience as the "the most secret core and sanctuary of a man. There he is alone with God, Whose voice echoes in his depths."[55] Milton Gonsalves describes conscience as "a person's reason, making a practical concrete judgment about the morality of an action that the

51. Pope John Paul II, "Address to the Participants in the International Congress on Life-Sustaining Treatments on Vegetative State: Scientific Advances and Ethical Dilemmas" [March 20, 2004], in *Catholic Health Care Ethics,* ed. Furton, Cataldo, and Moraczewski, no. 4.

52. Greg F. Burke, "Advanced Dementia," *Ethics and Medics* 26, no. 3 (March 2001): 1–3.

53. Ignatius Perkins, "Feed the Sick, Nourish the Person," *Ethics and Medics* 29, no. 9 (September 2004): 1–5.

54. Edmund D. Pellegrino, *The Philosophy of Medicine Reborn: A Pellegrino Reader,* ed. Tristram Engelhardt Jr. and Fabrice Jotterand (Notre Dame, Ind.: University of Notre Dame Press, 2008).

55. Vatican Council II, *Gaudium et Spes, Pastoral Constitution on the Church in the Modern World,* December 7, 1965, no. 16.

person is about to perform (or has already performed)."[56] The Catholic Church has always taught that one must follow one's conscience, but cautions that the conscience must be formed according to objective standards. Those objective standards come from the Magisterium, the teaching authority of the Church, which includes papal and Vatican documents.

The *Ethical and Religious Directives for Catholic Health Care Services*, developed by the U.S. Conference of Catholic Bishops (USCCB), provides additional direction on a variety of health-care issues. The National Catholic Bioethics Center, through its publications, consultations, and bishops' conferences, is also considered an authoritative and authentic guide to Catholic medical moral teaching. The writings of individual theologians and priests may be helpful, but these do not carry the authority of the Magisterium for one who is sorting through bioethical issues.

In addition to the teachings on PVS by John Paul II and the Congregation for the Doctrine of the Faith, which we have already considered, directive 58 of the *Ethical and Religious Directives* states:

In principle, there is an obligation to provide patients with food and water, including medically assisted nutrition and hydration for those who cannot take food orally. This obligation extends to patients in chronic and presumably irreversible conditions (e.g., the "persistent vegetative state") who can reasonably be expected to live indefinitely if given such care. Medically assisted nutrition and hydration become morally optional when they cannot reasonably be expected to prolong life or when they would be excessively burdensome for the patient or (would) cause significant physical discomfort, for example, resulting from complication in the use of the means employed. For instance, as a patient draws close to inevitable death from an underlying progressive and fatal condition, certain measures to provide nutrition and hydration may become excessively burdensome and therefore not obligatory in light of their very limited ability to prolong life or provide comfort.[57]

The USCCB also provides guidance about conscience regarding some conflicts that can arise between patients and Catholic institutions:

Within a pluralistic society, Catholic health-care services will encounter requests for medical procedures contrary to the moral teachings of the Church. Catholic health care does not offend the rights of individual conscience by refusing to provide or permit medical procedures that are judged morally wrong by the teaching authority of the Church.[58]

Though this statement was directed to Catholic hospitals and health-care services in general, it is also applicable to the physician's individual recommendations to patients, both Catholic and non-Catholic.

56. Quoted in Rev. Germain Kopaczynski, "Conscience," in *Catholic Health Care Ethics*, ed. Furton, Cataldo, and Moraczewski, 32.

57. USCCB, *Ethical and Religious Directives for Catholic Health Care Services*, dir. 58.

58. Ibid., pt. 1, intro.

Conversations about Faith and Sacraments in the ICU:
A Physician's Perspective

A 75-year-old-man presents with severe non-ischemic cardiomyopathy with an ejection fraction of 10 percent both by echo and by nuclear medicine stress testing. He is functionally impaired and experiences dyspnea even at rest (NYHA Class IV). He is in the ICU because of ongoing dyspnea despite medical therapy. His cardiologist wants to try a dobutamine infusion for a few days. His code status remains full. He has declined suggestions that he visit a tertiary care center to see if he is a candidate for transplant or a left ventricular assist device.

The patient's physician, who is Catholic, notices on his demographic sheet that he is also Catholic. The physician discloses her own faith and inquires whether he has had any spiritual support from the local parishes; he says he has not, since his infirmities made attendance at church difficult. The physician explains that the patient is eligible to receive the sacrament of the Anointing of the Sick, and offers to contact a priest. The patient accepts the offer, and the priest visits him that day.

This simple interaction brings up several questions: Is it appropriate for physicians to bring up matters of faith in the critical care setting? The short answer is a resounding "yes," but several factors should be considered. The first is the potential medical benefits patients may realize through recognition and discussion of faith matters. In his book *Spirituality in Patient Care*, Harold G. Koenig points out that "no fewer than 90 percent of patients believe in God, that over 90 percent [of patients] pray, nearly 70 percent are church members, and over 40 percent have attended church, synagogue, or temple within the past seven days."[59] He cites numerous studies in which religious beliefs are related to better health outcomes and quality of life. The vast majority of patients with religious beliefs and active faith practice believe that their faith helps them cope. In fact, 40 percent of patients indicate that "religion is *the most important factor*" in helping them cope.[60] Daniel Sulmasy, in his book *A Healer's Calling*, also recognizes the physical health benefits of faith, regarding it as a bonus.[61] The fundamental point is that religion matters a great deal to most patients, and if doctors are to respect patients as persons, they have a duty also to respect what matters to them.[62]

---

59. Harold G. Koenig, *Spirituality in Patient Care: Why, How, When, and What* (Philadelphia: Templeton Foundation Press, 2002), 6.

60. Ibid.

61. Daniel P. Sulmasy, *A Healer's Calling: A Spirituality for Physicians and Other Health Care Professionals* (Mahwah, N.J.: Paulist Press, 1997), 58.

62. Ibid., 64.

Taking the Spiritual History

Several authors offer tools for obtaining a patient's spiritual history, notably T. A. Maugans, C. M. Puchalski, and the aforementioned Sulmasy and Koenig.[63] A conscientious physician can determine the patient's religious preference even before entering the room, from reading the demographic sheet on his or her chart. This information may be accurate but should not be considered definitive. Many patients tell the interviewer in the admitting department that they have no religious preference, and this statement usually follows them around for the entire admission. Gentle inquiry, however, can unearth additional history: "I was brought up Catholic." "I used to be atheist, but now I'm a Muslim." "I'm Buddhist." "I'm Christian, but I'm not a churchgoer." Dr. Koenig recommends that a spiritual history be taken as part of the social history. This seems a natural extension of other questions that establish the patient's support system. The literature shows that most patients want to be asked about their spiritual beliefs or nonbelief and that many consider it rude if health-care professionals do not consider this important piece of their well-being. Ely wrote that the question should be asked out of respect and in a completely nonjudgmental manner (as one might take a sexual history: "Do you have sex with men, women, both, or neither?").[64] Thus, a physician can ask, "Do you have any spiritual values that you want me to know about that might influence your medical decisions?" Other ways a doctor can broach the subject of spiritual values are through such questions as:

- Is faith a part of your life?
- Do you have a faith tradition? How are you dealing with this illness in a spiritual sense?
- I know faith is important to many people, including myself, especially at times of illness. Is that true for you, too?
- Do you have any values we should be aware of that might influence your care?
- Are there any spiritual or pastoral needs that we can help you with?

Some physicians may find it more natural to make spiritual inquiries after they have finished the nuts and bolts of the consult and have presented recommendations to the patient. This tends to be a more relaxed point in the interview and exam, when the inherent inequalities of the doctor-patient relationship have been somewhat leveled. If the physician reveals his or her own faith to the patient, that revelation can level the relationship further. A useful approach is to ask a sequence of questions and allow time to gauge the patient's response to each one in turn: "I noticed on your registration information that you are Catholic. I'm also Catholic. Are you a parishioner at one of the local churches?" By treading lightly, listening sensitively, and

---

63. See C. M. Puchalski, "Spirituality and End-of-Life Care: A Time for Listening and Caring," *Journal of Palliative Medicine* 5 (2002): 289–94; T. A. Maugans, "The Spiritual History," *Archives of Family Medicine* 5 (1996): 11–16; Sulmasy, *A Healer's Calling*; Koenig, *Spirituality in Patient Care*.

64. See E. Wesley Ely, "What I Learned from a Dying Patient," *Wall Street Journal*, December 19, 2014, http://www.wsj.com/articles/wesley-ely-what-i-1419032604.

following the patient's lead, the doctor can judge how best to assist in ministering to the patient's spiritual needs, along with medical needs. The patient's initial responses should guide the subsequent direction of this conversation, and the main thing is to demonstrate absolute respect and love in handling every patient's answer to the spiritual history. If they do have a particular spiritual path, then be sure to offer to get them a professional and not ever to proselytize or attempt to be their spiritual advisor unless they drive that component of the relationship. This approach to the spirituality and faith preferences of our patients promotes a more personal doctor-patient relationship, which implies that the doctor is concerned about the patient in an eternal context, not just a temporal one, and wants what is best for the patient at all levels.

Sacraments in the Critical Care Setting

Sacrament of the Anointing of the Sick

The *Catechism of the Catholic Church* describes the purpose of the Sacrament of the Sick: "By the sacred anointing of the sick and the prayer of the priests, the whole Church commends those who are ill to the suffering and the glorified Lord, that he may raise them up and save them. And indeed she exhorts them to contribute to the good of the People of God by freely uniting themselves to the Passion and death of Christ."[65] Canon law further explains the indications for the sacrament:

The anointing of the sick can be administered to a member of the faithful who, having reached the use of reason, begins to be in danger due to sickness or old age. This sacrament can be repeated if the sick person, having recovered, again becomes gravely ill or if the condition becomes more grave during the same illness.[66]

And the *Catechism* gives guidance on the appropriate time to administer the sacrament: "The Anointing of the Sick is not a sacrament for those only who are at the point of death. Hence, as soon as anyone of the faithful begins to be in danger of death from sickness or old age, the fitting time for him to receive this sacrament has certainly already arrived."[67]

Once it has been confirmed that the patient is Catholic, and seems receptive, the physician can offer to arrange for celebration of the sacrament. This offer can still acknowledge an expectation that the patient will get through this illness, if such is the case. If the patient seems a bit hesitant, the doctor may reassure him or her that it is an easy process to ask the priest assigned to the hospital to come over. Explaining what the Anointing of the Sick involves, and that it can bring graces for spiritual and perhaps physical healing, may help the patient desire to receive it. The doctor can also mention that the sacrament offers an opportunity for Confession and Holy Communion (which

65. *Catechism of the Catholic Church*, 2nd ed. (Washington, D.C.: United States Catholic Conference, 1997), no. 1499.

66. John P. Beal, James A. Coriden, and Thomas A. Green, eds., *New Commentary on the Code of Canon Law* (Mahwah, N.J.: Paulist Press, 2000), can. 1004.

67. *Catechism of the Catholic Church*, no. 1514.

is called "Viaticum" if it is expected to be the last Holy Communion before death). If the patient is receptive to the sacrament, the hospital staff should notify either the chaplain, the priest assigned to the hospital, or the hospital's liaison with pastoral ministers.

Many patients in critical care are on mechanical ventilators, in a coma, or sedated for other reasons. Canon law says that the Sacrament of the Sick "is to be conferred on the sick who at least implicitly requested it when they were in control of the faculties."[68] The Rite of Anointing from the Sacred Congregation for Divine Worship reinforces this teaching: "The sacrament of anointing is to be conferred on sick people who, although they have lost consciousness or the use of reason, would, as Christian believers, have at least implicitly asked for it when they were they in control of their faculties."[69]

Holy Communion

Holy Communion is the most common sacrament conferred in the ICU. Typically, the ministers of Holy Communion arrive in the unit with a list of Catholic patients, checking with the charge nurse to see who is capable of receiving Holy Communion. Though there may be some restrictions based on a patient's medical condition, the main criterion for reception of Holy Communion is the same for the able-bodied and the disabled: namely, that the person be able to distinguish the Body of Christ from ordinary food. This recognition is valid even if evidenced only through manner, gesture, or reverential silence rather than verbally.[70] If a patient is unresponsive due to sedation or other malady, it is not proper to place Holy Communion in the mouth, because the patient cannot distinguish what is being received. There are clearly circumstances in which a patient may be unable to receive the Body and Blood of the Lord as Holy Communion, but one can be mindful of a spiritual communion that may be present by the patient uniting his or her sufferings with those of the Lord.

In their essay "Communion for NPO Patients," Greg Burke and Robb McIlvried make reference to their survey of physicians in the Geisinger Health System on opinions about receiving Communion and the NPO status.[71] They remind us that even the smallest particle of a consecrated host contains the entire divinity and humanity of the risen Christ. In fact, the majority of the physicians surveyed agreed that patients with NPO orders could safely receive a small portion of the Eucharistic host. It is, after all, likely that this small fragment of the host will dissolve in the mouth before it moves down the digestive tract. The one exception to this allowance would be a patient with intractable vomiting.

In the acute setting in an ICU, many conscious patients will have feeding tubes or breathing tubes in their mouths, and offering Eucharist in such situations does

---

68. Beal, Coriden, and Green, eds., *New Commentary on the Code of Canon Law*, can. 1006.

69. *Rites of the Catholic Church*, vol. 1 (New York: Pueblo Publishing Company, 1990), "Pastoral Care of the Sick," no. 14.

70. See National Conference of Catholic Bishops, "Guidelines for the Celebration of the Sacraments with Persons with Disabilities" [June 16, 1995], http://www.ncpd.org/views-news-policy/policy/church/bishops/sacraments.

71. Greg F. Burke and Robb McIlvried, "Communion for NPO Patients," *Ethics and Medics* 35, no. 5 (May 2010): 1–2.

not seem prudent. Although every reasonable attempt should be made to meet the patient's desire for reception of Holy Communion, if the Body or Blood of Christ could not be fully consumed because it might adhere to the plastic tubing, or be subsequently suctioned out of the patient's stomach, for example, then the sacredness of the sacrament would be compromised.

A person with a tracheostomy who is clearly able to swallow would be able to receive Communion, but many patients with a tracheostomy are not able to swallow and would have a high risk of aspiration. In the latter circumstance, obviously the patient could not safely receive the Communion host. In a patient who does demonstrate the ability to swallow food and liquids safely without aspiration, the Eucharistic host or a drop of the Precious Blood could be administered.

If a person has an extremely dry oral mucosa, the host may not dissolve in a timely manner. There are no relevant liturgical norms to deal with a host not progressing down the alimentary tract, so judgment is necessary. Similarly, for patients who can receive food and drink only through feeding tubes, there may be a tendency to think that one could place a small particle of bread or a drop of wine in the tube and propel it into the patient's stomach. In their essay "The Eucharist and Tube Feeding," Br. Ignatius Perkins and Fr. Peter Cameron point out that this situation needs further study by ethicists, bishops, clinicians, and others.[72] The sacramental signs of Communion, the bread and wine, may no longer be recognizable as such upon dilution. The authors call for continued discussion by all those who serve in the health-care ministries, toward a better understanding of the need for the Eucharist by the sick and the establishment of liturgical norms, policies, and procedures to respond to these needs.

Conclusion

Patients in the critical care unit are often the sickest patients in the hospital. Given the critical nature of an illness or the sometimes fast-paced intensity of medical care necessary for such critically ill patients, they—as well as the health-care staff in the unit—many times experience high stress. This stress may be further intensified by any of a number of medical-ethical dilemmas that may arise in a particular case. While only a small percentage of ICU patients may present an ethical dilemma that requires specific consideration, it is important to be prepared for the commonly encountered dilemmas that present themselves, and for the Catholic physician and caretaker to understand important underpinnings for practicing medicine with authentic Catholic witness. There is a spiritual dimension to every person, whether or not that dimension is evident, acknowledged, or expressed. Many times it seems that caring for patients while recognizing their spiritual dimension will elicit in some way, whether well formed or rudimentary in expression, that patient's spirituality. The richness of the Catholic faith provides practitioners in the critical care setting with

---

72. Ignatius Perkins and Peter John Cameron, "The Eucharist and Tube Feeding," *Ethics and Medics* 30, no. 11 (November 2005), 2, see also 1.

abundant opportunity to gently yet powerfully touch the lives of patients and families in ways that complement intensive medical care.

Bibliography

Beal, John P., James A. Coriden, and Thomas A. Green, eds. *New Commentary on the Code of Canon Law.* Mahwah, N.J.: Paulist Press, 2000.

Berger, J. T. "The Ethics of Deactivating Implanted Cardioverter Defibrillators." *Annals of Internal Medicine* 142, no. 8 (2005): 631–34.

Black, Lisa Gasbarre. "The Danger of POLST Orders." *Ethics and Medics* 35, no. 6 (June 2010): 1–2.

Brugger, Christian, Louis C. Breschi, Edith Mary Hart, Mark Kummer, John I. Lane, Peter T. Morrow, Franklin L. Smith, et al. "The POLST Paradigm and Form: Facts and Analysis." *Linacre Quarterly* 80, no. 2 (2013): 103–38. http://www.cathmed.org/assets/files/LNQ59%20FINAL.pdf.

Burke, Greg F. "Advanced Dementia." *Ethics and Medics* 26, no. 3 (March 2001): 1–3.

Burke, Greg F., and Robb McIlvried. "Communion for NPO Patients." *Ethics and Medics* 35, no. 5 (May 2010): 1–2.

Catechism of the Catholic Church. 2nd edition. Washington, D.C.: United States Catholic Conference, 1997.

Catholic Conference of Illinois. "CCI Provides Answers on POLST." September 8, 2014. http://www.ilcatholic.org/cci-provides-answers-on-polst.

Connor, Steve. "Vegetative Patients May Be More Conscious of the World Than We Think." *Independent* (U.K.), October 16, 2014. http://www.independent.co.uk/news/science/vegetative-patients-may-be-more-conscious-of-the-world-than-we-think-9799650.html.

Connors, Russell B., Jr. "The ICU as Holy Ground." In *Ethics in Critical Care Medicine*, ed. James P. Orlowski, 235–52. Hagerstown, Md: University Publishing Group, 1999.

Cronin, D. A. *The Moral Law in Regard to Ordinary and Extraordinary Means of Conserving Life.* Rome: Gregorian University, 1958.

DelVecchio Good, M. J., N. M. Gadmer, P. Ruopp, M. Lakoma, A. M. Sullivan, E. Redinbaugh, R. M. Arnold, and S. D. Block. "Narrative Nuances on Good and Bad Deaths: Internists' Tales from High-Technology Work Places." *Social Science and Medicine* 58 (2004): 939–53.

Diamond, Eugene F. *A Catholic Guide to Medical Ethics.* Palos Park, Ill.: Linacre Institute, 2001.

Ebell, Mark H., G. R. Bergus, L. Warbasse, R. Bloomer. "The Inability of Physicians to Predict the Outcome of in-Hospital Resuscitation." *Journal of General Internal Medicine* 11 (1996): 16–22.

Ehlenbach, William J., A. E. Barnato, J. R. Curtis, W. Kreuter, T. D. Koepsell, R. A. Deyo, and R. D. Stapleton. "Epidemiologic Study of In-Hospital Cardiopulmonary Resuscitation in the Elderly." *New England Journal of Medicine* 361 (2009): 22–31.

Ely, E. Wesley. "What I Learned from a Dying Patient." *Wall Street Journal*, December 19, 2014. http://www.wsj.com/articles/wesley-ely-what-i-1419032604.

Furton, Edward J., Peter J. Cataldo, and Albert S. Moraczewski, OP, eds. *Catholic Health Care Ethics: A Manual for Practitioners.* 2nd edition. Philadelphia: National Catholic Bioethics Center, 2009.

Ghoshal, S., and D. M. Greer. "Why Is Diagnosing Brain Death So Confusing?" *Current Opinion in Critical Care* 21 (2015): 107–12.

Goodlin, S. J. "Palliative Care in Congestive Heart Failure." *Journal of the American College of Cardiology* 54 (2009): 386–96.

Greer, D. M., P. N. Varelas, S. Haque, and E. F. Wijdicks. "Variability of Brain Death Determination Guidelines in Leading US Neurologic Institutions." *Neurology* 70 (2008): 284–89.

Jennett, B., and F. Plum. "Persistent Vegetative State after Brain Damage. A Syndrome in Search of a Name." *Lancet* 1 (1972): 734–37.

John Paul II, Pope. *Evangelium Vitae, On the Value and Inviolability of Human Life.* Encyclical Letter. March 25, 1995.

——. *Fides et Ratio, On the Relationship between Faith and Reason.* Encyclical Letter. September 14, 1998.

———. "Address to the Eighteenth Congress of the Transplantation Society" [August 29, 2000]. In *Catholic Health Care Ethics*, ed. Furton, Cataldo, and Moraczewski, 386–88.

———. "Address to the Participants in the International Congress on Life-Sustaining Treatments on Vegetative State: Scientific Advances and Ethical Dilemmas" [March 20, 2004]. In *Catholic Health Care Ethics*, ed. Furton, Cataldo, and Moraczewski, 401–2.

Koenig, Harold G. *Spirituality in Patient Care: Why, How, When, and What*. Philadelphia: Templeton Foundation Press, 2002.

Lampert, R., D. L. Hayes, G. J. Annas, et al. "HRS Expert Consensus Statement on the Management of Cardiovascular Implantable Electronic Devices (Ceids) in Patients Nearing the End of Life or Requesting Withdrawal of Therapy." *Heart Rhythm* 7 (2010): 1008–26.

Lewis, W. R., D. L. Luebke, N. J. Johnson, M. D. Harrington, O. Costantini, and M. P. Aulisio. "Withdrawing Implantable Defibrillator Shock Therapy in Terminally Ill Patients." *American Journal of Medicine* 119 (2006): 892–96.

Maugans, T. A. "The Spiritual History." *Archives of Family Medicine* 5 (1996): 11–16.

Moschella, M., and M. L. Condic. "Symposium on the Definition of Death: Summary Statement." *Journal of Medicine and Philosophy* 41 (2016): 351–61.

Mueller, P. S., C. C. Hook, and D. L. Hayes. "Ethical Analysis of Withdrawal of Pacemaker or Implantable Cardioverter-Defibrillator Support at the End of Life." *Mayo Clinic Proceedings* 78 (2003): 959–63.

Murphy, D. J., D. Burrows, S. Santilli, A. W. Kemp, S. Tenner, B. Kreling, and J. Teno. "The Influence of the Probability of Survival on Patients' Preferences Regarding Cardiopulmonary Resuscitation." *New England Journal of Medicine* 330 (1994): 545–49.

National Conference of Catholic Bishops. "Guidelines for the Celebration of the Sacraments with Persons with Disabilities." June 16, 1995. http://www.ncpd.org/views-news-policy/policy/church/bishops/sacraments.

National Conference of Commissioners on Uniform State Laws. *Uniform Determination of Death Act*. Chicago: National Conference of Commissioners on Uniform State Laws, 1980.

Peberdy, M. A., W. Kaye, J. P. Ornato, G. L. Larkin, V. Nadkarni, M. E. Mancini, R. A. Berg, G. Nichol, and T. Lane-Trultt. "Cardiopulmonary Resuscitation of Adults in the Hospital: A Report of 14720 Cardiac Arrests from the National Registry of Cardiopulmonary Resuscitation." *Resuscitation* 58 (2003): 297–308.

Pellegrino, Edmund D. "Decisions to Withdraw Life-Sustaining Treatment: A Moral Algorithm." *Journal of the American Medical Association* 283 (2000): 1065–67.

———. *The Philosophy of Medicine Reborn: A Pellegrino Reader*. Edited by Tristram Engelhardt Jr. and Fabrice Jotterand. Notre Dame, Ind.: University of Notre Dame Press, 2008.

Perkins, Ignatius. "Feed the Sick, Nourish the Person." *Ethics and Medics* 29, no. 9 (September 2004): 1–5.

Perkins, Ignatius, and Peter John Cameron. "The Eucharist and Tube Feeding." *Ethics and Medics* 30, no. 11 (November 2005): 1–3.

Pinnock, Hilary, M. Kendall, S. A. Murray, A. Worth, P. Levack, M. Porter, W. MacNee, and A. Sheikh. "Living and Dying with Severe Chronic Obstructive Pulmonary Disease: Multi-perspective Longitudinal Qualitative Study." *BMJ* 342, January 24, 2011: d142.

Pius XII, Pope. "The Prolongation of Life." In *Catholic Health Care Ethics*, ed. Furton, Cataldo, and Moraczewski, 299–301.

Plum, F., and J. Posner. *The Diagnosis of Stupor and Coma*. 3rd edition. Philadelphia: F. A. Davis, 1996.

Podrid, Philip J., Morton F. Arnsdorf, and Jie Cheng. "Outcome of Sudden Cardiac Arrest." *UpToDate*, 2010.

Puchalski, C. M. "Spirituality and End-of-Life Care: A Time for Listening and Caring." *Journal of Palliative Medicine* 5 (2002): 289–94.

Rites of the Catholic Church. Vol. 1. New York: Pueblo Publishing Company, 1990.

Sulmasy, Daniel P. *A Healer's Calling: A Spirituality for Physicians and Other Health Care Professionals*. Mahwah, N.J.: Paulist Press, 1997.

——— "Within You/Without You: Biotechnology, Ontology, and Ethics." *Journal of General Internal Medicine* 23, Supplement 1 (2008): 69–72.

Travaline, John, Robert Ruchinskas, and Gilbert D'Alonzo. "Patient-Physician Communication: Why and How." *Journal of the American Osteopathic Association* 105 (2005): 13–18.

Tuoley, John. "POLST Orders Are Not Dangerous." *Ethics and Medics* 35, no. 10 (October 2010): 3–4.

United States Conference of Catholic Bishops (USCCB). *Ethical and Religious Directives for Catholic Health Care Services.* 5th edition. Washington, D.C.: USCCB, 2009.

Vatican Council II. *Gaudium et Spes, Pastoral Constitution on the Church in the Modern World.* December 7, 1965.

Volandes, Angelo. *The Conversation: A Revolutionary Plan for End-of-Life Care.* New York: Bloomsbury USA, 2015. https://lisa-wang-p49c.squarespace.com/the-conversation.

Wahlster, S., E. F. Wijdicks, P. V. Patel, D. M. Greer, J. C. Hemphill III, M. Carone, and F. J. Mateen. "Brain Death Declaration: Practices and Perceptions Worldwide." *Neurology* 84 (2015):1870–79.

Weinhouse, Gerald L. "Hypoxic-Ischemic Brain Injury." *UpToDate*, 2010. http://www.uptodate.com/contents/hypoxic-ischemic-brain-injury-evaluation-and-prognosis.

Wijdicks, E. F. M. "The Diagnosis of Brain Death." *New England Journal of Medicine* 344 (2001): 1215–21.

Wijdicks, E. F., A. Hijdra, and G. B. Young. "Practice Parameter: Prediction of Outcome in Comatose Survivors after Cardiopulmonary Resuscitation (an Evidenced-Based Review): Report of the Quality Standards Subcommittee of the American Academy of Neurology." *Neurology* 67 (2006): 203–10.

Wijdicks, E. F., P. N. Varelas, G. S. Gronseth, D. M. Greer. American Academy of Neurology. "Evidence-Based Guideline Update: Determining Brain Death in Adults: Report of the Quality Standards Subcommittee of the American Academy of Neurology." *Neurology* 74 (2010): 1911–18.

Wood, Gordon, Elizabeth Chaitin, and Robert Arnold. "Communication in the ICU: Holding a Family Meeting." *UpToDate.* Last updated June 24, 2016. http://www.uptodate.com/contents/communication-in-the-icu-holding-a-family-meeting.

You, John J., Robert A. Fowler, and Daren K. Heyland, on behalf of the Canadian Researchers at the End of Life Network (CARENET). "Just Ask: Discussing Goals of Care with Patients in Hospital with Serious Illness." *Canadian Medical Association Journal* 186, no. 6 (April 1, 2014): 425–32.

Zandbergen, D. G., J. H. Koelman, R. J. de Haan, A. Hijdra; PROPAC-Study Group. "SSEPs and Prognosis in Postanoxic Coma: Only Short or Also Long Latency Responses?" *Neurology* 67 (2006): 583–86.

Zandbergen, D. G., R. J. de Haan, and A. Hijdra. "Systematic Review of Prediction of Poor Outcome in Anoxic-Ischemic Coma with Biochemical Markers of Brain Damage." *Intensive Care Medicine* 27 (2001): 1661–67.

Zandbergen, D. G., Rob J. de Haan, Christiaan P. Stoutenbeek, Johannes H. T. M. Koelman, Albert Hijdra. "Systematic Review of Early Prediction of Poor Outcome in Anoxic-Ischemic Coma." *Lancet* 352 (1998): 1808–12.

Leonard P. Rybak and Christopher Perro

9. CHALLENGES FOR CATHOLIC SURGEONS

Drs. Rybak and Perro discuss the parts of the *Ethical and Religious Directives* that pertain in a particular way to surgeons. Additionally they review listening, good communication, informed consent, and the importance of truth and honesty. From there they move into two challenging, though rare, case studies: transgender surgery and facial transplantation. Although Catholic surgeons may not participate in transgender surgery, they may and should be compassionate toward the patient, as well as refer for psychological or psychiatric care. Sexuality is intrinsic to the person, not merely biological; surgery does not change this, but rather mutilates and sterilizes the body. The guiding principle here is the principle of totality: the human being is not merely a psyche in a body but rather a unity of body and soul, and the body is the physical manifestation and expression of the person. Surgery does not change the person's gender; it only creates an appearance of the other sex. So-called "sex reassignment" surgery is neither ethically nor medically appropriate; it violates basic medical and ethical principles, requires mutilation of a healthy body, and incurs unnecessary risks. Different ethical questions and medical risks are involved in facial transplant surgery for severe facial deformities. Some may consider euthanasia, but this is not an option for Catholics, for patients with facial deformities or for any patient. At this time the surgery is still experimental and must be approached with caution. The concerns and risks include tissue rejection with the possibility that the patient is worse off afterwards, ascertaining the death of the donor, the ability of the patient to comply with medical advice, the availability of other options, the expected degree of functional recovery, and psychological concerns of the patient both about the deformity and about the post-operation new look. The face post-surgery will be an amalgam of the original and the donor faces. However, while the look of the face will change, it is only an accidental change, and the person will not change. At this time, the risks are high; nevertheless, facial transplantation may be an ethical option for those with severe deformities who have exhausted all other options.—*Editors*

Introduction

This chapter lays out general moral and ethical principles to guide Catholic surgeons and discusses two illustrative cases that apply these principles to the ethical and moral issues involved in the cases.

The *Ethical and Religious Directives for Catholic Health Care Services* provide guidelines for health-care institutions and caregivers to follow in treating and caring for their patients. These guidelines remind the surgeon to be compassionate and sensitive to the needs of the patient (dir. 2). This respect should extend to the marginalized, the uninsured, and persons with disabilities (dir. 3). The Catholic surgeon should help Catholic patients to receive pastoral care and the sacraments when hospitalized or in preparation for surgery (part 2). Patients facing potentially life-threatening surgery should be encouraged to receive the Sacrament of the Sick. Surgeons must respect the dignity of the human person regardless of the health problem or the social status of the patient (dir. 23). The surgeon may not honor an advance directive that is contrary to Catholic teaching (dir. 24). Free and informed consent must be obtained prior to performing surgery (dirs. 26–28). Surgical patients must protect and preserve integrity of the body and its functions except when necessary to sacrifice integrity for maintaining health if no other morally acceptable option exists (dir. 29). *In vitro* fertilization, abortion, and sterilization are not morally acceptable (dirs. 38–41, 45, 53, 70). Patients may refuse extraordinary or disproportionate treatments to extend life (dir. 57). The surgeon should make every effort to relieve pain. Dr. Benestad provides a detailed discussion on human suffering in chapter 1. He proposes the Good Samaritan from the Gospel of St. Luke as a model for the physician and surgeon to try to alleviate pain in the suffering patient.

Ethical Issues in Surgery

Listening and good communication are critical aspects of the physician-patient relationship. The busy surgeon may tend to neglect these obligations in order to move on to the next patient in his office or to rush off to perform surgery on another patient. Instead, taking the time to listen and communicate will avoid errors in understanding on the part of both the surgeon and the patient. Not doing so can lead to unnecessary complications and lack of informed consent on the part of the patient. To deny the patient proper informed consent diminishes the inherent dignity that he possesses as articulated in chapter 1. This dignity is not lost by the severely or terminally ill patient. It must be respected by the surgeon regardless of the patient's medical condition.

Informed consent is a critical part of patient care provided by the surgeon. The surgeon must be truthful with the patient and the family. The surgeon is obliged to tell the patient the risks and the benefits of proposed surgical procedures, including the options of nonsurgical treatments or the choice of no treatment, so that the patient or his or her surrogate can make a truly informed decision. The concept of informed consent includes disclosure, competence, and voluntariness. Besides providing information about the pros and cons of various surgical or nonsurgical options, the surgeon must explain these concepts in a way that the patient understands, and give the patient time to weigh the various options so that his or her decision is voluntary and free of coercion.

In the complex case of donation of a kidney, the donor must be thoroughly educated regarding the risks, both to the donor and to the recipient. The donor must be aware that the kidney could be rejected by the recipient. Therefore, the donor should be given accurate data on the success of kidney transplants in the particular center where this procedure would take place.

There is a lot of publicity encouraging people to become organ donors, including having this information on their driver's license. If a surgeon talks to his or her patients about becoming an organ donor, he or she should mention the basic principles of organ donation from a Catholic perspective. As stated in the *Ethical and Religious Directives for Catholic Health Care Services*, directive 30:

The transplantation of organs from living donors is morally permissible when such a donation will not sacrifice or seriously impair any essential bodily function and the anticipated benefit to the recipient is proportionate to the harm done to the donor. Furthermore, the freedom of the prospective donor must be respected and economic advantages should not accrue to the donor.[1]

Delivering bad news is part of the job of the surgeon. If a biopsy shows cancer, the patient has a right to know. However, the disclosure must be done in a tactful manner and with proper consideration of the impact of such news on the patient.

The surgeon also has the obligation to deliver the truth about surgical outcomes. Complications and poor outcomes can occur with any surgical procedure. The surgeon must be truthful with the patient and the family so that they understand the outcome and potential interventions to minimize harm and to try to ameliorate the adverse event. He or she must not try to cover up a complication because of fear of litigation by the patient or the family.

The surgeon must be honest in coding for office visits, diagnoses, and surgical procedures. The surgeon must also insure that the proposed surgical procedure is appropriate for the disease that a patient is suffering from and not more complex and expensive than is necessary. The surgeon must develop virtues in order to properly serve his patient. Benestad points out in chapter 1 that the physician must resist the temptation to self interest in order to avoid indifference to the proper needs of the patient.

Challenging Cases

The rest of this chapter discusses in detail two intriguing, although somewhat rare, cases: transgender surgery and facial transplantation. These are two challenging

---

1. USCCB, *Ethical and Religious Directives for Catholic Health Care Services*, 5th ed. (Washington, D.C.: USCCB, 2009), dir. 30. See also dirs. 63–65 on donation after death.

instances of contemporary issues faced by Catholic surgeons. Each of these issues offers a number of moral and ethical dilemmas which the surgeon must consider when these patients present for consultation. The teachings of the Catholic Church's Magisterium, along with medical, ethical, and moral principles, are presented to clarify the appropriate decisions to be made by Catholic physicians and Catholic health-care institutions in treating these patients.

The first case deals with transgender surgery. Sex-change operations are not necessarily new; the first occurred in 1953 (Christine Jorgensen). But more and more people are seeking such operations now, along with adjunctive procedures. This has forced Catholic physicians and hospitals to address the morality of sex-change operations, since such procedures may become part of mandatory insurance coverage or legislative mandates requiring Catholic hospitals to perform these procedures.

The second case concerns the new and experimental procedure of facial transplantation to repair severe deformities of the face and facial skeleton. This type of surgical treatment, too, involves challenging moral and ethical issues, including proper treatment of potential donors and health risks associated with this surgery.

Case 1: Transgender Surgery

T. L. is a twenty-eight-year-old unmarried Caucasian woman planning to have "gender-reassignment" surgery. She feels that she is a man trapped in the body of a woman and desires to "become" male. She believes she has the right to do with her body as she wishes, and she is determined to have a series of medical and surgical procedures in order to achieve this end result.

The patient has consulted other physicians and surgeons who are willing to be part of the team providing the treatment program, and she comes to consult a Catholic physician who is an otolaryngologist (head and neck surgeon) as a potential member of this team. She wants to undergo facial plastic and laryngeal surgery to make her appear and sound more masculine, in conjunction with the series of other gender-change procedures. She is not willing to see a psychiatrist, declaring that doing so would not be productive and that she has no psychological issues worth pursuing. Furthermore, she states that no amount of counseling could deter her from proceeding with the desired medical and surgical transformation into a "man."

Catholic Teaching on Transgender Surgery

Transgender surgery is not morally acceptable by the standard of the *Catechism of the Catholic Church*. The *Catechism* teaches that God has created in His own image two genders, intended to complement each other as partners in marriage.

Man and woman have been *created*, which is to say, *willed* by God: on the one hand, in perfect equality as human persons; on the other, in their respective beings as man and woman. "Being man" or "being woman" is a reality which is good and willed by God: man and woman possess an inalienable dignity which comes to them immediately from God their Creator [see Gn 2:7, 22]. Man and woman are both with one and the same dignity "in the image of God." In their "being man" and "being woman," they reflect the Creator's wisdom and goodness.[2]

Physicians, especially Catholic physicians, should have sympathy for "transgender" persons, who are suffering, confused, and in need of real compassion. They should be referred for psychological or psychiatric care, not for endocrine manipulations and mutilating surgery. The patient's feeling that his or her gender is a mistake is a real cause of psychological pain and suffering. One must listen with compassion, but not exacerbate the patient's confusion and erroneous thinking. There is great potential for grace and healing if such persons are treated properly, but this treatment should not include surgery or hormone therapy to alter their God-given gender. Sexuality does not have merely functional significance, and sexual organs are not just raw materials that can be manipulated and changed to serve a perceived function contrary to the function intended by the Creator. The *Catechism* explains: "Except when performed for strictly therapeutic medical reasons, directly intended amputations, mutilations, and sterilizations performed on innocent persons are against the moral law."[3] Clearly, the surgical procedures involved in "gender reassignment" surgery are mutilating and cause sterility.

Opponents of the Magisterium argue that persons have a right—even an obligation—to freely determine the meaning of their own behavior. However, Pope John Paul II argued that this is a misguided view of human freedom:

One has to consider carefully the correct relationship existing between freedom and human nature, and in particularly *the place of the human body in questions of natural law.*

A freedom which claims to be absolute ends up treating the human body as a raw datum, devoid of any meaning and moral values until freedom has shaped it in accordance with its design.[4]

Persons seeking "gender reassignment" surgery claim that their bodies are at variance with their sexual identities.[5] Donna Rose, a man who underwent male-to-female transgender surgery, described his story as "more than simply a journey across gender.... It is actually a much deeper journey of self-discovery, and of self-definition. It is a journey to revisit decisions made about her and for her the moment she was born, and to reclaim her own destiny."[6] This statement makes it clear that the desire for transsexual surgery is based on a distorted concept of freedom, divorced from truth and diminished to the person's mere ability to choose; the content of the choice is irrelevant. This represents an inappropriate abdication of the power of free will to choose the good over evil.[7]

---

2. *Catechism of the Catholic Church*, 2nd ed., trans. United States Conference of Catholic Bishops (Washington, D.C.: USCCB, 1997), no. 369; emphasis in original.

3. Ibid., no. 2297.

4. Pope John Paul II, *Veritatis Splendor, The Splendor of Truth* (Boston: St. Paul Books and Media, 1993), no. 48, emphasis in original.

5. See P. R. McHugh, "Surgical Sex," *First Things* 147 (2004): 34–38.

6. Donna Rose, "My Bio: Two Lives, One Lifetime," January 2004, http://www.donnarose.com/DonnaRoseOrig/bio.html.

7. See C. Gross, "Karol Wojtyla on Sex Reassignment Surgery: An Application of His Philosophical Anthropology," *National Catholic Bioethics Quarterly* 9 (2009): 711–23.

In his encyclical *Evangelium Vitae*, John Paul II wrote: "Freedom negates and destroys itself, and becomes a factor leading to the destruction of others, when it no longer recognizes and respects its *essential link with the truth*."[8] As C. Gross has pointed out, the "understanding of freedom contained in sex reassignment surgery does not harm others as much as it destroys the person undergoing the surgery."[9]

Sexuality is an intrinsic part of a person's being, not merely a biological function that can be separated from the intrinsic self or one's identity. This reality makes transgender surgery fundamentally different from blood or organ donation. Differences in gender identity should not be confused with stereotypical personality traits attributed to each gender by society. Body and soul form a unified whole, a psychosomatic unity; features of the body and soul influence each other. Heredity, not environment, makes a person male or female, through the clear and immutable chromosomal difference between males and females. Each individual's sex is encoded in the genes: females are XX, males are XY. Hormonal manipulation or surgery does not change this biological reality; it changes only the person's appearance. On the functional or biological level, individuals make their gender work in harmony with who they are. Maleness and femaleness are ontological realities integral to human nature. Moral norms are written into nature, which provides the starting point for morality. Natural law tells us that biological facts serve as symbols of the true, inner life of the person. Thus, male or female sexual biology is an outward expression of a deeper gender identity.

John Paul II spoke of the "language of the body," which illuminates the essence of a person's nature and is a basis for the person's intrinsic human dignity. The sacramental view of reality shows the intimate unity between the physical and spiritual. When transgender surgery is performed, the goodness of the human body is rejected.[10] In a speech to the Roman Curia, Pope Benedict XVI declared that the Church "has a responsibility to safeguard the created order" and to protect man against "the destruction of himself." He continued:

When the Church speaks of the nature of the human being as man and woman and asks that this order of creation be respected, it is not the result of an outdated metaphysic. It is a question here of faith in the Creator and of listening to the language of creation, the devaluation of which leads to the self-destruction of man and therefore to the destruction of the same work of God.[11]

---

8. Pope John Paul II, *Evangelium Vitae*, *The Gospel of Life* [Encyclical Letter, March 25, 1995] (Boston: Pauline Books and Media, 1995), no. 19, emphasis in original.

9. Gross, "Karol Wojtyla on Sex Reassignment Surgery," 720.

10. See ibid. There are chromosomal abnormalities such as XXY and XYY. XXY males have Klinefelter Syndrome and may have hypogonadism or infertility. XYY males may have increased height or developmental delay but have normal sexual development and normal fertility. Some individuals are born with both ovarian and testicular tissue. The external genitalia are often ambiguous, but only one set of gonads will be functional in children born with both male and female gonads. In cases of ambiguous genitalia, genetic testing may determine the true gender of the child.

11. Pope Benedict XVI, Address to the Roman Curia on the Occasion of Their Christmas Greetings, December 22, 2008, trans. Michael Campbell, http://www.lifesitenews.com/1dn/2008/dec/081223a.html.

The Principle of Totality

The Second Vatican Council's *Pastoral Constitution on the Church in the Modern World, Gaudium et Spes*, tells us:

Though made of body and soul, man is one. Through his bodily composition, he gathers to himself the elements of the material world; thus they reach their crown through him, and through him raise their voice in free praise of the Creator. For this reason man is not allowed to despise his bodily life, rather he is obliged to regard his body as good and honorable since God has created it and will raise it up on the last day. Nevertheless, wounded by sin, man experiences rebellious stirrings in his body. But the very dignity of man postulates that man glorify God in his body and forbid it to serve the evil inclinations of his heart.[12]

The Congregation for the Doctrine of the Faith, in *Donum Vitae*, adds:

It is only in keeping with his true nature that the human person can achieve self-realization as a "unified totality": and this nature is at the same time corporal and spiritual. By virtue of its substantial union with a spiritual soul, the human body cannot be considered as a mere complex of tissues, organs, and functions, nor can it be evaluated in the same way as the body of animals; rather it is a constitutive part of the person who manifests and expresses himself through it. The natural moral law expresses and lays down the purposes, rights, and duties which are based upon the bodily and spiritual nature of the human person. Therefore this law cannot be thought of as simply a set of norms on the biological level; rather it must be defined as the rational order whereby man is called by the Creator to direct and regulate his life and actions and in particular to make use of his own body.[13]

The debate here contrasts an integrated view of the human person with a separatist position. The integralist man would say, "I am a male person," whereas the separatist would argue, "I am a person who happens to be male." The separatist seeks to separate sexuality from the self, thus pitting the self against the body to redetermine the body's meaning. The separatist approach dissociates God's plan from human biology and leads to dualism, the separation and discord between the body and the soul. This is a Gnostic view, that the soul is good but the body is bad. The dualist declares that the human person should not be at the mercy of his or her biology; Catholic teaching responds that such a view ignores the person's freedom to transcend his or her mere nature.

A third position, that of the revisionist personalist, would agree with the dualist that man should avoid becoming a slave to biology, but should instead take control and manipulate biology at will to achieve supreme personhood. According to this view, one may use rational capacity to arbitrate over nature and the body, defining for oneself the meaning that lies within. Thus, "proportionate reason" would permit the violation of moral norms in the effort to find true sexuality. This violation comes about because of concupiscence, in which reason is directed by one's passions or in-

---

12. Vatican Council II, *Gaudium et Spes, Pastoral Constitution on the Church in the Modern World*, December 7, 1965, no. 14.

13. Congregation for the Doctrine of the Faith, *Donum Vitae, Instruction on Respect for Human Life in Its Origin and on the Dignity of Procreation* (Boston: Pauline Books and Media, 1987), intro., no. 3.

stinctual desires and is misapplied to allow the individual to decide whether or not to follow nature.

Physicalists, a fourth position, believe that human persons should direct their biology toward whatever they feel it should mean. In his encyclical *Veritatis Splendor*, John Paul II wrote:

A freedom which claims to be absolute ends up treating the human body as a raw datum, devoid of any meaning and moral values until freedom has shaped it in accordance with its design. Consequently, human nature and the body appear as *presuppositions or preambles*, materially *necessary* for freedom to make its choice, yet extrinsic to the person, the subject, and the human act. Their functions would not be able to constitute reference points for moral decisions, because the finalities of these inclinations would be merely "physical" goods, called by some "pre-moral." To refer to them, in order to find in them rational indications with regard to the order of morality, would be to expose oneself to the accusation of physicalism or biologism. In this way of thinking, the tension between freedom and a nature conceived of in a reductive way is resolved by a division within man himself.

This moral theory does not correspond to the truth about man and his freedom. It contradicts the *Church's teachings on the unity of the human person*, whose rational soul is *per se et essentialiter* the form of his body. The spiritual and immortal soul is the principle of unity of the human being, whereby it exists as a whole—*corpore et anima unus*—as a person. These definitions not only point out that the body, which has been promised the resurrection, will also share in glory. They also remind us that reason and free will are linked with all the bodily and sense faculties. *The person, including the body, is completely entrusted to himself, and it is in the unity of body and soul that the person is the subject of his own moral acts.* The person, by the light of reason and the support of virtue, discovers in the body the anticipatory signs, the expression and the promise of the gift of self, in conformity with the wise plan of the Creator. It is in the light of the dignity of the human person—a dignity which must be affirmed for its own sake—that reason grasps the specific moral value of certain goods towards which the person is naturally inclined. And since the human person cannot be reduced to a freedom which is self-designing, but entails a particular spiritual and bodily structure, the primordial moral requirement of loving and respecting the person as an end and never as a mere means also implies, by its very nature, respect for certain fundamental goods, without which one would fall into relativism and arbitrariness.[14]

The proper Catholic response to these dualistic arguments is that the human person has free will and thus is not a mere animal, driven by instinctual desires and at the mercy of biology. This is a truly personalistic approach. The *Catechism* instructs:

Everyone, man and woman, should acknowledge and accept his [or her] sexual *identity*. Physical, moral, and spiritual *difference* and *complementarity* are oriented toward the goods of marriage and the flourishing of family life. The harmony of the couple and of society depends in part on the way in which the complementarity, needs, and mutual support between the sexes are lived out.[15]

The *Charter for Health Care Workers* concurs:

---

14. John Paul II, *Veritatis Splendor*, no. 48, emphasis in original.
15. *Catechism of the Catholic Church*, no. 2333, emphasis in original.

One cannot prescind from the body and make the psyche the criterion and source of morality; subjective feelings and desires cannot replace or ignore objective corporal conditions. The tendency to give the former the pride of place over the latter is the basis for contemporary psychologization of ethics and law, which makes individual wishes (and technical possibilities) the arbiter of lawfulness of behavior and of interventions on life.[16]

Female-to-"Male" Surgery

Surgery to alter genitalia can be performed by a urologist, a gynecologist, a plastic surgeon, a specially trained general surgeon, or a team of surgeons. Otolaryngologists may be asked to alter the face and larynx to make the female person appear and sound more masculine. Clearly, the surgical procedures constitute significant mutilation, since normal (and healthy) organs and tissues are removed. The process usually requires several stages of destructive procedures. Genital surgery for the female-to-male patient may include hysterectomy, salpingo-oophorectomy, vaginectomy, metoidioplasty, scrotoplasty, urethroplasty, placement of a testicular prosthesis, and phalloplasty.[17] These mutilating procedures carry risks which include those associated with life-long hormone therapy, along with the rare incidence of gynecologic malignancy if the patient does not receive regular gynecologic care for retained genital organs.[18] Such patients, even though they appear to be male, require monitoring for cancer of the female organs.

Therapists who authorize a medical team to perform sex reassignment surgery encourage the team to feel they are doing something worthwhile, since their patients are grateful. However, this mindset ignores the reality that sex reassignment surgery "mutilates a healthy human body, results in significant physical pain and suffering, incurs real, unjustifiable health risks to patients, and does not address the real psychological problems."[19] As Dale O'Leary observes, "The 'sex change' surgeons know that they cannot change a person's sex; they can only create a non-functional appearance of the other sex. But they also know that they will be well paid for their skill, and so they go along with the deception."[20]

---

16. Pontifical Council for Health Pastoral Care, *Charter for Health Care Workers* (Boston: Pauline Books and Media, 1994), no. 41.

17. See M. Sohn and H. A. G. Bosinski, "Gender Identity Disorders: Diagnostic and Surgical Aspects," *Journal of Sexual Medicine* 4 (2007): 1193–1208.

18. See R. Urban, N. N. H. Teng, and D. S. Kapp, "Gynecologic Malignancies in Female-to-Male Transgender Patients: The Need of Original Gender Surveillance," *American Journal of Obstetrics & Gynecology* 204 (2011): e9–e12.

19. R. P. Fitzgibbons, P. M. Sutton, and D. O'Leary, "The Psychopathology of 'Sex Reassignment' Surgery: Assessing Its Medical, Psychological and Ethical Appropriateness," *National Catholic Bioethics Quarterly* 9 (2009): 97–125.

20. D. O'Leary, "Legalizing Deception: Why 'Gender Identity' Should Not Be Added to Anti- discrimination Legislation," *Catholic Exchange*, June 25, 2009, http://catholicexchange.com/legalizing-deception-why-%E2%80%9Cgender-identity%E2%80%9D-should-not-be-added-to-anti-discrimination-legislation/.

Male-to-"Female" Surgery

This process may include surgical modifications to feminize the voice, which can be accomplished by endoscopic laryngeal web formation, cricothyroid approximation and subluxation, and laser-assisted voice adjustment. The thyroid cartilage can be shaved to make the Adam's apple less prominent. Facial hair follicles can be ablated with a laser. Other facial plastic procedures can include feminization rhinoplasty and plastic surgery to alter the appearance of the forehead. Male-to-female transgender surgery also may require the placement of breast implants and genital surgery.

Hormonal Treatments and Their Risks

The treatment of female-to-male patients involves the administration of testosterone. Females undergoing transsexual surgery generally respond better to hormonal therapy than do males undergoing the opposite procedure; their voices get lower, beard growth occurs, and general muscle development increases.[21]

Male-to-female patients are administered anti-androgens and estrogens. The use of estrogen carries the potentially life-threatening risk of venous thromboembolism and strokes; this risk is higher in older patients and is increased with the use of oral ethinyl estradiol. Both steroid administration and surgery are important risk factors for venous thromboembolism, and this risk may continue for several weeks after major operations. Transsexual persons frequently have multiple operations, which can further increase the risks of blood clots. Furthermore, no guidelines exist to direct the timing of discontinuation and resumption of hormones in these patients before and after surgery.[22]

The overall mortality for sex-reassigned persons, particularly involving death from suicide, was higher than for controls of the same birth sex during a follow-up study. Sex-reassigned patients had elevated risks for suicide attempts and psychiatric inpatient care. Those who underwent female-to-male surgeries also had a higher risk for criminal convictions.[23] These findings indicate that sex reassignment surgery does not cure underlying psychiatric problems, but may actually exacerbate them.

When Dr. Paul McHugh interviewed men who were "changed" into "women" surgically, he found the claim that they were now women unconvincing. He wrote:

Those I met after surgery would tell me that the surgery and hormone treatments that made them "women" had also made them very happy and contented. None of these encounters were persuasive, however. The post-surgical subjects struck me as caricatures of women.

---

21. See Sohn and Bosinski, "Gender Identity Disorders."

22. See M. C. Meriggiola et al., "Endocrine Treatment of Transsexual Persons: An Endocrine Society Clinical Practice Guideline: Commentary from a European Perspective," *European Journal of Endocrinology* 162 (2010): 831–33.

23. C. Dhejne et al., "Long-term Follow-up of Transsexual Persons Undergoing Sex Reassignment Surgery: Cohort Study in Sweden," *PLoS ONE* 6, no. 2 (February 22, 2011): e16885, doi: http://dx.doi.org/10.1371/journal.pone.0016885.

They wore high heels, copious makeup, and flamboyant clothing; they spoke about how they found themselves able to give vent to their natural inclinations for peace, domesticity, and gentleness—but their large hands, prominent Adam's apples, and thick facial features were incongruous (and would become more so as they aged). Women psychiatrists [to] whom I sent them to talk with them would intuitively see through the disguise and the exaggerated postures. "Gals know gals," one said to me, "and that's a guy."[24]

While most sex-change patients interviewed said that they were happy with the outcomes, the surgery did not alter various existing psychological problems; they still had the same problems with relationships, work, and emotions.[25] McHugh concluded that these surgeries are misdirected, and that "to provide a surgical alteration of the body of these unfortunate people was to collaborate with a mental disorder rather than to treat it."[26] Mutilating surgery and hormone treatments can create the appearance of a male or female body, but they do not alter the reality that it is not possible to change a person's sex.[27] This is proven in those cases in which a woman was "changed" into a "man" and yet was still able to have children by in vitro fertilization. Whereas a man obviously cannot have children, a female who elects to retain her female reproductive organs preserves her capacity to have children as an apparent male.

So-called "sex reassignment" surgery is neither ethically nor medically appropriate; it violates basic medical and ethical principles, requires mutilation of a healthy body, and incurs unnecessary risks. It results in permanent sterility, which can be overcome only by the gravely immoral procedure of in vitro fertilization and artificial insemination. This surgery also violates the Hippocratic principle "First, do no harm" (*primum non nocere*). Candidates for transgender surgery may think that they are trapped in the body of the wrong sex, but this belief is irrational and delusional. The surgical change of the person's external appearance offers a surgical palliation for psychological problems. "Sex reassignment" surgery is a lie, since it does not provide what it purports to accomplish—changing a person's sex. Transgender surgery causes permanent changes in the person's body and is often an unsatisfying attempt to correct a potentially temporary psychological or psychiatric condition using the wrong approach—surgery instead of psychotherapy.[28] In the words of McHugh:

As for the adults who came to us claiming to have discovered their "true" sexual identity and to have heard about sex-change operations, we psychiatrists have been distracted from studying the causes and nature of their mental misdirections by preparing them for surgery and for a life in the other sex. We have wasted scientific and technical resources and damaged our professional credibility by collaborating with madness rather than trying to study, cure, and ultimately prevent it.[29]

---

24. McHugh, "Surgical Sex," 34.
25. See ibid.
26. Ibid., 35.
27. See R. P. Fitzgibbons, "The Desire for a Sex Change," *Ethics and Medics* 30, no. 10 (October 2005): 10–14.
28. See Fitzgibbons, Sutton, and O'Leary, "The Psychopathology of 'Sex Reassignment' Surgery."
29. McHugh, "Surgical Sex," 38.

McHugh has clearly pointed out the lack of empirical evidence to support trans-gender surgery. He writes:

One might expect that those who claim that sexual identity has no biological or physical basis would bring forth evidence to persuade others. But, as I've learned, there is a deep preju-dice in favor of the idea that nature is totally malleable. Without any fixed position on what is given in human nature, any manipulation of it can be defended as legitimate. A practice that appears to give people what they want—and some of them are prepared to clamor for—turns out to be difficult to combat with ordinary professional experience and wisdom. Even controlled trials or careful follow-up studies to ensure that the practice itself is not damaging are often resisted and the results rejected.[30]

In *Humanae Vitae*, Pope Paul VI reaffirmed the Church's teaching against direct sterilization, writing, "Equally to be condemned, as the Magisterium of the Church has affirmed on many occasions, is direct sterilization, whether of the man or of the woman, whether permanent or temporary."[31]

Properly understood, a person cannot change his or her sexual identity. A person is either male or female, the unity of soul and body; in this context, "soul" should be understood not as an immaterial self, but as that which makes the body be what it is, namely, a human person. We are either male or female persons, and nothing can change that, not even the mutilation of genitals.

Mutilation from "gender reassignment surgery" results in impotence or sterility and creates a lifelong dependence on a hormonal regimen that makes one appear to be other than what he or she is. The genitals removed in this surgery are not diseased, but are removed to conform to the patient's subjective belief about who he or she wants to be. Doing violence to one's body when there is nothing wrong with it is an unjustifiable mutilation.

It is not morally licit for Catholic hospitals to offer surgical breast implants to men who have been manipulated by hormones and mutilated by surgery to look like women. A recent court case in California involved a male-to-female transsexual pa-tient who sought breast augmentation surgery at a Catholic hospital. The hospital refused to allow the procedure and was sued for alleged violation of the California Unruh Civil Rights Act. The hospital administration subsequently developed a pol-icy for future cases of this sort: they decided that the same ethical standards which allow any woman to have breast implants would apply to men who had undergone transgender surgery. It was rationalized that since the mammoplasty was not part of the actual transgender surgical procedure, it could be considered morally licit. This argument is patently false, however, as mammoplasty in this situation is indeed part of the transgendering process. The procedure in this case is an evil action, and partici-pants in assisting the surgery who share the same intention are formally cooperating with evil. Others involved are materially cooperating as long as they do not share the same intention.

30. Ibid., 37–38.
31. Pope Paul VI, *Humanae Vitae, Of Human Life* [Encyclical Letter, July 25, 1968] (Boston: Pauline Books and Media, 1968), no. 14.

To avoid self-deception, one must also rely on natural law in order to find the truth. The nature of sexuality, which is known in the heart of human beings, tells us that sexuality is not merely a biological or functional entity. The sexual organs are not merely raw materials that can be manipulated or modified to fit the meaning that an individual thinks they should have, based on emotion or erroneous thinking. Sexual organs cannot be separated from our intrinsic self or identity; their removal is not like the donation of an organ or blood for transfusion.

Gender reassignment surgery raises numerous practical questions, many of which are raised by the case of Thomas Beatie, born a female, Tracy Lagondino. In the 1990s Lagondino underwent partial gender reassignment surgery to remove her breasts and alter her body to appear male, but she retained her uterus, vagina, and ovaries in the hope of becoming pregnant and delivering a child some day.[32] She changed her name to Thomas Beatie, was legally recognized as a man, and eventually "married" a woman who was infertile. Beatie stopped taking testosterone and twice underwent artificial insemination, giving birth to two children.

A woman who believes that having surgery and hormone treatments can transform her into a male is deceiving herself, since gender is defined by DNA in every cell of a person's body. Moreover, by retaining her female reproductive organs, Beatie indicated that she must have been keenly aware of her true sexuality. With the spread of information on the Internet and the use of social networks, more children may be born in the future to transgender "men."[33]

The Church has taken a clear stand in the debate over the moral issues involved in facilitating parenthood for men and women with nonstandard sexual identities or in unconventional relationships. In *Dignitas Personae*, the Church teaches:

Respect for that dignity is owed to every human being, because each one carries in an indelible way his own dignity and value. *The origin of human life has its authentic context in marriage and in the family*, where it is generated through an act which expresses the reciprocal love between a man and a woman. Procreation which is truly responsible vis-à-vis the child to be born "must be the fruit of marriage."[34]

A woman who has undergone gender-reassignment surgery cannot subsequently marry a woman in the Church: "People who have undergone a sex-change operation cannot enter into a valid marriage, either because they would be marrying someone of the same sex in the eyes of the Church or because their mental state casts doubt on their ability to make and uphold their marriage vows."[35] She also cannot be ordained to the priesthood or diaconate, as only men may be ordained priest or deacon.

---

32. See Gross, "Karol Wojtyla on Sex Reassignment Surgery."

33. See T. F. Murphy, "The Ethics of Helping Transgender Men and Women Have Children," *Perspectives in Biology and Medicine* 5 (2010): 46–60.

34. Congregation for the Doctrine of the Faith, *Dignitas Personae, Instruction on Certain Bioethical Questions* (Boston: Pauline Books and Media, 2008), no. 6, emphasis in original, quoting Congregation for the Doctrine of the Faith, *Donum Vitae*, II, A, no. 1.

35. John Norton, "Vatican Says Sex Change Operation Does Not Change a Person's Gender," *Catholic News Service*, January 14, 2003, quoted in Fitzgibbons, Sutton, and O'Leary, "The Psychopathology of 'Sex Reassignment' Surgery," 121.

In summary, transgender surgery is, for a variety of reasons, contrary to the teaching of the Church.

Case 2: Facial Transplantation

G. H. is a fifty-six-year-old woman who suffered extensive loss of soft tissue and bone from the face following a shotgun blast after an altercation. She has severe facial scarring and functional difficulties, including trouble with eating, loss of the sense of smell, and need for a tracheostomy for breathing. She has heard recent news stories from around the world about cases of facial transplants, and she asks to be considered as a candidate for facial transplantation.

History of the Transplant Procedure

A French woman, Isabelle Dinoire, received the world's first partial face transplant in 2005, after suffering severe facial disfigurement when she was mauled by a dog.[36] The second partial facial transplant was performed in China the following year on a recipient whose face had been mauled by a bear seventeen months earlier.[37] Since then, partial facial transplants have been carried out in several countries. The first partial facial transplant in the United States was performed at the Cleveland Clinic in December 2008.[38] The first total face transplant was said to have been carried out at Barcelona, Spain, in April 2010. The recipient was a thirty-year-old man who had suffered a gunshot wound five years earlier, sustaining severe facial deformities including severe facial scarring, acquired hypertelorism, bilateral orbital dystopia, and loss of lacrimal apparatus and medial canthal ligaments. His entire nose and part of his lips had been lost, and he had subtotal destruction of his maxilla, both zygomas, and mandible.[39] Recently, the first full face transplant in the United States was performed at Brigham and Women's Hospital in Boston on a twenty-five-year-old man from Texas, who suffered severe facial burns and was blinded after hitting a power line while painting a church in 2008. Though the patient said he hoped to be able to smile and feel kisses from his three-year-old daughter, his sight unfortunately will not be restored by the surgery.[40] Dr. Bohdan Pomahac, a plastic surgeon who led the team of surgeons during this fifteen-hour procedure, predicted that the transplant recipient will not resemble either his previous face or that of the donor, but that his facial appearance would be something between the two.[41]

Facial transplant surgery poses numerous ethical questions and medical risks. Al-

---

36. See J. M. Dubernard and B. Devauchelle, "Face Transplantation," *Lancet* 372 (2008): 603–4.

37. See Y. Chenggang et al., "Some Issues in Facial Transplantation," *American Journal of Transplantation* 8 (2008): 2169–72.

38. See C. Paradis et al., "Ethical Considerations in the First American Face Transplant," *Plastic and Reconstructive Surgery* 126 (2010): 896–901.

39. See J. P. Barret et al., "Full Face Transplant: The First Case Report," *Annals of Surgery* 254 (2011): 252–56.

40. See M. Marchione and R. Contreras, "Texas Man Gets First Full Face Transplant in U.S.," *MSNBC.com*, March 21, 2011, http://www.msnbc.msn.com/id/42192670/ns/health-health_care/.

41. See ibid.

though perceived benefits may warrant the risks, it should be remembered that facial deformities, unlike such conditions as kidney or liver failure, are not life threatening. Potential face transplant recipients may have undergone multiple previous attempts at facial reconstruction, including free flaps. These patients may suffer from multiple functional deficits, including impaired speech and smell, difficulty with feeding because of inadequate oral closure, scar contracture, and lack of an adequate oral airway; they may require gastrostomy tube feedings. They may have been hospitalized repeatedly for multiple surgical procedures, treatment of infections, and other complications,[42] and they may have undergone other reconstructive procedures. Some patients' facial deformities have had more than one hundred revision surgeries over the span of many years; this is in sharp contrast with facial transplantation, which may be accomplished with only a few surgeries.[43] Given the fact that few facial transplants—counting full and partial transplants, perhaps a dozen or so—have been performed worldwide at this writing, this procedure must still be considered experimental.

Benefits versus Risks, and Ethical Considerations

Facial transplantation raises complex ethical questions. One must consider the efficacy of alternative methods of facial reconstruction, along with psychological and social issues.[44] On the one hand, there is significant value to the patient in having a face that does not cause negative reactions in public; on the other, surgeons performing face transplantation have not yet fully examined the function of the transplanted organ. Potential facial transplant recipients will have hopes, anxieties, and questions about the stability of their personality, including the subjective experience of self-image, social acceptability, and sense of normalcy.[45]

Ethical codes, such as the Declaration of Helsinki and the Belmont Report, require analysis of risk/benefit relationships in assessing surgical research. As Wiggins et al. point out, according to the Declaration of Helsinki, "Every biomedical research project involving human subjects should be preceded by careful assessment of predictable risks in comparison with foreseeable benefits to the subjects or to others."[46] The Belmont Report echoes these concerns: "Many kinds of possible harms and benefits need to be taken into account. There are, for example, risks of psychological, physical, legal, social, and economic harm and the corresponding benefits."[47] The Declaration of Helsinki continues:

42. See Paradis et al., "Ethical Considerations in the First American Face Transplant."

43. See D. B. Chepeha et al., "Maxillomandibular-labial Reconstruction: An Autogenous Transplant as an Alternative to Allogenic Face Transplantation," *Plastic and Reconstructive Surgery* 126 (2010): 2007–11.

44. See ibid.

45. See O. P. Wiggins et al., "On the Ethics of Facial Transplant Research," *American Journal of Bioethics* 4 (2004): 1–12.

46. Ibid.; see World Medical Association, Declaration of Helsinki, 2008, sec. 17, http://www.wma.net/en/30publications/10policies/b3/index.html.

47. National Commission for the Protection of Human Subjects of Biomedical and Behavioral Research, "The Belmont Report: Ethical Principles and Guidelines for the Protection of Human Subjects of Research," April 18, 1979, http://www.hhs.gov/ohrp/humansubjects/guidance/belmont.html.

Where proven interventions do not exist or have been ineffective, the physician ... with informed consent from the patient ... may use an unproven intervention if, in the physician's judgment, it offers hope of saving life, reestablishing health, or alleviating suffering. Where possible, this intervention should be made the object of research, designed to evaluate its safety and efficacy.[48]

It may be difficult to predict results in facial transplantation surgery. As A. J. Alexander and colleagues point out, the patient should be the focus of any decision to perform an experimental surgical procedure; the first facial allograft transplant patient had no precedent on which to base her decision. Even when risks are poorly understood, Alexander argues, informed consent is possible so long as the unknowns are made clear to the potential transplant recipient.[49]

Risk/benefit analyses must be conducted on three levels by three different entities: the patient and the donor family, the surgical and medical team, and the institutional review board. Prior to the first partial facial transplant at the Cleveland Clinic, the clinic's institutional review board assembled a multidisciplinary subcommittee to examine the potential risks and benefits of the proposed transplant. Approval was granted even though it was impossible to quantify the risks and benefits for the patient. The team sought to minimize risks and maximize benefits for the procedure in these ways:

- Carrying out preliminary scientific work using animal models and cadavers
- Forming a skilled and experienced transplant team, including experts in microsurgery, facial reconstruction, transplantation biology, and infectious disease
- Ensuring meticulous protection of the patient's privacy from invasion by the media
- Providing psychological support for the patient
- Enforcing institutional review board review and oversight
- Utilizing long-term institutional support[50]

Risks and Concerns

It is worthwhile to examine in detail some of the most commonly cited potential risks or concerns associated with facial transplantation.[51]

Rejection and Drug Toxicity

Facial transplant recipients must deal with risks associated with the surgical procedure itself, as well as the risks of lifelong immunosuppressive medical treatment. Among the more rare complications is rhabdomyolysis. One patient with severe fa-

48. World Medical Association, Declaration of Helsinki, no. 37.

49. See A. J. Alexander et al., "Arguing the Ethics of Facial Transplantation," *Archives of Facial Plastic Surgery* 12 (2010): 60–63.

50. See Paradis et al., "Ethical Considerations in the First American Face Transplant."

51. C. J. Vercler has set forth an orderly account of these concerns; see his article, "Ethical Issues in Face Transplantation," *Virtual Mentor* 12 (2010): 378–82.

cial neurofibromatosis type 1 who received allogeneic facial transplantation suffered severe rhabdomyolysis and temporary oligoanuria in the early postoperative period. Fortunately, he recovered and was discharged after an extended hospitalization.[52]

The risks of immunosuppression include major rejection, diabetes, infections, the risk of the development of malignancy, and toxicity to end organs.[53] The risk to end organs was evident in the first face transplant recipient, who developed a rapid decline in renal function in the first year after her procedure. While her symptoms ameliorated by changing her drug regimen, long-term complications are likely.[54] Acute rejection has been reported in up to 85 percent of hand and face transplant recipients; these rejection episodes, however, were easily reversed with bolus injections of prednisone.[55] The adjunctive transplantation of bone marrow from the donor may help with long-term tolerance of the facial allograft. Transient low levels of chimerism have been reported.[56]

No facial transplant recipients have shown signs of chronic rejection, although the follow-up period has been relatively short.[57] Since the face transplant involves foreign tissue for the recipient, the potential for rejection at some point always exists. If rejection occurs and cannot be stopped, what can be done? Noted bioethicist Arthur Caplan proposed that such a case might call for physician-assisted suicide or euthanasia as a potential option to alleviate suffering. In his view, "insisting on a life with no face, as opposed to a horribly disfigured one, is too daunting a prospect to proceed ethically—if death is not an option."[58] Obviously, Caplan's proposal violates Catholic moral teaching. In *Evangelium Vitae*, John Paul II called euthanasia

a grave violation of the law of God, since it is the deliberate and morally unacceptable killing of a human person. This doctrine is based upon the natural law and the written word of God, is transmitted by the Church's tradition, and taught by the ordinary and universal Magisterium.

Depending on the circumstances, this practice involves the malice proper to suicide or murder.

Suicide is always as morally objectionable as murder. The Church's tradition has always rejected it as a gravely evil choice.[59]

Furthermore, according to Alexander, the fallback plan if a facial allograft fails would be to salvage the wound bed with the patient's own tissues. A transplant failure need not make the patient's condition worse than the pre-transplant state.[60]

---

52. See R. Hinojosa Pérez et al., "Severe Rhabdomyolysis after Allogeneic Transplantation of Facial Structures: A Case Report," *Transplantation Proceedings* 42 (2010): 3081–82.

53. See Wiggins et al., "On the Ethics of Facial Transplantation."

54. See J. M. Dubernard et al., "Outcomes 18 Months after the First Human Partial Face Transplantation," *New England Journal of Medicine* 357 (2007): 2451–60.

55. See Hinojosa Pérez et al., "Severe Rhabdomyolysis after Allogeneic Transplantation of Facial Structures."

56. See ibid.

57. See Vercler, "Ethical Issues in Face Transplantation."

58. A. Caplan, "Is Face Transplant Worth Risking Patient's Life?" *NBCNews.com*, December 17, 2008, http://www.msnbc.msn.com/id/28279182/ns/health-health_care/t/face-transplant-worth-risking-patients-life/#.UGt9ga5irN8.

59. John Paul II, *Evangelium Vitae*, nos. 65–66.

60. See Alexander et al., "Arguing the Ethics of Facial Transplantation."

As of March 2011, twelve face transplants had been performed worldwide.[61] One patient in China died after he stopped taking his medications and refused further medical treatment. A second transplant patient in France, who received a face and bilateral hand transplants for burn deformities, died of a myocardial infarction during surgery for an overwhelming infection of transplanted facial tissues.[62] Another patient died from an opportunistic infection two months after facial transplant.[63] Thus, the mortality rate for this procedure is 25 percent. The extremely high incidence of death after facial transplantation underscores the significant risks associated with this procedure. These risks should be made clear to potential face transplant recipients, so they can make a truly informed decision about this high-risk procedure.

Concerns for Donors and Their Families

Most reports provide little information about the status of the facial transplant donor, though when reported they are noted to be "brain-dead donors."[64] The donor for the first U.S. face transplant recipient was described as a brain-dead woman "who matched the patient in age, race, and skin complexion."[65] The privacy and confidentiality of both recipient and facial tissue donor need to be respected. The potential face transplant donor must meet the criteria of the Magisterium for "moral certainty" that he or she is dead in order to be considered a possible donor.

Nicanor Austriaco, OP, points out that "since the time of Pope Pius XII, the Catholic Church has explicitly supported the procurement of organs from the dead."[66] A person who agrees to donate organs, or one who gives consent for a family member to do so, exercises the virtue of charity.[67] Addressing the International Congress of the Transplantation Society, John Paul II explained: "Every organ transplant has its source in a decision of great ethical value: 'the decision to offer without reward a part of one's own body for the health and well-being of another person.'"[68] It is of critical importance that either the patient give informed consent in advance of death, or the patient's family give such consent, prior to the tissues being obtained for transplantation. In addition, the donor must be truly dead. It is morally unacceptable to harvest vital organs before the donor has died.[69] This formulation dates back to the time of Pope Pius XII, who wrote that "generally speaking, doctors should not be permitted to undertake

61. See Marchione and Contreras, "Texas Man Gets First Full Face Transplant in U.S."

62. See Vercler, "Ethical Issues in Face Transplantation."

63. C. R. Gordon et al., "The World's Experience with Facial Transplantation: What Have We Learned Thus Far?" *Annals of Plastic Surgery* 63 (2009): 572–78.

64. Ibid.

65. See M. Siemionow et al., "Near-Total Human Face Transplantation for a Severely Disfigured Patient in the USA," *Lancet* 374 (2009): 203–9.

66. N. P. G. Austriaco, "Presumed Consent for Organ Procurement," *National Catholic Bioethics Quarterly* 9 (2009): 247.

67. See John Paul II, *Evangelium Vitae*, no. 86.

68. Pope John Paul II, Address to the 18th International Congress of the Transplantation Society, August 29, 2000, no. 3, quoting his earlier Address to the Participants in a Congress on Organ Transplants, June 20, 1991, no. 3, http://w2.vatican.va/content/john-paul-ii/en/speeches/2000/jul-sep/documents/hf_jp-ii_spe_20000829_transplants.html.

69. See John Paul II, *Evangelium Vitae*, no. 15.

excisions or other operations on a corpse without the permission of those charged with its care, and perhaps even in the face of objections previously expressed by the person in question."[70] The *Catechism* outlines Church teaching on these prerequisites:

Organ transplants are in conformity with the moral law if the physical and psychological dangers and risks to the donor are proportionate to the good that is sought for the recipient. Organ donation after death is a noble and meritorious act and is to be encouraged as an expression of generous solidarity. It is not morally acceptable if the donor or his proxy has not given explicit consent. Moreover it is not morally admissible directly to bring about the disabling mutilation or death of a human being, even in order to delay the death of other persons.[71]

Recently, the issue of "presumed consent" for organ procurement, as a means to increase organ donor rates and to help potential transplant recipients, has raised some debate. Austriaco makes the argument that Catholic moral tradition cannot endorse a system of presumed consent for organ procurement.[72] He asserts that informed consent affirms and protects the intrinsic dignity and inviolability of the dead human person; it acknowledges that the cadaver of the human person deserves respect because it was made in the image and likeness of its Creator. Pius XII taught:

The human corpse deserves to be regarded entirely differently [from the dead body of an animal]. The body was the abode of a spiritual and immortal soul, an essential constituent of a human person whose dignity it shared. Something of the dignity still remains in the corpse. We can say also that, since it is a component of man, it has been formed 'to the image and likeness' of God.... Finally, the dead body is destined for the resurrection and eternal life. This is not true of the body of an animal.[73]

In addition, writes Austriaco, informed consent demonstrates that the human person is not the master of his or her own body, but only a steward. Thus, neither the dead person nor any other person, government, or society is free to treat the body or its organs at will, as items to be taken and given away arbitrarily.[74] Pius XII said, "God alone is the Lord of man's life and bodily integrity, its organs and members and faculties, those in particular which are instruments in the work of creation. Neither parents, nor husband or wife, not even the very person concerned, can do with these as he pleases."[75] Pope Benedict XVI reaffirmed this teaching:

With frequency, organ transplantation takes place as a completely gratuitous gesture on the part of the family member who has been certifiably pronounced dead. In these cases, informed consent is a precondition of freedom, so that the transplant can be characterized as being a gift, and not interpreted as a coercive or abusive act.[76]

---

70. Pope Pius XII, Allocution to a Group of Eye Specialists, May 14, 1956, quoted in Austriaco, "Presumed Consent for Organ Procurement," 247.

71. *Catechism of the Catholic Church*, no. 2296.

72. See Austriaco, "Presumed Consent for Organ Procurement."

73. Pius XII, Allocution to a Group of Eye Specialists, quoted in Austriaco, "Presumed Consent for Organ Procurement," 247–48.

74. See Austriaco, "Presumed Consent for Organ Procurement," 248.

75. Pius XII, Allocution to a Group of Eye Specialists, quoted in Austriaco, "Presumed Consent for Organ Procurement," 248.

76. Pope Benedict XVI, Address to the Participants in the International Congress "A Gift for Life: Con-

Austriaco continues:

A gift must be explicitly given by the giver in order for it to be a gift. Presumed consent would undermine this moral framework and as such has to be rejected.... Individual Catholics and Catholic institutions, especially Catholic hospitals, must reject presumed consent and not cooperate with an unjust and immoral system of organ procurement.[77]

John Paul II affirmed that "the technique of transplants has proven to be a valid means of attaining the primary goal of all medicine—the service of human life."[78] In *Evangelium Vitae*, he wrote that "the donation of organs [should be] performed in an ethically acceptable manner, with a view to offering a chance of health and even of life itself to the sick who sometimes have no other hope."[79] The late Holy Father stressed the need for informed consent, so that a free and conscientious decision may be made. Vital organs, he said, may be removed only after the donor is dead. Referring to the contemporary bioethical debate over ascertaining the fact of death, John Paul II cited the neurological criterion, which establishes the "complete and irreversible cessation of all brain activity (in the cerebrum, cerebellum, and brain stem). This is then considered the sign that the individual organism has lost its integrative capacity."[80]

Here it can be said that the criterion adopted in more recent times for ascertaining the fact of death, namely the complete and irreversible cessation of all brain activity, if rigorously applied, does not seem to conflict with essential elements of a sound anthropology. Therefore, a health-worker responsible for ascertaining death can use these criteria in each individual case as the basis for arriving at that degree of assurance in ethical judgment which moral teaching describes as "moral certainty." This moral certainty is considered the necessary and sufficient basis for an ethically correct course of action. Only where such certainty exists, and where informed consent has already been given by the donor or the donor's legitimate representatives, is it morally right to initiate the technical procedures required for the removal of organs for transplant.[81]

Therefore, if these criteria are rigorously met, the transplantation team may ethically and morally proceed to harvest facial tissues from a dead donor for transplantation. John Paul II's teaching on moral certainty with complete brain death has been reaffirmed recently by noted bioethicist John Haas, who draws the distinction between "moral certainty" and "absolute certainty." The latter is not required for tissue donation. The former is sufficient for the harvesting of organs for transplantation.[82]

Respect for the dead donor must also be observed. In France, the surgeons used a resin mask colored to resemble the donor's skin tone in order to restore the donor's face after tissue harvest.[83] Concerns that the transplant recipient's face will remind

---

siderations on Organ Donation," November 7, 2008, quoted in Austriaco, "Presumed Consent for Organ Procurement," 248.

77. Austriaco, "Presumed Consent for Organ Procurement," 249.

78. John Paul II, Address to the International Congress on Transplants, no. 1.

79. John Paul II, *Evangelium Vitae*, no. 86.

80. John Paul II, address to the International Congress on Transplants, no. 5.

81. Ibid.

82. See J. M. Haas, "Catholic Teaching Regarding the Legitimacy of Neurological Criteria for the Determination of Death," *National Catholic Bioethics Quarterly* 11 (2011): 279–99.

83. See J.-P. Meningaud et al., "Face Transplant Graft Procurement: A Preclinical and Clinical Study," *Plastic and Reconstructive Surgery* 122 (2008): 1383–89.

the family of the donor should be allayed. Studies using computer simulations and the results in previous facial transplant recipients show that the recipient face has a hybrid appearance between that of the donor and the recipient. The final appearance seems to be dictated primarily by the facial skeleton of the recipient.[84]

Patient Selection Criteria and Compliance

C. Paradis and associates have outlined selection criteria and their ethical justification:

- The potential transplant recipient must not be amenable to conventional facial reconstruction. Typically, such a candidate must have failed multiple attempts at facial reconstruction.
- The patient must be able to understand the risks of the surgery, including the risks of uncertainty about the outcome. This must be accomplished through ongoing discussions with the patient.
- The patient must have significant and severe functional deficits that could be ameliorated by facial transplantation. These may include impairment of nutrition, sense of smell, speech, and social acceptance, as well as severe pain and repeated infections.
- The potential transplant recipient should have realistic functional and physical goals that can be accomplished by facial transplantation. These could include the recovery of the ability to eat in public, the restoration of a nose with the sense of smell, and the ability to smile.
- The candidate should have good coping skills. He or she must have coped well with social situations despite the facial deformity and have been able to speak publicly about the facial injury.
- The patient must be compliant with medical treatment and have other indicators that minimize the risks. He or she must have demonstrated compliance with medical and surgical management in the past, must be age-appropriate, must have social support, and have no recent record of substance abuse.[85]

Availability of Other Options for Reconstruction

The patient must be informed that an alternative to facial transplantation exists for large mid- and lower-facial defects. A recent report demonstrated an alternative technique, which removes the risks of complications associated with allotransplantation of facial tissues. Two patients who were successfully reconstructed with free flaps from a single donor site experienced restored oral competence and swallowing comparable to that achieved by facial transplant recipients. No immune-suppression is required when the tissues are from the patient him- or herself.[86] If the patient has already failed previous attempts at facial reconstruction, then facial transplantation may be considered.

84. See Alexander et al., "Arguing the Ethics of Facial Transplantation."
85. See Paradis et al., "Ethical Considerations in the First American Face Transplant," 897.
86. See Chepeha et al., "Maxillomandibular-labial Reconstruction."

Degree of Functional Recovery

The first face transplant recipient in the United States was reported to have "excellent" functional outcome. Six months after surgery, the patient was described as being able to breathe through her nose, smell, taste, speak intelligibly, eat solid foods, and drink from a cup—all functions she was unable to perform prior to transplantation.[87] In another patient, some voluntary activity confirmed by electromyography was reported five months after transplantation.[88] Four facial transplant patients reported recovery of some sensory function, including pain sensation, mechanical sensation, and thermal sensitivity within three to twelve months.[89]

Psychological Concerns for the Transplant Recipient

Facial transplant patients must deal with such potential psychological risks as unrealistic hopes, fears of transplant rejection, guilt feelings about the death of the donor, and problems of compliance with medical treatment. The recipient must deal with his or her new appearance, which is closely associated with one's personal and social identity. The recipient may be subjected to excessive or prolonged publicity, which can severely invade privacy.[90] Emotional turmoil may result from a perceived change in "identity"; the patient may fear that a new face may make him or her into a new person.[91] Sr. Renée Mirkes has pointed out that

such predictions of identity change—change involving a person's very substance or self—are based on two alleged needs of the transplant recipients: 1) the need to incorporate the "non-self" of the transplanted organ into the recipient's own self, and 2) the need to accommodate the "living on" of the donor in the transplanted organ.[92]

"With the transplant of a visible organ, a deep identity split occurs, because one's self-image is modified substantially," wrote E. Carosella and T. Pradeu.

A transplant can be considered successful if it assures not only the function of the organ, but also the rebuilding of the recipient's identity. This difficult rebuilding work can be fruitful, because identity is characterized by a continuous evolution. The graft of a visible organ can lead to a full expression of one's identity, making the individual aware that to be oneself is to change constantly, and to accept oneself as changing.[93]

---

87. See Austriaco, "Presumed Consent for Organ Procurement."

88. See Meningaud et al., "Face Transplant Graft Procurement."

89. See M. Siemionow, B. B. Gharb, and A. Rampazzo, "Pathways of Sensory Recovery after Face Transplantation," *Plastic and Reconstructive Surgery* 127 (2011): 1875–89.

90. See Wiggins et al., "On the Ethics of Facial Transplantation."

91. See R. Mirkes, "Facial Transplantation and Self-identity," *National Catholic Bioethics Quarterly* 8 (2008): 51.

92. Ibid.

93. E. D. Carosella and T. Pradeu, "Transplantation and Identity: A Dangerous Split?" *Lancet* 368 (2006): 183; see also L. K. Kalliainen, "Supporting Facial Transplantation with the Pillars of Bioethics," *Journal of Reconstructive Microsurgery* 26 (2010): 547–54.

"In essence, then, the recipient experiences a reconstruction or transformation of the existing self."[94] As pointed out by Mirkes, predictions of an identity split in the face transplant recipient result from misconceptions about facial transplants and identity: "The Aristotelian distinction between substantial and accidental change reveals the error of thinking that facial transplantation results in a change in the recipient's very identity. Instead, a facial transplant recipient experiences what I will call a change in personality."[95]

Human beings do not just use their bodies; their bodies are an integral part of who they are. A facial transplant that becomes functional becomes a living part of the recipient. The donor's human soul has separated from his or her body and is no longer present in the grafted tissue. After it is incorporated into the recipient's body, it becomes an integral part of his or her body, and does not possess a separate identity. Thus, the donor does not continue to live in the person of the recipient. The functional integration of the transplanted facial tissues helps the recipient recognize that the transplant does not change his or her substantial self or identity. The transplant recipient remains the same person who existed prior to the transplant, despite the fact that he or she looks and functions differently. A person retains the same identity from birth until death; even a facial transplant and personality changes are incidental to his or her person.[96]

Although facial transplantation is not a life-saving procedure like transplantation of heart, kidney, or liver, it offers a number of anticipated benefits to the patient. The recipient could experience improved facial function and restoration of facial expression, oral feeding, and normal breathing without a tracheostomy. Aesthetic and psychological benefits can be substantial. In many cases, facial disfigurement may result in depression, social isolation, and risks of suicide.[97] Improved facial appearance and function would likely result in improved social interactions between the recipient and other persons. Since so few facial transplants have been performed to date, however, it is difficult to predict the functional and aesthetic outcome in individual patients.

Informed Consent

The potential face transplant recipient needs to consider whether participation in this procedure is consonant with his or her own values. Fully understanding the process takes time, and the patient should be given that time to consider the decision. The candidate should meet with members of the care team, including a psychiatrist and an infectious disease expert.[98] The potential transplant recipient must be made fully aware of the inherent risks involved with surgery and anesthesia, as well as risks of immunosuppression after surgery, loss of transplanted facial tissue, psychological read-

---

94. L. A. Sharp, "Organ Transplantation as a Transformative Experience: Anthropological Insights into the Restructuring of the Self," *Medical Anthropology Quarterly* 9 (1995): 379, quoted in Mirkes, "Facial Transplantation and Self-identity," 52.

95. Mirkes, "Facial Transplantation and Self-identity," 52.

96. See ibid., 49–56.

97. See J. H. Barker et al., "Patient Expectations in Facial Transplantation," *Annals of Plastic Surgery* 61 (2008): 68–72.

98. See Paradis et al., "Ethical Considerations in the First American Face Transplant."

justment, and potentially relentless media attention. The transplant recipient should be informed that the surgical outcomes are uncertain. Facial sensation, movement, speech, and ability to eat normally are not guaranteed; and the absolute requirements for strict compliance after surgery must be emphasized.[99] The surgeon who is proposing the surgery must be brutally honest about the number of such procedures he or she has performed in the past, the surgical team's strengths and weaknesses, and the medical care environment at the proposed institution.

These criteria correspond to the standards of the Belmont Report: "Respect for persons requires that subjects, to the degree that they are capable, be given the opportunity to choose what shall or shall not happen to them. This opportunity is provided when adequate standards for informed consent are satisfied."[100]

Seven key elements of informed consent have been proposed by Tom Beauchamp and James Childress:

1. Competence to understand and decide
2. Voluntariness in choice
3. Disclosure of material information by the physician or researcher
4. Recommendation of a plan
5. Understanding
6. Patient decision in favor of a plan
7. Authorization of a chosen plan[101]

A. Renshaw and colleagues have stated that the unknowns and ambiguities involved in facial transplantation do not preclude obtaining appropriate informed consent.[102]

Current recommended guidelines for face transplantation have been proposed by the Cleveland Clinic. The recipient should have the following characteristics:

• Strong desire to proceed with face transplantation
• Willingness to dedicate two to four years for postoperative rehabilitation
• Age between eighteen and sixty years old
• Minimal coexisting medical illness or trauma
• Elapsed injury-to-transplant time of more than six months
• All pertinent organ systems within normal limits
• Psychosocial stability according to transplant psychiatry
• Entire multidisciplinary face transplant team deems patient acceptable[103]

99. See ibid.

100. National Commission for the Protection of Human Subjects of Biomedical and Behavioral Research, "The Belmont Report," C.1

101. T. L. Beauchamp and J. F. Childress, *Principles of Biomedical Ethics*, 5th ed. (New York: Oxford University Press, 2001), 80.

102. A. Renshaw et al., "Informed Consent for Facial Transplantation," *Transplant International* 19 (2006): 861–67.

103. See M. Z. Siemionow and C. R. Gordon, "Institutional Review Board-Based Recommendations for Medical Institutions Pursuing Protocol Approval for Facial Transplantation," *Plastic and Reconstructive Surgery* 126 (2010): 1232–39.

It is important that, during the process of obtaining informed consent, a potential facial transplant recipient understand that facial transplantation will make only an incidental change. This would help the patient make the necessary mental and emotional adjustments required after facial transplantation. Mirkes has outlined a sample discussion between counselor and facial transplant candidate:

Your facial features will change, and if all goes well, could be dramatically improved. But you will continue to be the same person that you were before the transplant. Don't be fooled, then, by your reaction of "that's not me" or "I don't look at all like my old self" when you look into the mirror the first few times after receiving your new face. You've done the groundwork, carefully examining the whole question of the kind of accidental change produced by a facial graft. So you will be equipped to consistently temper your initial reactions by the realistic understanding that the "you" reflected in the mirror might have a new face, but not a new identity....

That your facial transplant changes you in a strictly accidental way is underscored by another possible outcome. Reconstructive facial surgeons have suggested that as your graft adjusts to the muscle and bone structure that you have retained, your new face will begin to shape itself around that structure. So, rather than looking completely unlike yourself, your new facial appearance could well turn out to be a cross between your uninjured face and that of your donor.[104]

Isabelle Dinoire, the partial face transplant patient in France, reported that her initial reaction was "that's not me." But as she adjusted to her new facial appearance and function, she became aware of how fortunate she was. "I have returned to the planet of human beings, those with a face, a smile, facial expressions that let them communicate," she said.[105]

In examining the psychological risks of facial transplantation, Mirkes has clarified the Aristotelian distinction between substantial and accidental change, in order to help clinicians provide potential recipients with correct information for informed consent. Examples of substantial changes are a person dying or a block of marble being chiseled into a statue. Accidental changes would be the skin color of a human being or cutting one's hair. Instead of causing a substantial change in the person, facial transplants may help the patient achieve a change in personality by causing only accidental changes in the person. This approach can help the transplant candidate more precisely evaluate accidental changes in appearance and personality, and may help the recipient deal with this life-changing procedure's mental and emotional challenges.[106]

The Costs of Facial Transplantation

The first U.S. facial transplant recipient underwent twenty-three separate conventional reconstructive procedures at a cost of about $353,000 prior to being consid-

104. Mirkes, "Facial Transplantation and Self-identity," 55–56.

105. L. Kowalczyk, "Brigham Doctors Will Do Rare Face Transplants," *Boston Globe*, July 29, 2007, http://www.boston.com/yourlife/health/diseases/articles/2007/07/29/brigham_doctors_will_do_rare_face_transplants/.

106. See Mirkes, "Facial Transplantation and Self-identity," 54.

ered for facial transplantation. The face transplant cost was about $350,000, with a post-transplant cost of $115,000. This suggested that in the United States, the costs of face transplantation may be similar to that of conventional reconstructive procedures, although there are additional ongoing costs for immunosuppressive medications.[107] The costs for such medications can be considerable for a young patient, such as the recipient in Texas who was only twenty-five at the time of his face transplant. If he lives a long life, the costs for immunosuppression and future medical treatments may be considerable. The face transplant procedure in China was said to cost only $80,000, and immunosuppression was estimated at $600 per month.[108] Despite the comparatively high costs, the benefits in alleviating physical and psychological suffering and providing both functional recovery and hope for social reintegration may be worth the cost.[109]

Ethical Debate

A number of arguments have been raised against facial transplantation; immunosuppression risk is among them. The possibility of chronic rejection is thought to be less than 5 percent for five years; the risk of developing diabetes is predicted at 5–15 percent. The risk of developing hypertension is put at 5–10 percent, and the danger that the patient will develop skin cancer is broadly estimated at 10–50 percent.[110] Long-term follow-up will be needed to assess the risks of complications, including graft loss.[111]

Concerns have been raised that the procedure will be broadened to include cosmetic enhancement. However, this is unlikely to become a widely used surgical procedure because of both the technical demands on the surgical teams and the huge amount of medical resources that must be marshaled. Also, the risks do not justify performing this procedure for purely cosmetic purposes. The goals of facial transplant recipients to date seem to be quite reasonable; they wish not to draw attention to their appearance, but rather to blend in with others.[112]

While the use of autologous tissues from the patient has been proposed for use in reconstruction, in many cases such procedures may not be adequate. Some of the patients who have received a facial transplant had previously undergone numerous attempts at reconstruction with tissues from other parts of their own bodies. The results were completely unsatisfactory in terms of appearance, function, and chronic pain.[113]

107. See M. Siemionow et al., "Cost Analysis of Conventional Facial Reconstruction Procedures Followed By Face Transplantation," *American Journal of Transplantation* 11 (2011): 379–85.

108. See Chenggang et al., "Some Issues in Facial Transplantation."

109. See Siemionow et al., "Cost Analysis of Conventional Facial Reconstruction Procedures Followed by Face Transplantation."

110. See D. Vasilic et al., "Risk Assessment of Immunosuppressive Therapy in Facial Transplantation," *Plastic and Reconstructive Surgery* 120 (2007): 1210–14.

111. See Kalliainen, "Supporting Facial Transplantation with the Pillars of Bioethics."

112. See ibid.

113. See ibid.

The potential failure of the donor graft could certainly have an adverse effect on the recipient. Excision of scar tissue with subsequent failure of transplanted tissues could result in a worse defect than the one that existed before the surgery. A back-up plan in the event of graft failure should be provided to the patient; this could include a second face transplant or reconstruction with autologous tissues. It should be noted that face transplant recipients have expressed the feeling that, even if the graft should fail, they would not be worse than they were prior to the transplant procedure.[114]

Some experts worry that this procedure may be attempted by medical centers that lack sufficient facilities to provide care for transplant patients. This procedure should be performed only in centers that participate in legitimate organ donation and harvesting networks. Such centers must also have adequately trained surgeons who are able to carry out these complex procedures. The potential transplant recipient would need to meet strict criteria established by institutional review boards and ethics committees.[115]

Absence of truly informed consent and risk of death from the procedure, or from infections after the surgery, are also serious concerns. Out of twelve reported facial transplants at this writing, three patients have died, providing an extremely high mortality rate of 25 percent.

Principles that Support Facial Transplantation

Autonomy is defined as the right of a patient to make decisions about his or her health care without coercion, after being given a reasonable amount of information and education.[116] The principle of autonomy is rooted in society's respect for an individual's ability to make informed decisions. In the last several decades, autonomy has become more important, as societal values have shifted to define medical quality in terms of outcomes that are important to the patient rather than those of medical professionals.[117] The patient must be able to give informed consent after weighing the risks and benefits of a proposed procedure, and must have realistic expectations. In the case of transplantation of life-saving organs, the patient may be willing to accept the risks of life-long immunosuppression. However, autonomy is not absolute. The facial transplant procedure is not viewed as a life-saving procedure. The facial deformity of potential transplant patients may cause them to be emotionally fragile, rendering them less capable of making a free and informed decision without duress. Although transplant candidates are under stress and vulnerable, this does not necessarily preclude them from being able to make an autonomous decision about a proposed transplantation procedure.[118]

---

114. See Dubernard et al., "Outcomes 18 Months after the First Human Partial Face Transplantation."

115. See Kalliainen, "Supporting Facial Transplantation with the Pillars of Bioethics."

116. See S. E. Johnson and M. J. Corsten, "Facial Transplantation in a New Era: What Are the Ethical Implications?" *Current Opinion in Otolaryngology and Head and Neck Surgery* 17 (2009): 274–78.

117. See ibid.

118. See Kalliainen, "Supporting Facial Transplantation with the Pillars of Bioethics."

The principle of justice requires that medical resources be provided in a fair manner, free of discrimination. Facial transplantation is technically demanding and expensive, requiring a huge number of resources which are available in a limited number of medical centers. The initial costs for facial transplantation in the United States have been estimated to range between $300,000 and $600,000, which does not include the costs of lifelong immunosuppression or subsequent surgical procedures. L. K. Kalliainen states:

Insofar as we have the ability to provide the service of facial transplantation, we have the ability to provide effective immunosuppression, we have documented that facial transplantation can be efficacious in relieving suffering, we effectively communicate the risks of the procedure, and the patient desires to accept the risks, an argument can be made that providing this service is just.[119]

The principle of beneficence refers to the moral obligation to do good, and is related to the requirement that health-care providers avoid evil. The maxim of *primum non nocere* (first, do no harm) must be a guiding principle. Health care seeks to ameliorate suffering, an act of beneficence. One could argue that severely disfigured appearance is as crippling as any other disability,[120] and so such disfiguration may be in the purview of health care to attempt to alleviate. On the other hand, there are the risks as discussed above. A. C. Grayling argues that the risks of immunosuppression, potential technical failure, and psychological problems among transplant recipients can be balanced against the perceived optimization of the patient's quality of life.[121] And so care must be taken in each individual case in determining if the act of beneficence lies with facial transplantation or not.

Bibliography

Alexander, A. J., Daniel S. Alam, Patrick J. Gullane, Benoît G. Lengelé, and Peter A. Adamson. "Arguing the Ethics of Facial Transplantation." *Archives of Facial Plastic Surgery* 12 (2010): 60–63.

Austriaco, N. P. G. "Presumed Consent for Organ Procurement." *National Catholic Bioethics Quarterly* 9 (2009): 245–52.

Barker, J. H., L. A. Furr, S. McGuire, M. Cunningham, O. Wiggins, B. Storey, C. Maldonado, and J. C. Banis Jr. "Patient Expectations in Facial Transplantation." *Annals of Plastic Surgery* 61 (2008): 68–72.

Barret, J. P., J. Gavaldà, J. Bueno, X. Nuvials, T. Pont, N. Masnou, M. J. Colomina, et al. "Full Face Transplant: The First Case Report." *Annals of Surgery* 254 (2011): 252–56.

Beauchamp, T. L., and J. F. Childress. *Principles of Biomedical Ethics.* 5th edition. New York: Oxford University Press, 2001.

Benedict XVI, Pope. Address to the Roman Curia on the Occasion of Their Christmas Greetings. December 22, 2008. Translated by Michael Campbell. http://www.lifesitenews.com/ldn/2008/dec/08122a3a.html.

Caplan, A. "Is Face Transplant Worth Risking Patient's Life?" *NBCNews.com.* December 17, 2008. http://www.msnbc.msn.com/id/28279182/ns/health-health_care/t/face-transplant-worth-risking-patients-life/#.UGt9ga5irN8.

119. Ibid., 549.
120. See A. C. Grayling, "Face Transplantation and Living a Flourishing Life," *Lancet* 371 (2008): 707–8.
121. See ibid.

Carosella, E. D., and T. Pradeu. "Transplantation and Identity: A Dangerous Split?" *Lancet* 368 (2006): 183.

Catechism of the Catholic Church. 2nd edition. Translated by the United States Conference of Catholic Bishops (Washington, D.C.: USCCB, 1997).

Chenggang, Y., H. Yan, Z. Xudong, L. Binglun, et al. "Some Issues in Facial Transplantation." *American Journal of Transplantation* 8 (2008): 2169–72.

Chepeha, D. B., K. M. Malloy, J. S. Moyer, E. J. Chanowski, and S. S. Khariwala. "Maxillomandibular-labial Reconstruction: An Autogenous Transplant as an Alternative to Allogenic Face Transplantation." *Plastic and Reconstructive Surgery* 126 (2010): 2007–11.

Congregation for the Doctrine of the Faith, *Donum Vitae, Instruction on Respect for Human Life in Its Origin and on the Dignity of Procreation*. Boston: Pauline Books and Media, 1987.

———. *Dignitas Personae, Instruction on Certain Bioethical Questions*. Boston: Pauline Books and Media, 2008.

Dhejne, C., P. Lichtenstein, M. Boman, A. L. Johansson, N. Långström, and M. Landén. "Long-term Follow-up of Transsexual Persons Undergoing Sex Reassignment Surgery: Cohort Study in Sweden" *PLoS ONE* 6, no. 2 (February 22, 2011): e16885. doi: http://dx.doi.org/10.1371/journal.pone.0016885.

Dubernard, J. M., and B. Devauchelle. "Face Transplantation." *Lancet* 372 (2008): 603–4.

Dubernard, J. M., B. Lengelé, E. Morelon, et al. "Outcomes 18 Months after the First Human Partial Face Transplantation." *New England Journal of Medicine* 357 (2007): 2451–60.

Fitzgibbons, R. P. "The Desire for a Sex Change." *Ethics and Medics* 30, no. 10 (October 2005): 10–14.

Fitzgibbons, R. P., P. M. Sutton, and D. O'Leary. "The Psychopathology of 'Sex Reassignment' Surgery: Assessing Its Medical, Psychological and Ethical Appropriateness." *National Catholic Bioethics Quarterly* 9 (2009): 97–125.

Gordon, C. R., M. Siemionow, F. Papay, et al., "The World's Experience with Facial Transplantation: What Have We Learned Thus Far?" *Annals of Plastic Surgery* 63 (2009): 572–78.

Grayling, A. C. "Face Transplantation and Living a Flourishing Life." *Lancet* 371 (2008): 707–8.

Gross, C. "Karol Wojtyla on Sex Reassignment Surgery: An Application of His Philosophical Anthropology." *National Catholic Bioethics Quarterly* 9 (2009): 711–23.

Haas, J. M. "Catholic Teaching Regarding the Legitimacy of Neurological Criteria for the Determination of Death." *National Catholic Bioethics Quarterly* 11 (2011): 279–99.

Hinojosa Pérez, R., M. Porras López, A. M. Escoresca-Ortega, A. Herruzo Avilés, A. León, J. A. Noval, T. Gómez-Cía, D. Sicilia, and J. D. González Padilla. "Severe Rhabdomyolysis after Allogeneic Transplantation of Facial Structures: A Case Report." *Transplantation Proceedings* 42 (2010): 3081–82.

John Paul II, Pope. *Veritatis Splendor, The Splendor of Truth* [Encyclical Letter. August 6, 1993]. Boston: St. Paul Books and Media, 1993.

———. *Evangelium Vitae, The Gospel of Life* [Encyclical Letter. March 25, 1995]. Boston: Pauline Books and Media, 1995.

———. Address to the International Congress on Transplants. August 29, 2000. http://www.vatican.va/holy_father/john_paul_ii/speeches/2000/jul-sep/documents/hf_jp-ii.

Johnson, S. E., and M. J. Corsten. "Facial Transplantation in a New Era: What Are the Ethical Implications?" *Current Opinion in Otolaryngology and Head and Neck Surgery* 17 (2009): 274–78.

Kalliainen, L. K. "Supporting Facial Transplantation with the Pillars of Bioethics." *Journal of Reconstructive Microsurgery* 26 (2010): 547–54.

Kowalczyk, L. "Brigham Doctors Will Do Rare Face Transplants." *Boston Globe*, July 29, 2007. http://www.boston.com/yourlife/health/diseases/articles/2007/07/29/brigham_doctors_will_do_rare_face_transplants/.

Marchione, M., and R. Contreras. "Texas Man Gets First Full Face Transplant in U.S." *MSNBC.com*. March 21, 2011. http://www.msnbc.msn.com/id/42192670/ns/health-health_care/.

McHugh, P. R. "Surgical Sex." *First Things* 147 (2004): 34–38.

Meningaud, J.-P., A. Paraskevas, F. Ingallina, E. Bouhana, and L. Lantieri. "Face Transplant Graft Procurement: A Preclinical and Clinical Study." *Plastic and Reconstructive Surgery* 122 (2008): 1383–89.

Meriggiola, M. C., E. A. Jannini, A. Lenzi, M. Maggi, and C. Manieri. "Endocrine Treatment of Transsexual Persons: An Endocrine Society Clinical Practice Guideline; Commentary from a European Perspective." *European Journal of Endocrinology* 162 (2010): 831–33.

Mirkes, R. "Facial Transplantation and Self-Identity." *National Catholic Bioethics Quarterly* 8 (2008): 49–56.

Murphy, T. F. "The Ethics of Helping Transgender Men and Women Have Children." *Perspectives in Biology and Medicine* 5 (2010): 46–60.

National Commission for the Protection of Human Subjects of Biomedical and Behavioral Research. "The Belmont Report: Ethical Principles and Guidelines for the Protection of Human Subjects of Research." April 18, 1979. http://www.hhs.gov/ohrp/humansubjects/guidance/belmont.html.

O'Leary, D. "Legalizing Deception: Why 'Gender Identity' Should Not Be Added to Anti-discrimination Legislation." *Catholic Exchange*, June 25, 2009. http://catholicexchange.com/legalizing-deception-why-%E2%80%9Cgender-identity%E2%80%9D-should-not-be-added-to-anti-discrimination-legislation/.

Paradis, C., M. Siemionow, F. Papay, R. Lohman, E. Kodish, C. Gordon, R. Djohan, K. Coffman, S. Bernard, and D. Alam. "Ethical Considerations in the First American Face Transplant." *Plastic and Reconstructive Surgery* 126 (2010): 896–901.

Paul VI, Pope. *Humanae Vitae, Of Human Life* [Encyclical Letter. July 25, 1968]. Boston: Pauline Books and Media, 1968

Pontifical Council for Health Pastoral Care. *Charter for Health Care Workers*. Boston: Pauline Books and Media, 1995.

Renshaw, A., A. Clarke, A. J. Diver, R. E. Ashcroft, and P. E. Butler. "Informed Consent for Facial Transplantation." *Transplant International* 19 (2006): 861–67.

Rose, Donna. "My Bio: Two Lives, One Lifetime." January 2004. http://www.donnarose.com/DonnaRoseOrig/bio.html.

Siemionow, M., J. Gatherwright, R. Djohan, and F. Papay. "Cost Analysis of Conventional Facial Reconstruction Procedures Followed by Face Transplantation." *American Journal of Transplantation* 11 (2011): 379–85.

Siemionow, M., B. B. Gharb, and A. Rampazzo. "Pathways of Sensory Recovery after Face Transplantation." *Plastic and Reconstructive Surgery* 127 (2011): 1875–89.

Siemionow, M. Z., and C. R. Gordon. "Institutional Review Board-Based Recommendations for Medical Institutions Pursuing Protocol Approval for Facial Transplantation." *Plastic and Reconstructive Surgery* 126 (2010): 1232–39.

Siemionow, M., F. Papay, D. Alam, et al. "Near-Total Human Face Transplantation for a Severely Disfigured Patient in the USA." *Lancet* 374 (2009): 203–9.

Sohn, M., and H. A. G. Bosinski. "Gender Identity Disorders: Diagnostic and Surgical Aspects." *Journal of Sexual Medicine* 4 (2007): 1193–1208.

United States Conference of Catholic Bishops. *Ethical and Religious Directives for Catholic Health Care Services*. 5th edition. (Washington, D.C.: USCCB, 2009).

Urban, R., N. N. H. Teng, and D. S. Kapp. "Gynecologic Malignancies in Female-to-Male Transgender Patients: The Need of Original Gender Surveillance." *American Journal of Obstetrics and Gynecology* 204 (2011): e9–e12.

Vasilic, D., R. R. Alloway, J. H. Barker, A. Furr, R. Ashcroft, J. C. Banis Jr, M. Kon, and E. S. Woodle. "Risk Assessment of Immunosuppressive Therapy in Facial Transplantation." *Plastic and Reconstructive Surgery* 120 (2007): 1210–14.

Vatican Council II. *Gaudium et Spes, Pastoral Constitution on the Church in the Modern World*. December 7, 1965. http://www.vatican.va/archive/hist_councils/ii_vatican_council/documents/vat-ii_cons_19651207_gaudium-et-spes_en.html.

Vercler, C. J. "Ethical Issues in Face Transplantation." *Virtual Mentor* 12 (2010): 378–82.

Wiggins, O. P., J. H. Barker, S. Martinez, et al. "On the Ethics of Facial Transplant Research." *American Journal of Bioethics* 4 (2004): 1–12.

World Medical Association. Declaration of Helsinki. 2008. http://www.wma.net/en/30publications/10policies/b3/index.html.

José A. Santos

10. A SPIRITUAL PERSPECTIVE IN REHABILITATION MEDICINE

As a devoutly Catholic physician practicing rehabilitation medicine, Dr. Santos provides a largely spiritual perspective to his work. Dr. Santos takes the reader through the salient features of caring for a person during the rehabilitative phase of their illness, and weaves together insightful observations about patients with acute and chronic pain, tapping into a patient's spirituality, and witnessing in truth and love to patients with impaired states of consciousness and other challenges commonly encountered in this area of clinical medicine. While steeped in Catholic spirituality, his presentation does not require assent to the Catholic tradition; it stands alone as a nicely articulated reflection about witness to truth found in the Gospel and shared in the everyday experience of caring for sick, injured, and disabled patients.—*Editors*

Many people will experience a disabling illness during their lifetime. In youth it may come through an accident, childhood cancer, or acute infectious illness. In middle age, patients experience degenerative conditions and chronic conditions caused by hypertension and diabetes, including strokes and amputations. It can also be the result of autoimmune events causing weakness, such as Guillian-Barré syndrome. In the golden years, patients become more susceptible to weakening structures and broken long bones. Any of these causes can lead to rehabilitation hospitalization in an acute care setting.

A rehabilitation doctor is called to carry out assessment of the patient, keeping in mind that the illness that brought him or her to the hospital now interferes with an immediate return to the home environment. A number of specific assessment components separate this area of specialization from others. Neurological information is collected to see how the patient can interact with the home environment, looking at all aspects: the perception or intake of the patient's senses, the processing or cognition of the information received, and the patient's ability to report, respond, or act on that information toward some intended goal. That goal may be provided by some internally driven source or by some external source, such as a therapist, physician, or family member. An orthopedic assessment demonstrates how the body's external frame—including the axial component, from which all limbs extend, and the appendages, which typically perform the action—is able to work against the forces of gravity. The connections between the subcomponents rely on several factors: ligaments to hold them together, joint surfaces to make them glide upon each other, and muscular components to effectively and precisely move them against the forces of gravity in order to hit their intended target.

A psychological and cognitive picture helps determine if the patient possesses the understanding, motivation, and desire to overcome whatever setback resulted in hospitalization. Rehabilitation care providers recognize that patients are influenced by forces outside themselves which give a sense of purpose, of belonging, of family and community. Both internal and external forces can propel the patient toward recovery, or repel him or her toward stagnation when faced with the daunting task of reintegrating with the home environment. If a task is overwhelming to the patient, the rehabilitation team's job is to look for subtasks that are attainable and measurable. The more concrete the measured task, the easier it is to convince someone to try and try again.

Physicians already possess the skills to carry out such an assessment of the natural forces that drive the physiology of recovery. The question is, how can the rehabilitation doctor now layer upon this assessment process the final part, the spiritual and supernatural components? Physicians are trained to involve the appropriate therapist for the appropriate deficit, such as an occupational therapist for loss of fine motor skills needed for an activity of daily living. By the same token, they can expand on that rationale to introduce a priest or hospital chaplain for healing through religious or spiritual practices. Priests serve to administer sacraments to people and to bring people to the sacraments. Rehabilitation professionals then working with Catholic patients should be capable of bringing their patients to the priest when they see a deficit in the sacramental life of the patient, in order to begin the rebuilding of the deficits in the patient's interior life.

The Gospels offer a clear example of a patient being led to spiritual healing in the story of the paralytic, who is brought on a stretcher to Jesus when he arrives for a visit to Capernaum.

He entered a boat, made the crossing, and came into his own town. And there people brought to him a paralytic lying on a stretcher. When Jesus saw their faith, he said to the paralytic, "Courage, child, your sins are forgiven." At that, some of the scribes said to themselves, "This man is blaspheming." Jesus knew what they were thinking, and said, "Why do you harbor evil thoughts? Which is easier, to say, 'Your sins are forgiven,' or to say 'Rise and walk'? But that you may know that the Son of Man has authority on earth to forgive sins"—he then said to the paralytic, "Rise, pick up your stretcher, and go home." He rose and went home. (Mt 9:1–7)

St. Thomas explains in his commentary on St. Matthew that the paralytic did not possess full belief in the healing powers of Jesus. He did, however, trust his friends enough to allow them to bring him to Christ.

This paralyzed man symbolizes the sinner lying in his sin. Just as the paralytic is unable to move, so too is the sinner helpless by himself. Those who carry the man immobilized by his paralysis represent those who, with their advice, lead the sinner towards God.[1]

Like the paralytic's friends, Catholics should have faith in the role of the sacraments and of the priest, acting in *persona Christi*, as part of the overall healing process. Physicians act as friends to their patients in bringing them to Christ when they see a need for spiritual healing. While this chapter highlights how Catholic witness in rehabilitation medicine may look when the patient is Catholic, non-Catholic Christians, and even non-Christian patients, remain subjects for the faithful physician to witness the Gospel.

In the physical rehabilitation world, therapists working as a team look at the patient from their vocational perspectives and develop a treatment plan in collaboration with the patient, the patient's family, and the other team members. This team approach tackles the disability task and shares the burden of the suffering among the patient and caregivers. Such teamwork keeps this task of sharing the burden tolerable. If the onus falls on just one individual, such as the patient, one family member or caregiver, or a member of the medical treatment team, the weight of the responsibility can be crushing. One way to maintain perspective on the improvement and the outcome that any patient obtains is to be mindful that three separate parties work in unison toward the healing process. These groups include the patients and all significant others who are part of their support community; the physician and all the members of the rehabilitation team; and finally, and most importantly, our Lord Jesus Christ. The outcome belongs in the hands of God, who already knows the patient's future, which is always one of hope, love and promise. Patients and physicians alike need to ask for God's grace and for patient endurance and trust in him who always loves his children.

The Catholic physician can rely on faith as a therapeutic tool, using it to place the burden of suffering on the strong shoulders of Christ. If the patient is receptive, the doctor can introduce the element of faith into the conversation in this way: "We will do what we can through our therapies and our medications to improve your recovery. You and we must keep in mind that, in addition to our best efforts, we must have faith in God's divine plan for us. Let us ask for his grace to maintain a patient endurance through the journey toward recovery. May our free will accept the challenge to improve. May our faith in him accept his will for our recovery."

Every person experiences times in their spiritual lives when they fall and they suffer. Catholics have the opportunity to use religious practices to seek redemption and to obtain rehabilitation again and again. A parallel exists between this spiritual rehabilitation and the world of physical rehabilitation medicine. In both worlds, it helps when the patient knows his or her deficits and weaknesses, so that attention can be focused on strengthening those areas. Awareness allows the patient to work on the

---

1. Quoted from Francisco Fernandez-Carvajal, *In Conversation with God*, vol. 1, *Advent and Christmastide* (New Rochelle, N.Y.: Scepter Publishing, 2007), 9.2.

correction. In both worlds, the training of an expert can guide the person through the rehabilitation process.

The Rehabilitation Team

In a hospital setting, a physical therapist will work on the big movements: how to get into and out of bed, how to come to a stand, how to balance, and how to propel oneself forward safely. That forward propulsion may require an assistive device, which could range from a single-tip cane all the way to a motorized wheelchair. An occupational therapist looks at the fine motor movements typically managed by the hands as they relate to activities of daily living: grooming, dressing, feeding, and meal preparation. A speech and language pathologist (which is essentially synonymous with a speech therapist) can assess deficits in communication (reception, comprehension, and production), cognition, and deficits in swallowing and articulation of speech. Most speech therapists have had additional training in treatment of swallow deficits using thermal and electrical stimulation to quicken the swallow reflex. Most can train the patient and family members on swallow strategies to minimize aspiration risks present because of swallow deficits.

The rehabilitation nursing staff has the most continuous job, that of monitoring the health status and managing the needs of persons who are physically unable to move themselves into or out of bed, who are recovering bowel and bladder control, who are frequently in pain, and who are frequently afraid of what the future will hold for them. The nursing staff usually has the closest proximity to the patient's interaction with visiting family members. Because nursing is a 24/7 service, nurses serve as the "listening post," observing and reporting these interactions. Social services are involved from the start of hospitalization to assess and to plan for discharge options, based on the patient's degree of recovery and on the family's capacity to care for someone with increased needs. A hospital chaplain serves to support the patient in religious and spiritual practices, as a source of coping and healing and as a connection to the home parish. All team members, including the nursing staff and physician, are constantly looking for reversible physical and cognitive deficits in the patient, seeking corrections to these deficits, and notifying the appropriate discipline to share their observations. A team approach is standard in a rehabilitation hospital setting.

In the interior life it is easy to overlook spiritual deficits. There may be a subconscious awareness of weaknesses, but the person often chooses to ignore them. Catholics are called to examine their consciences nightly, in order to practice acknowledgment and to ask forgiveness from God through Jesus Christ. The deficits thus discovered can be properly addressed, and the best way to do so is to rely on the proper therapist. In the mental health world, this would typically be a counselor, a behavioral psychologist, or a psychiatrist. In the Catholic spiritual world, one can seek the assistance of a spiritual director, who may be a priest or a lay person trained in this discipline. The physician who discovers the role of a spiritual director in his or her personal life will find it easier to see the need to refer a patient for this same healing.

Clinical Vignette 1

A 76-year-old man with history of hypertension presents with a diagnosis of lacunar brainstem cerebrovascular accident (CVA) resulting in a left hemiparesis. He has no dysarthria and no dysphagia. He requires moderate to maximum assistance for his transfers and mobility, and moderate assistance for basic activities of daily living. During the assessment of home support, he reports that he lives alone. He has adult children and an ex-wife in the vicinity, but he has lost contact with them during the past 10 to 15 years, largely as a result of his IV drug abuse habit. He describes himself as a lapsed Catholic, saying that he fell away as a result of that habit, which led to his divorce and the loss of contact with his wife and children. He lived for a time with a girlfriend and stopped going to Mass and receiving the sacraments, but says that he has since discontinued all IV drug abuse. He has not attempted reconciliation with his family or with the Catholic Church.

One typical response that many health professionals might have to such a history is to write off this man as unfortunate or beyond the scope of medical and social support services. However, the Catholic physician must strive always to see the suffering Jesus in the suffering patient. Seeing one's patients as the image of Christ motivates the physician to do all for him, for Christ told us that what we do for the least of our brothers, we do for him (Mt 25:40). Seen through the eyes of faith, this history offers an opportunity for spiritual healing of the patient's self-imposed alienation from family and Church. If the physician is practiced at evangelizing, the dialogue that offers personal testimony and experience as a Catholic who has fallen and returned for reconciliation may come easily. For other Catholic physicians, such a concept may be uncomfortable; it can feel like imposing oneself or proselytizing instead of evangelizing. But Catholics are called to share the Good News with all they encounter. Archbishop José H. Gomez describes this call in his pastoral letter "You Will Be My Witnesses":

The greatest love and service we can show to others is to share the Good News that they are loved by God and offered his salvation. We cannot neglect to tell others that in Jesus Christ they can find the answers to their questions about the fundamental meaning of existence and the purpose of life.[2]

He goes on to quote St. Teresa of Calcutta, who described how best to share her faith in a culture that did not know Christianity except in small pockets or minority groups: "I love all religions, but I am in love with my own. Naturally, I would like to give the treasure I have to you, but I cannot. I can only pray for you to receive it."[3]

The patient described above was invited to make use of local support offered in the Catholic hospital by the pastoral care department. He accepted all offers of intervention: he agreed to see a priest to make his confession, receive absolution, and receive

---

2. Most Rev. José H. Gomez, STD, "You Will Be My Witnesses," Pastoral Letter to the People of God of San Antonio, February 15, 2010, http://www.la-archdiocese.org/archbishop/Documents/2010-2006/2010-0215_Anv_Pastoral_Letter_SA.pdf.

3. Ibid.

Holy Communion. Once he was reconciled with the Lord through both healing sacraments and the Church, he unilaterally contacted his family to begin to reconcile with them as well. Like the prodigal son, he was accepted back into the family by his children and their mother. Perhaps this outcome would have happened without any specifically Catholic intervention, but the hospital staff extended the opportunity, sowing the seeds and letting the Holy Spirit do the rest.

All rehabilitation treatment team members develop the plan for a patient's recovery and keep their "eyes on the prize," the restoration of better health. That restoration waits down the road, in the future. It requires faith to imagine what improvement patients could achieve in the future, and it requires faith and determination to guide them there. If the physician's personal faith has weakened, he or she is called to faith practices that can lead to its restoration. If doctors are obliged to continue their medical education to improve the art and science of their medical practice, how much more are they called to continue enriching their faith practices with interior formation, so that their compassion for the injured and the fallen will constantly grow.

In the spiritual life, Catholics use prayer to connect with God and his will in their lives. They receive the sacrament of Reconciliation to be restored to a state of grace, which allows reception of the Lord in the sacrament of the Eucharist for further enrichment. The guidance of a priest or spiritual director is essential to correct weakness and to advance strengths. St. Josemaría Escrivá considered advancement in interior formation without a spiritual director analogous to building a house without the assistance of an architect:

It's good for you to know this doctrine, which is always sound: your own spirit is a bad advisor, a poor pilot to steer you through the squalls and storms and across the reefs of the interior life. That's why it is the will of God that the command of the ship be entrusted to a master who, with his light and knowledge, can guide us to a safe port.[4]

In daily existence, people can use physical and mental exercises to improve their ability to overcome gravity and to negotiate society. In a similar way, the Catholic rehabilitation physician's job is to assist patients in overcoming the weight of two types of gravity, physical and moral. The moral life has an impact on the spiritual life; a person's moral choices, exercised with free will, can be deadly and can remove the person from a state of grace. The choice to mortally sin is a willing choice to break off the relationship with God.

Pope Benedict XVI compares the weight of moral gravity with our desire to overcome it:

The Fathers of the Church maintained that human beings stand at the point of intersection between two gravitational fields. First, there is the force of gravity which pulls us down—towards selfishness, falsehood and evil; the gravity which diminishes us and distances us from the heights of God. On the other hand there is the gravitational force of God's love: the fact that we are loved by God and respond in love attracts us upwards. Man finds himself betwixt

4. St. Josemaría Escrivá, *The Way-Furrow-The Forge* (New Rochelle, N.Y.: Scepter Publishing, 2008), "The Way," no. 59.

this twofold gravitational force; everything depends on our escaping the gravitational field of evil and becoming free to be attracted completely by the gravitational force of God, which makes us authentic, elevates us and grants us true freedom.[5]

In order to appreciate the effects of physical gravity on those with physical limitations, it is helpful to imagine oneself on the surface of Jupiter, which has 2.5 times the gravitational strength of the earth. Imagine the difficulty of attempting to sit up from a prone position. Imagine trying to stand up, trying to take a step, trying to carry something or someone. Now imagine walking on Earth, climbing a steep hill: every effort is focused on going up. How long can the effort be maintained before exhaustion sets in?

These are the kinds of struggles that patients with physical weakness face every second as they challenge gravity. The job of the rehabilitation team is to help them cheat the downward pull of gravity without injury, and it is important that the team do all in its power to help them circumvent these forces. The job of Catholic caregivers is to fight the other gravity we all face, whether injured or not: escaping from the moral gravitational field of evil toward the gravitational force of God.

Acute Pain Management in a Rehabilitation Hospital Setting

Patients who arrive at the doors of a hospital rehabilitation unit or an outpatient clinic have earned their admission through a physical loss or the acquisition of an acute and persistent pain. The loss may be the result of a neurological event, such as a stroke or spinal cord injury that causes secondary loss of movement and function, or it may be the loss of a limb through trauma or vascular insufficiency. The patient may be in pain caused by injury or by the aftereffects of a needed surgery, and that pain may be severe or persistent enough to make the patient and the family agitated.

Once the source of pain is ascertained through the history collection and physical examination, the physician can address the use of analgesic agents to assuage the pain and secondary suffering. The physician can, over time, develop skill in distinguishing the difference between a patient's request for analgesics for pain and a patient's need for something more, such as alleviation of one's suffering. A request for analgesia may be only a partial expression of a request for a need such as relief of suffering, which, because it is a more complex reality touching upon more than just the physical dimension of a person, a patient may not be able otherwise to articulate. It can be helpful to educate the patient concerning his or her perception of the signal (pain) and the reaction to that signal (suffering). A numerical pain scale can be a helpful tool here: if the scale is 0 to 10, with 10 being the worst pain possible, and the patient rates the pain at 15, then the patient's suffering is probably compounding the pain. If the patient is overly sedated from the analgesic and still rating the pain after medication at 10, suf-

---

5. Pope Benedict XVI, Homily, St. Peter's Square, Palm Sunday, April 11, 2011, http://w2.vatican.va/content/benedict-xvi/en/homilies/2011/documents/hf_ben-xvi_hom_20110417_palm-sunday.html.

fering should be suspected. If the patient rates the pain level at 10 even in the absence of all physiologic markers that suggest increased physical stress (such as elevated pulse rate and blood pressure), suffering may be the underlying difficulty in controlling the pain with medication alone.

The treatment for suffering requires a different set of tools than the treatment of pain. When a patient suffers from a physical hurt, physical means can be used to reduce the stress of suffering. Suffering, though, can have both a physical component and a moral component; Pope John Paul II addressed the difference between the two in his apostolic letter *Salvifici Doloris*:

A certain idea of this problem comes from the distinction between physical suffering and moral suffering. This distinction is based upon the double dimension of the human being and indicates the bodily and spiritual element as the immediate or direct subject of suffering. Insofar as the words "suffering" and "pain," can, up to a certain degree, be used as synonyms, *physical suffering* is present when "the body is hurting" in some way, whereas *moral suffering* is "pain of the soul." In fact, it is a question of pain of a spiritual nature, and not only of the "psychological" dimension of pain which accompanies both moral suffering and physical suffering The vastness and the many forms of moral suffering are certainly no less in number than the forms of physical suffering. But at the same time, moral suffering seems as it were less identified and less reachable by therapy.[6]

Treatment options for physical suffering may involve psychological counseling from a trained therapist, or the counseling may be in the hands of the treating physician. One way to help patients derail the cycle of pain is to help them acknowledge and address the first typical thoughts that begin when pain starts. Upon feeling a pain signal, an internal conversation begins. Past pain is recalled ("Oh, not again!"). The current pain is acknowledged ("I really am hurting"). Fears about future pain or loss of function arise ("How will this affect my ability to work?"). The physician can ask the patient to review such internal thoughts, choosing a time to initiate the discussion when the patient is not overly sedated and is able to absorb the concept. The physician can ask the patient how much of the current suffering is compounded by the pain of the past or of the future. The patient should be reminded that most analgesics are effective only for the present pain, and so should be requested for that present pain only. The physician should be mindful that a patient's maladaptive coping strategy cannot usually be removed successfully without introducing a better adaptive strategy.

The Catholic understanding of human suffering calls us to join our suffering with that of Christ for the redemption of our sins and reparation for sins of others. It is important to remind suffering Catholic patients that, in uniting their own suffering with Christ's, they suffer in his company instead of alone. It is suffering while alone that can be truly unbearable. *Salvifici Doloris* tells us:

6. Pope John Paul II, *Salvifici Doloris, On the Christian Meaning of Human Suffering*, Apostolic Letter, February 11, 1984, no. 5, http://www.vatican.va/holy_father/john_paul_ii/apost_letters/documents/hf_jp-ii_apl_11021984_salvifici-doloris_en.html.

Every man has *his own share in the redemption*. Each one is also *called to share in that suffering* through which the redemption was accomplished. He is called to share in that suffering through which all human suffering has also been redeemed. In bringing about the redemption through suffering, Christ *has* also *raised human suffering to the level of the redemption*. Thus each man, in his suffering, can also become a sharer in the redemptive suffering of Christ.[7]

Catholic patients may have this understanding of suffering; for those who do not, however, and for non-Catholic patients, simply expressing this view of suffering to them at least provides a witness to this important dimension of suffering.

The profession of rehabilitation prides itself on using the parts that function to "work around" the parts that do not. If the patient's left side is weak, the therapist works on the left side to improve it but also works on helping the right side take up more of the work in the meantime. In order to work around physical pain and suffering, the rehabilitation team can address moral suffering with the work-around of shared redemption, while continuing to address the physical pain.

We Are Mind, Body, and Soul

Members of the rehabilitation team also pride themselves on looking at the whole person. Whereas many physicians profess a commitment to balance the mind and body when evaluating and treating patients, they often neglect the third element of the human person, the soul. Team members are accustomed to looking for the psychological coping skills that can aid patients in overcoming the physical challenges they face. How can they also integrate the spiritual realm, especially if they have no spiritual training?

Christina Puchalski, MD, of the George Washington Institute for Spirituality and Health, along with a group of primary care physicians, developed the FICA tool to assist with integrating a history of a patient's spirituality and faith practices and beliefs:

F = Faith and Belief (What is your belief or faith?)
I = Importance (What influence does your belief play in how you live or in how you recover your health?)
C = Community (Do you belong to a religious or faith community which is important in your support and recovery?)
A = Address in Care (How would you like for me, your health-care provider, to address these issues with you?)[8]

This tool was created to help health-care providers build an environment of trust by opening the door to discussion of spiritual issues with patients. The suggested questions can uncover coping mechanisms and support systems and can help identify

---

7. Ibid., no. 19, emphasis in original.
8. Christina Puchalski, "FICA Spiritual History Tool," https://smhs.gwu.edu/gwish/clinical/fica/spiritual-history-tool.

cases that need referral to a chaplain and or priest. Physicians can integrate the FICA questions into their history collection during the initial physical examination.

Once a patient has met the rehabilitation hospital's admission criteria, health-care providers are duty-bound to accept the patient, no matter their condition on arrival. In the course of examining and assessing the patient, obtaining a medical history, and reviewing medical records, team members may discover personal choices and practices that have been detrimental to the patient's health. The onset of treatment may not be the optimum time to address every risk-taking behavior; more frequently, the physician must await the proper moment to offer correction. It takes time to establish sufficient trust in a doctor-patient relationship to advise and guide a patient out of detrimental practices that require a change in lifestyle choices.

The Catholic physician should not hesitate to discuss patients' habits or practices that can be detrimental to either spiritual or physical health. This should in some ways be familiar as an outgrowth of standard medical practice, in which the physician observes the malady and lays out a plan for correction and recovery by verbalizing a change from current behavior. Catholic doctors must extend their concern for patients beyond their earthly health to include eternal and moral health, which is more durable and permanent than the physical body. Fr. Francisco Fernandez-Carvajal, a priest of the Opus Dei prelature, offers this advice:

Amongst the excuses that can lodge themselves in our mind, so that we do not make or so that we put off making fraternal correction, is the fear of offending the person we have to warn. It seems paradoxical that a doctor should not fail to tell a patient that if he wants to be cured he must undergo a painful operation, and that we Christians should be reluctant to tell people around us that the health of their soul—of how much greater value this is than bodily health—is at risk![9]

The Catholic physician has an opportunity in such moments to improve an eternal life. If the FICA tool is applied early, and a trusting fraternal connection has been established through dialogue, the doctor can broach the subject in several ways. The doctor can relate a story of one of his or her own life mistakes. Or, perhaps, the doctor can say something like, "In my personal friendships, I have had the opportunity to offer corrective advice to my friends. Although you and I met only recently and have not had time to develop such a friendship, I can offer you some advice if you wish to hear it." Another approach is to say, "Sometimes we know what we have done is wrong but we dare not think about it."

Patients will frequently offer their own observations or those of their family concerning their mistakes in moral judgment. The Catholic physician must always be attentive to such moments of grace when they appear. Even if the patient is not immediately receptive to discussion, the physician can leave the door open by saying, "Let me know when you are ready to talk about that choice you made, and I will share my observations with you then."

---

9. Francisco Fernandez-Carvajal, *In Conversation with God*, vol. 3, *Ordinary Time, Weeks 1–12* (New Rochelle, N.Y.: Scepter Publishing, 2007), 24.2.

This does not mean that the physician must be the direct provider of all services and corrective actions. If the physician discovered a medical condition requiring surgery, he or she would consult and refer to a surgeon, as the need for surgery exceeds the physician's area of expertise. Similarly, a fault in the moral or faith status and practices of a patient should be referred to the proper expert. The physician's duty is to know how to recognize the problem and how to refer the patient to a pastor, a chaplain, or a trained provider of pastoral care.

Chronic Pain Management in a Rehabilitation Setting

The team approach to rehabilitation for a patient with chronic pain includes nursing staff, therapy staff, and pastoral care. In the Catholic perspective, resources include not only pharmacological, psychological, and physical modalities, but also sacramentals and the sacraments. The litany of saints provides Catholic physicians and their patients with still more "team members."

In the case of a long-term disabled patient seeking an evaluation, the physician must review all that has been tried up until that time. Previous evaluations, tests, attempted treatments and their outcomes, diagnostic testing and referrals should all be investigated. In addition, the physician needs to know what problem has not been sufficiently improved and thus has driven the patient to seek reevaluation.

This is also an appropriate time to apply the FICA questions and make inquiries into the patient's supernatural life and interventions. If the patient identifies as Catholic, it is appropriate to ask whether he or she is receiving the sacraments, particularly the sacraments of healing: Reconciliation and the Sacrament of the Sick. Frequently, these questions will uncover more history, which may include an event that led to the patient's estrangement from the Church. Doctors frequently hear stories of loss of faith resulting from anger or heartache, from unanswered prayer for healing, or from a relationship that had an undesired outcome. They hear of attempts to seek priestly guidance or assistance that resulted in effects or responses different from those desired. Patients may leave the Church for other faith practices, or they may abandon faith practice entirely, saying "I just pray to God directly." Such a departure may indicate a poor faith formation, through which a person fails to understand the role of humility and faith in receiving healing as a grace from God.

The Catholic faith is rich in resources for forgiveness and healing, but it does require two things of Catholic physicians. First, it requires them to ask patients to submit to God's will, following the example of Christ's prayer at Gethsemane: "My Father, if it is possible, let this cup pass from me; yet, not as I will, but as you will.... My Father, if it is not possible that this cup pass without my drinking it, your will be done!" (Mt 26:39, 42). Second, it requires that physicians renew and acknowledge their faith in the healing power of Christ. This is the faith Jesus required when he was approached by the two blind men seeking a cure:

And as Jesus passed on from there, two blind men followed [him], crying out, "Son of David, have pity on us!" When he entered the house, the blind men approached him and Jesus said to them, "Do you believe that I can do this?" "Yes, Lord," they said to him. Then he touched their eyes and said, "Let it be done for you according to your faith." And their eyes were opened. (Mt 9:27–30)

The visionary St. Maria Faustina Kowalska wrote in her diary of the conversations between Christ and other souls that she heard in her visions; among these was a conversation with the suffering soul. This conversation in particular reveals much insight into the anguished heart a person in chronic pain brings to the clinical evaluation:

Poor health detains me on the way to holiness. I cannot fulfill my duties. I am as useless as an extra wheel on a wagon. I cannot mortify myself or fast to any extent, as the saints did. Furthermore, nobody believes I am sick, so that mental pain is added to those of the body, and I am often humiliated. Jesus, how can anyone become holy in such circumstances?[10]

We can acknowledge, as did Jesus, that sometimes we are not understood; however, this does not preclude openness to God's mercy.

One more thing, Lord. What should I do when I am ignored and rejected by people, especially by those on whom I had a right to count in times of greatest need?[11]

St. Faustina reports that Our Lord provides the final recommendation to the suffering soul:

My child, make the resolution never to rely on people. Entrust yourself completely to My will saying, "not as I want, but according to Your will, O God, let it be done unto me." These words, spoken from the depths of one's heart, can raise a soul to the summit of sanctity in a short time. In such a soul I delight. Such a soul gives me glory. Such a soul fills heaven with fragrance of her virtue. But understand that the strength by which you bear sufferings comes from frequent Communions. So approach this fountain of mercy often, to draw with the vessel of trust whatever you need.[12]

Managing the Resistant Rehabilitation Patient

After the records review and interview process results in a complete assessment, the next step is development of a treatment plan. Frequently these treatments involve other specialists, such as physical therapists or speech and language pathologists. However, a patient may insist on trying to recover without external help. The physician should recognize that pride of self-sufficiency may be the compelling factor in such a case. The physician may allow the patient to try going it alone, but should take care to advise him or her about the potential for undue frustration or the development of some maladaptive pathway during this solo process. The role of the therapist here should be that of a guide toward better adaptation to the existing physical deficit being treated.

In a similar manner, a patient may not be willing to accept the physician's frater-

---

10. St. Faustina Kowalska, *Divine Mercy of My Soul*, 3rd ed. (Stockbridge, Mass.: Marian Press, 2005), notebook V, verse 1487, p. 527.

11. Ibid., 528.

12. Ibid., 529.

nal correction for the moral choices that may contribute to their chronic pain and suffering. At such times, the physician should, for a Catholic patient, apply his or her referral skills to guide the patient toward spiritual healing through the sacraments and through spiritual direction from a priest. Ultimately, of course, the physician must accept the patient's decision to accept or to reject guidance. Not every attempt to restore a patient's spiritual health will be successful on the first encounter with the priest. The referring physician must be prepared to support patients who do not experience a sense of recovery or improvement. This applies also to the physician's own attempts at improving his or her interior life. The observation is put in perspective by Fr. Carvajal:

> As we make our way towards Our Lord, we cannot expect to be victorious all the time. Many of our defeats will be of only limited importance, but even when they are really important, reparation and contrition will bring us closer to God more than ever. And with Our Lord's help, we will begin again. We will not give way to discouragement or pessimism, which always spring from pride. With patience and humility, we can start all over again once more, even though we see no results.[13]

Rehabilitation of Persons with Impaired Comprehension

Not every lack of response to a treating physician's request is voluntary. For example, a left cerebral hemispheric injury may result in a disorder of communication affecting comprehension of spoken words. Injury to the speech center of the dominant hemisphere can produce impairment in the patient's reception, comprehension, and production of speech. In order to be understood by an aphasic patient, the physician must convert from verbal communication to "speaking" instead with symbolic gestures in order to achieve understanding. In the physical examination of someone who is aphasic (or who speaks a language in which the physician is not fluent), the physician must still communicate commands to carry out a task, such as "take a deep breath." Most aphasic persons will respond to the instruction "take a deep breath" when the examiner makes a very specific hand, arm, and mouth signal in front of the patient. If this gesture is done with the stethoscope around the physician's ears and the bell on the patient's chest, most patients will naturally respond by taking the deep breath. Symbolic gesture interpretation is maintained in portions of the brain other than the speech centers.

This description of a nonverbal gesture command makes clear that even nonverbal actions convey a message to the patient during an examination. The physician can convey acknowledgment of the patient's full dignity even through mere facial gestures. Going face-to-face with an attentive but non-communicative patient allows the doctor's face and eyes to speak clearly to the patient. In this way, the Catholic physician can, without words, convey happiness at seeing the face of Christ in the patient's face.

---

13. Fernandez-Carvajal, *In Conversation with God*, vol. 1, *Advent and Christmastide*, 12.2.

How can a physician tell if an aphasic patient might be Catholic? A scapular attached to the patient's gown or a rosary strung around a hospital bed rail, Marian objects on the bed stand or posted on the wall, or a television tuned to EWTN, may offer evidence of the patient's faith.

Impaired Alertness or Consciousness

Traumatic brain injury (TBI) from an external concussive force is a global injury, typically caused by a sudden deceleration of the exterior or skull with a delayed deceleration of the brain matter due to the momentum. This leads to a collision of the brain with the internal cranial vault. There are typically multiple micro shear disruptions at the interface of brain tissue of different densities, such as the transition of grey matter and white matter. Frequently the brain-injured person may manifest a predominant malfunction pattern suggesting greater injury to left or right cerebral hemispheres; however, the suspicion of probable bilateral hemispheric injury should be maintained. The concussive energy must be dispersed within the brain vault, and the greatest concentration of energy dispersal is in the central core, where the hippocampus resides; the hippocampus can incur structural injury. Hippocampus functions are critical for acquisition, storage, and retrieval of memory, and so persons with TBI frequently have difficulty with new memory even though they may recall events that happened prior to the TBI. The physician treating a TBI patient should be prepared to repeat him- or herself and not take it personally that the patient is repeating questions for the umpteenth time. Many rehabilitation centers will provide the forgetful patient with a "memory book" to record frequently asked questions and their answers. A typical memory book in a head injury program may include the patient's name, the date, and the patient's location within the facility. The book may also contain written reminders such as "take blood pressure pill at 11:30 am" or it may log daily activities that were completed. The purpose of the memory book is to keep the person with the memory deficit oriented to important daily tasks to be completed. The book is a helpful tool to which the forgetful questioner can refer if a specific question posed has been asked before.

Some conditions can result in complete loss of consciousness without disruption of respiration, heart function, or gastrointestinal function; this condition is called a coma. The National Institute of Neurological Disorders and Stroke describes coma in this way:

A coma, sometimes also called persistent vegetative state, is a profound or deep state of unconsciousness. Persistent vegetative state is not brain-death. An individual in a state of coma is alive, but unable to move or respond to his or her environment. Coma may occur as a complication of an underlying illness, or as a result of injuries, such as head trauma. Individuals in such a state have lost their thinking abilities and awareness of their surroundings, but retain non-cognitive function and normal sleep patterns. Even though those in a persistent vegetative state lose their higher brain functions, other key functions, such as breathing and circulation, remain relatively intact. Spontaneous movements may occur, and the eyes may open in response to external stimuli. Individuals may even occasionally grimace, cry, or laugh. Although individuals in a persistent vegetative state may appear somewhat normal, they do not speak and they are unable to respond to commands.[14]

Persons in coma are not typically managed in an acute rehabilitation setting; however, they deserve mention here since their families will seek the advice of rehabilitation practitioners on how best to maintain or stimulate the person in persistent vegetative state. Families can be instructed how to maintain proper routine in nutrition, hydration, and auditory, tactile, and proprioceptive stimulation. In such cases, it is important to convey to the family that their loved one remains a person even in a persistent vegetative state, with the full complement of human dignity inherent in a person created in God's image. Catholic physicians are called to continue administration of nutrition and hydration through ordinary means, which includes a feeding tube.

As we saw in chapter 2, Pope Benedict addressed the dignity of the patient in coma in a 2011 televised question-and-answer session, drawing the comparison to "a guitar whose strings have been broken and therefore can no longer play. The instrument of the body is fragile like that; it is vulnerable, and the soul cannot play, so to speak, but remains present.... [T]his hidden soul feels your love deep down, even if he is unable to understand the details."[15] Regarding rehabilitation medicine, what we can stress in this exchange is the pope's emphasis on the importance of the role of the patient's family:

Your presence, therefore, dear parents, dear mother, next to him for hours and hours every day, is the true act of a love of great value because this presence enters into the depth of that hidden soul. Your act is thus also a witness of faith in God, of faith in man, of faith, let us say, of commitment, to life, of respect for human life, even in the saddest of situations.... [C]arry on, to know that you are giving a great service to humanity with this sign of faith, with this sign of respect for life, with this love for a wounded body and a suffering soul.[16]

The level of alertness or consciousness in the comatose patient is directly related to the function of the reticular activating system (RAS), which is predominantly dispersed in the area adjacent to the lateral ventricles of the two hemispheres. Decreased alertness is most commonly seen when both hemispheres have suffered an injury or lesion. This bi-hemispheric involvement can be seen in conditions such as TBI, multiple stroke syndromes, or systemic induced process, which lead to loss of oxygen, circulation, or nutritional support to the entire brain. It can also be a result of medications that have a sedating effect. Another common etiology in a hospital setting is disruption of the sleep-wake cycle, so that patients are more alert and awake at night and more somnolent in daytime.

14. National Institute of Neurological Disorders and Stroke, "NINDS Coma Information Page," accessed December 12, 2016, https://www.ninds.nih.gov/Disorders/All-Disorders/Coma-Information-Page.

15. Pope Benedict XVI, "Where Is the Soul of a Comatose Person?" April 22, 2011, https://w2.vatican.va/content/benedict-xvi/en/speeches/2011/april/documents/hf_ben-xvi_spe_20110422_intervista.html

16. Ibid.

Impaired Memory Function

Loss of memory or difficulty recalling recent events is a common presenting complaint of rehabilitation patients. Normal memory acquisition requires a sequence of factors: alertness, attentiveness, reception of the message, interpretation of the message content, storage of the message content, and retrieval or recall of message content when internally or externally asked to produce it. In the normal population, most failures to recall new events are a function of decreased alertness due to physical or mental fatigue, or decrease in attentiveness due to physical distraction (somatic pain signals, for example) or mental distraction (such as obsessive thought or worry). People also tend to ignore those signals which they find uninteresting or annoying. Excessive pride can also cause inattention when the message, or the person delivering the message, are deemed of little value.

Patients with Difficulty Expressing Themselves

Counseling a patient in a rehabilitation setting frequently can be difficult when the prognosis differs from the patient's desired outcome. Often the reaction is anger or tears, but the physician is called to witness a patient's angst, even when he or she has difficulty putting words to it. The physician's response to these reactions can be a teachable moment for both patient and rehabilitation professional. For example, a patient may declare, "You wouldn't know what it feels like to be missing a leg or to have constant pain." The physician can, in turn, acknowledge the patient's loss with a response like, "You're right, I don't know and I can't know how you feel. What can you tell me about your experience with this so I can learn from you?" Or the physician can share experiences collected from earlier patients with a similar condition: "You are right, I don't know what *you* feel like in this situation, or how I would feel in your shoes. But I have listened carefully to many patients with a condition like yours. I'd be glad to share with you what I've learned from them whenever you feel ready to hear about it."

Adjusting the Pace of Recovery

Rehabilitation physicians are charged with helping to design the therapeutic blueprint for their patients' recovery, mapping out a plan that allows the patient to focus on the components of recovery in a simplified, "paint by numbers" way. The physician must guide patients who have lost their way after some major injury or surgery, who may be so overwhelmed by their change in physical capability that they cannot begin to see past their present brokenness. Rather than setting an arbitrary pace, the physician must lay out the landmarks and mark the trail so that the patient can stay on course, pausing as necessary for reflection and reassessment. Time is required to process change, and the rehabilitation specialist is required to monitor the processing of change for patients. Is the patient stuck, in need of help in stepping into the next stage (such as learning some different technique for bowel or bladder continence)? Is the patient moving too fast, glossing over the current challenge with denial and skipping the early, foundational lessons that will be necessary for the next step? Such moments provide an opportunity for the physician's own expertise and experience in Catholic formation to guide patients toward appealing to our Lord for assistance and healing, for sacramental cleansing and reinforcement in the faith.

A life-changing injury or illness offers a person the opportunity to assess the foundation on which that life is built, what serves as its cornerstone. Is that cornerstone Jesus Christ, the great builder and healer?

Selecting the Right Crutch and Opiate

Jesse Ventura once called organized religion "a sham and a crutch for weak-minded people who need strength in numbers."[17] Marx called religion the "opium of the people." Neither of these assertions is the Catholic view. The religion of a patient can, though, be used like a crutch to help that patient. Crutches and analgesics are tools of the trade in rehabilitation, and they serve the vital purpose of expanding the patient's physical and emotional world. Rehabilitation professionals are in the business of evaluating patients for the right crutch or assistive device, whether it be a single-tip cane, a fully equipped walker or something in between. Even if personal faith in God is nonexistent, weak, lukewarm or resistant, should any physician object to a well-fitted "crutch" that aids in the ambulation toward eternity?

In the case of pain, the physician works to assess the patient's physical and psychological pain and to determine its cause. The next step is to try to reduce the pain generator whenever possible, or to offer a palliative measure of analgesia so that the patient can carry on with the activities of daily life. Every physician has seen a patient paralyzed by pain or the fear of pain, and has witnessed how that same patient becomes more comfortable and mobile when provided with a proper dose of analgesic. The astute physician understands the positive effect of opiates, and, when they are indicated, chooses and prescribes them carefully, based on their potency and side-effect profile for specific patients. Always, the preference is for those with limited side effects and for dosages that stay clear of toxic levels. In the same way, no physician should hesitate to employ religious faith to help put pain and suffering in supernatural perspective.

The Role of Forgiveness in the Recovery Process

Forgiveness is helpful in the healing process. Since patients rely on their community to support them and assist them, resolving the barriers to connection with that community is important. Frequently these barriers include unresolved anger and resentment, which is sometimes nurtured by patients or their families even though the

17. Jesse Ventura, interview, http://en.wikipedia.org/wiki/Jesse_Ventura#Religion.

event that sparked these feelings occurred long ago. Forgiveness can help the patient and caregivers move through and away from the negative feelings that hinder emotional and spiritual progress and growth.[18]

The process of recovery usually requires the assistance of family or friends. If among these relationships with the patient there are unresolved tensions, it is best if they are resolved, or at least approached in an honest, open, and charitable way. Frequently this involves forgiveness, and when forgiveness is withheld there can be unnecessary tension. The stress of being unforgiven can reduce the degree and the rate of the patient's recovery. Whenever it is possible and appropriate, the physician should consider gently encouraging forgiveness.

The patient who then chooses to enter into the process of forgiveness moves along the steps to being reconciled. First, one reflects on the action that has offended or hurt someone; one recognizes the error in one's choice of action, recounts the action that was offensive or hurtful, reports one's error or offense, and acknowledges one's role in committing it; one expresses remorse for the action, requests forgiveness, and offers to repair the damage created. The act of forgiveness is completed when those who must forgive those actions acknowledge or offer their forgiveness to the offender. The complete conversation can be as succinct as: "Please forgive me; it is all my fault, I am sorry."

Typically, two persons are involved in an act of forgiveness, the offender and the offended. Each person has a role in completing the act of forgiveness. In the rehabilitation setting, the two involved are typically the patient and the one who will be involved with helping the patient in their rehabilitation. Sometimes, though, there are situations in which the patient must forgive himself for past actions, and perhaps even for actions that contributed to his present state of illness or injury. Forgiveness in these situations is sometimes better handled with the aid of a clinical psychologist, priest, or minister.

Sexuality, Fertility and Sanctity of Life

All Catholics are called to respect life at all stages and to respect the role of marriage as a covenant and a sacrament between one man and one woman.

Clinical Vignette 2

A 24-year-old college graduate has sustained an aortic injury secondary to a collision with a tree while snow skiing. He requires emergency surgery for repair of the aorta, which required cross clamping. He has ischemic injury to the spinal cord and awakens from surgery stating that he cannot move his legs. In addition, he has loss of bowel and bladder function. He is classified as a man

---

18. See Christina Puchalski, "Forgiveness: Spiritual and Medical Implications," *Yale Journal for Humanities in Medicine*, September 17, 2002, http://couples-families.com/forgiveness-spiritual-medical-implications-christina-puchalski/.

with T6 complete motor, incomplete sensory paraplegic and is admitted for rehabilitation services. He has many questions concerning his prognosis, especially about his fertility and sexual function, since he is engaged to be married in the coming year.

Physicians often bow to the technology of artificial contraception and barrier methods when counseling patients about sexuality, or they treat erectile dysfunction without regard to the patient's marital status. In counseling the unmarried person with spinal cord injury who lacks erectile function, the physician discusses alternatives that include pharmacologic agents which allow erection to take place by increasing naturally occurring nitric oxide levels. This disregards Church teaching that the sexual act is limited to the purpose of procreation, must be open to life, and is reserved for a couple married to each other. Pope Paul VI outlines this reality:

This particular doctrine, often expounded by the Magisterium of the Church, is based on the inseparable connection, established by God, which man on his own initiative may not break, between the unitive significance and the procreative significance *which are both inherent to the marriage act*.[19]

In a similar way, physicians often counsel patients on using barrier contraceptive methods for prevention of sexually transmitted diseases, even though this practice renders the sexual act no longer open to life. Since even the correct use of a condom, though, does not completely prevent the spread of HIV, counseling its use gives patients a false sense of hope and protection. The only appropriate advice a Catholic physician can give patients is to recommend sexual abstinence. No physician would hesitate to counsel an active smoker on the ills of smoking, advising cessation—abstinence—over reduction of substance intake, as the only effective prevention of disease. It is just as important for physicians to recommend abstinence to sexually active patients who are not in a marital relationship as the only dependable disease preventive. Just as smoking can lead to early separation from loved ones, sex outside of marriage may lead to eternal separation from heavenly happiness. Just as a doctor may offer a smoker medications for nicotine withdrawal, the patient urged to practice continence should be encouraged to seek the virtue of chastity, as defined by the *Catechism*:

Chastity means the successful integration of sexuality within the person and thus the inner unity of man in his bodily and spiritual being. Sexuality, in which man's belonging to the bodily and biological world is expressed, becomes personal and truly human when it is integrated into the relationship of one person to another, in the complete and lifelong mutual gift of a man and a woman. The virtue of chastity therefore involves the integrity of the person and the integrality of the gift.[20]

Chastity is fortified by temperance, or discipline and self-control. Temperance in the exercise of sexual appetites can be strengthened through the exercise of temper-

---

19. Pope Paul VI, *Humanae Vitae, Of Human Life*, Encyclical Letter, July 25, 1968, no. 12, emphasis in original.

20. *Catechism of the Catholic Church* (New York: Dell Publishing, 1995), no. 2337.

ance in use of food and drink. The more a person learns to strengthen the will by occasional self-denial of licit pleasures through such practices as fasting, the more likely the person will succeed in the temperance that supports chastity.

The practice of mortification disciplines the person's body through deprivation of pleasure, to gain mercy for the person's own sins and for the sins of others. Such mortification can be voluntary or involuntary. This means that a burden which the patient has not willingly chosen can be transformed into a source of grace. Disabled patients have many opportunities to offer up the challenges of their physical limitations as involuntary mortification to gain grace for themselves and their loved ones.

Summary through Prayer

The rehabilitation physician's calling finds parallels in, and can be juxtaposed on, the Lord's Prayer:

Our Father Who art in Heaven, Hallowed be thy name:
    (We should keep in mind him whom we love and glorify.)

Thy Kingdom come, Thy will be done, on earth as it is in Heaven:
    (Remember who is in charge of the recovery process. Request his assistance in all things.)

Give us this day our daily bread:
    (Help your patients with both bodily and spiritual nourishment. When possible, help them have access to the Eucharist.)

Forgive us our trespasses as we forgive those who trespass against us:
    (We should seek reconciliation for ourselves, and we should aid our patients in seeking the sacrament of Reconciliation, along with reconciliation with family members and caregivers.)

Lead us not into temptation, but deliver us from evil:
    (There will be much temptation to despair for one who is struggling with pain, paralysis, or both. Ask for deliverance from our Lord through the intercession and prayers of the saints and through the sacrament of Anointing of the Sick.)

For thine is the Kingdom, the power, and the Glory:
    (Remember from whom the healing comes and remember to give proper credit where credit is due. Glory to God in all things.)

    Amen.

Bibliography

Benedict XVI, Pope. Homily, St. Peter's Square, Palm Sunday. April 17, 2011. http://w2.vatican.va/content/benedict-xvi/en/homilies/2011/documents/hf_ben-xvi_hom_20110417_palm-sunday.html.

———. "Where Is the Soul of a Comatose Person?" Television interview. April 22, 2011. https://w2.vatican.va/content/benedict-xvi/en/speeches/2011/april/documents/hf_ben-xvi_spe_20110422_intervista.html.

Catechism of the Catholic Church. New York: Dell Publishing, 1995.

Escrivá, Josemaría. *The Way-Furrow-The Forge.* New Rochelle, N.Y.: Scepter Publishing, 2008.

Fernandez-Carvajal, Francis. *In Conversation with God.* 7 vols. New Rochelle, N.Y.: Scepter Publishing, 2007.

Gomez, José H. "You Will Be My Witnesses." A Pastoral Letter to the People of God of San Antonio on the Christian Mission to Evangelize and Proclaim Jesus Christ. February 15, 2010. http://www.la-archdiocese.org/archbishop/Documents/2010-2006/2010-0215_Anv_Pastoral_Letter_SA.pdf.

John Paul II, Pope. *Salvifici Doloris, On the Christian Meaning of Human Suffering.* Apostolic Letter. February 11, 1984. http://www.vatican.va/holy_father/john_paul_ii/apost_letters/documents/hf_jp-ii_apl_11021984_salvifici-doloris_en.html.

Kowalska, Faustina. *Divine Mercy of My Soul.* 3rd edition. Stockbridge, Mass.: Marian Press, 2005.

Paul VI, Pope. *Humanae Vitae, Of Human Life.* Encyclical Letter. July 25, 1968. http://w2.vatican.va/content/paul-vi/en/encyclicals/documents/hf_p-vi_enc_25071968_humanae-vitae.html.

Puchalski, Christina. "FICA Spiritual History Tool." https://smhs.gwu.edu/gwish/clinical/fica/spiritual-history-tool.

———. "Forgiveness: Spiritual and Medical Implications." *Yale Journal for Humanities in Medicine*, September 17, 2002. http://couples-families.com/forgiveness-spiritual-medical-implications-christina-puchalski/.

Wanda Skowronska

11. CATHOLIC PSYCHOLOGISTS AND THE SPIRITUAL DIMENSION

The human person has bodily, intellectual, and spiritual dimensions. The spiritual has, in the past, been seen as outside the realm of psychology. However, psychology has early roots in Christianity, and in the 1950s the spiritual dimension of counseling was rediscovered. A Catholic psychologist must possess a Catholic understanding of the human person, and it is proper for Catholic psychologists to integrate a Catholic perspective in counseling. In this chapter, Dr. Skowronska offers precisely this perspective. She discusses the rich Christian tradition on suffering and the meaning that can be found in it. She presents a perspective on marriage and the family when there is breakdown, and takes up the matter of abortion grief counseling. Dr. Skowronska also reminds her reader that forgiveness is an important ingredient of the healing process. This chapter provides—as do the other chapters in part 2—a clear, concise, and practical treatment of authentic Catholic witness in the care of others.—*Editors*

Catholic psychologists alive today have lived through a momentous "clash of humanisms," a central theological issue at the Second Vatican Council which preoccupied theologians and philosophers in a post-war, capitalist, Marxist, and postmodern context. It was a clash which Pope John Paul II, in *Christifideles Laici*, described as the false humanisms of atheist secularism and idolatry of the individual on the one hand, and a true Christian humanism on the other, a humanism that rightly acknowledges "the greatness and misery of individuals" and never loses sight of the "total dignity of the human person."[1] It was a clash with the prevailing hyper-individualism of current society to which Pope Benedict XVI referred in his encyclical *Caritas in Veritate*, saying, "A humanism which excludes God is an inhuman humanism."[2] It was a clash

1. Pope John Paul II, *Christifideles Laici, On the Vocation and Mission of the Lay Faithful in the Church and the World*, Apostolic Exhortation, December 30, 1988 (Boston: St. Paul Books and Media, 1988), no. 5.
2. Pope Benedict XVI, *Caritas in Veritate, On Integral Human Development in Charity and Truth*, Encyclical Letter, June 29, 2009 (Vatican City: Libreria Editrice Vaticana, 2009), no. 78.

over the retrieval of a true humanism to which Pope Francis referred in saying, "Each one of us is invited to recognize in the fragile human being the face of the Lord."[3] He evocatively portrays our postmodern world as a "field hospital" because of the tragic fallout of the ideological battle of humanisms which has left so many scarred in its aftermath—among them, those suffering from family breakdowns, post-abortion grief, confused gender identity, and lost hopes. His depiction of the spiritual nuclear fallout of the past century is especially relevant to psychologists, for, as he says, there is a pressing need to "heal the wounds.... And you have to start from the ground up."[4]

The *Charter for Health Care Workers*, issued by the Pontifical Council for Pastoral Assistance to Health Care Workers, echoes this Christian humanism, seeing the role of the psychologist or anyone working in the area of health as a "form of Christian witness."[5] That is, a Catholic psychologist cannot forget that the human person is a body-soul unity, whose end is eternal life with God. The charter calls for psychologists to be " 'guardians and servants of human life,' "[6] to serve life in its totality and to see their profession as "an actualized continuation of the healing love of Christ," adding that the work of all health-care workers "is love for Christ: He is the sick person."[7] The " 'service to man's spirit cannot be fully effective except it be service to his psycho-physical unity,' " and all in the healing professions " 'are called to be the living image of Christ and of his Church in loving the sick and the suffering' " in witnessing to the gospel of life.[8] Thus for a Catholic psychologist, healing and Christian witness go hand in hand in a thoughtful, sensitive integration, even if his or her secular training told him or her otherwise.

Solidarity and Rediscovered Roots among Christian Psychologists

American psychologist Paul Vitz recalls his psychological training, saying that anti-religious thought was part of "a predominant public assumption," and in psychology departments, "to refer to God in any serious way would bring the legitimacy of one's scholarship into question."[9] In *Faith of the Fatherless: The Psychology of*

---

3. Vatican Information Service, "Francis: No Human Life Is More Valuable than Another," Vatican Information Service, September 20, 2013, http://visnews-en.blogspot.com.au/2013/09/francis-no-human-life-is-more-valuable.html.

4. Antonio Spadaro, SJ, "A Big Heart Open to God," *America* 209, no. 8 (September 30, 2013): 24.

5. Pontifical Council for Pastoral Assistance to Health Care Workers, *Charter for Health Care Workers*, 1995, no. 1, http://www.ewtn.com/library/curia/pcpaheal.htm, quoting John Paul II, Address on a Visit to Mercy Maternity Hospital in Melbourne, November 28, 1986.

6. Ibid., no. 1, quoting Pope John Paul II, *Evangelium Vitae, On the Value and Inviolability of Human Life*, Encyclical Letter, March 25, 1995, no. 89.

7. Pontifical Council for Pastoral Assistance to Health Care Workers, *Charter for Health Care Workers*, no. 4.

8. Ibid., no. 5, quoting John Paul II, Address to the World Congress of Catholic Doctors, October 3, 1982; and John Paul II, Address to the Participants at the International Congress for Assistance to the Dying, March 18, 1992.

9. Paul Vitz, *Faith of the Fatherless: The Psychology of Atheism* (Dallas: Spence Publishing Company, 1999), xii, xiii.

Atheism (1999), he reflected generally on the anti-spiritual tenor of the past century in the following terms:

Only as it starts to fade can we see how strange the modern world has been. It is natural that some distance is needed for the characteristics of the "modern" to become obvious, and nothing has been more typical of public life especially than the presumption of atheism. God has been banished from public discourse.... atheism is a recent and distinctively Western phenomenon ... no other culture has manifested such a widespread public rejection of the divine.[10]

Beginning in the middle of last century, however, there arose a new solidarity among Christian psychologists who critiqued secular psychological approaches and rediscovered the spiritual dimension in counseling, also realizing what a Christian, indeed Catholic, profession psychology has been, even in the early modern periods.[11] Here I will put in an autobiographical note, for it may resonate with some readers.

As an Australian counseling psychologist trained in the standard secular way, studying research methods and delivering up evidence-based research at the end of each course, I realized there was something missing when I was pronounced a "psychologist." But I had no idea what was missing, for I did not know what I did not know. It is not that studying cognitive behavioral therapy and psychopathology and writing my master's thesis, "How Children Cope with Sadness" were not interesting for me—they were. But there was a kind of elephant in the room, which was the lack of any explanation of the implicit ideas behind many therapies I was assigned to study. Looking back, it seemed I had studied an ahistorical and philosophical course. This changed for me when, more than fifteen years ago, I came across the writings of some American psychologists. I can only describe the discovery as a "Eureka" moment from which I have never looked back; their writings led me to further study, this time at the John Paul II Institute in Melbourne. Suddenly I saw the elephant in the room and the herds on the horizon. Psychology had a story (we studied no "history of psychology" at all in my training), and the Judeo-Christian understanding of the human person was integral to it. When I read *Psychological Seduction* by William Kilpatrick—and later, *Psychology and Christianity* by Eric L. Johnson and Stanton L. Jones, *Religion and the Clinical Practice of Psychology* by Edward P. Shafranske, and *Psychology as Religion* by Paul Vitz—there began a journey that helped me realize who and what a psychologist is.[12] I understood that as psychologists we have a narrative too, a genealogy of ideas.

10. Ibid., xii–xiii.

11. Some critiques can be found in Paul Vitz, *Psychology as Religion: The Cult of Self-Worship* (Grand Rapids, Mich.: Eerdmans, 1977); Don Browning, *Religious Thought and the Modern Psychologies: A Critical Conversation in the Theology of Culture* (Philadelphia: Fortress Press, 1987); William Kilpatrick, *The Emperor's New Clothes: The Naked Truth about the New Psychology* (Ridgefield, Conn.: Roger A. McCaffrey, 1985); Robert Roberts and Mark Talbot, eds., *Limning the Psyche: Explorations in Christian Psychology* (Grand Rapids, Mich.: Wm. B. Eerdmans, 1997); Paul Vitz and Susan Felch, eds., *The Self: Beyond the Postmodern Crisis* (Wilmington, Del.: ISI Books, 2006).

12. William Kilpatrick, *Psychological Seduction: The Failure of Modern Psychology* (Nashville, Tenn.: Thomas Nelson Publishers, 1983); Eric L. Johnson and Stanton L. Jones, eds., *Psychology and Christianity: Four Views* (Downers Grove, Ill.: InterVarsity Press, 2000); Edward Shafranske, ed., *Religion and the Clinical Practice of Psychology* (Washington, D.C.: American Psychological Association, 1996); and Vitz, *Psychology as Religion*.

And telling the story of individuals and societies persists, for it is deeply embedded in our nature to do so. So, when I discovered the Christian roots of early modern psychology, it was like being an Indiana Jones going into a psychological Grand Canyon and discovering priceless treasures of psychology's lost ark—and being amazed and forever changed by it. Among the Christian roots, I found Catholic pioneers of modern psychology—Johannes Müller, Fr. Edward Pace, Albert Michotte, Fr. Verner Moore, Kazimierz Twardowski, Rudolf Allers, Sister Hilda, Emile Peillaube, Agostino Gemelli—among many others—not to mention Conrad Baars and Anna Terruwe and the subsequent Catholic psychologists who integrated Christianity's extraordinary legacy into their work. Catholic psychologists/psychiatrists will not hear about them in their mainstream courses, but they are part of *our story*.

The Assumptions of Catholic Psychology

From early modern times a psychologist could be experimenter or healer, or both. Two visions of psychology are reflected in this history. This first vision of psychology/psychiatry, the biological view (including neuroscience) focuses on the quantification and understanding of the brain's activity, the impact of psychic distress and medication. The second vision focuses more on the psychosocial dimension of the patient's life and how to apply psychological knowledge to ease distress. While the second vision—the psychologist as healer—is the focus of this chapter, both visions of psychology can overlap, and both entail a theory of the human person and the nature and purpose of human life which needs to be made explicit to Catholic psychologists.[13] Though there is no specific Catholic therapy as such, a Catholic psychologist needs to inform his or her therapeutic approach with the theological anthropology that uniquely arose from Christian history. Before proceeding to specific issues in counseling, it is therefore important to outline the parameters of this Catholic understanding of the human person.

In his article "Anthropological Foundations for a Clinical Psychology: A Proposal," Christian Brugger gives a coherent theological anthropology for all psychologists.[14] He begins by saying that every psychologist implicitly assumes some kind of stable concept of human nature:

13. Edward Shorter sees these two visions of psychology/psychiatry as a "tension between the Enlightenment of the eighteenth century as a social and intellectual movement stressing reason, and the Romantic movement of the late eighteenth and early nineteenth centuries stressing feeling and sentiment." He observed that what he called the "Romantic" psychiatrists preferred to "spend long hours talking to their patients about their subjective experiences." The Enlightenment-influenced ones usually gave factual, moral lectures to their patients and ordered them to observe strict, rational behaviors until they were healed. The two visions were not mutually exclusive, and their boundaries often overlapped. Most current psychologists, unless they are involved in pure research, are a blend of the two. (Edward Shorter, *A History of Psychiatry: From the Era of the Asylum to the Age of Prozac* [New York: John Wiley and Sons, 1997], 30.)

14. E. Christian Brugger, "Anthropological Foundations for Clinical Psychology: A Proposal," *Journal of Psychology and Theology* 36, no. 1 (Spring 2008): 3–15. Material reprinted with permission. Brugger is senior fellow of ethics and director of the Fellows Program at the Culture of Life Foundation.

[A]n implicit consent to a conception of human nature amenable to therapeutic influence is presupposed by all who undertake the therapeutic task. Such a conception is implied in the very concepts of mental disorder and dysfunction. There can only be disorder because there is departure from right order; and dysfunction by definition implies a concept of right function.[15]

There is a stability at the heart of any explanation of how the human person is viewed, and clinical psychology assumes this stability. We are not humans one day and zebras the next. This does not imply, Brugger continues, that human nature is static and unchanging. But its changes do not imply a change in the kind of *being* the human person is. The changes are developments in the possible actualizations of which human nature is capable. We are not free to become eight legged, to acquire wings or a tail. We are free to try to increase the practice of the virtues and lessen our vices. We have an enduring set of capacities that help us to identify the human person and to recognize when inaccurate versions of the person are imposed on individuals and societies.

Brugger proceeds to outline his assumptions of a Catholic understanding of psychology, taking into account that "human life is the accumulation of an historical inheritance in which there is always a dialogue between old traditions and the present endeavor to understand."[16] Brugger refers to Martin Seligman in this regard, saying that his positive psychology is an example of the revival of this consideration of tradition's links with the present.

The following is a summary of this comprehensive account of the primary assumptions for a Catholic psychology:

1. "*Human persons are unified wholes* . . . in relation to their bodily and spiritual dimensions. . . . [Thus] every person from the first moment of existence is a complete, wholly unified, living being constituted *of* a material body and an immaterial, incorruptible, and immortal soul. [The soul here is understood as] the body's 'animating principle.' . . . Although the whole person comes into existence when his or her living body comes into existence, . . . the multiple capacities of human nature [are] subject to development over time. . . . This premise provides support for the increasing consensus in clinical psychology that cognitional, emotional, behavioral, and interpersonal dimensions of people need to be holistically addressed in order to deal most effectively with psychological disorder and promote flourishing."

2. "*Human persons are bodily* [*beings*]. This means bodies are fully personal and persons fully embodied. . . . As bodily, humans are organic, living beings capable of bodily health and wellbeing, and possessing a natural inclination to preserve and promote bodily wellbeing. Persons as bodily are also either male or female: [as such they] are complementary embodiments of the one category of being we call the human person."

---

15. Ibid., 4.

16. Ibid., 8. Some fascinating outlines of this historical inheritance include Joseph Ratzinger, "Retrieving the Tradition: Concerning the Notion of Person in Theology," *Communio: International Catholic Review* 17 (Fall 1990): 439–54; and Hans Urs Von Balthasar, "On the Concept of Person," *Communio: International Catholic Review* 13 (Spring 1986): 18–26.

3. *"Human persons are interpersonally relational. . . .* Recognizing the primordial role that interpersonal relationships play both in human flourishing and in the developing and remediation of mental disorder, a central aim of clinical psychology is better understanding and contributing to the question of what constitutes healthy human relationship[s] for clients."

4. *"Human persons are rational.* At a certain point in their development, if free of significant pathology, humans become capable of knowing themselves, others, and the existence of God, and of expressing thoughts and affections in language. . . . Unique among other animals, humans as rational beings seek to find meaning in their lives and for their circumstances. In communities of meaning, they acquire the capacity to conceptually formulate and linguistically express their knowledge and understanding of themselves and the world around them."

5. *"Human persons are volitional and free.* At a certain point in their development, if unhindered by significant pathology, humans become capable of initiating and carrying through deliberate behavior of which they, and not factors external to them, are the originating cause. This brings them into the realm of moral responsibility and the development of character. It also makes them creative insofar as they become capable of conceiving of and deliberately bringing into existence things that once did not exist. They also become capable of love for natural and divine goods and persons. . . . Love here refers . . . to [an act of the will for] the authentic good of another."

6. *"Human persons are created by God 'in the image of God.'* As created by a good God, human nature is good, as is the nature of everything created by God. Humans however possess a special dignity and value not shared by non-human creation insofar as they are not only created by God, but created in God's image. . . . Moreover as God is a knowing and loving communion of persons (a Trinity of persons), humans, in God's image, are created as persons, to know truth, especially about God and to live in loving communion with God and other persons. This premise provides a transcendent ground for positing, even in the midst of severe clinical disorder, the fundamental goodness of human life and human nature."

7. *"All human nature is weakened by sin* . . . The realities of sin, physical and moral weakness, death and relational disorder are constitutive of human temporal existence, although secondary to the goodness of God's creation. Disorders, including mental illness, are manifestations of the disorder introduced into [the] world as a result of sin. . . . [This does not mean] that all mental disorder is the direct result of someone's sinning. Rather it is meant to provide a transcendent ground for understanding the origins of the problem of evil and human suffering."

8. *"Human nature, because of the life, death, and resurrection of Jesus of Nazareth, is 'redeemed' and restored to a rectified relationship with God* . . . . The entire created order and all the good fruits of human nature and enterprise, weakened

and marred by sin, are elevated by Jesus' redemption to a new end, an end above nature (i.e., a supernatural end).... The newness of the New Creation is a newness that suffuses the 'old fallen' [creation], ... [a] restoration and reorientation of the first creation, ... a dynamic vindication of God's original creation."[17]

Although the above assumptions form the basis from which a Catholic psychologist would begin to practice his or her profession, it is another question entirely as to *how* to integrate these principles into professional practice. Does one become a biblical counseling psychologist—as some are—and quote the Bible as a cure for each presented ailment? Or does one hold to these principles in a parallel universe, one that never sees the light of day in a counseling office? Or does one seek to integrate the discoveries of psychology and the above theological anthropology in an appropriate, thoughtful way? Most tend to the latter integrated, balanced approach using the best of psychological research in the light of their understanding of the human person, which necessarily entails some insight into the Christian understanding of suffering.

Psychology and Suffering

In an era of family breakdown, violence, war, social engineering, terrorism, and the exploitation of men, women, and children, psychologists try to help those who suffer, whatever their approach. The Catholic psychologist approaches this differently, however, inasmuch as there is a rich tradition of writing about suffering in the Judeo-Christian legacy, which informs what he or she may say in a counseling situation, for it affects the search for meaning at a deep level—which inevitably becomes an issue in itself in such situations.

In *Psychology as Religion: The Cult of Self-Worship*, American psychologist Paul Vitz points out the glaring omission of suffering particularly in humanistic (i.e., "selfist") psychology, which flourished in various forms from the 1960s onward:

A final profound conflict between Christianity and selfism centers around the meaning of suffering. The Christian acknowledges evil—with its consequent pain and ultimately death—as a fact of life.... By contrast selfist philosophy trivializes life by claiming that suffering ... is without intrinsic meaning. Suffering is seen as some sort of absurdity.[18]

The ignoring of suffering implies devaluation of the universal human search for the meaning of evil and suffering, of which Benedict XVI says in *Spe Salvi*: "none of us is capable of eliminating the power of evil, of sin which, as we plainly see, is a constant source of suffering."[19] Thus a Catholic psychologist needs to incorporate into his or her practice a deeper understanding of suffering than a typical secular training has given.

For the Christian, an openness to accept God's revelation and grace transforms the harsh realities of evil and suffering of this life into an unexpected new narrative,

---

17. Brugger, "Anthropological Foundations for Clinical Psychology," 9–12.

18. Vitz, *Psychology as Religion*, 103.

19. Pope Benedict XVI, *Spe Salvi, On Christian Hope*, Encyclical Letter, November 30, 2007 (Sydney: St. Paul's Publications, 2007), no. 36.

in which suffering is the prelude to an extraordinary new world of understanding. Christianity starts with suffering and ends with joy, whereas the secular psychologist's approach, by contrast, starts with optimism but ends with pessimism. Cardinal Ratzinger, in *The Yes of Jesus Christ,* observes that the optimism of secular liberalism, which humanistic psychology shares, represses real anxiety for the future, which must be created by the self, for "[secular] optimism is something we must ultimately produce ourselves."[20] The dark reality at the heart of humanistic psychology and secular humanism in general is that building a happy, secular utopia is an impossible burden for any self, and in fact it destroys the self.

A comprehensive synthesis that articulates the Catholic approach to suffering—and one that all psychologists might well read and reflect in their work—is John Paul II's encyclical *Salvifici Doloris.* John Paul II observes that suffering "is a universal theme that accompanies man at every point on earth: in a certain sense it co-exists with him in the world, and thus demands to be constantly reconsidered."[21] He avoids textbook definitions, using simple language saying that "[m]an suffers in different ways . . ." and that suffering "evokes respect and in its own way it intimidates. For in suffering is contained the greatness of a specific mystery."[22] John Paul II reveals a non-judgmental, compassionate, empathic approach to the subject. He begins by not presuming to understand every individual form of suffering. He says that suffering remains an intangible mystery and "seems almost inexpressible and not transferable,"[23] not only in the essence of the suffering itself, but in the sense of God's "silence" in "permitting" horrors which have pervaded human history in a "Gospel of Suffering" that touches some human lives more than others.

Thus a Catholic psychologist will listen with that "special respect for every form of human suffering," psychological, moral, or spiritual; and this silent, listening respect "must be set at the beginning of what will be expressed . . . by the deepest need of the heart and also by the deep imperative of the faith."[24] A Catholic psychologist is attuned to hear the depths of this inner world.

In referring to the suffering of Job as one of the central "narratives" of Western civilization (as J. Brian Benestad has pointed out earlier in this volume), John Paul II makes clear that it is undeserved suffering, the suffering of the innocent, which particularly disturbs us.[25] It is not adequate to state that Job's suffering is a consequence of deserved evil, as the three visitors tell Job when they "advise" him that he must have done something to deserve the loss of family and all he held dear in life. Their "blame the victim" approach finds new expression in today's secularist and New Age attitudes, which imply that those who fail to attain the bliss of self-fulfillment are to blame for their failure, or those who suffer have deserved "karma" from a previous

---

20. Joseph Ratzinger, *The Yes of Jesus Christ* (New York: Crossroad, 1991), 48ff.

21. Pope John Paul II, *Salvifici Doloris, On the Christian Meaning of Human Suffering,* Apostolic Letter, February 11, 1984 (Sydney: Pauline Books and Media, 1984), no. 2.

22. Ibid., nos. 3, 4.

23. Ibid., no. 5.

24. Ibid., no. 4.

25. See ibid., nos. 10–12.

life. *Salvifici Doloris* notes that although the "book of Job is not the last word on this subject in Revelation," it does ask the "why" of suffering, and it identifies with the innocent victim of suffering, praising Job's faithfulness and endurance when God seems silent and to have forsaken him.[26]

Noting the spiritual hunger of our age for answers beyond reductive ideologies, John Paul II's reflections constitute a more *spiritually empathic* response than Carl Rogers's *socially empathic* manner of dealing with his clients.[27] John Paul II's mode of hearing "listens" to the soul, which demands more of the listener. John Paul II also draws distinctions between levels of pain, pointing to a deeper spiritual, that is, moral, suffering.

In fact, it is a question of pain of a spiritual nature, and not only of the "psychological" dimension of pain which accompanies both moral and physical suffering. The vastness and the many forms of moral suffering are certainly no less in number than the forms of physical suffering. But at the same time, moral suffering seems as it were less identified and less reachable by therapy.[28]

The distinction between a psychological dimension and a moral dimension reminds us of the limits of psychology and the need to acknowledge the spiritual dimension of the person. It was the spiritual dimension that helped Viktor Frankl survive when he was confronted with immense evil in a concentration camp. Frankl (who lost his parents, brother, and pregnant wife in the Holocaust) realized very quickly that he had to jettison much of what he had learned about psychoanalysis if he was to survive. Psychoanalysis did not answer his search for meaning—his previous life, family, and accomplishments, and the meaning he found in them were gone. Frankl recalls that he carried into the camp the only manuscript for a book he had written: it was destroyed on his first day in Auschwitz. Later, when forced to sort the clothes of gassed victims, he found a scrap of paper amidst the striped shirts on which was written the Shema Yisrael.[29] Henceforth this scrap became something of greater importance than any personal accomplishment. Frankl states:

there is purpose in that life which is almost barren of both creation and enjoyment .... Not only creativeness and enjoyment are meaningful. If there is a meaning in life at all, then there must be a meaning in suffering. ... The way in which a man accepts his fate and all the suffering it entails, the way in which he takes up his cross, gives him ample opportunity—even under the most difficult circumstances—to add a deeper meaning to his life .... Such men are not only in concentration camps. Everywhere man is confronted with fate, with the chance of achieving something through his suffering.[30]

26. Ibid., nos. 11, 12.

27. Carl Rogers (1902–1987), along with Abraham Maslow (1908–1970), was one of the pioneers of humanistic psychology. Humanistic psychology (or "human potential psychology") was seen in the 1950s and 1960s as a "third force," a reaction to the reductionism of behaviorist psychology and the pessimism of Freud. Rogers placed emphasis on listening to the client in an empathic, non-judgmental way. He excluded, however, any religious considerations, especially Christian ones, from such empathic listening, for he viewed the Judeo-Christian legacy and its effects on human development in negative terms. Paul Vitz's *Psychology as Religion* is an excellent account and critique of Rogers and other humanistic psychologists.

28. John Paul II, *Salvifici Doloris*, no. 5.

29. The Shema is the foundational prayer of Judaism; Dt 6:4, "The Lord is our God, the Lord is one."

30. Viktor Frankl, *Man's Search for Meaning* (New York: Pocket Books, 1985), 89. Originally published as *Ein Psychologe erlebt das Konzentrationslager* (Vienna, 1946).

Being stripped of his accomplishments, Frankl comes to understand that, even with nothing at all, his life and suffering have meaning. In saying that "suffering has a meaning in itself" not only does he use the word "spiritual" in relation to suffering but also, unexpectedly, given his Jewish background, he uses the Christian understanding of the "cross" to describe its ultimate reality.[31]

Frankl's understanding of self-sacrificing love points to a Judeo-Christian understanding of the "Suffering Servant" and echoes John Paul II's reflection in *Salvifici Doloris*:

Suffering seems to belong to man's transcendence: it is one of those points in which man is in a certain sense "destined" to go beyond himself, and he is called to this in a mysterious way.[32]

God has given human suffering an extraordinary dignity: first, in its being acknowledged; second, in highlighting the suffering of the innocent; third, in underlining an eternal meaning for suffering; and fourth, in showing that all sufferings offered in union with Christ's have an invisible, profound impact on the spiritual fate of those who are prayed for, as if those uniting their sufferings with Christ's, exist within an underground cloister enduring till the end of time.[33]

For the Christian, suffering can be offered as a gift. Von Balthasar describes it as the "mysterious osmosis between the members of the 'Body of Christ' which does not stop at the interchange of external goods but extends to a sharing in what is most personal."[34] He points out a simultaneous "loneliness" and "communion" in suffering,

a paradoxical reality of a community of the cross that represents innermost loneliness and innermost communion at the same time.... The loneliness of the cross, archetypically and once for all in the death of Jesus, gives birth to community, which will continue to be created anew in the grace of the Church.

There are moments when a solitary Christian undergoes suffering that is unknown to others or not understood by them; he offers it to the Lord for him to use as he thinks fit.[35]

With those suffering grief and loss, it is appropriate for psychologists to refer to Catholic wisdom, in order to connect the suffering person to others with whom he or she may feel solidarity. Suffering calls on the counseling psychologist not only to be there on the journey with the suffering person but also to invite reflection and to en-

---

31. Ibid., 89. Mathew Scully, who interviewed Frankl when he was ninety years old, noted a crucifix in his apartment; Frankl married a Catholic after the war (Mathew Scully, "Viktor Frankl at 90: An Interview," *First Things* [Spring 1995]: 39–43).

32. John Paul II, *Salvifici Doloris*, no. 2.

33. French writer Martin Coudou explores this notion of a hidden cloister of suffering offered by those who are vulnerable in *Le monastère invisible de Jean Paul II* (Paris: Editions Salvator, 2008). Courdou himself has worked with disabled children who have joined this hidden cloister of prayer.

34. Hans Urs von Balthasar, *In the Fullness of Faith: On the Centrality of the Distinctively Catholic*, trans. Graham Harrison (San Francisco: Ignatius Press, 1988), 67; originally published as *Katholische* (Einsiedeln, Switzerland: Johannes Verlag, 1975).

35. Ibid, 73.

able the connection of that person to a wider horizon of understanding. This accompaniment of the suffering person by the psychologist does not involve an idolization of suffering, nor does it avoid remedying situations that can be remedied. Rather, it helps provide a transformation of perspective, particularly where unavoidable suffering is concerned, and it invites the person to see his or her suffering as a mission, a *vocation*, which journeys to a certain, future hope.

Family Breakdown

Having looked at some of the assumptions of a Catholic psychology and its understanding of suffering, we turn to some of the issues psychologists inevitably deal with in their practice. The Catholic Church does try to prepare young people for marriage, teaching them the meaning of the sacrament, but the inescapable reality is that family breakdown permeates our society and every counseling psychologist will deal with it at some stage, whether in trying to keep a marriage from breaking up, dealing with children caught in situations of separation and divorce, dealing with issues of young persons with gender identity problems, or helping couples who find it difficult to accept not being able to have children, to mention a few. The Church is surrounded by various toxic secular messages that offer "solutions" that compete with its clear, consistent teaching on love and life.

Pope Francis sees our current society as locked in a battle for the souls of the young, poor, and vulnerable. Much of this revolves around the attempted destruction of the family, the elimination of masculinity and femininity in favor of "gender preferences," the push for "gay marriage," and the promotion of adoption of children by gay couples:

We know that today marriage and the family are in crisis. We now live in a culture of the temporary, in which more and more people are simply giving up on marriage as a public commitment. This revolution in manners and morals has often flown the flag of freedom, but in fact it has brought spiritual and material devastation to countless human beings, especially the poorest and most vulnerable.[36]

He decries the deceptive "revolution in manners and morals" and exposes the moral horror of ideological engineering, which surrounds us from conception to death. The Catholic counseling psychologist needs to be aware of this increasing moral toxicity and be clear about the Church's teaching on marriage, divorce, contraception, abortion, homosexuality, and in vitro fertilization (IVF), always offering healing and hope. That clarity is no easy task when a person is distressed or confused, but it is the task of the psychologist nonetheless, to remind the one seeking help of the larger psychological and spiritual parameters of problems in the above areas.

As a school psychologist I had one 16-year-old boy come to me saying that he thought he was "gay." I could very easily have given him the phone number of the

---

36. Pope Francis, Opening Address to the Colloquium on the Complementarity of Man and Woman, *Zenit*, November 17, 2014, http://www.zenit.org/en/articles/pope-francis-address-at-opening-of-colloquium-on-complementarity-of-man-and-woman.

gay-lesbian hotline and left it at that. He was from a troubled background, his parents were elderly, had many children, and were unable to give him the attention he needed. He drifted to anyone he could find for company and found some younger boys paid him attention because he was a little older than they (two to three years difference). Having listened to his story, I used a variant of narrative therapy and retold the boy's story, suggesting to him that he was lonely and was desperately looking for someone to give him attention and affection. He did not deny this. I suggested that his search was taking him into places in which he might be looking for love in the wrong places, that there might be other ways of looking at this. To my surprise he was listening. I suggested to him that he was not gay at all, he just thought he was and that he might learn some social skills for communicating with others his own age. I continued the therapy and can say, many years down the track, he is not gay; in fact, he is now an adult, married man. What would have happened had I given that boy the gay-lesbian hotline phone number?

Of course there are many more complex situations than this, and Joseph Nicolosi and Gerard J. M. van den Aardweg have written comprehensively on them, but the point I am making is that the Catholic psychologist looks beyond the secular horizons and tries to deal with situations according to the theological anthropology on which he or she bases counseling.[37]

Of all the situations, it is perhaps in the area of family breakdown that we see the world's field hospital in its full, raw detail. The best prevention is to grow up in a good family, and have adequate preparation for marriage and an understanding of the Church's message of love and life. Not all, however, are thus prepared. Also, some families do break down for tragic reasons (mental illness, violence, immaturity at marriage) and others for not so tragic reasons (desire for a "change," inability to resolve conflict, desire to escape responsibility). Whatever the reason, though, the effect of family breakdown is always tragic for the children. American psychologist Judith Wallerstein et al. reminded us that the family

is the theater of our lives—our first and most important school for learning about ourselves and all others. From this we extrapolate the interactions of human society. The images of each family are imprinted on each child's heart and mind becoming the inner theater that shapes expectations, hopes, and fears.[38]

And again, looking at children from divorced families after twenty-five years:

I realized that adults raised in divorced families carry within them a unique kind of history. They are the product of two distinct families and the transition between them. Their lives

---

37. Joseph Nicolosi and Gerard van den Aardweg have described their integrated psychological-spiritual counseling approaches with homosexual persons in Joseph Nicolosi, *Healing Homosexuality* (Lanham, Md.: Rowman and Littlefield, 1993), and Gerard J. M. van den Aardweg, *The Battle for Normality: A Guide for Self-Therapy for Homosexuality* (San Francisco: Ignatius Press, 1997); also see Sr. Lydia Allen, RSM, "Psychological Principles for Vocation Directors and Seminary Formators as Applied to Persons with Homosexual Tendencies," *Seminarium* 47, no. 3 (2007): 840–72.

38. Judith Wallerstein, Julia M. Lewis, and Sandra Blakeslee, *The Unexpected Legacy of Divorce: The 25 Year Landmark Study* (New York: Hyperion, 2000), 32.

begin with an intact family that one day vanishes. This is replaced by a series of upheavals that leave them confused and frightened.[39]

In her pioneering study that spanned three decades, Wallerstein, saying things that no one wanted to hear nearly fifty years ago, gave a unique psychological insight into the world of children in situations of family breakdown. In essence, experience of divorce for children is very different from that of their parents. Some adults feel relief, but children rarely do. Because of their age and life experience, adults have some resilience (unless they suffer from some mental illness or personality disorder), but, because of their age, children are vulnerable. Adults focus on altering their relationship to one person, but for a child there is as yet no similar ability to alter life circumstances: the adults have a major change in one relationship, the children have major changes in their entire world.[40]

Thus in the aftermath of family breakdown, there is a need to address the child's sense of loss, which often the parents are too fragile to deal with. The child's known universe has disappeared, and so a child of divorce may quickly become attuned to paradox, to suffering, and even to deep questions of faith. They may hear biblical stories differently—when they hear of the Prodigal Son, they may think that the father or mother left the home, not the child. It is extremely important to address this sense of being alone, looking at practical, familial, and spiritual support. When the immediate details of custody are dealt with, children may ask "why" and may need to hear that, in Christian terms, family breakup is not the end of the story: God is the Father whom they can truly trust; they are of inestimable dignity in God's eyes; their ultimate homeland is in heaven. In counseling children in situations of divorce, I have found it necessary to "frame" the situation of loss, to remind them of their uniqueness, to acknowledge and search with them for points of resilience in their lives. The Catholic psychologist acknowledges the tragedy but always gives future hope.

According to Elizabeth Marquardt, who grew up in a family divided by divorce, the child needs security and ongoing contact with both parents (unless a parent is abusive and harms the child). In some cases this may involve being at both homes, but for most children it is having one home with regular visits to the other parent. Children from broken families often "approach marriage with complex, sometimes dissonant emotions—from hope to fear to cynicism."[41] Given that there are a significant proportion of children from such families in our contemporary Western context, it is necessary to address these dissonant emotions, as well as the possibility of higher

39. Ibid., xxxviii.

40. Some research on long-term effects of divorce include the following: P. Amato and J. Cheadle, "The Long Reach of Divorce: Divorce and Child Well-Being across Three Generations," *Journal of Marriage and Family* 67, no. 1 (2005): 191–206; A. J. Cherlin, K. E. Kiernan, and P. L. Chase-Lansdale, "Parental Divorce in Childhood and Demographic Outcomes in Young Adulthood," *Demography* 32 (1995): 299–318; A. J. Cherlin, P. L. Chase-Lansdale, and C. McRae, "Effects of Parental Divorce on Mental Health throughout the Life Course," *American Sociological Review* 63 (1998): 239–49.

41. Elizabeth Marquardt, *Between Two Worlds: The Inner lives of Children of Divorce* (New York: Crown, 2005), 187.

rates of depression, loss of interest in school, and loss of a sense of trust and reason for future hope. In particular:

1. The Catholic counseling psychologist will attempt to enter the territory of the child in order to validate his or her sense of loss. The psychologist listens to the heart and the soul of the child and if need be can gently draw out the child's thoughts by telling third person stories—"A girl whose family broke up once told me she felt like . . . "

2. The Catholic psychologist would emphasize the connections in the child's life, even if not as the child had hoped for. "Your father and mother both love you, though they're apart," or, in the case of unresolved grief due to abandonment, something like, "Your father has gone away. One day, when you grow older you may meet him and tell him how you missed him." Again, telling third person stories in a gentle way, of how some children coped with such loss, is a way of framing what might be an incomprehensible experience.

3. Having acknowledged the loss and the existing connections in a child's life, the Catholic psychologist would focus on reestablishing routine and would look for potential sources in the child's life which may afford him or her a greater capacity to work through the loss. What does the child like? For example, painting, music, sport, dancing.

4. While loss is acknowledged, connections and resilience focused on, the child needs to hear his or her spiritual story, to know of God's immense love, of his unfailing care, that he or she is a child of God, that God can be trusted, even though this world is imperfect and full of broken situations.

As the consequences of IVF unfold, there is becoming manifest the need for the Catholic psychologist to consider the emotions of children in such anomalous family situations. Alana, for example, was conceived through IVF and has never known her father; she expressed her feelings in this way:

I am indeed a human being. My liver, heart, hair, and enzymes all work the same. I've discovered it is my psychology that is different and not-quite-right, due to my conception. It's not a matter for doctors to fix; it's a spiritual problem. My father accepted money, and promised to have nothing to do with me. My mother was wonderful, and I have always loved her deeply, as she has loved me. But my journey is a battle against the void left by my father's absence, and a particular disability in understanding the difference between sacred and commercial, exploitation and cooperation. Those torments for me far outweigh any social stigma or momentarily painful gossip I've endured from ignorant people.[42]

This account, written in support for Domenico Dolce and Stefano Gabbana, gays themselves, who say each child needs a mother and father and who oppose gay adoptions, aroused tsunamis of international ire, which would have worsened the grief of Alana and others like her.

42. Hattie Hart and Alana Newman, "We Are 'Synthetic Children' and We Agree with Dolce & Gabbana," *The Federalist*, March 19, 2015, http://thefederalist.com/2015/03/19/we-are-synthetic-children-and-we-agree-with-dolce-gabbana/.

Catholic psychologists need to listen most acutely to all the dimensions of suffering that arise from current social engineering; they need always to offer words of healing for children who suffer because of the engineering, no matter what political correctness tells us. Never before has the language of healing been so urgently needed, language that integrates the sense of tragic loss with hope, language that is suited suited to children and to the current needs of our age. For the children in situations of family breakdown, of anomalous family structures, the Christian narrative is one of unfailing hope.

Abortion Grief

For the Catholic counseling psychologist, abortion grief counseling has become ever more significant in the decades since abortion became widespread. While secular society may downplay it, many women have stated that they have suffered severe psychological consequences in the aftermath of abortion. Dr. Julius Fogel, an American obstetrician who performed many abortions from the 1970s onward, was honest enough to observe:

Every woman, whatever her background or sexuality, has a trauma at destroying a pregnancy.... [Abortion] is not as harmless and casual an event as many in the pro-abortion crowd insist.[43]

This grief, sometime termed post-abortion syndrome (PAS), appears to have many features similar to those of PTSD (post-traumatic stress disorder).[44] If it is generally accepted that one can be traumatized by a severe threat to oneself or a close family member, then it is understandable that women who lose their child to abortion can suffer a range of traumatic reactions (intrusive thoughts, being on "high alert," or numbing any feeling at all) that affect their day-to-day lives.

It is not only women who may need counseling, but the fathers, brothers, sisters, and grandparents of the child who has been lost to abortion. Abortion may also affect the woman's bonding with her subsequent children, and it affects the social order, since the human being is the "heart of the whole social order."[45] The sense of loss is profound, and the lost child persists in memory. Subsequent children in particular, who realize that it could well have been them, may have difficulties in establishing trust with others. Such children—abortion sibling survivors—need reassurance regarding their situation in familial and spiritual terms, for it is the spiritual ecology that is harmed after such events. The challenge facing Christian psychologists is the inclusion

43. Julius Fogel, quoted in *Aborted Women Silent No More*, ed. David Reardon (Chicago: Loyola University Press, 1987), 141.

44. See V. Rue, "Post-Abortion Syndrome: A Variant of Post-Traumatic Stress Disorder," in *Post Abortion Syndrome*, ed. Peter Doherty (Cambridge: Cambridge University Press, 1995), 16. This book contains a wide selection of articles by psychologists, doctors, and allied professionals on post-abortion syndrome.

45. An expression used by Pope Benedict XVI in his Address to the Pontifical Academies of Sciences and the Social Sciences, November 21, 2005, http://w2.vatican.va/content/benedict-xvi/en/speeches/2005/november/documents/hf_ben_xvi_spe_20051121_academies.html.

of the child in a wider spiritual ecology, for his or her place is unique. This perspective, if brought into play early enough, can even help to avert an abortion. When one mother rang me to say she wanted to arrange an abortion for her teenage daughter, I invited her to consider that she was already a grandmother of a young child. Fortunately, this intervention aroused her sense of connection to the unborn child and changed her mind, and the girl had the baby and received family support. In most situations of pro-life counseling it is not so easy, but it remains of prime importance to attempt to create a social and spiritual "ecological," support network for the young girl, who is often frightened and feeling disconnected from everything. The Catholic psychologist will aim to reconnect the young person to warm, friendly support and social services that value the mother and child, and to God as creator of human life—the wider spiritual ecology as underlined by Pope Francis in his recent encyclical *Laudato Si*.[46]

As regards post-abortion grief, it is often helpful to share with the mother the accounts of the women who have suffered in this way. In the 1980s an American woman, Nancyjo Mann, began an organization called Women Hurt by Abortion in response to her doctor's indifference to her abortion trauma. Sadly, post-abortion counseling has grown in response to the times, with the founding of Rachel's Vineyard and other groups, and Women Hurt by Abortion is another spiritual network that speaks eloquently to suffering women and to the wider society.[47]

The approach of secular counselors to post-abortion counseling may be to give a white rosebud and to express regret, after reframing the sense of trauma as just another "event." The Catholic psychologist realizes the nature and depth of the psychological and spiritual wounds and therefore takes a very different approach. Initially, the process of recovery and healing cannot begin in human beings until the trauma is acknowledged and then processed, that is, given some meaning in the life story of that person. Many women (and men) realize, after trying to "tough it out" themselves, that they do need help in overcoming the effects of trauma and need some intervention that can mitigate the constant "high alert" or "numbing the emotions" state.

Sometimes, however, it is difficult to detect abortion grief. After an abortion, some people suffer depression and engage in substance abuse without realizing the source of their grief. Thus it is appropriate for a counselor who is assisting someone with depression to ask tactfully if there are life events that might have been a trigger for the depression—going through a list one by one—for example, loss of a family member, relationship breakdown, abortion. In the process of counseling this is very important. Canadian psychiatrist Phillip Ney found that there may be not only an abortion in the woman's past but also abuse of one kind or another in childhood, and

---

46. Pope Francis, *Laudato Si', On Care for Our Common Home*, Encyclical Letter, May 24, 2015.

47. Counselor Anne Lastman gives a moving account of the psychological and spiritual aspects of post-abortion grief in *Redeeming Grief* (Leominster, Herefordshire, U.K.: Freedom Press, 2008); and Melinda Tankard Reist has written the accounts of women who have had abortions in *Giving Sorrow Words* (Sydney: Duffy and Snellgrove, 2000). There are also many accounts and research links on the Elliott Institute's site: http://afterabortion.org/. Philip Ney and Marie Peeters outline the effects on doctors who have performed abortions in the past and no longer do so in *The Centurion's Pathway* (Victoria, B.C., Canada: Pioneer Publishing, 1997).

the abuse has been a factor in the woman's abortion. There are multiple issues here—in the situation of abuse, the woman may feel dehumanized and thus go on to "dehumanize" her own child. Given this, Ney's effective form of psychotherapy, which he has used for more than thirty years, attempts to *rehumanize* the woman who has had the abortion, that is, enable her to regain a sense of dignity.[48] This involves remembering dehumanizing experiences of the past and grieving the loss of innocence. It is important, he says, to mourn the self lost in the lonely times of childhood abandonment and neglect. The experiences can be difficult to understand, as the victim can blame him- or herself, thinking that he or she was not worthy enough to prevent the abuser from abusing.

The purpose of Ney's recasting of the narrative is to strengthen the woman who is overwhelmed and helpless when thinking of past experiences. The act of stating and trying to understand the experiences shapes the narrative of the person's life in such a way that the counselor can point out that self-negating judgements are inadequate accounts of the whole person. This process of untangling the threads reveals what Ney calls "the wounded pilgrim."[49] This process involves pulling away the false selves or "dances" used by the person to cover up the pain, to pretend everything is ok, to deny that they have suffered and are in need of help. The wounded pilgrim, after acknowledging past hurts, does not deny these things any longer but can face the past with increased resilience. He or she does not try to bury the true self in hyperactivity or numbness and avoidance of life. Ney speaks of farewelling childhood dreams—mourning the original blueprint of life and the lost child. That grief is handed over to God, and the person begins to make plans for the "alternative" blueprint. This has been a highly effective incorporation of the Christian narrative into post-abortion counseling. Another aspect of Ney's approach is the "forgiving" of perpetrators of past abuse—through letters written to the perpetrator. This is entirely voluntary, and is not to reestablish friendship but to state the past hurt and sincerely offer forgiveness by rising above it and being internally strong enough to forgive. This is not easy for the people involved, but it has had quite dramatic psychological and spiritual effects in some circumstances. (The next section deals with forgiveness in greater detail.)

Ney's account points to the unavoidable fact that post-abortion syndrome calls for a spiritual healing alongside psychological counseling. Full-time post-abortion counselor Anne Lastman, in an address to Catholic priests at a 1998 pro-life conference in Melbourne, exhorted priests to speak about this issue, to offer from the pulpit, or in any other way, their encouraging support to anyone who needs it.[50] She pointed out that such spiritual support was needed as never before. Lastman herself has counseled thousands of women, many referred to her by psychiatrists who "got nowhere," and she has found in the end that nothing could heal as effectively as draw-

48. See Philip Ney, *Deeply Damaged: An Explanation for the Profound Problems Arising from Infant Abortion and Child Abuse* (Victoria, B.C., Canada: Pioneer Publishing, 1997), 1.45ff; 2.16 ff.

49. Ibid., 2.56 ff. This paragraph is adapted from Ney's work.

50. John Dillon's *A Path to Hope* (New York: Resurrection Press, 1990) is very useful for priests and others involved in this area.

ing on the spiritual dimension for true healing of the post-abortion wounds—with the priest offering Christ's healing mercy through the sacrament of Reconciliation. In Lastman's regular newsletter, *Broken Branches*, the words of a young woman are recounted: "I killed my baby, and I didn't mean to. I didn't want to be pregnant, but I didn't want to kill my baby. Do you think I will ever forget?"[51] In answer to such a plea, St. John Paul II went beyond the therapeutic in addressing the following consoling words to every woman who has had an abortion, words that can be transmitted by the counseling psychologist:

The Father of mercies is ready to give you his forgiveness and his peace in the Sacrament of Reconciliation. You will come to understand that nothing is definitely lost, and you will be able to ask forgiveness from your child, who is now living in the Lord.[52]

Ultimately, many of those who have suffered trauma in various forms have come to understand that "It is better to trust in the Lord than to trust in princes" (Ps 118:9). For those whose "bones have been crushed" (Ps 51:10), and whose hearts have been broken, who have endured horrors beyond measure, there is the consolation that each person is precious in God's sight and that in the end "every tear will be wiped away" (Rev 21:4).

Forgiveness

It is not only major bioethical issues—post-abortion grief, IVF, euthanasia, and gender issues—that a Christian/Catholic psychologist will see in terms of spiritual-psychological integration. Something that has generated increasing psychological interest in recent years is the role of *forgiveness in psychological healing*. One would think this is not a controversial issue, but on the contrary, it has generated considerable debate and conflicting responses. How could this be so? Isn't forgiveness just a matter of saying "I forgive you"?

Every Christian knows that the words of the "Our Father" enjoin forgiveness on those who say it: "Our Father ... forgive us our trespasses, as we forgive those who trespass against us." And in Mark 11:25, Jesus urges his disciples to "forgive anyone against whom you have a grievance, so that your Father in heaven may in turn forgive you your transgressions" and exhorts us to forgive "seventy times seven." Christians understand this in everyday life—the thoughtless word, the snide remark, the lack of consideration in a work or home event—when the transgression hurts but forgiveness is possible.

There are situations, however, which cut so deeply that forgiveness seems impossible. They produce lifelong consequences. The core of the person is attacked in such a way that the ability to trust others is often destroyed. Consider parents whose child is

---

51. Anne Lastman, *Broken Branches*, Issue 13 (October 2000): 2.

52. John Paul II, *Evangelium Vitae*, no. 99. This quote is apparently contained in the original text from which modern language translations were made, and was deleted from the official Latin text as published in the *Acta Apostolicae Sedis*. See Jeffrey Mirus, "Limbo Again: Clarifying Evangelium Vitae No. 99," *Catholic Culture Commentary*, May 30, 2005, https://www.catholicculture.org/commentary/otc.cfm?id=42.

murdered, victims of physical, sexual, and emotional abuse, betrayal in business and marriage, destruction of families in war and holocausts, living with drug addiction in one's parents and/or children. Is it not arrogant of an outsider even to think of forgiveness in such situations? Examination of situations in which forgiveness seems "impossible" strikes deeply at the heart of universal human events and confronts us emotionally and spiritually. For such events have permeated human life from its out-set—whether on a personal, group, or societal, or even religious level.

As an indication of the increasing interest of this issue of forgiveness, the American Psychological Association had an annual national meeting in August 2000 in which there were twelve presentations on forgiveness; this was a new direction for the association. Some conferences now include "basics of forgiveness training."[53] And it is to be expected that forgiveness is an issue increasingly facing Christian psychologists as revenge, angst, and terror increase in our world. The interpersonal and social dimensions of forgiveness may well affect the well-being of nations.

So, what is forgiveness? Does it condone the crime and excuse the wrongdoer? Is not this an insult to the victim, and moreover an insult to the wrongdoer—to deprive him or her of the moral freedom to choose how to act? Forgiveness, according to Catholic psychologist Kevin Culligan, can be approached initially by what it is not. Thus true forgiveness:

- does not condone violence, abuse or injustice
- is not pardoning, condoning, excusing, forgetting, denying or even reconciling
- does not release others from the consequences of their behavior
- is essentially a unilateral, private choice, a necessary first step in freeing oneself from carrying the heavy burden of resentment over past hurts
- sets the basis for future possibilities in reconciliation, restoring broken relationships although psychological forgiveness does not require this.
- focuses on forgiving others, not on asking others for their forgiveness or on forgiving oneself, though these are related.[54]

Thus forgiveness is more than simply accepting or tolerating injustice—about "moving on" or "putting the past behind us."

Robert Enright gives an outline of the complexity of forgiveness, saying that first, it fully recognizes the depth of the hurt and pain, but it is also other-directed and reflects on the wrong and the wrongdoer. Second, forgiving is not the same as forgetting, for "a deep injustice suffered is rarely, if ever, wiped from consciousness."[55] When a person forgives, he or she remembers but in different ways from pre-forgiveness times. Third, forgiveness is more than ceasing our anger—it is not a neutral stance toward our injurer but a full recognition of what he or she has done. Fourth, forgiving is more

53. Kevin Culligan, "Prayer and Forgiveness: Can Psychology Help?" *Spiritual Life* 89 (2002): 78.

54. See ibid., 81–2.

55. Robert Enright, Suzanne Freedman, and Julio Rique, "The Psychology of Interpersonal Forgiveness," in *Exploring Forgiveness*, ed. Robert Enright and Joanna North (Madison: University of Wisconsin Press, 1998), 47. Much of this section is taken from chapter 5, 46–62, of the book.

than making ourselves feel good. It is not just creating a more peaceful atmosphere at home or at work. Enright calls this a pseudo-forgiveness, of which there are many kinds. For example, a person may say "I forgive you" yet harbor resentment; or a person may say sweetly, "I forgive you" but then remind the wrongdoer of the past hurt at every opportunity—as Oscar Wilde said, "Always forgive your enemies—nothing annoys them so much." It is possible to think of numerous variations on this theme, for human beings are capable of deceiving themselves in many different ways. Nietzsche viewed Christians as weaklings because of their tendency to forgive, saying that only weaklings practice forgiveness; but in Enright's view, Nietzsche described a pseudo- or false forgiveness and did not take into account what true forgiveness entails.[56]

It is important to understand that forgiveness is not just a "self-help" technique aimed at feeling better. Nor is it a question of simply changing our attitudes, for this does not confront the real harm done by the wrongdoer (terrorist, abuser). This approach may in fact become a second injury for the injured person, who will blame him- or herself for feeling bad or hurt. Enright points to the inadequacy of saying, "If only I could alter my view of the incest, I wouldn't feel so bad."[57] This emphasis on subjectivity denies the objective wrong, the full depth of the evil and harm done to the injured person, and the moral agency of the injurer. That is to say, there is an injurer, an injured person, and a wrong act. After considering its complexities, Enright (with a Human Development Study Group) defined forgiveness as:

A willingness to abandon one's right to resentment, negative judgement, and indifferent behavior toward one who unjustly injured us, while fostering the undeserved qualities of compassion, generosity, and even love toward him or her.[58]

The offended person makes a deliberate choice to forgive, *not with grim resignation*, but as a positive and free choice. This act, however, entails a long personal journey, often a collaborative task involving the counselor and the injured person. The decision involves changing affect; it involves overcoming condemnation with respect, resentment with compassion, and indifference with goodwill. This forgiveness involves reaching out to the offender, in a manner consistent with the Christian view of the world.

It is important to note that if a counselor proposes the journey of forgiveness, the injured person is entirely free to accept or not accept it. Some are not ready or able, or may not understand what it is or what its consequences are. Still, there is useful information that may be given to a person which may influence his or her decision. Forgiveness does not resolve all the emotional pain consequent on injury; the pain may remain for a lifetime. Nor does it need to be understood or accepted by the injurer—although acceptance of course would be desirable. Some who have been injured have had the experience of having the injurer reject their forgiveness and not admit to any wrongdoing. Thus there are degrees to which the process of forgiveness is achieved,

56. Ibid., 49.
57. Ibid., 51.
58. Ibid., 46–7.

but despite this, "forgiveness journeys" unleash forces that affect the injured person, the injurer (even if limited), and the social and spiritual environment.

U.S. Catholic psychiatrist Richard Fitzgibbons, basing his therapy on Enright's insights, outlined these stages of the "forgiveness journey":

1. *Uncovering*. This involves discussion of the nature of the incident, the anger ensuing from it, and the nature of anger itself. The therapist attempts to assess the depth of the injured person's anger, whether it is being "covered up" and denied, and whether it needs to be fully acknowledged.
2. In the *decision phase* the injured person hears accounts of forgiveness from the therapist—what it is, what it is not. There is movement toward a decision to forgive.
3. The *work phase*—the injured person explores ways of enacting forgiveness.
4. The *outcome phase*—the injured person forgives the injurer and may share this experience with the counselor.[59]

Each of these phases takes a long time and starts the therapist and the injured person on a journey that has no guarantee of success but offers a path that is different from the typical worldly narrative. It may involve other therapies (e.g., cognitive behavioral therapy or dialectical behavioral therapy) to deal with immediate distress, along with exploration of psychological and spiritual resilience.

Perhaps telling a story of forgiveness in "impossible circumstances" may help. One of the most haunting recent examples of forgiveness is that of Immaculée Ilibagiza, a young Catholic woman who lived through the Rwandan genocide and the murder of virtually all of her family. A young Tutsi of Catholic background, she recounts how, in 1994, a kind of collective evil took hold of former Hutu groups that, with incitement from leaders of the Hutu tribe, were propelled to behead, stab, and massacre more than a million of their Tutsi countrymen.

Immaculée describes her story in a simple, unadorned way, threading the narration of turbulent events with her own profound reflection.[60] Her book recounts her survival and spiritual odyssey that led her to forgive her family's killers, after experiencing evil on a scale beyond the experience of most people.

She was born into an affectionate, loving family with three brothers, Damascene, Aimable, and Vianney. Her parents pass their deeply lived Catholic faith on to their children, who befriend and help many of their Hutu neighbors. While Immaculée is at university in the capital, Kigali, she hears that war has started with the incursion of Tutsi refugees, who had been expelled years before to exile in Uganda and who now have crossed back into Rwanda to reclaim homes and land confiscated in the massacres of 1959 and 1973. Immaculée returns to her parents' house only to find that they are all trapped, surrounded by Hutus bent on exterminating the entire Tutsi tribe.

59. See Richard Fitzgibbons, "Anger and the Healing Power of Forgiveness," in *Exploring Forgiveness*, ed. Enright and North, 68–74.

60. Immaculée Ilibagiza with Steve Irwin, *Left to Tell: Discovering God amidst the Rwandan Holocaust* (Carlsbad, Calif.: Hay House, 2006).

When she hears a government minister on the radio inciting all Hutus to kill all the Tutsis, sparing none, she knows what faces her family and tribe.

Immaculée's father tells his daughter to hide in the house of a nearby Hutu Protestant pastor who offers to help at great risk. At the house, she is led to a tiny bathroom whose entrance is hidden by a wardrobe. She and seven other Tutsi women hide there for months, lying one atop the other, hearing Hutus outside the house boast how they have burned churches full of people, raped women, and killed families. The women, in terrorized silence, develop sign language to communicate. They are fed at night by the pastor. In the continuing horror, Immaculée seeks spiritual solace, retreating within saying: "I found a small part of the bathroom to call my own: a corner of my heart."[61] While lying crouched on the ground, with bodies above her, she talks to God the entire day, after fitful sleep, praising His goodness. She dreams that Jesus tells her that nearly all her family have been killed—which proves to be correct. One night, when the pastor enters with food, she asks for a Bible, which opens at Psalm 91:

> This I declare, that He alone is my refuge, my place of safety: He is my God, and I trust Him. He rescues you from every trap and protects you.... He will shield you with His wings! They will shelter you. His faithful promises are your amour.... Though a thousand fall at my side, though ten thousand are dying around me, evil will not touch me.

Immaculée's closeness to God in prayer helps her to console the other women. One day, they learn that the French army has entered Rwanda, setting up safe houses around the country. They have to try to reach one, as a young Hutu has become suspicious about possible hideouts in the pastor's house. The pastor selects some trusted men to surround the gaunt women as they walk to a safe, French area. Along the road they pass Hutu militias, who bypass them, but the women's protectors then flee, leaving them exposed and forcing them to run the final five hundred meters to the French camp.

In time, Immaculée learns that most of her family have died in the massacre. One brother, who had been studying in Senegal during the conflict, survives. She tries to make sense of this living nightmare which has taken hold of her entire life, realizing, as Holocaust survivor Primo Levi said, "he who loses all often easily loses himself."[62] She concludes that her life is over, as the memory of this evil will forever haunt her and destroy her, if she cannot find a way of releasing herself from it. She calls on spiritual help, reflecting that the hold of evil, anger, and pain in those who cannot forgive continues the triumph of that evil, stealing a person's life. She comes to understand that she must see the killers as God's creatures, souls who fell prey to evil but are nonetheless His children. She realizes that she must forgive the Hutu killers. Forgiveness is the only way of leaving the hollowness of despair, the prison of revenge. After the war, Immaculée travels to a jail to meet her family's killer, Felicien, whose children she had played with; now in a prison cell, he crouches before her in shame. She writes:

---

61. Ibid., 95.
62. Primo Levi, *If This Is a Man* (New York: Penguin, 1971), 33.

Felicien had let the devil enter his heart, and the evil had ruined his life like a cancer in his soul. He was now the victim of victims, destined to live in torment and regret. I was overwhelmed with pity for the man.[63]

She says, slowly, sincerely—"I forgive you"—to Felicien. She realizes that the people who had hurt her family "had hurt themselves more," seeing the situation in a wider, spiritual perspective. She quietly turns to go, leaving the prison guard indignant and uncomprehending, for he had expected revenge. She describes how, after this momentous event, she is gradually able to reconnect with people and to look at life with hope again. Without forgiveness, she says this would have been impossible.

Immaculée's experiences have become the basis of a life mission in speaking about forgiveness, touching the hearts of many victims of injustice. Her story is not only about Rwanda but about any soul suffering injustice, abuse, and horror—rising above sufferings, trusting the power of grace, of divine mercy, to transcend the unforgivable and the unforgettable.

On a societal level, there is a need to validate the stories of victims in a world of wars and horrors where the techniques of destruction are continually being improved. There are many victims whose stories are simply not heard and who live with enormous burdens of painful memory, some hoping for redress. Martha Minow writes in *Vengeance and Forgiveness*:

Traumatized people imagine that revenge will bring relief even though the fantasy of revenge simply reverses the roles of perpetrator and victim, continuing to imprison the victim in horror, degradation, and the bounds of the perpetrator's violence.... [B]y seeking to lower the perpetrator in response to his or her infliction of injury, does the victim ever master the violence or instead become its tool?[64]

Psychologists have realized that in the affirmation of human dignity, there is an urgent need to explore alternatives to vengeance, not only for the healing of individuals but for the healing of the wider society. Minow states that it is important that national commissions give some public voice to those injured on a wider scale—thus the Nuremberg trials and truth commissions, however imperfect they may have been, did listen to and validate the victims' suffering. The important thing from a psychological point of view here is that public recognition of the wrong can help survivors reestablish the capacity to trust and begin the journey to forgiveness, even if only to some extent. Though not everyone can and will forgive, those who do often have a hidden impact on those around them and find healing where they thought there was none.

Conclusion

There are many other issues confronting Catholic psychologists beyond those mentioned in this chapter, but psychology's legacy, its understanding of the human person and consequent assumptions, point the way to an authentic faith-psychology bal-

---

63. Ilibagiza, *Left to Tell*, 204.
64. Martha Minow, *Vengeance and Forgiveness* (Boston: Beacon Press, 1998), 13.

ance. No culture, no psychology, can account for itself without humanity's legacy of engagement with the transcendent, a theological dimension that engages each mind and heart in ongoing exploration of the compelling questions, so eloquently stated in *Veritatis Splendor*:

What is man? What is the meaning and purpose of our life? What is good and what is sin? What origin and purpose do sufferings have? What is the way to attaining true happiness? What are death, judgement, and retribution after death? Lastly, what is that final, unutterable mystery which embraces our lives and from which we take our origin and towards which we tend? [65]

A Catholic psychologist cannot avoid these questions in integrating an authentic humanism with his or her therapeutic approaches "in a way that answers the needs of our time."[66] As Vitz has put it in an essay titled "Experiencing the Supernatural," "the question of spiritual experience" is of utmost relevance to the "social and moral dilemmas of our postmodern age" for without it, "there is no way to deal with our crisis."[67] Catholic psychologists possess, along with valuable psychological research, a spiritual legacy of inestimable value, and they can call on it and apply it to the pressing need for healing in our age. As St. John Paul II stated: "[h]uman longing and the need for religion ... are not able to be totally extinguished." The psychological reality was and remains that people, including psychologists, will always want to know "the truth about God, about man, and about the meaning of life itself."[68]

Bibliography

Allen, Lydia. "Psychological Principles for Vocation Directors and Seminary Formators as Applied to Persons with Homosexual Tendencies." *Seminarium* 47, no. 3 (2007): 840–72.

Amato, P., and J. Cheadle. "The Long Reach of Divorce: Divorce and Child Well-Being across Three Generations." *Journal of Marriage and Family* 67, no. 1 (2005): 191–206.

Benedict XVI, Pope. Address to the Pontifical Academies of Sciences and the Social Sciences. November 21, 2005. http://w2.vatican.va/content/benedict-xvi/en/speeches/2005/november/documents/hf_ben_xvi_spe_20051121_academies.html.

——. Address to the Roman Curia Offering Them His Christmas Greetings. December 22, 2005. http://w2.vatican.va/content/benedict-xvi/en/speeches/2005/december/documents/hf_ben_xvi_spe_20051222_roman-curia.html.

——. *Spe Salvi, On Christian Hope*, Encyclical Letter. November 30, 2007. Sydney: St. Paul's Publications, 2007.

65. John Paul II, *Veritatis Splendor, The Splendor of Truth* (1993), no. 30, quoting Vatican Council II, *Nostra Aetate*, no. 1.

66. Benedict XVI, Address of His Holiness Benedict XVI to the Roman Curia Offering Them His Christmas Greetings, December 22, 2005, http://w2.vatican.va/content/benedictxvi/en/speeches/2005/december/documents/hf_ben_xvi_spe_20051222_roman-curia.html.

67. Paul Vitz, "Experiencing the Supernatural," in *Things in Heaven and Earth* ed. *Harold Fickett* (Orleans, Mass.: Paraclete Press, 1988), 81; cf. Benedict XVI's call to acknowledge that in all cultures lies a "respect for that which another group holds sacred, especially respect for the sacred in the highest sense, for God." Pope Benedict XVI and Marcello Pera, *Without Roots: The West, Relativism, Christianity, Islam* (New York: Basic Books, 2006), 78.

68. Pope John Paul II, *Redemptoris Missio, Mission of the Redeemer*, Encyclical Letter, December 7, 1990 (Boston: Pauline Books and Media, 1990), no. 3.

———. *Caritas in Veritate, On Integral Human Development in Charity and Truth*, Encyclical Letter. June 29, 2009. Vatican City: Libreria Editrice Vaticana, 2009.

Benedict XVI, Pope, and Marcello Pera. *Without Roots: The West, Relativism, Christianity, Islam*. New York: Basic Books, 2006.

Browning, Don. *Religious Thought and the Modern Psychologies: A Critical Conversation in the Theology of Culture*. Philadelphia: Fortress Press, 1987.

Brugger, Christian. "Anthropological Foundations for Clinical Psychology: A Proposal." *Journal of Psychology and Theology* 36, no. 1 (Spring 2008): 3–15.

Cherlin, A. J., P. L. Chase-Lansdale, and C. McRae. "Effects of Parental Divorce on Mental Health throughout the Life Course." *American Sociological Review* 63 (1998): 239–49.

Cherlin, A. J., K. E. Kiernan, and P. L. Chase-Lansdale. "Parental Divorce in Childhood and Demographic Outcomes in Young Adulthood." *Demography* 32 (1995): 299–318.

Coudou, Martin. *Le monastère invisible de Jean Paul II*. Paris: Editions Salvator, 2008.

Culligan, Kevin. "Prayer and Forgiveness: Can Psychology Help?" *Spiritual Life* 89 (2002): 81–89.

Dillon, John. *A Path to Hope*. New York: Resurrection Press, 1990.

Doherty, Peter, ed. *Post Abortion Syndrome*. Cambridge: Cambridge University Press, 1995.

Enright, Robert. "The Psychology of Interpersonal Forgiveness." In *Exploring Forgiveness*, ed. Robert Enright and Joanna North, 46–62. Madison: University of Wisconsin Press, 1998.

Fitzgibbons, Richard. "Anger and the Healing Power of Forgiveness: A Psychiatrist's View." In *Exploring Forgiveness*, ed. Robert Enright and Joanna North, 63–74. Madison: University of Wisconsin Press, 1998.

Frankl, Viktor. *Man's Search for Meaning*. New York: Pocket Books, 1985. Originally published as *Ein Psychologe erlebt das Konzentrationslager* (Vienna, 1946).

Francis, Pope. Opening Address to the Colloquium on the Complementarity of Man and Woman. *Zenit*, November 17, 2014. http://www.zenit.org/en/articles/pope-francis-address-at-opening-of-colloquium-on-complementarity-of-man-and-woman.

———. *Laudato Si', On Care for Our Common Home*. Encyclical Letter. May 24, 2015.

Hart, Hattie, and Alana Newman. "We Are 'Synthetic Children' and We Agree With Dolce & Gabbana." *The Federalist*, March 19, 2015. http://thefederalist.com/2015/03/19/we-are-synthetic-children-and-we-agree-with-dolce-gabbana/.

Ilibagiza, Immaculée, with Steve Irwin. *Left to Tell: Discovering God amidst the Rwandan Holocaust*. Carlsbad, Calif.: Hay House Inc., 2006.

John Paul II, Pope. *Salvifici Doloris, On the Christian Meaning of Human Suffering*. Apostolic Letter. February 11, 1984. Sydney: Pauline Books and Media, 1984.

———. *Christifideles Laici, On the Vocation and Mission of the Lay Faithful in the Church and the World*. Apostolic Exhortation. December 30, 1988. Boston: St. Paul Books and Media, 1988.

———. *Redemptoris Missio, Mission of the Redeemer*, Encyclical Letter. December 7, 1990. Boston: Pauline Books and Media, 1990.

———. *Veritatis Splendor, The Splendor of Truth*. Encyclical Letter. August 6, 1993.

———. *Evangelium Vitae, On the Value and Inviolability of Human Life*. Encyclical Letter. March 25, 1995. http://w2.vatican.va/content/john-paul-ii/en/encyclicals/documents/hf_jp-ii_enc_25031995_evangelium-vitae.html.

Johnson, Eric L., and Stanton L. Jones. *Psychology and Christianity: Four Views*. Downers Grove, Ill.: InterVarsity Press, 2000.

Kilpatrick, William. *Psychological Seduction: The Failure of Modern Psychology*. Nashville, Tenn.: Thomas Nelson, 1983.

———. *The Emperor's New Clothes: The Naked Truth about the New Psychology*. Ridgefield, Conn.: Roger A. McCaffrey Publishing, 1985.

Lastman, Anne. *Broken Branches*, Issue 13 (October 2000).

———. *Redeeming Grief*. Leominster, Herefordshire, U.K.: Freedom Press, 2008.

Levi, Primo. *If This Is a Man*. New York: Penguin, 1971.

Marquardt, Elizabeth. *Between Two Worlds: The Inner Lives of Children of Divorce*. New York: Crown, 2005.

Minow, Martha. *Vengeance and Forgiveness*. Boston: Beacon Press, 1998.

Ney, Phillip. *Deeply Damaged: An Explanation for the Profound Problems Arising from Infant Abortion and Child Abuse*. Victoria, B.C., Canada: Pioneer Publishing, 1997.

Ney, Philip, and Marie Peeters. *The Centurion's Pathway*. Victoria, B.C., Canada: Pioneer Publishing, 1997.

Nicolosi, Joseph. *Healing Homosexuality*. Lanham, Md.: Rowman and Littlefield, 1993.

Pontifical Council for Pastoral Assistance to Health Care Workers. *Charter for Health Care Workers*. 1995. http://www.ewtn.com/library/curia/pcpaheal.htm.

Ratzinger, Joseph. "Retrieving the Tradition: Concerning the Notion of Person in Theology." *Communio: International Catholic Review* 17 (Fall 1990): 439–54.

———. *The Yes of Jesus Christ* New York: Crossroad, 1991.

Reardon, David. *Aborted Women Silent No More*. Chicago: Loyola University Press, 1987.

Roberts, Robert, and Mark Talbot, eds. *Limning the Psyche: Explorations in Christian Psychology*. Grand Rapids, Mich.: Wm. B. Eerdmans, 1997.

Rue, V. "Post-Abortion Syndrome: A Variant of Post-Traumatic Stress Disorder." In *Post Abortion Syndrome*, ed. Peter Doherty, 15–28. Cambridge: Cambridge University Press, 1995.

Scully, Mathew. "Viktor Frankl at 90: An Interview." *First Things* (Spring 1995): 39–43.

Shafranske, Edward. *Religion and the Clinical Practice of Psychology*. Washington, D.C.: American Psychological Association, 1996.

Shorter, Edward. *A History of Psychiatry: From the Era of the Asylum to the Age of Prozac*. New York: John Wiley and Sons, 1997.

Spadaro, Antonio. "A Big Heart Open to God." *America* 209, no. 8 (September 30, 2013): 15–38.

Tankard Reist, Melinda. *Giving Sorrow Words*. Sydney: Duffy and Snellgrove, 2000.

van den Aardweg, Gerard J. M. *The Battle for Normality: A Guide for Self-Therapy for Homosexuality*. San Francisco: Ignatius Press, 1997.

Vatican Information Service. "Francis: No Human Life Is More Valuable Than Another." Vatican Information Service. September 20, 2013. http://visnews-en.blogspot.com.au/2013/09/francis-no-human-life-is-more-valuable.html.

Vitz, Paul. *Psychology as Religion: The Cult of Self-Worship*. Grand Rapids, Mich.: Eerdmans, 1977.

———. "Experiencing the Supernatural." In *Things in Heaven and Earth,* ed. Harold Fickett, 81–92. Orleans, Mass.: Paraclete Press, 1988.

———. *Faith of the Fatherless: The Psychology of Atheism*. Dallas: Spence Publishing Company, 1999.

Vitz, Paul, and Susan Felch, eds. *The Self: Beyond the Postmodern Crisis*. Wilmington, Del.: ISI Books, 2006.

von Balthasar, Hans Urs. *In the Fullness of Faith: On the Centrality of the Distinctively Catholic*. Translated by Graham Harrison. San Francisco: Ignatius Press, 1988. Originally published as *Katholische* (Einsiedeln, Switzerland: Johannes Verlag, 1975).

———. "On the Concept of Person." *Communio: International Catholic Review* 13 (Spring 1986): 18–26.

Wallerstein, Judith, Julia M. Lewis, and Sandra Blakeslec. *The Unexpected Legacy of Divorce: The 25 Year Landmark Study*. New York: Hyperion, 2000.

Reverend Patrick Flanagan and
Robert A. Mangione

12. THE CATHOLIC PHARMACIST

From the earliest times in the history of medicine, those whom we have come to refer to as pharmacists have been an integral part of the practice of the healing arts. In this chapter Drs. Flanagan
and Mangione help us to appreciate many of the challenges facing the Catholic pharmacist
today. Adopting an approach similar to that taken by authors of other chapters in this book, they
show the basis of authentic Catholic witness rooted in Scripture, magisterial documents, and
other authoritative writings from experts. Their presentation raises awareness of important contemporary issues facing pharmacists, and offers insightful connections between Church teachings and proposed approaches to handling these important issues. Pharmacists are sure to find
this chapter unique and interesting; other health-care providers, in recognizing the challenges
for pharmacists and their potential responses, also will be enriched.—*Editors*

Introduction

Pharmacists have historically been important providers of health care. The practice
of their profession has continually evolved to meet changing societal needs, resulting in new and expanded roles for these health-care professionals. Although historically pharmacists have focused primarily on providing a product to the patient, the
scope of practice has expanded significantly, particularly during the last fifty years.
Today pharmacists are providers of pharmaceutical care that goes far beyond the traditional role of accurately filling a prescription.[1] Pharmaceutical care is essentially the
responsible provision of drug therapy for the purpose of achieving definite outcomes
to improve a patient's quality of life.[2] These outcomes include the cure of disease;

1. See G. F. Higby, "Professional Socialization of Pharmacists," in *Social and Behavioral Aspects of Pharmaceutical Care*, ed. N. M. Rickles, A. I. Wertheimer, and M. C. Smith (Sudbury, Mass,: Jones and Bartlett
Publishers, 2010), 109–19.
2. See C. D. Hepler and D. M. Angaran, "The Nature of Caring," in *Pharmaceutical Care*, ed. C. H.
Knowlton and R. P. Penna (New York: Chapman and Hall, 1996): 155–75.

elimination or reduction of a patient's symptoms; the arresting or slowing of a disease process; and preventing a disease or symptomatology.[3] It is noteworthy that a fundamental principle of pharmaceutical care is the development of a covenantal relationship between the patient and the pharmacist.[4]

The educational requirements associated with becoming a pharmacist have also evolved, in order that practitioners may be prepared for their expanded roles. Pharmacy education has progressed from the apprentice model of colonial times to the sophisticated, rigorous doctor of pharmacy curriculum mandated today. Colleges and universities that offer doctor of pharmacy programs, along with their specific pharmacy curricula, are subjected to careful external evaluation by the Accreditation Council on Pharmacy Education (ACPE) to ensure that they meet ACPE accreditation requirements and are worthy of designation as nationally accredited programs.

Pharmacy and the Catholic Tradition

The practice of pharmacy has a strong foundation in the history of the Catholic Church. The extraordinary care provided by third-century saints Cosmas the physician and his brother Damian, who is believed by many to have been an apothecary, is an important historic example of collaborative patient care. St. Damian is among the saints who have been associated with the pharmacy profession; these saints include St. Raphael the Archangel, identified in the Old Testament (Tobit 12:15) and whose name means "medicine of God"; St. Luke the physician (died ca. 84); St. Martin de Porres (1579–1639); and St. Hildegard of Bingen (1098–1179). The patron saint of pharmacists, St. John Leonardi, was identified by Pope Benedict XVI during a general audience in October 2009. St. John, an Italian saint canonized by Pope Pius XI in 1938, studied pharmacy before changing his focus to theology. Although St. John ultimately became a theologian, he reportedly never lost his passion for pharmacy and, as Pope Benedict noted, he was convinced that " 'the medicine of God,' which is the Crucified and Risen Jesus Christ, [is] 'the measure of all things.' "[5]

Catholic colleges and universities are important providers of pharmacy education. In the United States today, ten institutions with a Catholic identity or tradition offer doctor of pharmacy programs (see table 12-1).

The Oath of the Pharmacist

It is a tradition that graduates of doctor of pharmacy programs take an oath, just as do newly minted practitioners in other professions, that will guide them in their

---

3. See American Society of Hospital Pharmacists, "ASHP Statement on Pharmaceutical Care," *American Journal of Hospital Pharmacy* 50 (1993): 1720–23.

4. See C. D. Hepler and L. M. Strand, "Opportunities and Responsibilities in Pharmaceutical Care," *American Journal of Hospital Pharmacy* 47 (1990): 533–43.

5. Pope Benedict XVI, General Audience, October 7, 2009, http://www.vatican.va/holy_father/benedict_xvi/audiences/2009/documents/hf_ben-xvi_aud_20091007_en.html.

Table 12-1. **Institutions of Higher Learning Self-Identifying as Catholic, or in the Catholic Tradition, with Pharmacy Schools**

Creighton University

Duquesne University

D'Youville College

Notre Dame of Maryland University

Regis University

St. John Fisher College

St. John's University (New York)

University of St. Joseph (Connecticut)

University of the Incarnate Word

Xavier University of Louisiana

professional practice. The Oath of the Pharmacist adopted by the American Association of Colleges of Pharmacy calls the graduating pharmacist to nine important ideals, including the promise to "hold myself and my colleagues to the highest principles of our profession's moral, ethical, and legal conduct."[6] The profession's Code of Ethics also dictates, as one of its eight principles, that pharmacists must act "with honesty and integrity in professional relationships."[7] Although these directives are independent of any faith-based teaching, they provide important ideals that guide practice and set a strong foundation for the pharmacist's professional commitment to providing ethical, competent, and compassionate health care.

Challenges for the Catholic Pharmacist

When we consider that the practice of pharmacy is a significant and highly integrated aspect of health care in the United States, it is not surprising that Catholic pharmacists face the same ethical challenges encountered by other health-care professionals. The specific challenge may manifest itself differently in each profession, but the fundamental principle that guides its resolution remains essentially the same. This has become particularly evident as the role of the pharmacist has focused increasingly on pharmaceutical care.

Pharmacists face many dilemmas in their practice. And increasingly, pharmacists are more and more under duress to ignore their consciences. A Catholic pharmacist's

6. AACP, "Oath of a Pharmacist," July 2007, http://www.aacp.org/resources/studentaffairspersonnel/studentaffairspolicies/Documents/OATHOFAPHARMACIST2008-09.pdf.

7. American Pharmacists Association, "Code of Ethics for Pharmacists," October 1994, http://www.pharmacist.com/code-ethics.

response to these challenges is driven by the teachings of the Church. Among the most significant concerns are:

- issues related to contraception (such as the sale of condoms, the dispensing of contraceptive or abortifacient drugs, patient age, and matters of privacy);
- providing oral syringes to individuals who are addicted to or abusing illegal parenteral drugs;
- preparing injections of lethal drugs for the execution of convicted criminals;
- the just cost of pharmaceuticals (including subsidizing the cost of pharmaceuticals for the poor in the United States and in developing nations);
- the use of experimental drugs in children; and
- the sale of cigarettes in a pharmacy, in view of their effects on patient health.

Catholic pharmacists must also understand their right to refuse to engage in certain activities as a right of conscience, and they should be aware of the relevant legal mandates of the state in which they practice. The guidance of the Church is very important in today's complex health-care delivery system. The significance of that guidance will continue in the future, as advances in genetics, pharmacogenomics, and other scientific fields lead to dramatic changes in the provision of health care.

The Nobility of the Pharmacist's Profession

The Roman Catholic Church understands pharmacists as participating in a noble healing profession. The dignity of the pharmacist's calling is rooted in a concern that extends beyond the filling and dispensing of medication to the attentive care of the human person. Working in cooperation with other dignified medical professionals, the pharmacist assists the human person in sustaining his or her health.

For the Catholic, pharmacy practice is caught up in a continuum of salvation, whereby through his or her own work the pharmacist continues the work of God. Pope John Paul II made this clear in *Laborem Exercens*, his 1981 encyclical on human labor. He wrote that the human person is "the image of God partly through the mandate received from his Creator to subdue, to dominate, the earth. In carrying out this mandate, . . . every human being reflects the very action of the Creator of the universe."[8] The pharmacist carries on the divine mission that was begun by God at the beginning of history, illuminated in the pages of the Bible, and culminates in the mission of Jesus Christ.

The Judeo-Christian Sacred Scriptures contain a rich cache of narratives confirming God's attentive concern for the sick and suffering. In the Old Testament, a number of people are healed from the ravages of leprosy and other serious diseases, among them Miriam (Nm 12:1–15); Jeroboam, who had a withered hand (1 Kgs 13:4–6); King Hezekiah, who had a terminal illness (2 Kgs 20:1–11); and Naaman the Syrian

---

8. Pope John Paul II, *Laborem Exercens, On Human Work*, Encyclical Letter, September 14, 1981, no. 4, http://www.vatican.va/holy_father/john_paul_ii/encyclicals/documents/hf_jp-ii_enc_14091981_laborem-exercens_en.html.

(1 Kgs 5). In one instance, the whole nation of Israel is relieved of the burden of the plagues (the account appears in Exodus at 23:25 and in Numbers at 16:14–50 and 21:5–9). Pericopes from Leviticus (3:7–8) and Proverbs (15:4, 30) offer prescriptions for medical care and healthy living.

In the New Testament, the gospel writers give testimony to Jesus' healing powers. The catalogue of sicknesses and diseases that Jesus cured is legion. A sampling of the list includes blindness (told in Matthew 20:29–34 and John 9:1–7), a withered hand (Mk 3:1–5), leprosy (Mt 8:2–4, 20:29–34; and Mk 1:40–44), deafness (Mk 7:32–35), and chronic hemorrhage (Mt 9:20–22; Mk 5:25–34; and Lk 8:43–48). Each of the evangelists records the power that Jesus had to transform the human person's condition of illness and to restore health. Jesus' outreach to the compromised was marked by a compassion that his followers and onlookers had not encountered in other healers. In his healing ministry, Jesus sought not only to treat the medical condition, but also to transform the sick person and to reintegrate the person into the community, which might otherwise have shunned him or her.

These Scripture passages attest to the magnificent transformation experienced by those who approached Jesus or were approached by him. There are myriad other examples of healing stories, but these should suffice to give Catholic pharmacists a real appreciation for the rich tradition of which they are a part. The patient who approaches pharmacists should find in them the same disposition that would be found in the person of Jesus Christ.

Sick people should experience in the pharmacist "some counsel, a reason for hope, or a path to follow."[9] Catholic pharmacists are called to imitate Jesus Christ, their Savior, and to reflect his mission in their attitudes and activities with their patients. This awesome responsibility builds upon their primary vocation as Christians, begun in the sacrament of Baptism, attested to in the sacrament of Confirmation, and strengthened by the Eucharist. It is fortified by the grace of these sacraments of initiation, together with Confession and its graces.

The Catholic pharmacist's task prompts him or her to first develop or deepen a relationship with Jesus Christ. This exhortation is rarely heard by Roman Catholics and is more often associated with Christians of fundamentalist traditions. Yet, this relationship is critically important; developing it and plumbing its depths cannot be bypassed if Catholic pharmacists truly want to know, follow, and imitate Jesus in their profession. Catholic pharmacists can find in the Church's tradition a rich appreciation for both who Jesus is and how relationships with Jesus have been lived out historically by others. The Church's tradition also relies on philosophical concepts that enhance and extend its positions.

9. Pope John Paul II, Address to the Federation of Catholic Pharmacists, November 3, 1990, no. 3, http://www.pfli.org/papalpharmacyallocutions.html#Section2.

Reconsidering the Role of the Catholic Pharmacist

Before we examine these philosophical underpinnings and their critical import to a pharmaceutical morality, it is important to further clarify the Catholic pharmacist's role as an integral part of the larger healing process for the sick person. Pharmacists stand alongside other health-care professionals, with all their scientific and technological skill, also to serve as instruments of the Divine Healer, Jesus Christ, in attending to their patients.

While some outside the profession might mistakenly perceive pharmacists as mere educated businesspeople, their role is far greater. The interaction between a pharmacist and his or her patient must be more than a sterile and anonymous commercial transaction, or this misconception will be reinforced. The pharmacist-patient relationship is often challenged by a lack of continuity; frequently the patient does not have the same pharmacist in the same pharmacy for an extended time. Making an effort to ensure a stable community practice environment will help to build the patient's trust. Although in many communities pharmacies have changed from small local establishments to large corporate entities, the need for outstanding personal patient care and the obligation to provide it remain the same. Pharmacists must embrace their role in the larger schema of healing. If they find that their practice environment does not enable them to exercise their personal and professional values, they may strive to transform the corporate mindset into one of more attentive personal care, one that is more in harmony with the teachings of the Church and of professional organizations.

This undertaking can prove a bit of a challenge in light of the pharmacist's myriad responsibilities. Pharmacists may find themselves tempted to abandon the personal approach for the strictly commercial transaction, but the Church calls them to a higher standard. Catholic pharmacists are to be neighbors, not strangers, to their patients, who expect and need pharmacists to be more than dispensers of medication, but true providers of comprehensive pharmaceutical care.

The Church uses the image of the Good Samaritan as found in Sacred Scripture (Lk 10:25–37) to describe her appreciation for the role of the Catholic pharmacist,[10] who is called to have a respect for the patient that transcends cultural, philosophical, or other differences. Further, the sick person's needs may be deeper and less obvious than can be reached by the medication itself. Certainly it is important for the Catholic pharmacist to fill prescriptions accurately, but the pharmacist should also be encouraged to check in on patients in some way as they are taking their medicine.

The *Code of Ethics for Pharmacists* adopted by the American Pharmacists Association (APhA) at its October 27, 1994, meeting uses the word "covenant" in its preamble to describe the relationship between pharmacist and patient. The APhA explains that this relationship is based on trust placed in the individual pharmacist by society as a whole. While the wording may be unintentional and go unnoticed by

---

10. Ibid., no. 5.

the secular reader, for the believer, this wording resonates as true and accurate. The notion of "covenant" is deeply rooted in the Judeo-Christian Scriptures. It is an agreement between God and humanity in which both parties promise to give each other love and friendship.

Reconsidering the Role of the Pharmacy Patient

The authors of the books of Genesis (1:26–27) and Psalms (8:5–7) emphasize the reality that each and every human life is inherently sacred, from the moment of conception to natural death. Life's dignity is imprinted on the human person and is not something for which the person has to work. The Church teaches that human dignity forms the foundation for all its moral teaching on human rights and responsibilities, justice, and the common good. This foundation should inspire reverence and evoke a sincere desire to affirm and work toward attitudes, speech, and policies that protect the dignity of others. The affirmation may begin with a simple acknowledgment on the part of the Catholic pharmacist that the person seeking product and counsel is not a mere consumer of goods but is rather a person in need of care. The patient is a reflection of God, endowed with a profound dignity.

Life is always to be understood as an end in itself and never a means. Pope John Paul II, in *Evangelium Vitae*, declared with uncompromising clarity that the Church has a profound respect for the life and dignity of the human person from conception to natural death.[11] When popular opinion seeks to negotiate around questions of when life begins, the Christian should stand firm in promoting a "culture of life." As for death, the Church yields to the medical community's definition of death, but does not hedge, even at the point of demise, on the value of life. The Church expects that pharmacists will underscore this teaching on human life as they dispense medication and counsel patients. Some might argue that science and technology offer greater appreciation for human life than does the Church. But in reality, Church teaching values science and technology, but not at the expense of her own moral tradition.

Patients in pharmacies will differ, but the pharmacist must maintain a consistently dignified disposition toward each patient, no matter what culture, color, or creed. This is also something that the APhA highlights in the preamble to its *Code*:

> III. A pharmacist respects the autonomy and
> dignity of each patient.

A pharmacist promotes the right of self-determination and recognizes individual self-worth by encouraging patients to participate in decisions about their health. A pharmacist communicates with patients in terms that are understandable. In all cases, a pharmacist respects personal and cultural differences among patients.

---

11. Pope John Paul II, *Evangelium Vitae, On the Value and Inviolability of Human Life*, Encyclical Letter, March 25, 1995, http://www.vatican.va/holy_father/john_paul_ii/encyclicals/documents/hf_jp-ii_enc_25031995_evangelium-vitae_en.html.

IV. A pharmacist acts with honesty and integrity
in professional relationships.

A pharmacist has a duty to tell the truth and to act with conviction of conscience. A pharmacist avoids discriminatory practices, behavior, or work conditions that impair professional
judgment, and actions that compromise dedication to the best interests of patients.[12]

The Church's understanding of dignity differs from the understanding of the wider
pharmacy community. For the Church, the person standing in line is just that: a person, an *imago Dei*, and thus entitled to be accorded the treatment consonant with
the dignity of that status. This treatment involves attentiveness to the patient, good
counsel and direction, and concern for larger moral questions that may be elicited in
conversation with the patient. The Catholic pharmacist, in order to offer this kind of
care, must keep abreast of changes in the field and of the Church's updated guidance
about those changes.

In its reflections on human dignity, the United States Conference of Catholic
Bishops (USCCB) states that "the measure of every institution is whether it threatens
or enhances the life and dignity of the human person."[13] Building on this appreciation of dignity and the natural law tradition, the Church would then be quick to encourage Catholic pharmacists to choose wisely where and how they work and to be
guided by their consciences.

To Act with Conviction of Conscience

The consciences of Catholic pharmacists are taxed more and more as they must contend with laws mandating the dispensing of emergency contraception, such as Plan B
medication, to interrupt fertilization or ovulation, and intrauterine devices (IUDs),
which are used primarily as a contraceptive but are also employed for emergency contraception. In addition to these highly publicized, controversial medico-pharmaceutical
issues, Catholic pharmacists face other troubling decisions related to dispensing
medication to repeat abusers and preparing drugs for investigational studies, particularly in children. End of life issues, such as use of drugs in capital punishment and
physician-assisted suicide, can occupy a Catholic pharmacist's conscience, because he
or she believes in a different valuation of life. Questions of conscience in these instances can weigh heavily on Catholic pharmacists as they see the quest for scientific and
technological progress trump opportunities for reflection on underlying values and
significant outcomes.

The common postmodern understanding of conscience describes it as a "feeling,"
"private opinion," or "personal peace." Even the American College of Obstetrics and
Gynecology's definition of conscience as "the private, constant, ethically attuned part

---

12. American Pharmacists Association, "Code of Ethics for Pharmacists."

13. USCCB, *Themes of Catholic Social Teaching* Washington, D.C.: USCCB, 2005; available online at
http://www.usccb.org/beliefs-and-teachings/what-we-believe/catholic-social-teaching/themes-of-catholic-
social-teaching.cfm.

of the human character" fails to convey the richness of what conscience is.[14] While surely conscience involves a combination of these elements, they do not define it fully. These incomplete descriptions fail to acknowledge the importance of objective truth that the Church provides for Catholic pharmacists. They yield instead a subjective morality and a relativism contrary to the Church's teaching. Conscience is not a private inner voice telling one what should be done, nor is it an intuition about moral matters.

Rather, a proper understanding of conscience tells us that conscience is first an act of human will oriented toward truth, that is, what is objectively morally good. Second, conscience necessarily also has a view toward moral action. Accordingly, Daniel Sulmasy defines conscience as having two interrelated parts: "(1) a commitment to morality itself; to acting and choosing morally according to the best of one's ability, and (2) the activity of judging that an act one has done or about which one is deliberating would violate that commitment."[15]

The Second Vatican Council, in *Lumen Gentium*, precisely defined conscience:

Deep within his conscience man discovers a law which he has not laid upon himself but which he must obey. Its voice, ever calling him to love and to do what is good and to avoid evil, sounds in his heart at the right moment.... For man has in his heart a law inscribed by God.... His conscience is man's most secret core and his sanctuary. There he is alone with God whose voice echoes in his depths.[16]

In the *Catechism of the Catholic Church*, the Church teaches about the connection of conscience with the objective truth revealed by God:

In the formation of conscience the Word of God is the light for our path; we must assimilate it in faith and prayer and put it into practice. We must also examine our conscience before the Lord's Cross. We are assisted by the gifts of the Holy Spirit, aided by the witness or advice of others and guided by the authoritative teaching of the Church.[17]

In the USCCB's November 2007 document *Forming Consciences for Faithful Citizenship*, the formation of conscience is outlined:

First, there is a desire to embrace goodness and truth. For Catholics this begins with a willingness and openness to seek the truth and what is right by studying Sacred Scripture and the teaching of the Church as contained in the *Catechism of the Catholic Church*. It is also important to examine the facts and background information about various choices. Finally, prayerful reflection is essential to discern the will of God. Catholics must also understand that if they fail to form their consciences they can make erroneous judgments.[18]

14. ACOG Committee, "The Limits of Conscientious Refusal in Reproductive Medicine, *Obstetrics and Gynecology* 110 (2007): 1203–8.

15. Daniel P. Sulmasy, "What Is Conscience and Why Is Respect for It So Important?" *Theoretical Medicine and Bioethics* 29, no. 3 (2008): 135–49.

16. Vatican Council II, *Lumen Gentium, Dogmatic Constitution on the Church, November 21, 1964*, no. 16, http://www.vatican.va/archive/hist_councils/ii_vatican_council/documents/vat-ii_const_19641121_lumen-gentium_en.html.

17. *Catechism of the Catholic Church*, 2nd ed. (Washington, D.C.: United States Catholic Conference, 2000), no. 1785.

18. United States Conference of Catholic Bishops, *Forming Consciences for Faithful Citizenship: A Call*

Formation of conscience is a formidable activity. Catholic pharmacists should desire to know and follow God's will using their God-given gifts of reason and will. God's plan for salvation is found in the divine law, revelation, tradition, and Church teaching. Catholic pharmacists believe that the Church, founded by Jesus Christ and sustained by the Holy Spirit, offers indispensable moral truths. Integrating those truths after discernment leads to a well-formed conscience.

Conscience formation is a process that requires a great deal of prayer, study, reflection, and conversation. Considering the intense efforts involved in forming a conscience, the beliefs or decisions a well-formed conscience renders must be respected as sacred. A conscience clause in law allows Catholic pharmacists to be excused from medical procedures they deem immoral (e.g., preparing injections of lethal drugs to be used for the execution of convicted criminals, or participating in the preparation of blind pharmaceutical studies of children) and from providing medication that can ultimately end a life (e.g., abortifacient drugs). In turn, conscience clauses protect individuals from any resultant employer action against the objecting pharmacist. Some pharmacies uphold this conscience clause when it involves birth control medication; however, they also require a Catholic pharmacist to inform the patient of where the medication can be obtained without a delay in treatment. And, this can be ethically problematic.

Planned Parenthood and other "freedom of choice" organizations, however, consider these conscience clauses inconsistent with *Roe v. Wade,* and they continue to lobby Congress to abandon them. These groups also target Catholic hospitals for their consistent and unapologetic extension of Church belief into the realm of health care. Obviously, within a Catholic environment there generally would be no need to appeal to conscience clauses, unless a member of another religion is bound in conscience to step aside from a procedure. These exempted employees, however, would be the exception rather than the rule.

While Catholic pharmacists' consciences must be respected, Catholic moral theology also holds that patients' consciences should be accorded similar respect. This is the essence of the informed consent clause. No patient can be forced to take medication or undergo a medical procedure against his or her conscience, even if refusal of the medication or procedure ignores or rejects the best and most reasoned medical opinion. This fact requires of the Catholic pharmacist a high esteem for honesty and for the value of conscience over the powers of manipulation.

Formal and Material Cooperation

In some unfortunate instances, because of unjust laws and increasing threats to religious liberties, Catholic pharmacists may find themselves in compromising professional situations, in which they may be forced to participate in an immoral action

---

to Political Responsibility (Washington, D.C.: USCCB, 2007), no. 18, http://www.usccb.org/faithfulcitizenship/FCStatement.pdf.

contrary to God's law or else risk disciplinary action from their employer. In *Evangelium Vitae*, Pope John Paul II admits this painful reality:

Sometimes the choices which have to be made are difficult; they may require the sacrifice of prestigious professional positions or the relinquishing of reasonable hopes of career advancement. In other cases, it can happen that carrying out certain actions, which are provided for by legislation that overall is unjust, but which in themselves are indifferent, or even positive, can serve to protect human lives under threat. There may be reason to fear, however, that willingness to carry out such actions will not only cause scandal and weaken the necessary opposition to attacks on life, but will gradually lead to further capitulation to a mentality of permissiveness.[19]

The pontiff admits the reality that Catholic pharmacists encounter when they are required to participate in or, better, tolerate immoral actions, such as those found in phases of consultation, preparation, and execution of acts against life. Participation in such actions could result in either personal or institutional scandal. In their 2009 *Ethical and Religious Directives for Catholic Health Care Services*, the U.S. bishops amplify the importance of carefully applying these principles to lessen risk of scandal:

The possibility of scandal must be considered when applying the principles governing cooperation. Cooperation, which in all other respects is morally licit, may need to be refused because of the scandal that might be caused. Scandal can sometimes be avoided by an appropriate explanation of what is in fact being done at the health care facility under Catholic auspices. The diocesan bishop has final responsibility for assessing and addressing issues of scandal, considering not only the circumstances in his local diocese but also the regional and national implications of his decision.[20]

John Paul II also teaches that it is a moral duty to abstain from any immoral activity. Denial of this right to abstain violates a basic human right, and this violation of religious rights is unconstitutional in the United States under the First Amendment.

There are certain situations, however, in which Catholic pharmacists attempting to do good participate in some evil. The Church offers us guidance with respect to participation in certain acts where an evil is done, and it helps us to distinguish between principles of "formal" and "material" cooperation. These principles provide a basis for moral discernment about involvement with the action and the degree of sharing in the intention of the principal agent's immoral act. Further distinguishing formal and material cooperation into explicit and implicit and immediate and mediate, respectively, helps us to understand the gravity of the act and the moral complicity of the cooperator. As a caution, these principles should never be used for the purpose of finding creative ways to bypass proper moral obligations.

A pharmacist who cooperates formally in an immoral action is one who does so freely and shares in the intention of the immoral actor. Such cooperation, whether

19. John Paul II, *Evangelium Vitae*, no. 74.

20. United States Conference of Catholic Bishops, *Ethical and Religious Directives for Catholic Health Care Services*, 5th ed. (Washington, D.C.: USCCB, 2009), http://usccb.org/issues-and-action/human-life-and-dignity/health-care/upload/Ethical-Religious-Directives-Catholic-Health-Care-Services-fifth-edition-2009.pdf.

explicit or implicit, is never morally licit. An example of explicit formal cooperation would be a Catholic hospital allowing the dispensing of oral contraceptives in its pharmacy, in order to stave off the risk of pregnancy, or permitting pharmaceutical sterilization in a Catholic health-care setting. An example of implicit formal cooperation would be a Catholic pharmacy, in the interest of saving money, sharing a common laboratory and storefront with a pharmacy that regularly dispenses a spectrum of drugs that are inconsistent with the valuation of life as understood by the Catholic Church (e.g., assisted suicide regimens, fertility drugs, and abortifacients, to name a few).

Pharmacists who act as material cooperators are ones who do so freely, but do not share in the intention of the immoral actor, yet are involved in the performance of an immoral action (the cooperator's action must be good or neutral). Material cooperation may be either immediate or mediate. In the instance of immediate material cooperation, a Catholic pharmacy might consider itself to be acting virtuously in providing pharmaceutical ingredients to another pharmacy that has run short. Those very same ingredients (materials) then could be used by the recipient pharmacy for immoral actions such as contraception, sterilization, euthanasia, and similar actions deemed immoral by the Catholic Church. As for mediate material cooperation, a Catholic pharmacist might donate pharmaceuticals or even manufacturing equipment to, say, an IVF center, clearly engaging in moral activity contrary to Catholic moral teaching. In this example of mediate material cooperation, however, the immoral actions stemming from the recipient center still could have occurred without the help of the Catholic pharmacy's benevolent action.[21]

The Influence of Business on Pharmacy

No one can deny that business has an impact on the Catholic pharmacist, even if he or she is not the business proprietor or works for a large corporation, such as a chain pharmacy. Whether they are self-employed or working for others, Catholic pharmacists must be committed to engaging in just business practices in the pharmacy, and must work toward correcting any perceived deviation from these practices. In conformity with Church teaching on human dignity, the human person should never be treated as an object, but always as a subject. This applies not only to patients, but also to pharmacists, particularly in the areas of price gouging and wages.

Prescription drug prices are rising faster now than they were in recent years, as the Government Accountability Office announced in its February 2011 report.[22] Patients are keenly aware of this frightening truth, and they rightly question the profit margins achieved by drug manufacturers based on prices charged at the point of

---

21. See NCBC Ethicists, "Cooperating with Non-Catholic Partners," in *Catholic Health Care Ethics*, 2nd ed., ed. Edward J. Furton, Peter J. Cataldo, and Albert S. Moraczewski (Philadelphia: National Catholic Bioethics Center, 2009), 266–69; J. F. Keenan and T. F. Kopfensteiner, "The Principle of Cooperation: Theologians Explain Material and Formal Cooperation," *Health Progress* 76, no. 3 (1995): 23–27; and Sulmasy, "What Is Conscience and Why Is Respect for It So Important?"

22. U.S. Government Accountability Office, "Trends in Usual and Customary Prices for Commonly Used Drugs" (GAO-11-306R), February 10, 2011, http://www.gao.gov/products/GAO-11-306R.

dispensing. Pharmacists are also mindful of this price rise from their own histori-cal exposure to pricing schedules, their growing role as arbiters between doctors and insurance companies, and the frustration and distrust they hear from their patients. Some patients turn to international sources for their medications, since they often offer prices significantly lower than those in the United States This practice, however, involves a huge risk, as there is limited regulatory oversight to insure that the medica-tion received is the one prescribed. There is also a great danger that the drugs may be adulterated, counterfeit, or both.

While the government sorts out its concerns, the Church has its own wisdom, which Catholic pharmacists can proffer to the medical community. The Church frames its argument against price-gouging within the framework of seventh com-mandment. In the *Catechism of the Catholic Church*, it teaches:

Even if it does not contradict the provisions of civil law, any form of unjustly taking and keep-ing the property of others is against the seventh commandment: thus, deliberate retention of goods lent or of objects lost; business fraud; paying unjust wages; forcing up prices by taking advantage of the ignorance or hardship of another.[23]

In the Church's understanding, "forcing up prices" (that is, price gouging) is an im-moral act. The price of pharmaceuticals should be a "just price," as Thomas Aquinas defines it:

if either the price exceed the quantity of the thing's worth, or, conversely, the thing exceeds the price, there is no longer the equality of justice: and consequently, to sell a thing for more than its worth, or to buy it for less than its worth, is in itself unjust and unlawful.[24]

Temptation is real, however, and both pharmaceutical manufacturers and pharma-cists may be inclined to raise prices illegitimately. While grieving unjust price in-creases may place an employee pharmacist at risk for violating corporate policy or may compromise his or her employment, that should not be a deterrent to upholding Christian values. This may be difficult when such values oppose the pharmacy's estab-lished policies, especially in light of personal economic circumstances and the need for one's job. However, the Church charges its own members to be examples to others and to act in accord with the moral law.

A just price charged by the pharmaceutical company would account for research and development costs associated with the discovery, development, manufacture, and distribution of a drug, as well as for the generation of a profit for stakeholders. The pharmacy, for its part, must determine a just price to be charged to the patient; this price takes into account the pharmacy's cost in purchasing and dispensing the drug, as well as the actions taken by competing pharmacies. There is the risk, however, that additional monetary accretion, outside of an emergency, has the potential to grow to a point of theft.

One often-overlooked group of stakeholders to be considered in setting a just

---

23. *Catechism of the Catholic Church*, no. 2409.

24. Thomas Aquinas, *Summa theologiae*, trans. Fathers of the English Dominican Province (New York: Benziger Brothers, 1947), II-II, q. 77, a. 1.

price consists of the employees at various levels of drug manufacture and sales. In all its social teaching, the Church has taught consistently that workers are entitled to a just wage. Due compensation provides a living wage, which the bishops of the National Catholic Welfare Conference (precursor to the USCCB), in its 1940 *Statement on Church and Social Order* defined:

The first claim of labor, which takes priority over any claim of the owners to profits, respects the right to a living wage. By the term living wage we understand a wage sufficient not merely for the decent support of the workingman himself but also of his family. A wage so low that it must be supplemented by the wage of wife and mother or by the children of the family before it can provide adequate food, clothing, and shelter together with essential spiritual and cultural needs cannot be regarded as a living wage.

Furthermore, a living wage means sufficient income to meet not merely the present necessities of life but those of unemployment, sickness, death, and old age as well.[25]

Pope John XXIII, in his 1961 encyclical *Mater et Magistra*, taught that the notion of the living wage is connected with justice:

We therefore consider it Our duty to reaffirm that the remuneration of work is not something that can be left to the laws of the marketplace; nor should it be a decision left to the will of the more powerful. It must be determined in accordance with justice and equity; which means that workers must be paid a wage which allows them to live a truly human life and to fulfill their family obligations in a worthy manner. Other factors too enter into the assessment of a just wage: namely, the effective contribution which each individual makes to the economic effort, the financial state of the company for which he works, the requirements of the general good of the particular country—having regard especially to the repercussions on the overall employment of the working force in the country as a whole—and finally the requirements of the common good of the universal family of nations of every kind, both large and small.[26]

In a time of delicate economic maneuvering, the employee's wage must not be sacrificed. Catholic pharmacists in managerial positions have a certain insight and wisdom and should exercise whatever influence they may have to ensure that all subordinate employees, including employee pharmacists, receive a just wage for their positions.

A Catholic Pharmacist in a Postmodern World

The postmodern world is not a homogenous environment. This can present poignant challenges to Catholic pharmacists who desire to be faithful to their religious tradition and live out this fidelity in the workplace. Apart from those working in an ecclesial institution, Catholic pharmacists will find themselves working in pharmacies alongside professionals of other faiths or of no faith.

---

25. Archbishops and Bishops of the Administrative Board of the National Catholic Welfare Conference, *The Church and Social Order* (New York: Paulist Press, 1940), nos. 40–41; currently available in *Pamphlets on the Catholic Church*, vol. 2, *1836–1940* http://books.google.com/books/about/Pamphlets_on_the_Catholic_Church_The_chu.html?id=sU5pAAAAIAAJ.

26. Pope John XXIII, *Mater et Magistra, On Christianity and Social Progress*, Encyclical Letter, May 15, 1961, no. 71, http://www.vatican.va/holy_father/john_xxiii/encyclicals/documents/hf_j-xxiii_enc_15051961_mater_en.html.

Catholic pharmacists may run a great legal risk if they choose to proselytize in their workplaces. Some might suggest that the practice of religion in a capitalistic economy can obfuscate the purpose of the business and interfere with the generation of profit. Religion, however, is not something ancillary to pharmacists, no matter what their faith tradition. For believers, it is part and parcel of their identity. It cannot be expected that Catholic pharmacists (or any religiously devout persons) should suspend their beliefs and values when entering the pharmacy. Can these two forces—business and religion—be reconciled? And if so, how? For Catholic pharmacists, the answer may lie in the Church's call to evangelize.

In 1975, Pope Paul VI promulgated the apostolic exhortation *Evangelii Nuntiandi*,[27] charging all Roman Catholics, not just ordained ministers, to find ways to disseminate the Catholic faith into society. Paul VI was mindful that the Church was losing its authoritative ground and moral voice in an increasingly secularized environment. Yet he also recognized that secularism's attractive enticements were ultimately empty, and that humanity hungered for something deeper. The good news of Jesus Christ, found in the Bible and in the tradition of the Church, offers a lived experience of the kingdom of God, partially manifested in this world and reaching its fulfillment in eternal life.

Some things, such as evangelism, are easier said than done. The pope acknowledged the political, economic, sociological, and even religious obstructions that challenge the promotion of the Catholic faith and its morals. Efforts in evangelization must be motivated by a sincere desire to bring others to the truth about God in Jesus Christ. Before Catholic pharmacists can evangelize, they must first be transformed by their own relationship with God, or their efforts will be mechanistic and empty.

While *Evangelii Nuntiandi* identifies particular venues for evangelization and encourages subsidiarity for application to local levels, Paul VI admitted that there is no specific methodology. However, some obvious principles guide the process. First and foremost, Catholic pharmacists must understand what they believe and appreciate why they believe it. Second, they must convey that understanding and appreciation through the use of sincere dialogue. These conversations must be fresh, not rehearsed or hinting at any arrogance. In the process of evangelizing, Catholic pharmacists are not asking co-workers or patients to join an organization, support a cause, or enroll in a learned society. They are inviting people to the kind of relationship with God and Jesus Christ that has enriched their own lives.

Although this task of evangelization might seem novel, it is far from it: for the Catholic pharmacist, it is nonnegotiable. This duty is rooted in the commission pronounced by Christ in the book of Matthew, bestowed on Catholics at their baptism, and strengthened in their confirmation: "Go, therefore, and make disciples of all nations, baptizing them in the name of the Father, and of the Son, and of the Holy Spirit, teaching them to observe all that I have commanded you" (Mt 18:19–20a). The

---

27. Pope Paul VI, *Evangelii Nuntiandi, On Evangelization in the Modern World*, Apostolic Exhortation, December 8, 1975, http://www.vatican.va/holy_father/paul_vi/apost_exhortations/documents/hf_p-vi_exh_ 19751208_evangelii-nuntiandi_en.html.

Acts of the Apostles describes how Peter, Paul, and other early Church leaders took this commission seriously and brought many people to God in Jesus Christ through repentance and baptism. John Paul II, in an address to the Catholic Union of Italian Pharmacists' national congress in 1994, emphasized this duty:

Your work ... is not limited to dispensing products destined for psychological and physical well-being. As Catholics working in the health-care sector, you are called to play an important human, social, and ethical role. Through contact with all those who rely on your competence, you have an opportunity to become advisers and even evangelizers, precisely because your profession implies trust in your skill and in your humanity.[28]

Such a clear directive should provide impetus for Catholic pharmacists to consider their expression of faith in the workplace with new insight.

Augustine of Hippo, in his fifth-century text *The City of God*, speaks of the disparity between the city of God and the city of Man. Christians live in the city of God, intently anticipating the New Jerusalem, the heavenly city.[29] The city of God has its own vision, values, and virtues, which, even today, compete with those of the city of Man, as they did in Augustine's day. Catholic pharmacists must abide by the legitimate legal and ethical constraints of the city of Man; however, that reality does not excuse them from seeking new, fresh ways to transform the city of Man with the richness of the city of God.

Organization for Solidarity

The challenges are growing for Catholic pharmacists who are trying to be faithful to Catholic moral teachings while working in an increasingly secular, and even anti-religious, marketplace. This is evident not only in the pharmacy field but in the wider health-care arena, most notably in the ongoing struggle between the federal government and the Little Sisters of the Poor over conscience rights.[30] With respect to a pharmacist's legal responsibility to fill a prescription that violates his or her conscience, these cases are informed by individual state governments and state pharmacy boards.[31] If, though, a Catholic pharmacist were to break the law, there is no question that that pharmacist would be subject to legal ramifications. In 2015, in a matter unrelated to health but helpful for understanding the increasing gravity of this matter, Kim Davis became famous for her refusal to issue marriage licenses to same sex couples in Kentucky. Davis contended it countered her own conscience. In turn, Davis joined a historical roll of other citizens who opted for civil disobedience over

---

28. Pope John Paul II, Address to Italian Pharmacists at the National Congress of the Catholic Union of Italian Pharmacists, January 29, 1994, Pharmacists for Life International, http://www.pfli.org/papalpharmacyallocutions.html.

29. Augustine, *City of God*, trans. Marcus Dods (New York: Random House, 1993).

30. Richard M. Doerflinger, "Washington Insider," *National Catholic Bioethics Quarterly* 14, no. 3 (2014): 409–18.

31. National Women's Law Center, "Pharmacy Refusals 101," http://www.nwlc.org/sites/default/files/pdfs/pharmacy_refusals_101.pdf. Accessed September 27, 2015.

compromising their religious beliefs, and was incarcerated for breaking the law.[32]

No matter how far negative feelings toward those matters contrary to the faith may extend, a pharmacist, as a health-care provider, has to recognize that the first responsibility she has toward her patients is telling the truth. The pharmacist then is responsible for helping a patient to understand, for example, the possible side effects and long-term effects of contraceptive drugs, keeping in mind that it could be inappropriate or unprofessional to engage in a conversation about proper moral action. Again, a pharmacist could risk litigation not because of any evangelizing efforts, but because the advice given was outside her professional competency. Finally, while the temptation to alert a parent or guardian is real, any legal aged patient is protected by the confidentiality clauses outlined in the Health Insurance Portability and Accountability Act (HIPAA) of 1996.[33] As painful as it might be religiously and personally to dispense the contraception, unless the pharmacist chooses conscientious objection and, in turn, possible legal consequences, she is legally obliged to fill the patients' prescriptions. It may be a difficult action with few options outside of leaving the industry or transferring to another sector of health care. The Catholic pharmacist, however, may want to be mindful of John Paul II's address to an international gathering of Catholic pharmacists where he speaks of a duty of Catholic pharmacists to be attentive counselors and offer moral help to those they may encounter in their profession.[34]

As Catholic pharmacists endeavor to make their voices heard in a contemporary milieu that pays little or no attention to faith concerns, they should seek out supportive organizations for solidarity. A number of professional groups offer Catholic pharmacists the encouragement and education they need to deepen their commitment to their faith. The International Federation of Catholic Pharmacists (FIPC) is a Church-recognized organization established in 1950.

[Serving] as a forum for debate and action, FIPC endeavors to address all the issues relating to the pharmacist's profession in the light of the Christian faith; it supports the creation of associations of Catholic pharmacists in countries where they do not already exist; it represents these associations before ecclesiastical authorities and international health agencies or entities operating in the fields of health care, economics, and medical ethics, and the training of pharmacists; in respect for the dignity of the human person and with the help and consultancy of constantly updated professionals, it strives to ensure that medicines are within the reach of everyone everywhere. FIPC has a bioethics committee, and develops programs for providing access to life-saving drugs; it encourages the ethical training of pharmacists; it works to alert authorities to the need for schools to provide pharmaceutical training and practice. It holds international congresses and study days at the national level to provide important training opportunities for the members of the member associations.[35]

---

32. See Mary Ellen Snodgrass, "Acts of Conscience and Civil Disobedience," in *Civil Disobedience: An Encyclopedic History of Dissidence in the United States* (New York: Routledge, 2015), 377.

33. See Brian A. Gallagher, "HIPAA Privacy in the Pharmacy," in *Pharmacy Law Desk Reference*, ed. Delbert D. Konnor (New York: Routledge, 2009): 309–38.

34. John Paul II, Address to the Federation of Catholic Pharmacists, 1990.

35. International Federation of Catholic Pharmacists, "Identity," accessed September 27, 2015, http://

On a national level, there was at one time a National Catholic Pharmacists Guild, established in 1962 and based in St. Louis, Missouri, which published the quarterly *Catholic Pharmacist* journal, but it appears that it is no longer active. Many other, more general Catholic medical societies can offer Catholic pharmacists support, but the only other organization that seems to deal specifically with Catholic pharmacists is Pharmacists for Life International. The website for this association of pro-life pharmacists contains a wealth of literature and interactive resources.[36] Additionally, where more than moral support is needed, the American Catholic Lawyers Association provides pro-bono assistance to pharmacists "needing legal assistance in matters of faith and conscience."[37]

There are great reasons to be optimistic for a future seasoned with the dynamism of the Catholic faith. As the third millennium unfolds, Catholic pharmacists are engaged in a renewal of faith and evangelization, firmly grounded in Church tradition and in the life and ministry of Jesus Christ. In a world so willing to jettison the values of faith for a world view guided by entitlement or empty beliefs, contemporary Catholic pharmacists witness to values that can challenge and transform the human condition. Catholic pharmacists offer a reason for hope.

Bibliography

American Association of Colleges of Pharmacy (AACP). "Oath of a Pharmacist." July 2007. http://www.aacp.org/resources/studentaffairspersonnel/studentaffairspolicies/Documents/OATHOFA PHARMACIST 2008-09.pdf.

American College of Obstetrics and Gynecology (ACOG) Committee. "The Limits of Conscientious Refusal in Reproductive Medicine." *Obstetrics and Gynecology* 110 (2007): 1203–8.

American Pharmacists Association. "Code of Ethics for Pharmacists." October 27, 1994. http://www.pharmacist.com/code-ethics.

American Society of Hospital Pharmacists. "ASHP Statement on Pharmaceutical Care." *American Journal of Hospital Pharmacy* 50 (1993): 1720–23.

Archbishops and Bishops of the Administrative Board of the National Catholic Welfare Conference. *The Church and Social Order.* New York: Paulist Press, 1940. Currently available in *Pamphlets on the Catholic Church*, vol. 2, *1836–1940.* http://books.google.com/books/about/Pamphlets_on_the_Catholic_Church_The_chu.html?id=sU5pAAAAIAAJ.

Augustine. *City of God.* Translated by Marcus Dods. New York: Random House, 1993.

Benedict XVI, Pope. General Audience. October 7, 2009. http://www.vatican.va/holy_father/benedict_xvi/audiences/2009/documents/hf_ben-xvi_aud_20091007_en.html. Accessed September 27, 2015.

Catechism of the Catholic Church. 2nd edition. Washington, D.C.: United States Catholic Conference, 2000.

Doerflinger, Richard M. "Washington Insider." *National Catholic Bioethics Quarterly* 14, no. 3 (2014): 409–18.

Gallagher, Brian A. "HIPAA Privacy in the Pharmacy." In *Pharmacy Law Desk Reference*, ed. Delbert D. Konnor, 309–38. New York: Routledge, 2009.

---

www.vatican.va/roman_curia/pontifical_councils/laity/documents/rc_pc_laity_doc_20051114_associazioni_en.html#INTERNATIONAL FEDERATION OF CATHOLIC PHARMACISTS.

36. Pharmacists for Life International, http://www.pfli.org/.

37. American Catholic Lawyers Association, "Faith and Justice," accessed September 27, 2015, http://www.americancatholiclawyers.org/.

Hepler, C. D., and D. M. Angaran. "The Nature of Caring." In *Pharmaceutical Care*, ed. C. H. Knowlton and R. P. Penna, 155–75. New York: Chapman and Hall, 1996.

Hepler, C. D., and L. M. Strand. "Opportunities and Responsibilities in Pharmaceutical Care." *American Journal of Hospital Pharmacy* 47 (1990): 533–43.

Higby, G. F. "Professional Socialization of Pharmacists." In *Social and Behavioral Aspects of Pharmaceutical Care*, ed. N. M. Rickles, A. I. Wertheimer, and M. C. Smith, 109–19. Sudbury, Mass.: Jones and Bartlett Publishers, 2010.

John Paul II, Pope. *Laborem Exercens, On Human Work*. Encyclical Letter. September 14, 1981.

——. Address to Italian Pharmacists at the National Congress of the Catholic Union of Italian Pharmacists. January 29, 1994. Pharmacists for Life International. Accessed September 27, 2015. http://www.pfli.org/papalpharmacyallocutions.html.

——. *Evangelium Vitae, On the Value and Inviolability of Human Life*. Encyclical Letter. March 25, 1995.

——. Address to the Federation of Catholic Pharmacists. November 3, 1990. Pharmacists for Life International. Accessed September 27, 2015. http://www.pfli.org/papalpharmacyallocutions.html#Section2.

John XXIII, Pope. *Mater et Magistra, On Christianity and Social Progress*. Encyclical Letter. May 15, 1961.

Keenan, J. F., and T. F. Kopfensteiner. "The Principle of Cooperation: Theologians Explain Material and Formal Cooperation." *Health Progress* 76, no. 3 (1995): 23–27

NCBC Ethicists. "Cooperating with Non-Catholic Partners." In *Catholic Health Care Ethics*, 2nd edition, ed. Edward J. Furton, Peter J. Cataldo, and Albert S. Moraczewski, 266–69. Philadelphia: National Catholic Bioethics Center, 2009.

Paul VI, Pope. *Evangelii Nuntiandi, On Evangelization in the Modern World*. Apostolic Exhortation. December 8, 1975.

Snodgrass, Mary Ellen. "Acts of Conscience and Civil Disobedience." In *Civil Disobedience: An Encyclopedic History of Dissidence in the United States*, 375–482. New York: Routledge, 2015.

Sulmasy, Daniel P. "What Is Conscience and Why Is Respect for It So Important?" *Theoretical Medicine and Bioethics* 29, no. 3 (2008): 135–49.

Thomas Aquinas. *Summa theologiae*. Translated by Fathers of the English Dominican Province. New York: Benziger Brothers, 1947.

United States Conference of Catholic Bishops. *Themes of Catholic Social Teaching*. Washington, D.C.: USCCB, 2005. Available online at http://www.usccb.org/beliefs-and-teachings/what-we-believe/catholic-social-teaching/themes-of-catholic-social-teaching.cfm.

——. *Forming Consciences for Faithful Citizenship: A Call to Political Responsibility*. Washington, D.C.: USCCB, 2007. Available online at http://www.usccb.org/faithfulcitizenship/FCStatement.pdf.

——. *Ethical and Religious Directives for Catholic Health Care Services*. 5th edition. Washington, D.C.: USCCB, 2009. Available online at http://usccb.org/issues-and-action/human-life-and-dignity/health-care/upload/Ethical-Religious-Directives-Catholic-Health-Care-Services-fifth-edition-2009.pdf.

Vatican Council II. *Lumen Gentium, Dogmatic Constitution on the Church*. November 21, 1964.

PART III

TOWARD A SHIFTING CULTURE

13. APPRENTICED TO CHRIST

The Formation of Catholic Medical Students

The necessary, though alone insufficient, stage through which every person called to be a physician must pass is a period of formal medical education in a medical school, and typically a period of post-graduate medical training in a particular discipline of the profession. With the aim of practicing medicine in truth and love, it is important that the medical student, and then trainee during these formative years of medical education be attuned to the richness of living in faith, and be aware of some of the Catholic thought and teaching underpinning authentically Catholic medical care. This chapter precisely unpacks some of the thought and catechesis essential to this mode of practice. Drawing from magisterial documents and relating the thoughts and teachings from these with the experience of medical education, the author, a medical student, provides a refreshing perspective on the formation of medical students disposed to being fully alive in their faith and professional life in medicine.—*Editors*

The eighth graders sat restlessly as the silver-haired physician took his place in the front of the room. As part of a unit on the vocation of the laity, he had been invited to speak about how he integrates his Catholic faith with his work as a physician.

"Who can name the corporal works of mercy?" he asked.

With some prompting the class eventually listed them: "Feed the hungry," "Shelter the homeless," "Clothe the naked," "Visit the sick and imprisoned," "Give alms," "Bury the dead."

"Who can name the spiritual works of mercy?"

Again, with some encouragement the children called them out: "Instruct the ignorant," "Counsel the doubtful," "Admonish the sinner," "Comfort the sorrowful," "Forgive the sinner," "Bear wrongs patiently," "Pray for the living and the dead."

The physician paused, lowered his head in a brief, silent prayer for mercy, and then began again: "Many think that the sum of my labors as a physician is a singular corporal work of mercy, visiting and, when I am able, healing the sick. In truth, I spend my life instructing, comforting, forgiving, and, at times, admonishing. I am asked to bear the wrongs of my patients and, at every moment, to offer a prayer for the sick and those who have died. Some people say that my duty as a Catholic physician is to evangelize my patient, and this is true. But it is an evangelization through witness. It is my prayer that, in every act I do as a physician, my patient may experience the love and healing touch of Christ, who is the Divine Physician."

The Call of Christ

Your vocation *is one which commits you to the noble mission of service to people in the vast, complex, and mysterious field of suffering.*[1]

Each academic year, interviewers listen to countless prospective medical students explain why they want to become doctors. Although each student will have a multitude of reasons, most will restrict themselves to conveying a single, defining event that clarified an as-yet-unspoken inner desire to become a physician. The savvy applicant will then use the description of this incident as a segue to listing his various honors and accomplishments as he attempts to distinguish himself as truly excellent in the matters of intelligence, academic ability, research, integrity, and community service. The entire discussion is framed around an applicant's self-determination to be a physician and whether he can prove himself worthy of acceptance to the profession. Yet, if we accept the words of John Paul II cited above, the practice of medicine is rooted fundamentally in a calling or vocation to the profession. It is not the applicant's decision to be a physician but rather a calling to the profession that he has chosen to follow that sets him on the course of application to medical school.

How would the parley between applicant and interviewer change if their discussion was one of vocational discernment and readiness to respond to a vocation to medicine? If such a discussion were the premise of medical school application, who would be the members of each incoming class of students? Would the pedigree of the class be diminished? Can we dare to hope that the words of St. Paul, "Those he predestined he also called; and those he called he also justified; and those he justified he also glorified" (Rom 8:30), will apply to medical school applicants? Can we not trust that God begins to prepare the one he will call to serve as a physician from the very moment he first places the call in his servant's heart? That he will lead him to academic excellence, compassionate service to others, research, medical experience, and thereby fulfill and far surpass even the most exacting admission requirements? Imagine the profile on an incoming class if each member came in response to an inner desire to make a sacrifice of his life for the sake of those who are sick and suffering.

---

1. John Paul II, Address to Representatives of the Italian Catholic Doctors, March 4, 1989, no. 2, in *Insegnamenti* XII/1, 480, emphasis added; quoted in Pontifical Council for Pastoral Care to Health Care Workers, *Charter for Health Care Workers* (Boston: St. Paul Books and Media, 1995), no. 3, note 8. Full text of the charter is available online at http://www.ewtn.com/library/CURIA/PCPAHEAL.HTM

Students would be those who asked to be formed in the profession of medicine so that they may, by the mercies of God, offer their bodies as a living sacrifice, holy and pleasing to God, and "be transformed through the renewal of [their] mind[s]" (Rom 12:1–2). Would that every patient know the care of such a physician.

The Vocation of the Physician

To speak of mission is to speak of vocation: the response to a transcendent call which takes shape in the suffering and imploring countenance of the patient.[2]

The vocation of the physician is at once both a witness to the effusive love of God for those who suffer, and an act of love for God who reveals himself in the person of the patient. The Church thus considers health care as an integral expression of her mission to humanity.[3] The Magisterium is therefore right to address the subject of medical formation and the authentic practice of medicine, so as to ensure that those called to follow Christ as physicians receive appropriate education and guidance as they participate in the ministry of the Church. This chapter describes the vocational discernment and formation of physicians in training, as detailed in the magisterial writings.

I turn first to the question of vocation and the application of this term to the work of the physician. The glossary of the *Catechism of the Catholic Church* defines vocation as "[t]he calling or destiny we have in this life and hereafter."[4] All people share a common vocation: God calls all people "to seek him, know him, and love him with all [their] strength";[5] and this is what it means to be holy. This common vocation to holiness has a unique expression in the life of each individual person. The laity—those not called to life as a religious brother, sister, or priest—fulfill their vocation through "engaging in temporal affairs and directing them according to God's will."[6] This call of every person to holiness may seem an unattainable, visionary ideal, yet this is not the case. In a pastoral diocesan visit to Venice, Pope Benedict XVI reminds us:

"Holiness" does not mean doing extraordinary things, but following the will of God each day, living one's own vocation really well with the help of prayer, the Word of God, the sacraments, and the daily effort for consistency. Yes, it takes lay faithful who are fascinated by the ideal of "holiness" to build a society worthy of man, a civilization of love![7]

Asserting holiness as the norm to which a medical student is held does not imply the formation of a new band of miracle-faith healers to be unleashed on the sick and

2. Pontifical Council for Pastoral Care to Health Care Workers, *Charter for Health Care Workers*, no. 3.

3. See ibid., no. 4.

4. *Catechism of the Catholic Church*, trans. USCCB, 2nd ed. (Washington D.C.: United States Catholic Conference, 1997), no. 903.

5. Ibid., no. 1.

6. Ibid., no. 898.

7. Pope Benedict XVI, Address to the Assembly for the Conclusion of the Pastoral Diocesan Visit to Aquileia and Venice, May 8, 2011. http://w2.vatican.va/content/benedict-xvi/en/speeches/2011/may/documents/hf_ben-xvi_spe_20110508_assemblea-chiusura.html.

suffering; rather, these physicians are called to orient the science of medicine to the dignity of the human person, so that the practice of medicine may be worthy of those it serves.

The introduction to the *Charter for Health Care Workers* provides a brief summary of the physician's vocation in the context of the general vocation of the laity. The introduction begins by affirming that "[l]ife is a primary and fundamental good of the human person" and those engaged in health care are engaged in a "service to life ... undertaken ... not only as a technical activity but also as [an expression] of dedication to and love of neighbor."[8] The technical competence of the physician is inseparable from his motivation and intention to use this competence to come to the aid of a patient in need, especially when this requires the physician's self-sacrifice.

Medical formation is a time for students to gain technical competence and to practice the gift of self that is required to practice medicine, recognizing that "[s]cientific and professional expertise are not enough; what is required is personal empathy with the concrete situations of each patient."[9] I myself remember first learning this concept during my preclinical years. I found that, when attempting to force myself to memorize in fine detail the contents of various lectures in anatomy, biochemistry, or physiology, I had little personal motivation to do so. In such moments, I found that I needed only to reflect on the purpose of my studies in order to renew my determination to master the material expected of me. I knew that I would one day be summoned to a patient's bedside because I was a physician, one who had applied herself to the study of medicine so that I could serve one who suffers. Faced with the countenance of Christ in a suffering patient, I could not help but renew my efforts to study, lest my own sluggishness cause me to fail my patient. In my clinical years, I continued to experience the dichotomy between my own listlessness and the urgent summons to place the gift of the medical knowledge and skills I was learning at the service of my patient. This experience was relived with every twilight page for a crash C-section, every eight-hour surgery, every painstaking phone call to obtain past medical records, and every literature search to answer yet another a question that had arisen in the care for a patient.

These repeated exercises of gift-of-self asked of medical students become a school of virtue whereby they learn to think and act as Christ the Divine Physician. They are an indispensable element of formation specific to medical school, a special time when students do not have full responsibility for patient care. This allows students the benefit of time to practice their response to a patient in need with minimal repercussions in patient outcome should the student fail in either knowledge of medicine or generosity of heart. While we do well in the teaching of medical science, it is also necessary to form a student in the generosity of heart required to follow Christ the Divine Physician. Without a basic understanding of vocational formation, a time when a student apprentices himself to the Divine Physician who will be both his

---

8. Pontifical Council for Pastoral Care to Health Care Workers, *Charter for Health Care Workers*, no. 1.
9. Ibid., no. 2.

model of holiness specific to a physician as well as the source of the grace needed to conform himself to this model, the self-sacrifice required in the practice of medicine becomes an unsustainable exercise in sheer personal will-power. To speak of medicine as a vocation removes it from the realm of a personal accomplishment or career and elevates it to a divine mission, intended and sustained through the will of God, for "to care lovingly for a sick person is to fulfill a divine mission, which alone can motivate and sustain the most disinterested, dedicated, and faithful commitment, and gives it a priestly value."[10]

We do medical students a disfavor if we do not approach their application to medical school and their time of education as an examination of vocation and vocational formation. The formation of medical students, like other types of formation, should be neither haphazard nor accidental; rather, it must be systematic and complete, including the essential elements needed to respond fully to the vocation of medicine. These critical elements are described in detail in the *Charter*:

The continuous progress of medicine demands of the health care worker a thorough preparation and ongoing formation so as to ensure, also by personal studies, the required competence and fitting professional expertise.

Side-by-side with this, they should be given a solid "ethico-religious formation" which "promotes in them an appreciation of human and Christian values and refines their moral conscience." There is need "to develop in them an authentic faith and a true sense of morality, in a sincere search for a religious relationship with God, in whom all ideals of goodness and truth are based."[11]

These words provide a road map for the journey of the medical student congruent with the exhortation of Romans 12 that the student be transformed through the renewal of his mind and discern the will of God for the human person.

In the following sections, I examine this journey more fully, beginning with the sincere search for God, then moving to the ideals of truth and goodness found in God and fulfilled through Christ. This leads to a profession of faith, which matures the student's understanding of the content of faith, teaches him to live in a religious relationship with God through prayer and sacraments, and refines his moral conscience. The integration of these essential elements of Christian life with the work of the physician then drive the student to professional and technical competence that confidently applies the norms of conscience to the practice of medicine, thus ensuring the ethical practice of medicine oriented to the true good of the human person recognized in the face of every patient.

---

10. Ibid., no. 6.

11. Ibid., no. 7, making reference to John Paul II, *Dolentium Hominum*, Motu Proprio, February 11, 1985; John Paul II, Address to the Association of Catholic Health Care Workers, October 24, 1986; and Synod of Bishops, Special Assembly for Europe, Concluding Statement, December 20, 1991.

I. The Evangelization of Medical Students

A Sincere Search

It is God who gives to everyone life and breath and everything. He made from one the whole human race to dwell on the entire surface of the earth, and he fixed the ordered seasons and the boundaries of their regions, so that people might seek God, even perhaps grope for him and find him, though indeed he is not far from any one of us. For "In him we live and move and have our being."

(Acts 17:25–28)

These words from the Acts of the Apostles echo in varied expressions of mankind's quest for God throughout history. Indeed, the desire for God is deeply engraved in the human heart, and only in God does the human person find the yearned-for source of truth and goodness.[12] Medical students, too, participate in this quest for God, and the decision to study medicine is, consciously or unconsciously, part of this search. God, in his never-ending love for humanity, responds to this search and draws near to medical students in this special time of formation.

Each student comes to medical school in a different stage of his or her search for God. Some have already found God to be the source of life and are developing a mature relationship with him; their medical education is the next logical response. For others, the search for God may have been forgotten, overlooked, or even explicitly rejected.

People find many reasons to reject the search for God. They may be lured by the cares and riches of the world; they may be distressed by the world's evil or scandalized by the bad example of so-called "believers." They may be ignorant of, indifferent to, or even hostile to religion, or they may simply be trapped in the "attitude of sinful man which makes him hide from God out of fear and flee his call."[13] But, as pointed out by the fathers of Vatican II in *Gaudium et Spes*, the decision to pursue the sciences or arts, including medical formation, reflects an openness to God as he may be found in creation; "the humble and persevering investigator of the secrets of nature is being led, as it were, by the hand of God in spite of himself, for it is God, the conserver of all things, who made them what they are."[14]

Led by God to the study of medicine, the student inevitably finds what the *Catechism of the Catholic Church* calls "converging and convincing arguments" leading to knowledge of God, through both the study of the human body and reflection on the human person encountered in the patient.[15] The study of the human body begins with understanding its function in the physical world and how the laws that govern the

---

12. See *Catechism of the Catholic Church*, no. 27.

13. See ibid., no. 29.

14. Vatican Council II, *Gaudium et Spes, Pastoral Constitution on the Church in the Modern World*, no. 36. All the quotes of Vatican Council II documents are taken from *Vatican Council II: The Basic Sixteen Documents*, ed. Austin Flannery (New York: Costello Publishing, 1996).

15. *Catechism of the Catholic Church*, no. 31.

physical world also govern the body. This study presents the student with concepts of movement, becoming, and contingency, which progressively reveal the world's order and beauty. By reflecting on these realities, the student can come to know God as the origin and the end of the universe.[16] As the medical student attempts to care for patients as human persons rather than just as bodies beset with illness, God's existence is further revealed. The student finds these persons open "to truth and beauty," possessing a conscience and a "sense of moral goodness," and "[longing] for the infinite and for happiness." "In all of this, [the student] discerns signs of [the human person's] soul," a spiritual entity that is "irreducible to the merely material and can have its origin only in God."[17] Thus the study of medicine naturally tends toward discovery and knowledge of God as the first cause and final end of the human person. It is right to pray that students of medicine will hasten along this path of discovery, led by wise and faithful teachers.

Basis for Ideals of Truth and Goodness

The practice of goodness is accompanied by spontaneous spiritual joy and moral beauty. Likewise, truth carries with it the joy and splendor of spiritual beauty.[18]

Physicians dedicate themselves to the pursuit of the truth of the human body and indenture themselves to the service of the good of the human person who is a composite of body and soul. Through the study of the basic sciences and their application in clinical practice, the medical student comes to recognize a master plan for the human body that constitutes "health," contrasting it with deviations that jeopardize physical life, which are the hallmarks of "disease." Medicine is widely thought to be purely scientific and thus philosophically and religiously neutral. The practice of medicine, however, depends on the fundamental philosophical dictum that health manifests the fundamental good and truth of the human body and disease manifests its antithesis. The care of the human body oriented toward the service and preservation of life is thus infused with an intrinsic morality the laws of which lie hidden within the human body. In stark contrast to the relativist tendencies of modern culture, there is little relativism in medicine. The body is unable to forgive the administration of a medicine which is in fact a poison. The existence of an ultimate truth and good of the human body remains uncertain not because it does not exist, but rather because it does exist and physician-scientists as yet know it only imperfectly and so are baffled by it. The study of the human body thus offers an opportune time for the student to ponder the basis of the ideals of truth and goodness, and that is why the *Charter* includes this discussion as an essential element in the formation of medical students.

16. See ibid., no. 32.
17. Ibid., no. 33.
18. Ibid., no. 2500.

The Ideal of Truth

Jesus answered, "For this I was born, and for this I have come into the world, to bear witness to the truth. Every one who is of the truth hears my voice." Pilate said to him, "What is truth?"

(Jn 18:37–38)

The practice of evidence-based medicine demands that every physician struggle to act in accord with the truth of the human body, as revealed by the most current, valid scientific evidence. The presently known truth of the body is, however, incomplete. Ongoing research labors to develop this knowledge so that it may conform more perfectly to the actual truth. Because errors in medical research pose a risk of harm to patients, this research is carefully scrutinized for bias, appropriateness of method, statistical accuracy, completeness of data, and clinical relevance to ensure accurate conclusions. Integrity in the search for the truth of the human body and obedience to this truth are fundamental to the physician's work; how can a doctor claim to serve patients if that service is based in falsehood?

As previously discussed, the knowledge of the science of medicine and technical expertise is not enough to sustain the practice of medicine, because the truth of the human body is rooted in the person of the patient whom the physician serves. For the physician, "the sick person is never merely a clinical case, an anonymous individual on whom to apply the fruit of their knowledge, but always a sick person towards whom they show a sincere attitude of empathy in the etymological sense of the term."[19] Beyond the truth of the human body, the student of medicine must be led to the question of the human person expressed through the body both in a general sense and in the specific person of his patient. The student finds that, at the limit of what medical science can teach, this progression leads to the contemplation of religious truth. John Paul II speaks of this progression from scientific to ultimate religious truths in his encyclical *Veritatis Splendor*. He says:

The development of science and technology, this splendid testimony of the human capacity for understanding and for perseverance, does not free humanity from the obligation to ask the ultimate religious questions. Rather, it spurs us on to face the most painful and decisive struggles, those of the heart and of the moral conscience.[20]

How then can the student learn the truth of the human person that the science of medicine cannot teach? The entirety of his medical studies has shown the student that truth can be known, and if it is not known it is because of the limitations of the one seeking truth. If only there was a person, composite of body and soul, who is the perfection of the human person, who can show man the way of truth and of the life for which he yearns! This thirst for a human model of the truth of the human person as a composite of body and soul changes the student's question from a generic reli-

19. Pontifical Council for Pastoral Care to Health Care Workers, *Charter for Health Care Workers*, no. 2.

20. Pope John Paul II, *Veritatis Splendor*, *The Splendor of Truth*, Encyclical Letter, August 6, 1993, no. 1, emphasis in original, http://www.vatican.va/holy_father/john_paul_ii/encyclicals/documents/hf_jp-ii_enc_06081993_veritatis-splendor_en.html.

gious question to a specific desire for Christ, God who becomes man, in whom the mystery of humanity truly becomes clear. "Christ fully reveals humanity to itself and brings to light its very high calling."[21] A catechesis on the reasons for the Incarnation and how the student comes to know and share in the mystery of Christ is beyond the scope of this discussion. It is enough simply to recognize how the search for the truth of the human body starts the student of medicine on a path that naturally leads to the discovery of the hope offered in Christianity, that there is indeed a Christ who reveals man to himself. In the next section, I will consider the hope that Christ also offers to man to fulfill this truth in himself. This hope forms the basis of the ideal of goodness accessible to every human person.

The Ideal of Goodness

Or what man of you, if his son asks him for bread, will give him a stone? Or if he asks for a fish, will give him a serpent? If you then, who are evil, know how to give good gifts to your children, how much more will your Father who is in heaven give good things to those who ask him!

(Mt 7:9–11)

Patients trust their physicians to work for their good, or at the very least to "do no harm." Although nearly everyone in health care, including patients, agrees that the goal of medical care is the patient's good, the good to be pursued is not always clear. Medical science has the potential to provide many "goods": preventing disease, prolonging life by managing chronic disease, preventing death by healing acute illness, and relieving pain. But how do patients and their physicians know which good to pursue when these goods are in conflict? Should medications be administered despite bothersome side effects? Should preventive care be continued beyond an age when the patient is likely to benefit from it? Should pain be relieved at the expense of a shortened life expectancy? In order to avoid harming the patient in the name of serving a "greater good," medical students must have a clear understanding of the true good of the human person, and of the role of medicine in pursuit of this good.

At this point, let me pause to address the experience of death. Physicians are powerless to alter the ultimate course marked by death. What, then, is the response of the physician to the final journey of his patient into the valley of death? Does he retreat and leave the patient in his final hours, afraid of the truth that death teaches man about his human condition? In an ancient funeral discourse, St. Ambrose exhorts:

Death was not part of nature; it became part of nature. God did not decree death from the beginning, he prescribed it as a remedy. Human life, because of sin … began to experience the burden of wretchedness in unremitting labor and unbearable sorrow. There had to be a limit to its evils; death had to restore what life had forfeited. Without the assistance of grace, immortality is more of a burden than a blessing.[22]

---

21. Vatican Council II, *Gaudium et Spes*, no. 22.

22. St. Ambrose, *De excessu fratris sui Satyri* [On the Decease of His Brother Satyrus], II, 47 (CSEL 73, 274), quoted in Pope Benedict XVI, *Spe Salvi, On Christian Hope*, Encyclical Letter, November 30, no. 10.

We hear in St. Ambrose's text an echo of the inner contradiction inherent in the practice of medicine: On the one hand, the patient and those who love him wish to postpone death as long as possible. On the other hand, no patient asks to live indefinitely,
for to live always in the present world seems monotonous and ultimately unbearable.
Death offers man a cure for this inner contradiction, and so death becomes a moment
of healing that the physician must embrace if he is truly to place his craft of medicine
in service to the human person.

What is it, then, that a patient ultimately seeks, not only from his physician but
in life? Certainly it is life without end, a blessed life, a life of unending happiness. In
his encyclical *Spe Salvi*, Pope Benedict XVI says that "we cannot stop reaching out
for [this life], and yet we know that all we can experience or accomplish is not what
we yearn for, . . . [and this] is the cause of all forms of despair."[23] Human experience
leads us to imagine eternal life as an unending succession of calendar days in a life
that we cannot bear to lose and yet that often brings more suffering than joy. Man
yearns for a life of perfect and unending joy that he cannot hope to attain while he
lives. Indeed, man's heart causes him to hope in the possibility of an eternal life that
will be an infinite moment of joy, when, as Jesus says in John's Gospel, "I will see you
again and your hearts will rejoice and no one will take your joy from you" (Jn 16:22).

If such a life exists, it cannot be known while living. Death opens the door to enter
into this blessed life and as such it is beyond the confines of scientific inquiry. What
then can the physician say to his patient who is faced with the moment of crossing
into a life the existence of which the physician's science can neither prove nor deny?
In times when religion played a more prominent role in society, the physician had the
freedom to yield to members of the clergy to guide patients and families through the
mystery of death. But as modern man seems to turn less and less to religion to help
him understand the mysteries of life and death, a void is left for patients and families
imminently facing these mysteries. This void is often recognized only by the physician, who is the first to see death's summons for a patient as a disease advances to its
final stages.

How is the physician to respond to those desperately seeking a shepherd for this
final journey? For patients and patient families who share a common hope in the eternal joy offered through death, these end-of-life discussions and decisions are simple.
The goals of medical care change, and the physician, rather than offering medicines
to cure or at least prolong life, instead offers medicines to give bodily comfort during the final hours. More difficult are the discussions with patients or families who
do not share this hope and instead fear the loss of life or loss of their loved one, even
if medical science is powerless to restore the life that is slowly slipping away. In such
cases, physicians often retreat to terms such as "futile care" and cost/benefit ratio.
But "futility" and "cost/benefit ratio" seem cold, inhuman, impersonal terms inappropriate to the discussion of the specific person of a patient to whom the physician
has vowed his self-giving love and service at all cost. What is left to consider, then, is

23. Benedict XVI, *Spe Salvi*, no. 12.

whether the advances of medical science will be exercised with the intention of staving off death as long as possible, thereby postponing the patient's passage into eternal beatitude. In such a circumstance, will the physician dare to speak freely of death and its role in human life, or will he turn his back and ask others, such as hospice workers, to help the patient or family "let go" so that he will not be reminded of his failure?

I do not mean to open the discussion of "futile care." I do, however, think that it is fundamental to the practice of medicine that death is understood as an essential moment in every patient's life that must be embraced, not feared or avoided no matter the cost. Hope allows the physician to comfort his patient and their family until the last breath. Without hope there is only fear and despair; the physician retreats, and the patient and family make this final journey alone. Javier Cardinal Barragán encourages physicians faced with the imminent death of a patient in his address "The Profile of the Catholic Medical Educator":

Death is not a frustration for physicians, but rather a triumph, as they accompanied their patients in such a way that they have been able to use their talents to the full at each stage of their life. When it has reached its end, the medical function ends, not with a cry of impotency but rather with the satisfaction of a mission fulfilled, both by the patient and by the physician.[24]

Having now strayed far from the original discussion of this section, namely that the desire for the absolute good of the human person drives the practice of medicine, let me draw the preceding discussion of the physician's encounter with the death of his patient into the pursuit of the absolute good of the human person. Medicine is irrational if it is not based on the hope that the human person can experience his own good and that medicine, through its service to the body, helps man to achieve this good in part, all the while pointing toward the complete fulfillment of this good in a life not yet known on earth. Just as the experience of the study of the human body leads to the discovery of the human person and the hope that, in Christ, this truth can be known by man, so likewise the study of the good of the human body leads naturally to the question of the good of the human person and the hope that this good can be attained.

Here again, Christianity offers to the student of medicine the hope that there exists not only an absolute truth of the human person that can be known through the person of Jesus Christ, but also that Christ makes it possible for each person to share in this truth and so fulfill his humanity. The end of the study of the human body is the human person, and the student of medicine is left with a choice of disposition: he may either despair that the good of the human person is limited to life on earth, or he can hope that the yearning of the human heart for a good unattainable in earthly life is not in vain. If the physician chooses despair, all that he can offer is the possibility of avoiding death as long as possible, thereby sentencing his patient to the monotony of daily life. The physician who dares to hope in the good offered to man through

---

24. Javier Lozano Barragán, "On Catholic Teachers of Medicine," *Zenit*, July 21, 2007, https://zenit.org/articles/on-catholic-teachers-of-medicine/.

Christ, however, assists his patients in attaining the good of their bodies, all the while cognizant that bodily life will culminate in an ultimate good of the human person, which can be experienced only when the body can no longer survive.

What value is there in caring for a body that will only pass away and return to dust? A similar question can be posed to the human conception of eternal happiness: In his earthly life, man can know happiness only through his body's perception of the good, so can eternal life really offer man the experience of the good apart from his body? In Christ, man is assured that he will share in eternal happiness in both body and soul. Christ, at the end of his earthly ministry, having suffered death and been resurrected from the dead, ascended body and soul into heaven. It is the essence of Christian hope, that we too will follow after him and that one day, our souls united with their bodies will rest in eternal joy. This hope of the resurrection of the body infuses the work of the physician with eschatological significance, linking the work of the physician with that of the priest, as Pope John Paul remarks:

> You are aware of the close relationship, the analogy, the interaction between the mission of the priest on the one hand and that of the health-care worker on the other: all are devoted, in different ways, to the salvation of the person, to the care of his health, to free him from illness, suffering, and death, to promote in him life, wellbeing and happiness.[25]

Although modern man may have forgotten the role of the clergy in the care of the human person, the physician must not. The human body shares in the dignity of the image of God because it is animated by a spiritual soul, and yet the soul does not perish when it separates from the body at death; instead, it will be reunited with the body at the final Resurrection.[26] Indeed, the human person is fundamentally an embodied person—while on earth he needs the care of both physician and priest.

II. The Catechesis of Medical Students

Those who accepted his message were baptized; some three thousand were added that day. They devoted themselves to the apostles' instruction and the communal life, to the breaking of bread and the prayers.

(Acts 2:42)

The only appropriate response to the recognition of Christ as the truth and the ultimate good of humanity, as well as the means to live according to this truth and so to attain eternal life, is a response of faith. The student who chooses to hope in the good offered through Christ must, in the end, proclaim, "I believe." This proclamation marks the beginning of a new moment in his formation, the time of catechesis. In our present context, the affirmation of Catholic health care, this also marks the point at which the formation of the medical student becomes specifically Catholic—the

---

25. John Paul II, Discourse for the 120th Anniversary of the Bambino Gesù Hospital, March 18, 1989, no. 2, in *Insegnamenti* XII/1, 605–8, quoted in Pontifical Council for Pastoral Care to Health Care Workers, *Charter for Health Care Workers*, 20, note 9.

26. See *Catechism of the Catholic Church*, nos. 364, 366.

catechesis offered to the student who has come to believe in Christ is the fullness of revelation as passed on through the Catholic tradition. This education is not, strictly speaking the responsibility of medical educators, although those formally trained in catechesis may also function in this capacity, but it is most properly overseen by those members of the Church whose duty it is to provide formal catechesis. This formation, carried out in conjunction with the formation required for medical expertise, assists the student in developing an authentic faith, a religious relationship with God that is lived through prayer and the sacraments, and a refined moral conscience capable of acting in conformity with what is truly good for the human person. There is no need in this chapter to provide a detailed account of the content of faith or the mystical theology of the Church; rather, I will highlight several key elements of catechesis of medical students that are of particular significance.

An Authentic Faith

Faith is man's response to God, who reveals himself and gives himself to man, at the same time bringing man a superabundant light as he searches for the ultimate meaning of his life.[27]

In a keynote address given at a medical research conference I attended as a resident, the speaker remarked, "We need research. Research is the key to breaking down the barriers of religion and politics." If the above discussion achieves nothing else, my hope is that it reveals the absurdity of the speaker's statement. In matters of faith, science and research, it may seem, can do nothing except remain silent. (Research may have a role in dissolving political barriers, but I will leave this discussion to scholars of law and government.) Despite the volumes of scholarly thought that continually affirm that there can be, and there exists in fact, no discrepancy between faith and reason in matters of truth, scientists seem rarely to have use for faith, operating instead according to the principle that research is the method by which reason ascertains what is true and there can be no other vehicle of truth. Only a clear understanding of the relationship between faith and reason can spare the student the task of painstakingly dividing his life into separate spheres: medicine, where research reigns supreme, and the remainder of life, where the truth that comes from faith directs the ebb and flow of life.

Let me be absolutely clear: medical research is indispensable to the authentic practice of medicine. The entirety of the content of medical science as it pertains to the raw matter of the human body, the diseases that beset the body, and the body's physiological response to various treatment modalities is the fruit of diligent medical research. Science alone, however, cannot fully uncover the meaning of the human body as it pertains to the fulfillment of the human person. This knowledge is the fruit of faith—both an act of faith and the content of faith to which a believer gains access through his act of faith. The *Catechism* reminds the student that it is "the same

27. Ibid., no. 26.

God who reveals mysteries and infuses faith, who has bestowed the light of reason on the human mind.... God cannot deny himself, nor can truth ever contradict truth ... [for in fact] the things of the world and the things of faith derive from the same God."[28] The student of medicine is thereby permitted, and in fact required, to integrate his seemingly disparate lives of faith and science with the confident expectation that reason governed by faith will lead him to the truth of the human body as integral to the truth of the human person.

In what does faith consist? Faith is an act by which the human person completely submits both intellect and will to the truth as it is revealed and "guaranteed by God, who is Truth itself."[29] The *Catechism* teaches that faith is a gift of God, a supernatural virtue infused by him, and yet faith remains an authentically human act that is not contrary to human dignity or to human reason.[30] What must be clearly stated, however, is that the impetus driving a student's act of faith is not the apparent truth and intelligibility of God's existence. The masterful catechist or medical educator may be able to convince a skeptical student of the plausibility of the existence of God, but he or she will never be able to summon the response of faith. This response can come only from an encounter with the living God. It is God's revelation of himself to the student as he who can neither deceive nor be deceived, the author of all that is true, that has the power to summon forth an act of faith.[31]

Such encounters belong to the designs of God's loving pursuit of each person and are not subject to the schedules of catechists or medical educators. The responsibility of catechists and medical educators is to ready the student for this encounter and then to assist the student in maturing the response of faith (*fides qua*) through the study of the deposit of faith (*fides quae*). This requires a systematic and complete catechesis, whereby the student comes to know more fully this God who has not only summoned him to the practice of medicine but has revealed himself and has drawn the student to himself through bonds of love that are capable of silencing the fears of uncertainty and the bonds of evil. What a wondrous time for the student called by God to the service of medicine, a time when he finds in Christ not only the fulfillment of the perfect physician who offers healing to all who come to him, but also a kind and gentle teacher who holds the secrets of life, who will fashion the student to resemble his teacher more closely in word and deed, that he too may learn to be a physician like his Divine Teacher. The authentic practice of medicine presupposes an understanding and assent to the entire deposit of faith. If the student is deprived of a full and complete presentation of the deposit of faith, how will he ever hope to know and serve the good of his patients?

28. Ibid., no. 159.
29. See ibid., no. 144.
30. See ibid., nos. 153–54.
31. See ibid., no. 156.

A Religious Relationship with God

What faith confesses, the sacraments communicate.[32]

Given the academic rigors of medicine, it is tempting to confuse knowledge of the deposit of faith in Sacred Scripture and tradition with adequate catechesis. However, the heart of catechesis is not a book, but rather a person, Jesus of Nazareth.[33] Full knowledge of God is possible only through an intimate relationship with Christ, the splendor of the Father, who promises that all who remain in him remain in the Father.[34] The authentic catechesis of medical students must lead the student to encounter and enter into communion with Christ, particularly in the sacramental life of the Church. This is of foremost importance, given that the aim of authentic Catholic medical formation is not only the education of physicians, but their transformation to think and act as Christ, the Divine Physician. Pope John Paul II, in his apostolic exhortation *Catechesi Tradendae*, points out, "[F]or it is in the sacraments, especially in the Eucharist, that Christ Jesus works in fullness for the transformation of human beings."[35] Thus medical students must be helped to understand the gift offered to them in the sacraments and be given opportunity to partake of these sacraments. For as John Paul II warns, "Sacramental life is impoverished and very soon turns into hollow ritualism if it is not based on serious knowledge of the meaning of the sacraments, and catechesis becomes intellectualized if it fails to come alive in the sacramental practice."[36] This may require creativity on the part of catechists and pastors, particularly as students take on clinical responsibilities that entail working long and odd hours that do not easily lend themselves to participation in traditional parish life. The hospital chaplain, who tends to the spiritual and sacramental needs of health-care workers as well as patients, can be of tremendous assistance in this regard. The chaplain's loving concern can provide a source of strength to students who are being asked to rise above their personal needs for sleep, food, and companionship, in order to serve their sick and suffering brethren.

The relationship with God forged through the sacraments is nurtured through the life of prayer. The mystery of faith requires that the Christian believe, celebrate, and live in a vital and personal relationship with the living and true God through prayer.[37] But many medical educators would likely admit that teaching a student medicine seems easier than teaching the student how to pray. The words of St. Paul are all too true: "we do not know how to pray as we ought" (Rom 8:26). The living tradition of the Church provides an inexhaustible treasury of spiritual wisdom on

---

32. Ibid., no. 1692.

33. See Pope John Paul II, *Catechesi Tradendae, On Catechesis in Our Time*, Apostolic Exhortation, October 16, 1979, no. 5, http://w2.vatican.va/content/john-paul-ii/en/apost_exhortations/documents/hf_jp-ii_exh_16101979_catechesi-tradendae.html.

34. See *Catechism of the Catholic Church*, no. 35.

35. John Paul II, *Catechesi Tradendae*, no. 23.

36. Ibid.

37. See *Catechism of the Catholic Church*, no. 2558.

prayer in its many forms; in the end, however, the believer relies on the Holy Spirit, who intercedes for Christians according to God's will.[38] The method of teaching is of less importance; it is essential only that students learn *to* pray. To do so, they will need the opportunity to pray, the example of others, and responsible guidance as they develop this relationship with God.

It is worth reflecting on why the formation of a religious relationship with God is critical to medical formation and why it is not merely a pious aspiration to imitate Christ. The physical and intellectual work of learning both the science of medicine and the clinical care of patients is daunting, requiring long hours and personal sacrifice. Added to this burden is the spiritual work of being present, as the mysteries of life, death, sickness, and suffering unfold in the lives of patients. In short, every day offers new questions and new tasks for the medical student; always there is the potential that the student's physical and spiritual strength will be overwhelmed. But a vibrant relationship with God, based on the sacraments and enriched through the spiritual life, connects the student with an inexhaustible source of strength and wisdom, refreshing the wearied soul and helping the student to carry out all God's work in medical practice.

A True Sense of Morality and a Refined Moral Conscience

By the sacraments of rebirth, Christians have become "children of God," "partakers of the divine nature." Coming to see in the faith their new dignity, Christians are called to lead henceforth a life "worthy of the Gospel of Christ." They are made capable of doing so by the grace of Christ and the gifts of his Spirit, which they receive through the sacraments and through prayer.[39]

Steeped in Christ's mystery and transformed by sacramental grace into a new creature, the student now "sets himself to follow Christ and learns more and more within the Church to think like Him, to judge like Him, to act in conformity with His commandments, and to hope as He invites us to."[40] A thorough and complete catechesis of medical students must necessarily "reveal in all clarity the joy and the demands of the way of Christ."[41] The *Catechism* lists eight essential elements of this catechesis. The formation of a true sense of morality and a refined conscience includes: (1) *"a catechesis of the Holy Spirit,* ... who inspires, guides, corrects, and strengthens this life"; (2) *"a catechesis of grace,"* through which mankind is saved; (3) *"a catechesis of the beatitudes* ... [as] the only path that leads to the eternal beatitude for which the human heart longs"; (4) *"a catechesis of sin and forgiveness"* whereby man admits that he is a sinner and comes to know the truth about himself and through the offer of forgiveness is able to bear this truth; (5) *"a catechesis of the human virtues* which

---

38. See Rom 8:26–27.

39. *Catechism of the Catholic Church*, no. 1692, quoting Jn 1:12; 1 Jn 3:1; 2 Pet 1:4; and Phil 1:27.

40. John Paul II, *Catechesi Tradendae*, no. 20.

41. See *Catechism of the Catholic Church*, no. 1697.

causes one to grasp the beauty and attraction of right dispositions towards goodness"; (6) *"a catechesis of the Christian virtues* of faith, hope and charity" which animate the human virtues; (7) *"a catechesis of the twofold commandment of charity* set forth in the Decalogue"; and finally (8) *"an ecclesial catechesis"* that opens to each person the manifold exchange of spiritual goods in the communion of saints that allows the "Christian life [to] grow, develop, and be communicated."[42]

As previously discussed, the work of the physician is the care of human persons. Thus a moral character is imparted to even the most menial of tasks carried out in the course of the physician's day. Each of the elements of catechesis listed is essential to the moral formation of a physician if he is to be conformed ever more to the image of Christ the Divine Physician. But perhaps this is too much to expect from a physician. It is easy to see how a physician whose lapse in response to a patient in dire need leads to the suffering or death of that patient is guilty of a moral atrocity. But if considered in the fullness of its implication, the same can be said of failure in even menial tasks, although often with less severe patient consequences. Neglect in filling out medical pre-authorizations from insurance companies, or the failure to return regularly to the body of medical literature to ensure that one offers the most appropriate treatment available to a patient, may attain to moral failure, since they may result in real injury to a patient. Further, they cause failure in one's vocation. In fairness, such failures are rarely done with mal-intent; rather, they are consequent upon other demands that are placed on the physician, either through no fault of his own or, at times, through personal choices that leave him indisposed to fulfill his responsibilities. The practice of medicine is a grueling school of virtue that rarely forgives a physician a moment of rest or repose, let alone moments of sloth, imprudence, cowardice, or gluttony. The formation of virtue is the only respite of the physician; he may rest assured that he has been granted strength through repeated acts in conformity with the good and through the gift of God, that he will choose what is good and not necessarily what is easy.

Virtue, however, is not enough. The physician is in dire need of conscience, which alone is able to scrutinize the moral dimensions of human behavior in light of the good as it is understood. The role of conscience in human behavior is not limited to those who profess a particular religion, as St. Paul affirms in his letter to the Romans:

When the Gentiles who do not have the law keep it as by instinct, these men, although without the law, serve as a law for themselves. They show that the demands of the law are written in their hearts. Their conscience bears witness together with the law, and their thoughts will accuse or defend them on the day when, in accordance with the gospel I preach, God will pass judgment on the secrets of men through Christ Jesus. (Rom 2:14–16)

The mere presence of conscience, however, does not guarantee the veracity of its judgments. Is this not the heart of the moral climate of modern day, wherein "what is right for you is not right for me"? If we accept the unity of truth and that an action cannot be at one time both good and evil, then the flaw in the discernment of what is truly good must lie not in the good itself, but in the person who is seeking the good.

---

42. See ibid.

In order to recognize a good and to act in conformity with it, conscience must be formed. The *Catechism* reminds us, "The education of conscience is indispensable for human beings who are subjected to negative influences and tempted by sin to prefer their own judgment and to reject authoritative teachings."[43] For the medical student, this education of conscience requires a thorough study of the dignity of the human person and the implications of this dignity for the care of the human body, beginning at the time of conception and persisting through the moment of death.

III. Vocational Formation

Thus far I have described the soil in which the seed of a vocation to medicine is planted. Important elements to help that seed flourish include the discovery of God as the source of truth and goodness, the profession of faith and the discovery, in Christ, of the fullness of truth about the human person, and the means of attaining eternal life. Now I turn to the formation specific to the student who is called to follow Christ the Divine Physician. I consider the question of what skills are essential to the practice of medicine. These include competence in the science and practice of medicine, professional expertise, and ethical-religious formation.

Required Competence

Health-care activity is based on an interpersonal relationship of a special kind. It is "a meeting between trust and conscience." The "trust" of one who is ill and suffering, and hence in need, who entrusts himself to the "conscience" of another who can help him in his need and who comes to his assistance to help and care for him and cure him.[44]

The nature of the health-care relationship as a meeting between trust and conscience elevates the acquisition of technical expertise and competence from that of a career requirement to that of an ethical mandate. A student who comes to medical school in response to an authentic vocation to medicine is ethically bound to commit fully to its required academic studies and clinical clerkships, thus fulfilling his or her vocation as a lay person. As John Paul II says, "To respond to their vocation, the lay faithful must see their daily activities as an occasion to join themselves to God, fulfill his will, serve other people, and lead them to God in Christ."[45] Indeed, those who have apprenticed themselves to Christ, the Divine Physician, should be role models for their classmates both by their commitment to excellence in their studies and by their loving care of their patients.

---

43. Ibid., no. 1783.

44. Pontifical Council for Pastoral Care to Health Care Workers, *Charter for Health Care Workers*, no. 2, quoting Pope John Paul II, Address to the Participants at Two Congresses of Medicine and Surgery, October 27, 1980.

45. John Paul II, *Christifidelis Laici, On the Vocation and the Mission of the Lay Faithful in the Church and in the World*, Apostolic Exhortation, December 30, 1988, http://w2.vatican.va/content/john-paul-ii/en/apost_exhortations/documents/hf_jp-ii_exh_30121988_christifideles-laici.html, no. 17.

The acquisition of medical competence is also important for the lay vocation's missionary aspect, which calls the medical student to go out into the Lord's vineyard and transform it according to God's plan. Just as Christ took on human nature to allow humans a share in divine nature, so too must medical students learn the culture of medicine if they are truly to transform medical culture and orient it toward the kingdom of God.[46] They must speak the language of medicine, learn its practices, and be one with their fellow physicians. Only thus can they gain the legitimacy that will be needed to effect the evangelization and conversion of medical culture. It is inexcusable for any student of medicine, particularly one who is responding to a vocation to medicine, to present himself to a patient as a physician without first having given himself fully to the study of medicine. The patient trusts that the physician is a master of his craft. The authentic physician returns day after day to the body of medical literature so that he may ever know more fully the truth of the human body and may better serve his patient.

Professional Expertise

I have no doubt that the *Charter*'s writers did not intend by "professional expertise" what the Accreditation Council for Graduate Medical Education (ACGME) meant by "professionalism" as a core competency of both resident and medical student education. It is worth noting however, that the fulfillment of the *Charter*'s criteria for authentic medical practice far exceeds the ACGME's requirement of professionalism, which is described as:

(1) compassion, integrity, and respect for others; (2) responsiveness to patient needs that supersedes self-interest; (3) respect for patient privacy and autonomy; (4) accountability to patients, society, and the profession; and (5) sensitivity and responsiveness to a diverse patient population.[47]

It is hard to imagine that any apprentice of Christ the Divine Physician would not embody each of these characteristics.

---

46. See Congregation for the Clergy, *General Directory for Catechesis*, 1998, no. 139, http://www.vatican.va/roman_curia/congregations/cclergy/documents/rc_con_ccatheduc_doc_17041998_directory-for-catechesis_en.html.

47. Accreditation Council for Graduate Medical Education, "Common Program Requirements," ACGME Outcome Project, July 1, 2016, http://www.acgme.org/Portals/0/PFAssets/ProgramRequirements/CPRs_07012016.pdf.

Ethical-Religious Formation

In fidelity to the moral law, health-care workers live out their fidelity to the human person, whose worth is guaranteed by the law, and to God, whose wisdom is expressed by the law.[48]

Medical students are trained to search the medical literature, critically appraise what is known about a clinical topic, and use this knowledge to guide patient care. Similarly, medical students must be taught a legitimate and systematic approach to bioethical questions. Every Catholic physician should be able to efficiently find and comprehend the bioethical teachings of the Magisterium. Before discussing how this can be accomplished, it is important to recognize that the bioethical teaching of the Magisterium is distinct from the academic discipline of bioethics, which proceeds according to its own rules and procedures to address bioethical questions. The discussions of bioethicists are not ethically binding; only the final conclusions of these discussions that are formally taught by the Magisterium have the authority to guide the actions of physicians.

But how is the physician to proceed when the advances of science and the therapies available to patients daily progress beyond the teaching of the Magisterium. Is the physician to stagnate his practice while the Magisterium considers the ethical implications of each new discovery? In this it is seen why the physician cannot content himself simply with knowledge of the body of the bioethical teaching of the Magisterium. Rather he must also have a working knowledge of bioethics that he may recognize when a medical advance broaches an ethical dilemma and seek appropriate guidance. While on the one hand, the Magisterium affirms that "[h]ealth-care workers, especially doctors, cannot be left to their own devices and burdened with unbearable responsibilities when faced with ever more complex and problematic clinical cases arising from bioethical possibilities,"[49] the bishops also require that "all health-care workers be taught morality and bioethics."[50] Since medicine is first and foremost a service to life, and since each act of medicine made in the name of service to life is at its heart a moral action, the physician's training finds its source and summit in his moral formation. The separation of the study of bioethics from the study of medicine is artificial and unsustainable. If the field of bioethics develops apart from actual service to a patient, it recedes into a body of abstract rules and principles that in each passing age becomes less accessible to the common physician, whose practice may then stray further and further from its intended purpose of serving the good of a patient. In mandating the bioethical formation of all future physicians, the Church reverences the service of physicians to their brethren. The physician then can freely submit his own moral considerations to the guidance of the Magisterium, knowing that he, too, shares the mission to help man achieve his final good.

---

48. Pontifical Council for Pastoral Care to Health Care Workers, *Charter for Health Care Workers*, no. 6.
49. Ibid., no. 8.
50. Ibid., no. 7.

The Role of Medical Educators

This search for God demands of man every effort of intellect, a sound will, "an upright heart," as well as the witness of others who teach him to seek God.[51]

Thus far we have focused on the medical student's own responsibility to engage his formation in a way that leads him to conform his vocation to medicine more perfectly. But medical students are not left to make this journey on their own and without the help of trusted guides. Catholic medical educators are entrusted with the responsibility to assist students on this journey of faith through the active witness of a medical practice fully informed by the Gospel. Pope Paul VI, in his apostolic exhortation *Evangelii Nuntiandi*, reflects on the potential for such witness,

Above all the Gospel must be proclaimed by witness. Take a Christian or a handful of Christians who, in the midst of their own community, show their capacity for understanding and acceptance, their sharing of life and destiny with other people, their solidarity with the efforts of all for whatever is noble and good. Let us suppose that, in addition, they radiate in an altogether simple and unaffected way their faith in values that go beyond current values, and their hope in something that is not seen and that one would not dare to imagine. Through this wordless witness these Christians stir up irresistible questions in the hearts of those who see how they live: Why are they like this? Why do they live in this way? What or who is it that inspires them? Why are they in our midst? Such a witness is already a silent proclamation of the Good News and a very powerful and effective one.[52]

Just as the physician reveals the face of Christ to patients, so too medical educators reveal Christ to their students. If the preceding discussion of medical education as an occasion for the evangelization of medical students is accepted, then those entrusted with their education function as de facto evangelists and catechists. Therefore, the documents of the Church that deal specifically with the discipline of catechesis provide insight into the work of forming medical students. John Paul II, in *Catechesi Tradendae*, reminds catechists that at the heart of catechesis is found in essence a Person, the Person of Jesus of Nazareth, who offers the student knowledge of God and of himself, and the means of transformation so that he too can learn to think and act like Christ and ultimately share in eternal life. Similarly, at the heart of medical education is a Person, the Person of Christ the Divine Physician, who calls students to follow after him, to see him in the face of every patient, and to care for each patient as Christ himself would tend to their needs.[53] It is the work of Catholic medical educators to guide their students to discover this person of Christ the Divine Physician, who will be their teacher and model throughout their time of medical education.

It is beyond the scope of this work to provide a complete instruction in catechesis as it applies to medical education, so I will limit myself to simply highlighting a com-

51. *Catechism of the Catholic Church*, no. 30.
52. Pope Paul VI, "Evangelization in the Modern World" [*Evangelii Nuntiandi*, Apostolic Exhortation, December 8, 1975], in *Teaching the Catholic Faith Today*, ed. E. Kevane (Boston: Daughters of St. Paul, 1982), no. 21.
53. See John Paul II, *Catechesi Tradendae*, no. 5.

mon theme among the catechetical documents of the Church—including the *General Directory for Catechesis*, its precursor the *General Catechetical Directory*, *Catechesi Tradendae*, and the *Catechism of the Catholic Church*. The theme is that the process of evangelization and catechesis is rooted in and based on the pedagogy of God. More simply, if we are to instruct others in such a way that they too will come to know the person of Christ and follow after him (thereby discovering the fulfillment of their own nature), we do well to follow the model by which God has chosen to instruct the human race.

How then does a medical educator assist a student in the progression from seeking truth about the human body to deeper questions about the truth of the human person? The answer lies in how God has chosen to reveal himself:

> He assumes the character of the person, the individual, and the community according to the conditions in which they are found. . . . To this end, as a creative and insightful teacher, God transforms events in the life of his people into lessons of wisdom, adapting himself to the diverse ages and life situations.[54]

The medical educator need not become a student again to relate to a medical student, but he must situate the gospel message he proclaims through the witness of his example and his words of instruction in the context of the medical student's experience. Physicians who have found in Christ the hope for mankind's salvation, are uniquely poised to assist students in recognizing the deeper questions of the meaning of life that daily present themselves in the work of the physician. This does not require proselytization; in fact, in the case of students who are still in the beginning stages of their search for God, a time referred to as pre-catechesis, the *General Directory for Catechesis* reminds catechists that the "proclamation of the Gospel [must] always be done in close connection with human nature and its aspirations, [showing] how the Gospel fully satisfies the human heart."[55]

Beyond the general pedagogy of God, Christ himself provides a living standard for the interaction between student and teacher. Christ first and foremost received others, especially the poor, the little ones, and sinners. He received them as persons loved and sought by God. He taught them both in word and deed of the love of God that liberates from evil and promotes life. He offered hope in the kingdom. He did all of this through "the use of all the resources of interpersonal communication, such as word, silence, metaphor, image, example, and many diverse signs. . . ."[56] The physician educator whom students witness receiving all patients with gentleness and charity; who receives every student with kindness and warmth; who reveals in the witness of his life and his practice of medicine the freedom offered through a life lived in accordance with the gospel; who engages each student and patient through word, silence, metaphor, image, and, at times, signs; who exposes the questions of the meaning of life that underlie the anguish of illness; who, with conviction that a physician's work

---

54. Congregation for the Clergy, *General Directory for Catechesis*, no. 139.

55. Ibid., no. 117.

56. Ibid., no. 140.

is an essential component of God's plan for the human person, fulfills his duty not only as a physician but also as a teacher who leads his students to know and follow Christ the Divine Physician. The role of the medical educator as witness to the truth of the gospel and the freedom offered to man through a life lived in conformity to the gospel cannot be underestimated. Pope Paul VI reminds all those entrusted with the task of evangelization and catechesis, "Modern man listens more willingly to witnesses than to teachers, and if he does listen to teachers it is because they are also witnesses."[57]

Conclusion

The preceding pages have occasioned the discussion of the elements of an authentic Catholic medical education. I have used the introduction to the *Charter for Health Care Workers* as the foundation for the discussion. In a spirit of disclosure, the discussion stems from my own reflections on my experience of medical education. It is my hope that these reflections can provide a point of discussion for students as well as medical educators, campus ministers, pastors, and all those who interact with medical students as they grow in their knowledge and practice of medicine. I close with a passage from Sirach that relays both the divine origin of medicine and its earthly limitations. Let us offer a prayer that young hearts will respond generously to the call of God to serve him through the practice of medicine and that each of us will strive each day more perfectly to follow Christ, the Divine Physician.

Honor the physician with the honor due him, according to your need of him, for the Lord created him; for healing comes from the Most High, and he will receive a gift from the king. The skill of the physician lifts up his head, and in the presence of great men he is admired. The Lord created medicines from the earth, and a sensible man will not despise them. Was not water made sweet with a tree in order that his power might be known? And he gave skill to men that he might be glorified in his marvelous works. By them he heals and takes away pain; the pharmacist makes of them a compound. His works will never be finished; and from him health is upon the face of the earth. My son, when you are sick do not be negligent, but pray to the Lord, and he will heal you. Give up your faults and direct your hands aright, and cleanse your heart from all sin. Offer a sweet-smelling sacrifice, and a memorial portion of fine flour, and pour oil on your offering, as much as you can afford. And give the physician his place, for the Lord created him; let him not leave you, for there is need of him. There is a time when success lies in the hands of physicians, for they too will pray to the Lord that he should grant them success in diagnosis and in healing, for the sake of preserving life. (Sir 38:1–14)

Bibliography

Barragán, Javier Lozano. "On Catholic Teachers of Medicine." *Zenit*, July 21, 2007. https://zenit.org/articles/on-catholic-teachers-of-medicine/.

Benedict XVI, Pope. *Spe Salvi, On Christian Hope*. Encyclical Letter. November 30, 2007.

———. Address to the Assembly for the Conclusion of the Pastoral Diocesan Visit to Aquileia and Venice.

---

57. Paul VI, "Evangelization in the Modern World," no. 41.

May 8, 2011. http://w2.vatican.va/content/benedict-xvi/en/speeches/2011/may/documents/hf_ben-xvi_spe_20110507_cittadinanza-venezia.html

Catechism of the Catholic Church. Translated by USCCB. 2nd edition. Washington D.C.: United States Catholic Conference, 1997.

Congregation for the Clergy. *General Directory for Catechesis*. 1998. http://www.vatican.va/roman_curia/congregations/cclergy/documents/rc_con_ccatheduc_doc_17041998_directory-for-catechesis_en.html.

John Paul II, Pope. *Catechesi Tradendae, On Catechesis in Our Time*. Apostolic Exhortation. October 16, 1979. http://w2.vatican.va/content/john-paul-ii/en/apost_exhortations/documents/hf_jp-ii_exh_16101979_catechesi-tradendae.html.

——. *Christifidelis Laici, On the Vocation and the Mission of the Lay Faithful in the Church and in the World*. Apostolic Exhortation. December 30, 1988. http://w2.vatican.va/content/john-paul-ii/en/apost_exhortations/documents/hf_jp-ii_exh_30121988_christifideles-laici.html.

——. *Veritatis Splendor, The Splendor of Truth*. Encyclical Letter. August 6, 1993. http://www.vatican.va/holy_father/john_paul_ii/encyclicals/documents/hf_jp-ii_enc_06081993_veritatis-splendor_en.html.

Paul VI, Pope. "Evangelization in the Modern World" [*Evangelii Nuntiandi*. Apostolic Exhortation. December 8, 1975]. In *Teaching the Catholic Faith Today*, ed. E. Kevane, 145–207. Boston: Daughters of St. Paul, 1982.

Pontifical Council for Pastoral Care to Health Care Workers. *Charter for Health Care Workers*. Boston: St. Paul Books and Media, 1995.

Vatican Council II. *Gaudium et Spes, Pastoral Constitution on the Church in the Modern World*. In *Vatican Council II: The Basic Sixteen Documents*, ed. Austin Flannery, 163–282. New York: Costello Publishing, 1996.

Deacon William V. Williams

14. ETHICS IN CLINICAL RESEARCH

Clinical research is an indispensable part of medical practice in today's world. In this chapter physician-scientist Williams first provides background for the development of ethical codes of conduct in clinical research which are essential for understanding the reasons underlying current clinical research practices. Williams then extends the discussion of ethics in clinical research by illuminating principles to which faithful Catholic researchers especially should adhere. These principles are truth, respect for life, respect for the integrity of persons, and the principles of generosity and justice. In the appendix to the chapter, Williams shows these principles imbedded throughout the foundational documents for ethical clinical research. Further, he provides practical sets of guidelines for each of the principles articulated in the chapter. All physicians and others engaged in any degree of clinical research would find this chapter useful for their work, and may appreciate the many opportunities in the research fields for witnessing to their faith in truth and love.—*Editors.*

Introduction

While clinical research has a long history, the ethics that guide it have evolved significantly in the last century, largely in response to abuse of research subjects. And while many codes have developed to guide research practice, they generally rest upon three basic principles—beneficence, autonomy, and justice. These terms are defined more fully in appendix 4 but can be briefly summarized in terms of their use in clinical research ethics: *Beneficence* refers to the obligation to maximize the possible benefits to a research subject while minimizing the possible harm. *Autonomy* refers to the right of subjects to enter into research freely and without coercion or undue influence and with adequate information to assess the risks and benefits. Since some research subjects are not capable of making autonomous judgments, or are in situations in which coercion is difficult to avoid (e.g., prisoners), autonomy is often coupled with the obligation to protect such vulnerable people under the broader obligation of *respect for persons*. *Justice* refers to the fair distribution of the burdens and benefits of a particular research study. This chapter will address these principles, as well as the unique challenges that confront the Catholic clinical researcher today, and it will mention some additional principles that have been put forward that address some of these challenges.

History of Clinical Research

The Greek and Roman empiricists were the first doctors to address clinical research,[1] stating that a medicine's efficacy should be judged by the actual results. The eleventh-century physician Avicenna expanded on this idea, proposing that to evaluate a medicine properly, one must apply the drug to two different cases: "Experimentation must be done on the human body, for testing a drug on a lion or a horse might not prove anything about its effect on man."[2] From this we can surmise that pre-clinical research was already being conducted in Avicenna's day, but its lack of predictive value led to forays into clinical research. Soon after, in the twelfth century, Maimonides proposed what is probably the first ethical guideline for clinical research: A physician should treat patients as ends in themselves, not as means for learning new truths. The violation of this principle is the basis for all abuses in clinical research. In a similar vein, Roger Bacon (1214–92) commented on the difficulty of performing clinical research:

> The … sciences which do their work on insensate bodies can multiply their experiments till they get rid of deficiency and errors, but a physician cannot do this because of the nobility of the material in which he works, … and so experience (the experimental method) is so difficult in medicine.[3]

This "nobility of the material" of the human research subject still presents challenges to clinical researchers today.

In the late eighteenth century, clinical experimentation became more widespread as germ theory gained acceptance and vaccines came into use. Edward Jenner, in 1789, performed the first experiment with cow pox vaccination against smallpox, inoculating his son, who was only one year old, as well as an eight-year-old neighbor, whom he then challenged with smallpox material. Jenner's success led other physicians to inoculate their own and their colleagues' children with cow pox; some of these doctors also challenged their subjects with smallpox exposure. As is typical in the recent history of clinical research, the success of this effort superseded any ethical concerns regarding the research methods used.

Throughout the nineteenth century, clinical researchers generally used themselves or their neighbors as research subjects. For example, James Simpson tested chloroform on himself; fortunately, he survived (awakening upon the floor). Louis

---

1. Most of the historical information is taken from David J. Rothman, *Strangers at the Bedside: A History of How Law and Bioethics Transformed Medical Decision Making* (New York: Aldine de Gruyter, 2003); and from John O'Grady and Otto I. Linet, *Early Phase Drug Evaluation in Man* (Boca Raton, Fla.: CRC Press, 1990).

2. Rothman, *Strangers at the Bedside*, 19.

3. Ibid., 19–20.

Pasteur, a biologist rather than a physician, tested his rabies vaccine in dogs, but then administered the vaccine to a nine-year-old boy who had been bitten fourteen times by a rabid dog. Despite Pasteur's great trepidation, the series of inoculations worked; and that rabies vaccine continues to be used to this day. Claude Bernard, writing in the late nineteenth century, posited that

morals do not forbid making experiments on one's neighbors or one's self.... The principle of medical and surgical morality consists in never performing on man an experiment which might be harmful to him to any extent, even though the result might be highly advantageous to science, i.e., the health of others.[4]

He reiterated Maimonides's principle that patients should be treated as ends in themselves, not as a means for others to gain knowledge.

The twentieth century saw many great advances in clinical research that engendered the development of more highly detailed ethical codes. Early in the century, hospital patients were used as clinical research subjects to evaluate anti-diphtheria serum in Germany, insulin therapy on diabetics in extremis, and a liver preparation for the treatment of pernicious anemia. These successes emboldened others to pursue human experimentation, sometimes with disastrous results, as in the case of Walter Reed. His first experiments evaluating transmission of yellow fever by mosquito bites were conducted on research team members, a practice that was stopped after two of the subjects died. Reed then solicited servicemen as volunteers, offering them one hundred dollars in gold for exposure and another one hundred dollars if they contracted yellow fever. Reed downplayed the risks and touted the potential benefits, thus tainting what limited success his research achieved.

During World War II, the prevailing spirit of volunteerism inspired many civilians to volunteer as clinical research subjects. Unfortunately, researchers at this time also began to use mentally impaired persons as research subjects, reasoning that they would volunteer if they could. As a result, residents of asylums and orphanages were subjected to exposure to live dysentery bacteria, influenza virus, and trials of sulfonamides as antibiotics, sometimes with very severe reactions. Despite the obvious lack of informed consent, these studies continued for some time. Finally, the failure of a clinical trial involving gonorrhea in prison inmates raised questions that sparked the development of standard informed-consent protocols.

Wartime research produced such spectacular successes as penicillin, a near-miraculous drug whose scarcity prompted ethical debate over how it was to be allocated. The proven efficacy of the influenza vaccine, in an era when many still remembered the 1918 epidemic, seemed similarly miraculous. Other war-related research involved survival studies in hardship conditions, conducted on conscientious objectors.

These wartime achievements stood in stark contrast to horrific abuses, especially in Nazi Germany and Japan.[5] Jewish people were subjected to death by exposure to

4. Ibid., 23.
5. See D. M. Pressel, "Nuremberg and Tuskegee: Lessons for Contemporary American Medicine," *Journal of the National Medical Association* 95 (2003): 1216–25.

study the limits of human endurance. Castration was carried out to study the effects of genital irradiation. People were subjected to intentional hypothermia and malarial infection; bones were deliberately broken or portions of them excised to study "bone regeneration." Hitler justified these atrocities with the decree that "as a matter of principle, if it is in the interest of the state, human experiments were to be permitted," noting that it was unacceptable that "someone in a concentration camp or prison to be totally untouched by the war, while German soldiers had to suffer the unbearable."[6]

Development of Clinical Research Ethical Codes

These terrible abuses led, in 1947, to the first modern statement of clinical research ethics, the Nuremberg Code, which stated that "the voluntary consent of the human subject is absolutely essential. This means that the person involved should have the legal capacity to give consent."[7] The Declaration of Helsinki, issued in 1964, was developed to codify the principles expounded in the Nuremberg Code.[8] Although it was a tremendous step forward for the international community, the Nuremburg Code was largely ignored by the American press, as the Nazi abuses were seen as unthinkable in the United States. Simultaneously, the National Institutes of Health (NIH), formed in the 1930s, was given an expanded role and a soaring budget, along with an NIH clinical research center in Bethesda, Maryland. However, the assumption that the patient-researcher relationship was the same as patient-doctor relationship meant that potential conflicts of interest were not acknowledged, and informed consent was unregulated and rarely used.

The tide began to turn in the United States with the revelation of thalidomide-induced birth defects.[9] Clinical trials with thalidomide had involved about twenty thousand Americans, including 3,750 women of childbearing potential and 624 pregnancies. Many of these subjects did not know they were in an experiment and that

6. Rothman, *Strangers at the Bedside*, 61.

7. *Trials of War Criminals before the Nuremberg Military Tribunals under Control Council Law No. 10*, vol. 2, *The Medical Case; The Milch Case* (Washington, D.C.: U.S. Government Printing Office, 1949), 181–82, available online at https://www.ushmm.org/information/exhibitions/online-exhibitions/special-focus/doctors-trial/nuremberg-code.

8. World Medical Association, Declaration of Helsinki, "Ethical Principles for Medical Research Involving Human Subjects," last amended October 2013, http://www.wma.net/en/30publications/10policies/b3/, adopted by the 18th WMA General Assembly, Helsinki, Finland, June 1964, and amended by the 29th WMA General Assembly, Tokyo, Japan, October 1975; 35th WMA General Assembly, Venice, Italy, October 1983; 41st WMA General Assembly, Hong Kong, September 1989; 48th WMA General Assembly, Somerset West, Republic of South Africa, October 1996; 52nd WMA General Assembly, Edinburgh, Scotland, October 2000; 59th WMA General Assembly, Seoul, Republic of Korea, October 2008, and the 64th WMA General Assembly, Fortaleza, Brazil, October 2013. Note of Clarification on Paragraph 29 added by the WMA General Assembly, Washington 2002. Note of Clarification on Paragraph 30 added by the WMA General Assembly, Tokyo 2004.

9. See A. E. Rodin, L. A. Koller, and J. D. Taylor, "Association of Thalidomide (Kevadon) With Congenital Anomalies," *Canadian Medical Association Journal* 86(1962): 744–46; A. L. Speirs, "Thalidomide and Congenital Abnormalities," *Lancet* 1 (1962): 303–5.

the drug had not been approved in the United States The incidence of phocomelia following thalidomide exposure during pregnancy led to the drug's withdrawal in Europe and to the authorization of the Food and Drug Administration to evaluate efficacy as well as safety in clinical trials (the Kefauver-Harris 1962 amendments).[10] However, this authorization left out the key Javits amendment, which required that "no such [experimental] drug may be administered to any human being in any clinical investigation unless that human being has been appropriately advised that such drug has not been determined to be safe in use for human beings."[11] Thus, truly informed consent was still not viewed as a top priority compared with the advancement of research goals.

Then in the mid-1960s a "whistle blower" emerged: Henry Beecher, the head of anesthesiology at the renowned Massachusetts General Hospital. In a 1965 address on ethics in clinical research, he cited specific cases of breaches of ethical conduct, which drew much interest from the media but only criticism from colleagues. Beecher published a paper on the same topic the following year in the *New England Journal of Medicine*, naming specific cases of ethics violations in clinical research. Interestingly, Beecher's arguments were at their basis very Catholic: he noted in his introduction, "According to Pope Pius XII, 'science is not the highest value to which all other orders of values ... should be subordinated.'"[12] Beecher concluded, "A far more dependable safeguard than consent is the presence of a truly *responsible* investigator."[13]

Beecher's cases included such ethical lapses as withholding therapy from patients with rheumatic fever or typhoid; injection of live cancer cells into subjects; and subjecting mentally impaired subjects and juvenile delinquents to a suspected hepatoxin for acne, among many others. He noted that informed consent was absent or inadequate in these studies, and that some subjects were incapable of informed consent or consented under duress. Beecher declared that procedures or treatments likely to be injurious to subjects should not be attempted at all, and he held journals accountable for publishing these unethical studies. "Any classification of human experimentation as 'for the good of society' must be viewed with distaste, even alarm," wrote Beecher.

There is no justification here for risking an injury to an individual for the possible benefit to other people. ... Such a rule would open the door wide to perversions of practice, even such as were inflicted by Nazi doctors on concentration-camp prisoners. ... The individual must not be subordinated to the community. The community exists for man.[14]

Other breaches of clinical research ethics in this era had a profound impact on the development of ethical codes in the field. One example is the 1960s case of the

10. See H. Edgar and D. J. Rothman, "New Rules for New Drugs: The Challenge of AIDS to the Regulatory Process," *Milbank Quarterly* 68 S1 (1990): 111–42.

11. Ibid.

12. Henry K. Beecher, "Ethics and Clinical Research," *New England Journal of Medicine* 274 (1966): 1354, quoting Pope Pius XII, Address to the First International Congress on the Histopathology of the Nervous System, September 14, 1952, http://www.papalencyclicals.net/Pius12/P12PSYCH.HTM.

13. Beecher, "Ethics and Clinical Research," 1355, emphasis in original.

14. Quoted in Rothman, *Strangers at the Bedside*, 82–83.

Willowbrook Children's Home, where mentally retarded children were deliberately injected with hepatitis virus to study the disease.[15] The researchers justified their actions with the reasoning that hepatitis was so common that the children probably would have contracted it anyway. From the 1940s through the 1970s, the U.S. military carried out experiments that involved exposing unsuspecting military and civilian subjects to radiation, using national security as their justification. A congressional document described these procedures:

The chief objectives of these experiments were to directly measure the biological effects of radioactive material; to measure doses from injected, ingested, or inhaled radioactive substances; or to measure the time it took radioactive substances to pass through the human body. American citizens thus became nuclear calibration devices.[16]

Perhaps the most widely known case was the Tuskegee syphilis observational trial, carried out by the U.S. Public Health Service from 1932 through 1972, the longest nontherapeutic experiment on humans in history.[17] Four hundred sharecroppers with untreated syphilis were recruited through the Tuskegee Institute, as well as through their communities and churches—the trial clearly targeted African-Americans. Diagnosis and treatment were withheld, even after penicillin became widely available; and more than one hundred subjects died from syphilis or related complications during the study. The outrage over the Tuskegee trials still echoes in a lingering distrust of medical research among members of minority groups.[18]

The revelation of these abuses illuminated the need for a clear differentiation between the roles of the physician and the investigator. In response, in 1966 the NIH issued new guidelines, which required any institution receiving a grant to assure and document informed patient consent. The guidelines also mandated an institutional review board consisting of institutional associates not directly associated with the investigator's project. The institutional review board is charged with addressing the study's treatment of the subjects' rights and welfare, the methods it employs to obtain informed consent, and its risks and potential benefits.

The FDA's response to the Kefauver and Javits resolutions was a regulation requiring informed consent for patients taking experimental drugs, "except where a conscientious professional judgment is made that this is not feasible or is contrary to the best interest of the patient."[19] Further guidelines were issued by the FDA in 1966, requiring informed consent for both therapeutic and nontherapeutic research;

---

15. See E. F. Diamond, "The Willowbrook Experiments," *Linacre Quarterly* 40 (1973): 133–37.

16. United States House of Representatives, Committee on Energy and Commerce, Subcommittee on Energy Conservation and Power, "American Nuclear Guinea Pigs: Three Decades of Radiation Experiments on U.S. Citizens," October 24, 1986, 99th cong., 2nd sess., http://nsarchive.gwu.edu/radiation/dir/mstreet/commeet/meet1/brief1/br11n.txt.

17. See G. Corbie-Smith, "The Continuing Legacy of the Tuskegee Syphilis Study: Considerations for Clinical Investigation," *American Journal of the Medical Sciences* 317 (1999): 5–8.

18. See V. L. Shavers, C. F. Lynch, and L. F. Burmeister, "Knowledge of the Tuskegee Study and Its Impact on the Willingness to Participate in Medical Research Studies," *Journal of the National Medical Association* 92 (2000): 563–72.

19. Rothman, *Strangers at the Bedside*, 93.

the only exceptions were situations in which consent was not feasible (for example, in a comatose patient) or if it was not in a patient's best interest (for example, a cancer patient whose physician did not want to divulge the diagnosis). The FDA said that subjects had the right to a fair explanation of the procedure, including potential inconveniences and risks, and information on the nature of placebo-controlled trials and on any alternative forms of therapy. Ultimately, the subject also had a right to choose whether or not to participate.

Yet in spite of all these reforms, and in spite of the existence of international standards for clinical good practice, abuses in the conduct of clinical trials continued, sometimes with disastrous and widely publicized outcomes. In 2004, the drug company Merck withdrew its anti-inflammatory drug Vioxx from the market when it became clear that it increased cardiovascular risk in long-term users, even though Merck had access to data indicating this risk several years earlier.[20] A similar situation occurred with the diabetes drug Avandia. Its maker, GlaxoSmithKline, knew the drug had a deleterious effect on lipid profiles, with the potential for an increased risk of cardiovascular events, but failed to make the data public.[21]

Catholics who participate in clinical research face additional challenges. For example, pharmaceutical company researchers who are evaluating drugs with unknown or known teratogenic risks commonly require subjects to use pre-specified contraceptive methods. These put the investigator in a position of requiring that research subjects engage in the immoral practice of contraception. Research on the similarly immoral practice of artificial insemination and in vitro fertilization may require an investigator to cooperate in or even encourage these practices. Other issues include embryonic stem-cell research, the failure of drug companies to publish negative trials, and clinical trials that are primarily promotional.

The Nuremberg Code

The Nuremberg Code was drafted to address several of the most egregious human rights violations of the Nazi and Japanese clinical researchers. Their clinical studies violated their subjects' autonomy and were performed without the interests of the research subjects in mind. In addition, the studies' potential benefits would not be available to the persons being studied or the groups they represented; for example, research carried out on Jewish concentration camp prisoners were meant to benefit German soldiers.

Among the Nuremberg Code's key principles is the provision that studies should avoid the use of human subjects unless it is absolutely necessary, and when they do, they should create no unnecessary risks. They must seek also knowledge intended for the good of society which is "unprocurable by other methods or means of study"

---

20. See J. S. Ross et al., "Pooled Analysis of Rofecoxib Placebo-Controlled Clinical Trial Data: Lessons for Postmarket Pharmaceutical Safety Surveillance," *Archives of Internal Medicine* 169 (2009): 1976–85.

21. See S. Philpott and R. Baker, "Why the Avandia Scandal Proves Big Pharma Needs Stronger Ethical Standards," *Bioethics* 24 (2010): ii–iii.

(n. 2). The voluntary consent of the subject is described in the code as "absolutely essential" (n. 1). The code also decreed, "No experiment should be conducted where there is a priori reason to believe that death or disabling injury will occur; except, perhaps, in those experiments where the experimental physicians also serve as subjects" (n. 5). The safety of the experimental subjects was thus defined as the highest consideration in any clinical trial.

See appendix 1 below for the text of the Nuremberg Code and the ethical principles that inform each of its directives.

The Declaration of Helsinki

The Declaration of Helsinki, first issued in 1964, was intended to codify the principles set forth in the Nuremberg Code. The declaration states the purpose of biomedical research: "to improve diagnostic, therapeutic, and prophylactic procedures and understanding of the etiology and pathogenesis of disease" (n. 3). While acknowledging the need to rely ultimately on human subjects, it clarifies the premise that the well-being of the human subject should take precedence over the interests of science and society. See appendix 2 for a paraphrase of the declaration.

Since its original issuance, the declaration has been amended five times, and the most recent amendment in 2000 was controversial enough to require notes of clarification in 2002 and 2004. See appendix 3 for a paraphrase of the most recent issuance of the Declaration of Helsinki.

The Belmont Report

The Belmont Report was created and issued in 1979 by the National Commission for the Protection of Human Subjects of Biomedical and Behavioral Research, in part to respond to the Tuskegee syphilis scandal.[22] As the most recent of these three major ethical codes, it builds upon the others and clarifies the underlying basis of their specific principles in terms of three ideals: respect for persons, beneficence, and justice.

Respect for persons requires that researchers treat their subjects as autonomous individuals and that they protect persons who have diminished autonomy. Respect for persons includes informed consent, which consists of three elements. The potential subject must have sufficient information on anticipated risks and benefits as well as on alternative therapies, and must be allowed to ask questions. In addition, the subject must fully comprehend this information; if necessary, it must be adapted to the subject's ability to understand. Last, the subject must agree voluntarily, without coercion, to participate.

The principle of beneficence involves respecting subjects' decisions, protecting

---

22. See appendix 4 below. For the full report, see National Commission for the Protection of Human Subjects of Biomedical and Behavioral Research, "The Belmont Report: Ethical Principles and Guidelines for the Protection of Human Subjects of Research," April 18, 1979, http://www.hhs.gov/ohrp/humansubjects/guidance/belmont.html.

them from harm, and working to assure their well-being. This principle outlaws bru-
tal or inhumane treatment of human subjects and requires that risks be minimized,
which may mean avoiding the use of human subjects if at all possible. If vulnerable
populations are to be used, it must be demonstrated that their use is appropriate.
Institutional review boards are required to assess a study's validity of hypothesis, the
nature and magnitude of risk, and whether such projected risk and probable benefits
are reasonable. They should also determine the justification for research involving
significant risk of serious impairment.

The principle of justice requires fairness in the distribution of research's benefits
as well as its burdens. This includes fairness in the selection of research subjects—
for example, not deliberately selecting undesirable subjects for risky research. Adults
must be selected before children, and some classes of subjects, such as the institutionalized, mentally infirm, or prisoners, should be used seldom, if at all, since obtaining
meaningful informed consent from them is problematic.

Beyond the Belmont Report

The Belmont Report's three principles, along with the specific provisions of both
the Nuremberg Code and the Declaration of Helsinki, have greatly influenced the
conduct of clinical research over the past forty years. Ethical guidelines continue to
develop, with newer provisions addressing protection of the environment, the treatment of experimental animals, and the ethical obligations of authors and publishers,
among others. Some of these do not cleanly fit into the Belmont Report's three categories, which suggests that additional principles may be at work.

Some of these protections have been codified into law. The primary U.S. legislation is Title 21 of the U.S. Code of Federal Regulations (21 CFR), which addresses
informed consent as well as financial disclosure, assuring that clinical investigators
are not biased by monetary factors in the outcome of their research.[23] The law also
deals with institutional review boards and with the processes governing investigational new drug applications. Documents, such as document E6, *Good Clinical Practice*, from the International Conference on Harmonization, have also been devised to
provide an objective international standard of practice.[24] Along with consent and institutional review board issues, this document addresses such issues as medical care of
trial subjects, randomization and unblinding of subjects, safety reporting, compensation of subjects, sponsor considerations, and contents of the clinical trial protocol.

Such regulations protect research subjects, but do they go far enough? As noted
above, some of the updated guidelines from Helsinki do not fit cleanly into the Bel-

---

23. Available at http://www.accessdata.fda.gov/scripts/cdrh/cfdocs/cfcfr/CFRSearch.cfm?CFRPart=
312&showFR=1.

24. U.S. Department of Health and Human Services, Food and Drug Administration, Center for Drug
Evaluation and Research (CDER), Center for Biologics Evaluation and Research (CBER), *Guidance for Industry*, E6, *Good Clinical Practice: Consolidated Guidance* (Rockville, Md.: ICH, 1996), http://www.fda.gov/
downloads/Drugs/GuidanceComplianceRegulatoryInformation/Guidances/ucm073122.pdf.

mont principles, indicating that other standards may be at work. Abuses continue to occur, in spite of the safeguards currently in place. New challenges have also arisen from the changes in the secular culture since the promulgation of these guidelines. When these ethical guidelines were first drafted, the range of medicinal products was limited chiefly to the treatment of disease. Over the past fifty years, many nontherapeutic medicinal products have come into widespread use, creating a new set of ethical issues for physicians who take seriously the admonition "above all do no harm." For example, hormonal contraceptives are used by millions of women; they address no underlying pathology, yet serious side effects have been documented with their use.[25] Financial conflicts of interest by research investigators have been the subject of intense scrutiny, along with other conflicts for investigators whose careers and reputations hinge on being the first to introduce new technologies into the clinic. Perhaps most seriously, the role of the physician as protector of life in the Hippocratic tradition has been greatly eroded by legalized abortion and euthanasia in many places. These and other transformations in the field of clinical research necessitate a fresh look at its underlying ethical principles and their application.

Development of a Catholic Guide for Ethical Clinical Research

In 2004 a group of individuals representing the Catholic Medical Association and the National Catholic Bioethics Center joined together to discuss and formulate basic ethical principles for the conducting of clinical research. This joint effort aimed to develop a reference guide for clinical researchers, in both academic and pharmaceutical industry settings, and to provide a resource for moral theologians in such matters. The group's work culminated in the 2007 publication of "Catholic Principles and Guidelines for Clinical Research," with Deacon Albert T. Derivan, MD, and Peter J. Cataldo, PhD, as primary authors.[26] Unsatisfied with the generalized nature of this document, the group continued to meet to develop hypothetical cases that could offer concrete examples to guide clinical researchers. This resulted in the 2008 publication of the combined "Principles and Guidelines" and "Case Studies in Clinical Research Ethics," newly titled *A Catholic Guide to Ethical Clinical Research*.[27] We will now

---

25. See, for example, J. M. Baeten et al., "Hormonal Contraception and Risk of Sexually Transmitted Disease Acquisition: Results from a Prospective Study," *American Journal of Obstetrics and Gynecology* 185 (2001): 380–85; Ø. Lidegaard et al., "Hormonal Contraception and Risk of Venous Thromboembolism: National Follow-up Study," *British Medical Journal* 13 (2009): b2890. For a brief summary, see M.-A. Boursiquot, "The Real Risks of Oral Contraceptives," *Linacre Quarterly* 78 (2011): 100–104.

26. Catholic Medical Association and National Catholic Bioethics Center, "Catholic Principles and Guidelines for Clinical Research," *National Catholic Bioethics Quarterly* 7, no. 1 (2007): 153–65. *Imprimatur* and *nihil obstat* from the Archdiocese of Philadelphia. The author of this chapter was also a collaborator on the document cited.

27. Catholic Medical Association and National Catholic Bioethics Center, *A Catholic Guide to Ethical Clinical Research* (Philadelphia: Catholic Medical Association and National Catholic Bioethics Center, 2008). Also published in Catholic Medical Association and the National Catholic Bioethics Center, "A Catholic Guide to Ethical Clinical Research," *Linacre Quarterly* 75 (2008): 181–224.

examine the basic elements of this document, particularly those which are distinct from the Nuremberg Code, the Declaration of Helsinki, and the Belmont Report.

Basic Principles and Rationale

A Catholic Guide to Ethical Clinical Research begins by declaring that science and technology should serve humankind; yet, of themselves, principles and guidelines cannot supply the moral vision and norms to assure that they are not being employed to humanity's detriment.[28] Such vision can and should come from the Church. *A Catholic Guide* makes it a point that "the Church's rejection of illicit ways of pursuing knowledge should not be confused with impeding the search for truth itself."[29] In other words, it is essential to safeguard the human person's intrinsic dignity in the pursuit of knowledge. *A Catholic Guide* cites the specific moral criteria for biomedical research described in Congregation for the Doctrine of the Faith's *Donum Vitae* (The Gift of Life): "the respect, defense and promotion of man"; "his 'primary and fundamental right' to life," "his dignity as a person who is endowed with a spiritual soul and with moral responsibility," and his calling "to beatific communion with God."[30] The principles and guidelines in *A Catholic Guide* are crafted to articulate specifically how these criteria should be applied to clinical research.

The guidelines of *A Catholic Guide* are based on four principles rooted in Catholic theology: truth, respect for life, respect for the integrity of persons, and the combined principles of generosity and justice. When applied to the current clinical research environment, these principles can assure that the dignity of human subjects as well as the consciences of researchers are respected, and that the study will promote the betterment of society as a whole. Although adherence to these principles does not guarantee that subjects will never suffer side effects or be injured, or that unwanted results will never occur, it still should minimize the risk of untoward consequences for subjects, research teams, and the communities which hope to benefit from the research.

The principles and guidelines from *A Catholic Guide to Ethical Clinical Research* are shown in appendix 5.

The Principle of Truth

This principle leads the others, because Catholics follow the teaching of Jesus Christ, who is himself the Truth (cf. Jn 14:6). Thus, truth is highly valued in the Catho-

---

28. Catholic Medical Association and National Catholic Bioethics Center, *A Catholic Guide*, citing Congregation for the Doctrine of the Faith, *Donum Vitae*, February 22, 1987, Introduction, no. 2. Also see Vatican Council II, *Gaudium et Spes*, December 7, 1965, no. 36.

29. Catholic Medical Association and National Catholic Bioethics Center, *A Catholic Guide*, quoting Pope Pius XII, "Moral Aspects of Genetics," Address to the First International Congress of Medical Genetics, September 7, 1953, *AAS* 44 (1953): 605.

30. Catholic Medical Association and National Catholic Bioethics Center, *A Catholic Guide*, quoting Congregation for the Doctrine of the Faith, *Donum Vitae*, Introduction, no. 1.

lic tradition and deserves prominence in any discussion of ethics. There is a great
need for the principle of truth in clinical research today, as recent violations against
truth in clinical research have abounded. For example, Korean investigator Woo-Suk
Hwang claimed to have developed human embryonic stem-cell lines from cloned human embryos, a claim he later retracted when it was found that the work was based
on fraudulent data.[31] The withdrawal of Vioxx and effective withdrawal of Avandia,
both of which involved the manufacturers' concealment or withholding of negative
data, are noted above.[32] These and other examples make upholding truth a crucial
ideal in both academic and industrial research.

Clinical research must be guided by a deep dedication to truthfulness and trans-
parency, from the inception of the research study through the publication of final
results.[33] The study's underlying motivation, its conduct, and the communication of
its results should all be directed by this principle. The research program "must be of
value and done for the good of society" (guideline 1a); any research subject would
implicitly assume this was the case. Otherwise, the researcher is misrepresenting the
study to prospective subjects. "Only scientifically qualified individuals should conduct clinical research" (guideline 1b); they should be trained in the area under investigation, knowledgeable about its scientific rationale, working with a testable hypothesis and familiar with International Conference on Harmonization's *Good Clinical
Practice*.[34] The design of a research protocol usually requires input from several disciplines. These might include a specialist in the disease area under investigation; a
clinical scientist; a pharmacokineticist; a statistician; a study operations expert; and
perhaps a radiologist or a pharmacodynamics expert. If the appropriate expertise is
not available, the study should be cancelled or delayed until it becomes available; otherwise researchers will be putting the research subjects at risk without the means to
achieve the study's goals.

A Catholic Guide also addresses the research protocol, the investigation's blueprint. It must clearly describe the known and potential risks for the research subjects,
as well alternative treatments, if they exist (guideline 1c). These risks and alternatives
must also be addressed in the informed consent form and any related documents
(guideline 1d). Patients must be told what will be required of them in terms of visits,
laboratory work, x-rays, and so on, and whether they will be compensated for their
time. For subjects unable to provide informed consent, such as dependent minors or
persons with limited intellectual capacity, a surrogate can provide informed consent
(guideline 1e). However, the interests of the subject, not those of the surrogate or the

31. W. S. Hwang et al., "Patient-Specific Embryonic Stem Cells Derived from Human SCNT Blastocysts,"
Science 308 (2005): 1777–83; erratum: *Science* 310 (2005): 1769. W. S. Hwang et al., "Evidence of a Pluripotent
Human Embryonic Stem Cell Line Derived from a Cloned Blastocyst," *Science* 303 (2004): 1669–74; D. Ken-
nedy, editorial retraction, *Science* 311 (2006): 335.

32. See Ross et al., "Pooled Analysis of Rofecoxib Placebo-Controlled Clinical Trial Data"; Philpott and
Baker, "Why the Avandia Scandal Proves Big Pharma Needs Stronger Ethical Standards."

33. See Catholic Medical Association and National Catholic Bioethics Center, *A Catholic Guide*, 6–7,
"The Principle of Truth."

34. U.S. Department of Health and Human Services et al., *Good Clinical Practice*.

researcher, must be the only consideration in such cases, as dependent subjects have a right to trust that their interests are being protected.

The dissemination of results from research has been the subject of much scrutiny in recent years, due in part to situations like GlaxoSmithKline's failure to publish negative results from research studies for Avandia and Paxil.[35] Legislation now requires U.S. pharmaceutical companies to make public their ongoing clinical studies and to post the results.[36] Publishing only positive results and concealing negative results violates the principle of truth; thus all results should be made available, particularly when they affect the assessment of a therapeutic intervention's safety (guideline 1f).

Several cases cited in *A Catholic Guide* illustrate the research dilemmas that test the application of the principle of truth. For example, in one case a nurse administering informed consent for a study is asked to put a certain "spin" on the consent, in order to boost enrollment.[37] While information is always subject to interpretation, the informed consent process must be as free from bias and hidden agendas as possible. Another case involves the results of a major drug study for a small company.[38] The chief executive officer of the company directs the researcher to split the study into two papers: one addressing the drug's positive efficacy, and another addressing some troubling safety issues. Further, the CEO directs that the latter paper's release be delayed until more is known about the safety issues. This is clearly unethical: all results from a study, including unfavorable ones, must be made public in a timely manner.

The Principle of Respect for Life

It might seem odd that this tenet should even be included in a list of principles for clinical research. After all, the purpose of clinical research is to further the understanding of disease and the development of new treatments, with the ultimate goal of preserving human life. Yet, in this era of post-Hippocratic medicine, where the adage to "do no harm" seems no longer to be in vogue, respect for life must be actively affirmed. This is especially true in clinical research, where the desire to understand disease and develop treatments for patients not involved in the research study may involve exposing research subjects to risks that directly violate this principle. This is all the more true when financial gain or the desire to enhance academic reputation and acclaim can cloud the researchers' judgment.

---

35. See Gardiner Harris, "Diabetes Drug Maker Hid Test Data, Files Indicate," *New York Times*, July 13, 2010, http://www.nytimes.com/2010/07/13/health/policy/13avandia.html; and Gardiner Harris, "Regulators Want Antidepressants to List Warning," *New York Times*, March 23, 2004, http://www.nytimes.com/2004/03/23/health/23DEPR.html?hp.

36. Ongoing clinical studies can be accessed at the U.S. National Institutes of Health website, http://clinicaltrials.gov/.

37. Catholic Medical Association and National Catholic Bioethics Center, *A Catholic Guide*, 23–25, case 1.1.

38. Ibid., 28–29, case 1.4.

The gift of life is from God, and the clinical researcher is a steward of this gift.[39] The gift's intrinsic dignity and nature must be respected, both in the research subjects at hand and in those to whom the fruits of the research are directed. This includes the human subject at every stage of development, from "its first formation to natural death."[40] At what point is the human first formed? As noted by Maureen Condic, the fusion of cell membranes of the sperm and ovum, which occurs in less than a second, forms a zygote, which is clearly distinct from either gamete and has a unique molecular composition.[41] The zygote then rapidly begins a series of changes that do not occur in sperm or ova. These include changes in ionic composition and in the zona pellucid, which block fusion with other sperm, culminating in breakdown of the nuclear membranes in preparation for the first cell division (syngamy). Thus, from a scientific perspective, the formation of the zygote, at the moment when the sperm's and ovum's cell membranes fuse, marks the creation of "a new cell with unique genetic composition, molecular composition, and behavior"; in short, a new organism.[42] This new organism, this new human being, possesses intrinsic dignity which is worthy of respect.

The human person's intrinsic dignity continues from this point to natural death, and in fact is so profound that it even extends beyond death. The controversy over use of body tissues post-mortem for medical research exemplifies this premise.[43] Typically, post-mortem human tissues and organs can be used for research only with the pre-mortem consent of the individual. This requirement helps guard against illicit means of procuring tissues, or even ending a person's life for the purpose of accessing the person's tissues. A Catholic Guide make this abundantly clear: "The medical researcher may never willfully destroy any living human being of any age whatsoever" (guideline 2a). It is worth recalling the atrocities conducted by the National Socialists in Germany during World War II, atrocities in which lives were deliberately endangered and people were killed for the purposes of research.

A more difficult problem is posed by the proliferation of "reproductive technologies" that do not respect the intrinsic dignity of the human person and that routinely end lives for the purpose of research. A brief literature search of PubMed (conducted in February 2017) for the title words "in vitro fertilization" limited to clinical research in humans returned 859 references; more than 90 of those references come from within the past five years.[44] Thus, this remains a very active area of clinical research, despite the fact that it clearly violates the dignity of the human person, who should be engendered through an act of mutual life-giving love in the context of mar-

---

39. See ibid., 7–8.

40. Ibid., 7, citing Pope John Paul II, *Evangelium Vitae, On the Value and Inviolability of Human Life,* Encyclical Letter, March 25, 1995, nos. 48 and 89, http://w2.vatican.va/content/john-paul-ii/en/encyclicals/documents/hf_jp-ii_enc_25031995_evangelium-vitae.html.

41. Maureen L. Condic, "When Does Human Life Begin? A Scientific Perspective," Westchester Institute White Paper Series 1, October 2008: 3, https://www.cedarville.edu/personal/sullivan/bio4410/condic_whitepaper.pdf.

42. Ibid., 5.

43. See Lori Andrews and Dorothy Nelkin, "Whose Body Is It Anyway? Disputes over Body Tissue in a Biotechnology Age," *Lancet* 351 (1998): 53–57.

44. http://www.ncbi.nlm.nih.gov/pubmed.

riage, not manufactured in a laboratory. Of equal concern is the vast area of research spawned by the in vitro fertilization industry: embryonic stem-cell research. This field of research has been fueled in large part by the ready availability of "surplus" frozen human embryos engendered through in vitro fertilization. Those who write in this area routinely use dehumanizing language, referring to human embryos in terms more frequently applied to inventory in manufacturing ("surplus"). Embryos, which contain the potential of the next Einstein, or Mother Teresa, or John or Jane Imagodei, are frozen for storage like produce in a supermarket, and then destroyed by dissection for the creation of cell lines for experimentation. No matter how great the advances achieved by research performed on human embryos, such research is never justified, because it is achieved through the evil means of a human being's destruction.

It is worthwhile to reflect on how the public perceives the utility of embryonic stem-cell research, and to compare this perception with the actual data available. A 2006 Virginia Commonwealth University survey found that more than half of Americans strongly or somewhat favored embryonic stem-cell research, and 37 percent strongly or somewhat opposed it.[45] The survey asked respondents which of three research options—embryonic stem cell, adult stem cell, or stem cells from other sources, such as an umbilical cord—offered, in their opinion, the greatest promise for new treatments for disease. Embryonic stem cells drew positive responses from 22 percent of respondents, an increase of 8 percent from a similar survey done the previous year. Other-sourced stem cells were favored by 25 percent of respondents, down 12 percent from the previous year, and adult cells were favored by only 17 percent, an increase of 10 percent from 2005.

In order to explore briefly the actual clinical utility of embryonic stem cells, the NCBI PubMed database was searched for the term "embryonic stem cells."[46] Fifty-three titles were returned and were read in full.[47] The same database was similarly searched for the term "stem cell." There were 6,977 titles returned. Therefore, the search was narrowed to include only human clinical trials. There were then 2,103 titles returned. This included more than 760 publications in cancers as well as numerous publications in autoimmune diseases, genetic diseases, and other diseases. In addition, six other clinical studies of adult stem-cell therapy were noted with sources from muscle, eye, adipose tissue, and umbilical cord blood with some promising results.[48]

---

45. David J. Urban, "2006 Virginia Commonwealth University Life Sciences Survey," http://www.vcu.edu/lifesci/images2/ls_survey_2006_report.pdf.

46. http://www.ncbi.nlm.nih.gov/sites/entrez.

47. Searched on May 25, 2011, with the following limitations: Field of search for "Embryonic Stem Cell": Title/Abstract. Limits: Humans only. Type of Article: All of the following were selected, Clinical Trial, Randomized Controlled Trial, Case Reports, Phase I Clinical Trial, Phase II Clinical Trial, Phase III Clinical Trial, Phase IV Clinical Trial, or Controlled Clinical Trial.

48. *Muscle:* See L. K. Carr et al., "1-year Follow-up of Autologous Muscle-Derived Stem Cell Injection Pilot Study To Treat Stress Urinary Incontinence," *International Urogynecology Journal and Pelvic Floor Dysfunction* 19 (2008): 881–83. *Eye:* See V. S. Sangwan et al., "Successful Reconstruction of Damaged Ocular Outer Surface in Humans Using Limbal and Conjuctival Stem Cell Culture Methods," *Bioscience Reports* 23 (2003): 169–74; erratum: *Bioscience Reports* 124 (2006): 1483. See also K. Tsubota et al., "Treatment of

In contrast, as of May 2011 only one case report of actual embryonic stem-cell therapy was noted.[49] The case involved the use of a differentiated embryonic stem-cell line to aid in tolerance induction in a transplant recipient. While this case was published in 2006, it is widely accepted that the first documented creation of a cloned embryo (blastocyst) from a terminally differentiated adult human cell was not reported until 2008, by the company Stemagen.[50] It is noteworthy that the Stemagen procedure was confirmed by DNA fingerprinting of the donor somatic-cell nuclear DNA and donor oocyte mitochondrial DNA, matching these to the embryonic DNA. Since this was not performed in the 2006 case, the results of this report are thrown into doubt. In any case, this is one dubious case report using embryonic stem cells, compared with more than a thousand papers documenting clinical trials with adult stem cells, many of them successful. Similar findings have recently been published by a group from the Institute of Life Sciences at the Catholic University of Valencia.[51] (Also, there has been publication of a study of embryonic stem-cell therapy in macular degeneration that reported limited success.[52] A trial in spinal cord injury was reported but later cancelled.)[53]

These findings show that, although embryonic stem-cell research has been effectively marketed to the public as a promising avenue for the development of new treatments, it in fact faces significant hurdles that must be overcome before it produces effective therapies; examples of the hurdles include the tendency of embryonic stem cells to form teratomas,[54] as well as their tendency to be rejected by the immune system. Induced pluripotent stem cells (IPS), which are a more recent innovation, show

---

Severe Ocular-Surface Disorders with Corneal Epithelial Stem-Cell Transplantation," *New England Journal of Medicine* 340 (1999): 1697–1703. *Adipose tissue*: See H. L. Trivedi et al., "Human Adipose Tissue-Derived Mesenchymal Stem Cells Combined with Hematopoietic Stem Cell Transplantation Synthesize Insulin," *Transplant Proceedings* 40 (2008): 1135–39. *Umbilical cord blood*: See H. Nishihira et al., "Unrelated Umbilical Cord-Blood Stem Cell Transplantation: A Report from Kanagawa Cord Blood Bank, Japan," *International Journal of Hematology* 68 (1998): 193–202; also P. D. Wadhwa et al., "Hematopoietic Recovery after Unrelated Umbilical Cord-Blood Allogeneic Transplantation in Adults Treated with In Vivo Stem Cell Factor (R-MetHuSCF) and Filgrastim Administration," *Leukemia Research* 27 (2003): 215–20.

49. See H. L. Trivedi et al., "Embryonic Stem Cell Derived and Adult Hematopoietic Stem Cell Transplantation for Tolerance Induction in a Renal Allograft Recipient: A Case Report," *Transplant Proceedings* 38 (2006): 3103–8.

50. See A. J. French et al., "Development of Human Cloned Blastocysts Following Somatic Cell Nuclear Transfer with Adult Fibroblasts," *Stem Cells* 26 (2008): 485–93.

51. J. Aznar and J. L. Sánchez, "Embryonic Stem Cells: Are Useful in Clinic Treatments? *Journal of Physiology and Biochemistry* 67 (2011): 141–44.

52. See S. D. Schwartz et al., "Embryonic Stem Cell Trials for Macular Degeneration: A Preliminary Report," *Lancet* 379, no. 9817 (February 25, 2012): 713–20.

53. See F. Bretzner et al., "Target Populations for First-in Human Embryonic Stem Cell Research in Spinal Cord Injury," *Cell Stem Cell* 8 (2011): 468–75; and D. Lukovic et al., "Concise Review: Human Pluripotent Stem Cells in the Treatment of Spinal Cord Injury," *Stem Cells* 30 (2012): 1787–92.

54. See N. Amariglio et al., "Donor-Derived Brain Tumor Following Neural Stem Cell Transplantation in an Ataxia Telangiectasia Patient," *PLoS Medicine* 6 (2009): e1000029; F. Erdö et al., "Host-Dependent Tumorigenesis of Embryonic Stem Cell Transplantation in Experimental Stroke," *Journal of Cerebral Blood Flow and Metabolism* 23 (2003): 780–85; B. E. Reubinoff et al., "Embryonic Stem Cell Lines from Human Blastocysts: Somatic Differentiation In Vitro," *Nature Biotechnology* 18 (2000): 399–404; erratum: *Nature Biotechnology* 18 (2000): 559.

much greater promise; M. Stadtfeld and K. Hochedlinger have performed a review of the research.[55] These cells are developed by transfection of human fibroblasts (which can be derived from a simple skin biopsy) with genes encoding four transcriptional regulators—(*Klf4*, *Sox2*, *c-Myc*, and *Oct4*).[56] Since these cells are derived from the individual patient, immune rejection is thought to be less of an issue. More importantly, these cells can be differentiated into various cell types with great therapeutic potential, just as ESCs can. No human is destroyed in this process, and none need be created.

A Catholic Guide clearly prohibits ethical researchers from participating in, or immorally cooperating with,[57] research that willfully destroys a human life (as does ESC research) or that engenders life outside the marital act, as does in vitro fertilization (guideline 2b). It also outlaws participating in or immorally cooperating with research that willfully hastens the end of life for those who are nearing it (guideline 2c). Since respect for life extends through the person's natural death, those who are near death or in states of persistent or permanent unconsciousness represent a vulnerable population that must be especially protected. Certainly research—such as trials of new pain-relieving medication in those with metastatic cancer, or trials of medications that may assist in awakening the persistently unconscious—may be acceptable, even welcome, for those in these states. However, the researcher must intend only the good of the patient and must never intend to hasten his or her demise. This is especially crucial in transplantation research, where the demand for organs far outstrips the supply. The debate regarding determination of death is important in discussions of the ethics of organ donation, but it is not the purpose here to enter into that debate;[58] for this chapter it is enough to be aware that the magisterial judgment is that either cardiopulmonary or neurological criteria can be used to determine death.[59] Further, researchers in organ transplantation are urged to remove organs only from those who have provided informed consent pre-mortem and only after consultation with the family and after death has indeed occurred.

A Catholic Guide cites several case studies that pose dilemmas centering on the respect for life. One such case examines development of a new medical abortifacient in the light of three research roles: the principal investigator, the clinical research

---

55. M. Stadtfeld and K. Hochedlinger, "Induced Pluripotency: History, Mechanisms, and Applications," *Genes and Development* 24 (2010): 2239–63.

56. See K. Takahashi et al., "Induction of Pluripotent Stem Cells from Adult Human Fibroblasts by Defined Factors," *Cell* 131 (2007): 861–72.

57. Note that certain forms of cooperation may be permissible and therefore not immoral, such as remote material cooperation where the immoral end is not intended and the role of the moral agent is not essential to the performance of the act. Forms of cooperation, and their moral implications, are discussed in *The Catholic Guide for Ethical Clinical Research*.

58. For more on the debate, see Scott Alessi, "Debate Continues on Whether Brain Death Signifies End of Life: Ethical and Medical Questions Persist as to Whether Brain Death Truly Marks the End of a Person's Life," *Our Sunday Visitor Newsweekly*, June 12, 2011, http://www.osv.com/tabid/7621/itemid/7993/Debate-continues-on-whether-brain-death-signifies.aspx.

59. See Pope John Paul II, Address to the Eighteenth International Congress of the Transplantation Society, August 29, 2000, http://w2.vatican.va/content/john-paul-ii/en/speeches/2000/jul-sep/documents/hf_jp-ii_spe_20000829_transplants.html.

monitor, and the statistician.[60] Both the principal investigator, who oversees all aspects of the study, and the research monitor, who assures that the study is being performed properly, are involved in immoral cooperation. The principle investigator's role is formal cooperation, since the intent is to develop the abortifacient drug.[61] The clinical research monitor's cooperation could also be formal; or, if the monitor's work contributes in an essential way to the research, even if the drug's development is not intended, it could be immediate material cooperation. Neither of these researchers should participate in the study. The statistician's involvement in data analysis, which would be considered mediate material cooperation, may be tolerated if there is a pressing need, such as employment to feed the statistician's family, but if there are any other alternatives for the statistician, they should be pursued.[62]

Two cases in *A Catholic Guide* address embryonic stem-cell research. One case centers on a technician at a biotechnology company, who is asked to retrain on a technique of harvesting cells from human blastocysts.[63] Another case is that of a patient with a neurodegenerative disease, who is considering entering a clinical study that would infuse him with embryonic stem cells directly derived from blastocysts.[64] As the first case requires the technician to directly kill a human being, and the second case requires the patient's complicity in direct killing, both procedures are prohibited. More can be read on these cases in *A Catholic Guide* itself. An additional case involves the use of cell lines derived from an elective abortion dating back several decades to develop the only available vaccine for rubella, which causes fetal malformations and spontaneous abortions.[65] Is it licit for a physician to develop this vaccine? In this case, it would be permissible, since no other alternative is available. This position has been challenged in recent years as additional cell lines have been developed from electively aborted fetuses. The situation emphasizes the urgent need for pharmaceutical companies to find new, morally derived cell lines for use in vaccine production.[66]

---

60. Catholic Medical Association and National Catholic Bioethics Center, *A Catholic Guide*, 29–30, case 2.1.

61. For a definition of formal cooperation, immediate material cooperation, and other terms used in this discussion, see ch. 12, "The Catholic Pharmacist," and appendix 5, "A Catholic Guide to Ethical Clinical Research" below.

62. Note that the case of the statistician could be considered proximate or remote mediate material cooperation, assuming that the evil of the development of the abortifacient drug is not intended by the statistician (which would make the cooperation formal) and the statistical analysis is not essential to development of the drug (which would constitute immediate material cooperation). Proximate mediate material cooperation has a direct causal influence on the act of the principle agent (the drug company) while remote mediate material cooperation has an indirect causal influence on the act of the principle agent. If the statistical analysis has a direct causal influence on the development of the abortifacient drug, for example, if it evaluates the effectiveness of the drug in terminating pregnancies and this information is used to help design the pivotal study for approval of the drug, then it would constitute proximate mediate material cooperation. If the statistical analysis has an indirect causal influence on development of the drug, for example, if it examines adverse events comparing the drug to a placebo, and this analysis does not favor the drug, this could constitute remote mediate material cooperation.

63. Catholic Medical Association and National Catholic Bioethics Center, *A Catholic Guide*, 30, case 2.2.

64. Ibid., 31–33, case 2.3.

65. Ibid., 33–34, case 2.4

66. See Debra L. Vinnedge, "Aborted Fetal Cell Line Vaccines and the Catholic Family: A Moral and Historical Perspective," Children of God for Life, updated October 2005. https://cogforlife.org/vaccines-

The final case, which involves in vitro fertilization, centers on a research coordinator assigned to recruit subjects into a study of an ovarian hyperstimulation agent for "egg" harvesting.[67] Participating in this research protocol would be immoral, as it promotes a technology that seeks to separate the unitive and procreative meanings of the marital act. Dividing these two meanings relegates the spouse to the role of an object being used as a means to an end, that of getting a child, and thus violates the dignity of both spouse and child. If the research coordinator did participate, his or her actions could be misinterpreted to indicate that the study is moral, creating an insurmountable scandal.

The Principle of Respect for the Integrity of Persons

Respect for persons extends beyond the research subject's life; the entire human person must be treated with the utmost respect and concern. The research subject must never be treated as an object or a means to an end, because the research subject is in fact the most important factor in every clinical trial or research study (guideline 3c). The research subject is obliged by natural law to conserve his or her own health, so the subject's health must never be compromised, particularly when children and other vulnerable populations are involved, whose well-being and safety must be carefully safeguarded (guidelines 3b and 3d). In every case, the researcher must seek to work only for the good of the subjects and must never cause deliberate harm (guideline 3f). The research subject's powers of intellect and free will, endowed by the Creator, imply the need for the subject's free and informed consent; performing research while circumventing this right would deny the subject the exercise of free will and intellect (guideline 3a).

These guidelines do not rule out subjects' participation in studies from which they expect to gain no benefit. Healthy human subjects are typically used in early-phase clinical trials to evaluate the safety and pharmacokinetics of a drug. However, in such studies the associated risks must be relatively insignificant for the healthy subjects (guideline 3e), and, of course, their free and informed consent must be obtained.

A Catholic Guide speaks directly to conscience rights and the spirituality and religious beliefs of both research subject and researcher. Researchers should strive to form their consciences properly, and they should never act against their conscience's certain judgment (guideline 3h). In accord with their own properly formed consciences, they must also respect the spirituality and religious beliefs of research subjects without compromising those beliefs, except when in doing so the investigator

---

abortions/. These principles regarding the use of aborted fetal cell lines for vaccines also apply to the use of similar cell lines in basic (bench) research. For example, the cell lines HEK293 and WI38 are commonly used in basic research in academia and in pharmaceutical research to test drugs in vitro. Their use should be avoided if at all possible, and other alternatives sought. However, if there are no viable alternatives, and the research is critically important in discovering new therapies for serious diseases, or in advancing understanding of mechanisms of disease that could lead to new therapies, then their use may be tolerated. Again, the potential for scandal also needs to be taken into account.

67. Catholic Medical Association and National Catholic Bioethics Center, *A Catholic Guide*, 34–35, case 2.5.

will fail in some moral duty of the natural law (guideline 3g). One example cited by *A Catholic Guide* deals with pregnancy prevention during clinical trials of drugs.[68] Prudence and common sense make it desirable that research subjects in clinical drug trials avoid becoming pregnant or fathering a child, since a new drug's effect on a fetus can rarely be predicted, even when there are benign results in preclinical animal studies. In addition, liability issues could arise if a female subject became pregnant and suffered a miscarriage or a fetal anomaly; it would be impossible to completely rule out the drug as the cause, leaving the drug company vulnerable to potential damages. *A Catholic Guide* leaves the specific method of preventing a pregnancy to the woman, her conscience, and her religious beliefs, with a key footnote:

In listing the permitted methods of avoiding pregnancy, abstinence should always be included and encouraged as the preferred method. Protocols should never require a physician to provide a method of birth control, nor should a subject in a study ever be required to use a method of birth control, contrary to their properly formed conscience in accord with the natural moral law. (Guideline 3g note 21)

This directive conflicts with the practice of many pharmaceutical companies, which "require" research subjects to use specific contraceptive methods, a problematic practice for a researcher wishing to follow his or her well-formed conscience. Finally, *A Catholic Guide* specifies that if a research subject does become pregnant and wishes to have an abortion, "it would not be morally licit for her to have one or for the investigator to recommend her having one" (guideline 3g).

This author has had personal experience with this ethical dilemma, when working as a research monitor after his conversion to the Catholic faith. The job required signing off on research protocols that required subjects to employ two barrier methods of birth control while participating in the study. As the author became more cognizant of the Catholic teaching on contraception, he conferred with a moral theologian, Reverend Monsignor James J. Mulligan, STL, who offered these insights:

Compliance with the protocol, which requires that researchers *direct* women of childbearing potential to use two contraceptives if they will not abstain from sexual intercourse, raises the added problem of the researchers' cooperation in moral evil. There are times when certain types or degrees of such mediate material cooperation might be morally justified, but that does not seem to be the case here. The justification of such cooperation usually depends on the fact that there is some sort of coercion or duress. Here, however, it appears that such duress would be ongoing and that the person under duress should be taking steps to remove himself from the situation entirely. Otherwise the researcher becomes involved in immediate material cooperation, and that is, for all practical purposes, indistinguishable from implicit formal cooperation.[69]

In the case presented in *A Catholic Guide*, the physician who signs off on the protocol, the investigator at the research site, and the research nurse who obtains informed consent from subjects are all cooperating with morally illicit behavior. On the other

---

68. Ibid., 35–39, case 3.1.
69. Reverend Monsignor James J. Mulligan to author, March 2004.

hand, a statistician analyzing the study data and contributing to the study protocol (apart from the contraception requirement) is not cooperating with the contraceptive act. Similarly, a medical writer who writes the protocol can avoid immoral cooperation if morally acceptable wording can be substituted in the protocol and consent forms; if not, the medical writer should excuse him- or herself from writing that part of the protocol. To make the protocol morally acceptable, subjects *may* be required to take appropriate precautions of a high level of certainty in avoiding pregnancy or fathering a child (e.g., 99 percent certainty) but *may not* not be required to use artificial contraceptives. "The subjects must be free to choose how they will avoid pregnancy or fathering a child," and it is permissible to inform them about the effectiveness of certain methods, and to prohibit the use of some methods. "Abstinence should always be included as an acceptable method"; "abortion is never permissible."[70]

A behavioral research case involving a technique of aversive conditioning to enhance language acquisition in young children with severe mental retardation is examined next.[71] The use of aversive conditioning, in which the children are given a brief, very painful electric shock, is not in and of itself immoral per se, but its use must respect the dignity and nature of the human subject. Because the child is not competent to provide informed consent, a surrogate must be employed who clearly represents the subject's best interests. The potential benefits must outweigh the risks, and these risks must be relatively insignificant.

Three cases of genetic modification are presented in *A Catholic Guide*; one involves a genetic modification technique, shown to reverse the effects of Alzheimer's disease in experimental animals, being applied to Down syndrome patients with Alzheimer's.[72] Informed consent is particularly challenging in this situation. Along with assent of a surrogate who truly acts in the subject's best interest, the subject's own assent should be obtained if possible. Such subjects also should not be excluded from these studies if they may benefit from participation, even if they cannot advocate for their own health, and their well-being must be safeguarded through the appointment of a patient advocate if a guardian or other surrogate is not available.

The next case involves gene insertion, a technique which the investigator has tested in animals and now wishes to attempt in humans without a specific therapeutic intent.[73] Such a research study may be permissible, but several conditions must be met. The information sought must be available only through study in humans; the risks must be relatively insignificant; and there must be some reasonable chance of future benefit. If these conditions are not met, the research would be frivolous and not in accord with the dignity of the human subjects involved.

The third case involves delivery of suppressor genes to a carcinoma in a cancer patient, using a technique that has never been tested in humans.[74] Potential benefits

70. Catholic Medical Association and National Catholic Bioethics Center, *A Catholic Guide*, 38–39.
71. Ibid., 39–40, case 3.2.
72. Ibid., 40–41, case 3.3.
73. Ibid., 41–42, case 3.4.
74. Ibid., 42–43, case 3.5.

and risks must be clearly conveyed to the patient, who might be desperate for any hope and vulnerable to coercion. Such subjects may be willing to take undue risks, and this must be avoided.

The Principles of Generosity and Justice

The principles of generosity and justice are inexorably linked, since they are rooted in the same premise: medical researchers are "instruments through which a loving God cares for his creation," so all they do must be directed toward serving the sick.[75] To remain ethical, clinical research must be necessary and potentially useful in furthering human health and combating disease. The researcher should avoid conflicts of interest that provide him or her with gain at the subject's expense and treat the subject as an object for unjust profit (guideline 4b). Both immoral cooperation with evil and the occasion of insurmountable scandal must be avoided (guideline 4c). Vulnerable subjects should be involved only in studies from which they may benefit, at least indirectly (guideline 4d). "Compensation to subjects should never be excessive or coercive [and] recruitment methods must not be misleading" (guideline 4e). In addition, "a medical researcher should not accept compensation that is disproportionate to the work performed" (guideline 4f), nor should research "be undertaken primarily for the purpose of enhancing the influence or reputation of the researcher" (guideline 4g).

A Catholic Guide illuminates these principles with several case studies, one of which involves a drug whose major action is enhancing cognition; it is targeted to normal individuals to improve their performance.[76] This raises the question of whether the drug may provide an advantage to certain populations who can afford it, at the expense of those who cannot. As this drug does not treat an illness, the risks undertaken in its development must be relatively insignificant, and its potential impact on the social order must be seriously considered.

In another case, healthy medical students are recruited into a study of a new brain imaging modality, for which they receive a large sum of money and course credits by the investigator.[77] This situation amounts to the immoral use of coercion. Another case discusses recruitment of subjects to donate oocytes for use in somatic cell nuclear transfer (cloning).[78] Several aspects of the case are troubling, including the immorality of the research itself, misrepresentation of the potential benefits of the research, and lack of proper informed consent, as the risks of such reactions as ovarian hyperstimulation syndrome are minimized or omitted.

Two drug development cases are discussed in *A Catholic Guide*.[79] The first involves little unmet medical need but an opportunity for significant financial gain

---

75. Ibid., 10.
76. Ibid., 43–45, case 4.1.
77. Ibid., 45–46, case 4.2.
78. Ibid., 46–48, case 4.3.
79. Ibid., 48–50, cases 4.4 and 4.5.

for the drug company. In the second, a post-marketing "research" study is intended primarily to promote prescription of the drug. Both cases are unethical if no valid scientific hypothesis is being tested or there is no measurable benefit for the sick.

A Catholic Guide addresses the case of a drug intended to treat a rare form of cancer; the drug is under development in a poor country where the cancer is more prevalent.[80] Conducting the research in the impoverished country speeds up the study, but the drug company does not plan to market the drug there if it is approved. This is an example of unethical exploitation of the impoverished for the benefit of those who ultimately will be able to afford the drug.

Another case describes a drug that is being removed from development because of hepatotoxicity.[81] An ongoing study evaluates the mechanism of action of the drug, and researchers propose continuing with more diligent monitoring of liver function, to gain more information. The ethical continuation of this study hinges on the risk-benefit ratio as well as proper informed consent, which must include the information that the drug will never be developed. In another case, the marketing company desires to conduct a placebo-controlled study of an off-label drug, even though it already represents the standard of care for a condition; however, the drug lacks formal approval, and the drug company hopes to be able to advertise it for use in this condition.[82] Since there is no other effective treatment for the condition, the use of placebo is problematic. *A Catholic Guide* suggests a single-arm study, in which all the subjects receive the active drug, as an ethical alternative.

Two other justice-related cases present scenarios in which the target disease population differs from the study group.[83] One case involves a drug for patients with systemic lupus erythematosus, who are primarily women, many of them African-American; early phase clinical studies, however, can be carried out only in a different population. This is likely permissible if limiting the study population would delay the development of a potentially efficacious therapy. The second case describes a drug in development for a disease that predominately affects men. Regulatory authorities, however, require that early phase clinical studies include women of child-bearing potential, and these women be obliged to use artificial contraceptive methods. This requirement involves the researchers in immoral cooperation with evil, which must be avoided.

Conclusion

Clinical research has developed rapidly over the past century, and new developments continue to pose ethical dilemmas for those involved. Yet despite the proliferation of ethical codes and laws governing clinical research, Beecher's premise rings true: the presence of a truly responsible investigator is still the best way to protect the safety

---

80. Ibid., 50–52, case 4.6.
81. Ibid., 52–53, case 4.7.
82. Ibid., 53–54, case 4.8.
83. Ibid., 55–57, cases 4.9 and 4.10.

and well-being of research subjects. It should be added that the truly responsible investigator is one with a well-formed conscience. It is hoped that *A Catholic Guide to Ethical Clinical Research*, and this chapter, will help investigators and all those involved in clinical research better to form their consciences.

Appendix 1: The Nuremberg Code[84]

To each of the directives below have been added in brackets the related ethical principle from the 1979 Belmont Report (see appendix 4). These principles are beneficence, respect for persons, and justice. These directives are excerpted from the sources noted without further modification.

Permissible Medical Experiments

The great weight of the evidence before us is to the effect that certain types of medical experiments on human beings, when kept within reasonably well-defined bounds, conform to the ethics of the medical profession generally. The protagonists of the practice of human experimentation justify their views on the basis that such experiments yield results for the good of society that are unprocurable by other methods or means of study. All agree, however, that certain basic principles must be observed in order to satisfy moral, ethical, and legal concepts:

1. The voluntary consent of the human subject is absolutely essential. [*Respect for Persons*]

This means that the person involved should have legal capacity to give consent; should be so situated as to be able to exercise free power of choice, without the intervention of any element of force, fraud, deceit, duress, over-reaching, or other ulterior form of constraint or coercion; and should have sufficient knowledge and comprehension of the elements of the subject matter involved as to enable him to make an understanding and enlightened decision. This latter element requires that before the acceptance of an affirmative decision by the experimental subject there should be made known to him the nature, duration, and purpose of the experiment; the method and means by which it is to be conducted; all inconveniences and hazards reasonably to be expected; and the effects upon his health or person which may possibly come from his participation in the experiment.

The duty and responsibility for ascertaining the quality of the consent rests upon each individual who initiates, directs, or engages in the experiment. It is a personal duty and responsibility which may not be delegated to another with impunity.

2. The experiment should be such as to yield fruitful results for the good of society, unprocurable by other methods or means of study, and not random and unnecessary in nature. [*Justice*]

3. The experiment should be so designed and based on the results of animal experimentation and a knowledge of the natural history of the disease or other problem under study that the anticipated results will justify the performance of the experiment. [*Beneficence*]

---

84. "The Nuremberg Code," in *Trials of War Criminals before the Nuremberg Military Tribunals under Control Council Law No. 10*, vol. 2, *The Medical Case; The Milch Case* (Washington, D.C.: U.S. Government Printing Office, 1949), 181–82, http://www.ushmm.org/research/doctors/Nuremberg_Code.htm.

4. The experiment should be so conducted as to avoid all unnecessary physical and mental suffering and injury. [*Beneficence*]

5. No experiment should be conducted where there is an a priori reason to believe that death or disabling injury will occur; except, perhaps, in those experiments where the experimental physicians also serve as subjects. [*Beneficence*]

6. The degree of risk to be taken should never exceed that determined by the humanitarian importance of the problem to be solved by the experiment. [*Beneficence*]

7. Proper preparations should be made and adequate facilities provided to protect the experimental subject against even remote possibilities of injury, disability, or death. [*Beneficence*]

8. The experiment should be conducted only by scientifically qualified persons. The highest degree of skill and care should be required through all stages of the experiment of those who conduct or engage in the experiment. [*Justice*]

9. During the course of the experiment the human subject should be at liberty to bring the experiment to an end if he has reached the physical or mental state where continuation of the experiment seems to him to be impossible. [*Respect for Persons*]

10. During the course of the experiment the scientist in charge must be prepared to terminate the experiment at any stage, if he has probable cause to believe, in the exercise of the good faith, superior skill, and careful judgment required of him, that a continuation of the experiment is likely to result in injury, disability, or death to the experimental subject. [*Beneficence*]

Appendix 2: Paraphrase of the Declaration of Helsinki[85]

The following specific statements are noted to serve "only as a guide."

1. Biomedical research must conform to scientific principles. [*Beneficence, Justice*]

2. Each experimental procedure should be formulated in an experimental protocol. [*Respect for Persons, Justice*]

3. Only qualified and properly supervised individuals should conduct the research. [*Beneficence*]

4. The importance of the research objective must be proportional to the inherent risk to the subject. [*Beneficence, Justice*]

5. Risks and benefits to the subject should be determined before the project begins; concern for the interests of the subject must be greater than concern for the interests of society. [*Respect for Persons, Beneficence*]

6. The right of the subject to safeguard his or her integrity must always be respected. [*Respect for Persons*]

7. Physicians should not engage in human research if the hazards involved are not predictable. [*Beneficence*]

8. Research reports should be accurate. [*Justice*]

9. Informed consent must be obtained from subjects in advance; subjects must always be free to withdraw from a given study. [*Respect for Persons*]

10. Care must be taken with regard to obtaining informed consent if the subject is in a dependent relationship with the investigator. [*Respect for Persons*]

85. The full text can be found at World Medical Association, Declaration of Helsinki, "Ethical Principles for Medical Research Involving Human Subjects," http://www.wma.net/en/30publications/10policies/b3/.

11. In case of legal incompetence or if the subject is a minor or otherwise incapacitated, informed consent should be obtained from the legal guardian in accordance with national legislation. [*Respect for Persons*]

12. The research protocol should always contain a statement of ethical considerations indicating that the principles of this declaration have been met. [*Respect for Persons*]

The following principles are noted to apply to clinical research wherein experimentation is combined with patient care:

1. In treating the sick, physicians are free to use new measures if they offer hope of saving life, reestablishing health, or alleviating suffering. [*Beneficence*]

2. The potential of "a new method should be weighed against the advantages of the best" current methods. [*Beneficence*]

3. In any study all patients including those in a control group should be assured of the best proven diagnostic and therapeutic methods. [*Beneficence, Justice*]

4. The refusal of a patient to participate must not interfere with the physician-patient relationship. [*Respect for Persons, Beneficence*]

5. If the physician does not obtain informed consent, the reason for this should be stated in the protocol for transmission to the review committee. [*Respect for Persons*]

6. Medical research and professional care can be combined only to the extent that the research is justified by its potential value to the patient. [*Beneficence, Justice*]

Additional principles are noted for non-therapeutic biomedical research involving human subjects:

1. In research that is purely scientific, the physician must remain the "protector of the life and health" of the person being studied. [*Beneficence*]

2. The subjects must be volunteers. [*Respect for Persons*]

3. The investigator should discontinue the study if there is evidence that it may be harmful. [*Beneficence*]

4. The interest of science and society should never take precedence over the well-being of the subject. [*Justice, Beneficence*]

Appendix 3: Paraphrase of the Amendment of the Declaration of Helsinki[86]

- It is the duty of the physician in medical research to protect the life, health, privacy, and dignity of the human subject. [*Beneficence, Respect for Persons*]
- Medical research involving human subjects must conform to generally accepted scientific principles, based on a thorough knowledge of the scientific literature, other sources of information, and adequate laboratory and animal experimentation. [*Beneficence, Justice*]
- Appropriate caution must be exercised if the research may affect the environment; the welfare of animals must be respected. [*Beneficence*]
- The design and performance of the study should be formulated in an experimental protocol [*Respect for Persons*]

86. The full text can be found at World Medical Association, Declaration of Helsinki, "Ethical Principles for Medical Research Involving Human Subjects," http://www.wma.net/en/30publications/10policies/b3/.

- submitted ... to a specially appointed ethical review committee, independent of the investigator, sponsor, or any undue influence.
  - Ethics committees should conform with laws and regulations of the country where the research is performed.
  - The committee has the right to monitor ongoing trials.
  - The researcher is obliged to provide monitoring information to the committee, especially serious, adverse events and information regarding funding, sponsors, institutional affiliations, other potential conflicts of interest, and incentives for subjects.
- Research protocols should contain a statement of the ethical considerations involved. [*Respect for Persons, Justice*]
- Medical research should be conducted only by scientifically qualified persons and under a clinically competent medical person. [*Beneficence, Justice*]
- There must be careful assessment of predictable risks and burdens and foreseeable benefits to the subject or to others. [*Beneficence*]
  - This does not preclude the participation of healthy volunteers in medical research.
  - Risks involved should be adequately assessed and satisfactorily managed.
  - The investigation must cease if the risks outweigh the potential benefits or conclusive proof of positive benefit is found.
  - The importance of the objective must outweigh inherent risks and burdens to the subjects, especially for healthy volunteer subjects.
- Medical research is only justified if the populations in which the research is carried out may benefit from the results. [*Justice*]
- The subjects must be volunteers and informed participants. [*Respect for Persons*]
- Respect subjects right to safeguard their integrity, privacy, and confidentiality, and minimize impact on the subject's physical and mental integrity and on the personality of the subject [*Respect for Persons*]
- Adequate informed consent, right to abstain or withdraw. [*Respect for Persons*]
- For dependent persons, need guardian's consent and subject's assent if possible. [*Respect for Persons*]
  - Specific reasons for involving research subjects unable to give informed consent should be stated in the protocol for consideration and approval of the review committee.
- Authors and publishers have ethical obligations [*Beneficence, Justice*]
  - accuracy of the results,
  - present positive and negative results,
  - possible conflicts of interest.

Additional principles are noted for medical research combined with medical care:

- May combine medical research with medical care only if there is potential prophylactic, diagnostic, or therapeutic value. [*Beneficence*]
- The benefits, risks, burdens, and effectiveness of a new method should be tested against those of the best current prophylactic, diagnostic, and therapeutic methods. [*Beneficence*]
  - —This does not exclude the use of placebo, or no treatment, in studies where no proven prophylactic, diagnostic, or therapeutic method exists [a footnote was added here as a note of clarification]
    - A placebo-controlled trial may be ethically acceptable, if, for compelling and scientifically sound methodological reasons, its use is necessary; or for a minor

condition and placebo patients are not subject to additional risk of serious or irreversible harm.

- At the conclusion of the study, every patient entered into the study should be assured of access to the best proven prophylactic, diagnostic, and therapeutic methods identified by the study [a footnote was added here as a note of clarification]. [*Justice, Beneficence*]

—or access to other appropriate care.

- The physician should inform the patient which aspects of the care are related to the research. [*Respect for Persons*]
- Where proven prophylactic, diagnostic, and therapeutic methods do not exist, the physician, with informed consent from the patient, must be free to use unproven or new prophylactic, diagnostic, and therapeutic measures, if in the physician's judgment it offers hope of saving life, reestablishing health, or alleviating suffering. [*Beneficence*]
- Where possible, these measures should be made the object of research, designed to evaluate their safety and efficacy. [*Beneficence, Justice*]
- In all cases, new information should be recorded and, where appropriate, published. [*Justice*]
- The other relevant guidelines of this declaration should be followed.

Appendix 4: Excerpt from the Belmont Report[87]

Ethical Principles and Guidelines for Research Involving Human Subjects

Scientific research has produced substantial social benefits. It has also posed some troubling ethical questions. Public attention was drawn to these questions by reported abuses of human subjects in biomedical experiments, especially during the Second World War. During the Nuremberg war crime trials, the Nuremberg code was drafted as a set of standards for judging physicians and scientists who had conducted biomedical experiments on concentration camp prisoners. This code became the prototype of many later codes[88] intended to assure that research involving human subjects would be carried out in an ethical manner.

The codes consist of rules, some general, others specific, that guide the investigators or the reviewers of research in their work. Such rules often are inadequate to cover complex situations; at times they come into conflict, and they are frequently difficult to interpret or apply. Broader ethical principles will provide a basis on which specific rules may be formulated, criticized, and interpreted.

Three principles, or general prescriptive judgments, that are relevant to research involving human subjects are identified in this statement. Other principles may also be relevant. These three are comprehensive, however, and are stated at a level of generalization that should assist scientists, subjects, reviewers and interested citizens to understand the ethical issues

87. National Commission for the Protection of Human Subjects of Biomedical and Behavioral Research, "The Belmont Report: Ethical Principles and Guidelines for the Protection of Human Subjects of Research," April 18, 1979, http://www.hhs.gov/ohrp/humansubjects/guidance/belmont.html. For a scan of the original text, see http://videocast.nih.gov/pdf/ohrp_belmont_report.pdf.

88. Since 1945, various codes for the proper and responsible conduct of human experimentation in medical research have been adopted by different organizations. The best known of these codes are the Nuremberg Code of 1947, the Helsinki Declaration of 1964 (revised in 1975), and the 1971 Guidelines (codified into Federal Regulations in 1974) issued by the U.S. Department of Health, Education, and Welfare. Codes for the conduct of social and behavioral research have also been adopted, the best known being that of the American Psychological Association, http://www.apa.org/ethics/code/index.aspx.

inherent in research involving human subjects. These principles cannot always be applied so as to resolve beyond dispute particular ethical problems. The objective is to provide an analytical framework that will guide the resolution of ethical problems arising from research involving human subjects.

This statement consists of a distinction between research and practice, a discussion of the three basic ethical principles, and remarks about the application of these principles.

A. Boundaries between Practice and Research

It is important to distinguish between biomedical and behavioral research, on the one hand, and the practice of accepted therapy on the other, in order to know what activities ought to undergo review for the protection of human subjects of research. The distinction between research and practice is blurred partly because both often occur together (as in research designed to evaluate a therapy) and partly because notable departures from standard practice are often called "experimental" when the terms "experimental" and "research" are not carefully defined.

For the most part, the term "practice" refers to interventions that are designed solely to enhance the well-being of an individual patient or client and that have a reasonable expectation of success. The purpose of medical or behavioral practice is to provide diagnosis, preventive treatment or therapy to particular individuals.[89] By contrast, the term "research" designates an activity designed to test an hypothesis, permit conclusions to be drawn, and thereby to develop or contribute to generalizable knowledge (expressed, for example, in theories, principles, and statements of relationships). Research is usually described in a formal protocol that sets forth an objective and a set of procedures designed to reach that objective.

When a clinician departs in a significant way from standard or accepted practice, the innovation does not, in and of itself, constitute research. The fact that a procedure is "experimental," in the sense of new, untested or different, does not automatically place it in the category of research. Radically new procedures of this description should, however, be made the object of formal research at an early stage in order to determine whether they are safe and effective. Thus, it is the responsibility of medical practice committees, for example, to insist that a major innovation be incorporated into a formal research project.[90]

Research and practice may be carried on together when research is designed to evaluate the safety and efficacy of a therapy. This need not cause any confusion regarding whether or not the activity requires review; the general rule is that if there is any element of research in an activity, that activity should undergo review for the protection of human subjects.

---

89. Although practice usually involves interventions designed solely to enhance the well-being of a particular individual, interventions are sometimes applied to one individual for the enhancement of the well-being of another (e.g., blood donation, skin grafts, organ transplants) or an intervention may have the dual purpose of enhancing the well-being of a particular individual, and, at the same time, providing some benefit to others (e.g., vaccination, which protects both the person who is vaccinated and society generally). The fact that some forms of practice have elements other than immediate benefit to the individual receiving an intervention, however, should not confuse the general distinction between research and practice. Even when a procedure applied in practice may benefit some other person, it remains an intervention designed to enhance the well-being of a particular individual or groups of individuals; thus, it is practice and need not be reviewed as research.

90. Because the problems related to social experimentation may differ substantially from those of biomedical and behavioral research, the Commission specifically declines to make any policy determination regarding such research at this time. Rather, the Commission believes that the problem ought to be addressed by one of its successor bodies.

B. Basic Ethical Principles

The expression "basic ethical principles" refers to those general judgments that serve as a basic justification for the many particular ethical prescriptions and evaluations of human actions. Three basic principles, among those generally accepted in our cultural tradition, are particularly relevant to the ethics of research involving human subjects: the principles of respect of persons, beneficence, and justice.

1. *Respect for Persons*. Respect for persons incorporates at least two ethical convictions: first, that individuals should be treated as autonomous agents, and second, that persons with diminished autonomy are entitled to protection. The principle of respect for persons thus divides into two separate moral requirements: the requirement to acknowledge autonomy and the requirement to protect those with diminished autonomy.

An autonomous person is an individual capable of deliberation about personal goals and of acting under the direction of such deliberation. To respect autonomy is to give weight to autonomous persons' considered opinions and choices while refraining from obstructing their actions unless they are clearly detrimental to others. To show lack of respect for an autonomous agent is to repudiate that person's considered judgments, to deny an individual the freedom to act on those considered judgments, or to withhold information necessary to make a considered judgment, when there are no compelling reasons to do so.

However, not every human being is capable of self-determination. The capacity for self-determination matures during an individual's life, and some individuals lose this capacity wholly or in part because of illness, mental disability, or circumstances that severely restrict liberty. Respect for the immature and the incapacitated may require protecting them as they mature or while they are incapacitated.

Some persons are in need of extensive protection, even to the point of excluding them from activities which may harm them; other persons require little protection beyond making sure they undertake activities freely and with awareness of possible adverse consequence. The extent of protection afforded should depend upon the risk of harm and the likelihood of benefit. The judgment that any individual lacks autonomy should be periodically reevaluated and will vary in different situations.

In most cases of research involving human subjects, respect for persons demands that subjects enter into the research voluntarily and with adequate information. In some situations, however, application of the principle is not obvious. The involvement of prisoners as subjects of research provides an instructive example. On the one hand, it would seem that the principle of respect for persons requires that prisoners not be deprived of the opportunity to volunteer for research. On the other hand, under prison conditions they may be subtly coerced or unduly influenced to engage in research activities for which they would not otherwise volunteer. Respect for persons would then dictate that prisoners be protected. Whether to allow prisoners to "volunteer" or to "protect" them presents a dilemma. Respecting persons, in most hard cases, is often a matter of balancing competing claims urged by the principle of respect itself.

2. *Beneficence*. Persons are treated in an ethical manner not only by respecting their decisions and protecting them from harm, but also by making efforts to secure their well-being. Such treatment falls under the principle of beneficence. The term "beneficence" is often understood to cover acts of kindness or charity that go beyond strict obligation. In this document, beneficence is understood in a stronger sense, as an obligation. Two general rules have been formulated as complementary expressions of beneficent actions in this sense: (1) do not harm and (2) maximize possible benefits and minimize possible harms.

The Hippocratic maxim "do no harm" has long been a fundamental principle of medical ethics. Claude Bernard extended it to the realm of research, saying that one should not injure one person regardless of the benefits that might come to others. However, even avoiding harm requires learning what is harmful; and, in the process of obtaining this information, persons may be exposed to risk of harm. Further, the Hippocratic Oath requires physicians to benefit their patients "according to their best judgment." Learning what will in fact benefit may require exposing persons to risk. The problem posed by these imperatives is to decide when it is justifiable to seek certain benefits despite the risks involved, and when the benefits should be foregone because of the risks.

The obligations of beneficence affect both individual investigators and society at large, because they extend both to particular research projects and to the entire enterprise of research. In the case of particular projects, investigators and members of their institutions are obliged to give forethought to the maximization of benefits and the reduction of risk that might occur from the research investigation. In the case of scientific research in general, members of the larger society are obliged to recognize the longer term benefits and risks that may result from the improvement of knowledge and from the development of novel medical, psychotherapeutic, and social procedures.

The principle of beneficence often occupies a well-defined justifying role in many areas of research involving human subjects. An example is found in research involving children. Effective ways of treating childhood diseases and fostering healthy development are benefits that serve to justify research involving children—even when individual research subjects are not direct beneficiaries. Research also makes it possible to avoid the harm that may result from the application of previously accepted routine practices that on closer investigation turn out to be dangerous. But the role of the principle of beneficence is not always so unambiguous. A difficult ethical problem remains, for example, about research that presents more than minimal risk without immediate prospect of direct benefit to the children involved. Some have argued that such research is inadmissible, while others have pointed out that this limit would rule out much research promising great benefit to children in the future. Here again, as with all hard cases, the different claims covered by the principle of beneficence may come into conflict and force difficult choices.

3. *Justice*. Who ought to receive the benefits of research and bear its burdens? This is a question of justice, in the sense of "fairness in distribution" or "what is deserved." An injustice occurs when some benefit to which a person is entitled is denied without good reason or when some burden is imposed unduly. Another way of conceiving the principle of justice is that equals ought to be treated equally. However, this statement requires explication. Who is equal and who is unequal? What considerations justify departure from equal distribution? Almost all commentators allow that distinctions based on experience, age, deprivation, competence, merit and position do sometimes constitute criteria justifying differential treatment for certain purposes. It is necessary, then, to explain in what respects people should be treated equally. There are several widely accepted formulations of just ways to distribute burdens and benefits. Each formulation mentions some relevant property on the basis of which burdens and benefits should be distributed. These formulations are (1) to each person an equal share, (2) to each person according to individual need, (3) to each person according to individual effort, (4) to each person according to societal contribution, and (5) to each person according to merit.

Questions of justice have long been associated with social practices such as punishment, taxation and political representation. Until recently these questions have not generally been associated with scientific research. However, they are foreshadowed even in the earliest reflections on the ethics of research involving human subjects. For example, during the nineteenth and early twentieth centuries the burdens of serving as research subjects fell largely upon poor ward patients, while the benefits of improved medical care flowed primarily to private patients. Subsequently, the exploitation of unwilling prisoners as research subjects in Nazi concentration camps was condemned as a particularly flagrant injustice. In this country, in the 1940s, the Tuskegee syphilis study used disadvantaged, rural black men to study the untreated course of a disease that is by no means confined to that population. These subjects were deprived of demonstrably effective treatment in order not to interrupt the project, long after such treatment became generally available.

Against this historical background, it can be seen how conceptions of justice are relevant to research involving human subjects. For example, the selection of research subjects needs to be scrutinized in order to determine whether some classes (e.g., welfare patients, particular racial and ethnic minorities, or persons confined to institutions) are being systematically selected simply because of their easy availability, their compromised position, or their manipulability, rather than for reasons directly related to the problem being studied. Finally, whenever research supported by public funds leads to the development of therapeutic devices and procedures, justice demands both that these not provide advantages only to those who can afford them and that such research should not unduly involve persons from groups unlikely to be among the beneficiaries of subsequent applications of the research.

Appendix 5: The Principles and Guidelines from
A Catholic Guide to Ethical Clinical Research[91]

1. The Principle of Truth

Everything a medical researcher does must be guided by truth; there is no place for intentional falsehoods, misleading statements, bias, and hidden agendas. The research protocol and the conduct of the research, as well as the preparation and publication of the research reports, must be done in an open and honest manner, maintaining the highest level of integrity.

Guidelines

a. All research programs must be of value and done for the good of society. Clinical research in particular should aim to relieve suffering and foster the health and well-being of humanity.

b. Only scientifically qualified persons should conduct clinical research. To engage in research without proper qualifications is deceptive, inappropriate, and misleading.

c. Research protocols must clearly and openly state all that will take place within a clinical study. They must be written in a complete, scientific, and understandable manner. All risks, side effects, consequences, and costs must be clearly communicated to the potential subject before the research is begun. Alternative treatments, including no treatment at all, must always be honestly and fairly described.[92]

d. Informed consent and related documents must be complete, clear, and communicated at a level that can be understood by the subjects in the research. Potential subjects

---

91. Catholic Medical Association and National Catholic Bioethics Center, *A Catholic Guide,* 6–11.

92. See United States Conference of Catholic Bishops, *Ethical and Religious Directives for Catholic Health Care Services,* 4th ed. (Washington, D.C.: USCCB, 2001), dir. 26.

who do not understand the nature of the study, or who otherwise lack capacity, cannot provide informed consent.

e. In the case of minors and others who lack the capacity to consent for themselves, a surrogate may provide permission for their participation in the study. In such cases the researcher must ensure that the surrogate represents the best interests of the subject and not only those of the surrogate.

f. Results of medical experiments, including negative results, must be made available promptly. They must always display and demonstrate a true and complete description of what took place during the experiment. They must be made reasonably available for all physicians to review. Conclusions and recommendations must be honestly portrayed.

2. The Principle of Respect for Life

God, our Creator and Father, is the author of life. God does not relinquish control over the gift of life but shares himself with the human being who receives this gift. Therefore, the clinical researcher must act as a steward of God's gift of life and respect the intrinsic dignity and nature of the gift.[93] It is the responsibility of everyone, especially a physician and a medical researcher, to respect the sacred and inviolable right to life of the human subject at every stage, from its first formation to natural death.[94] In this regard the obligations of the natural moral law and Catholic moral teaching must always be respected.

Guidelines

a. The medical researcher may never willfully destroy any living human being of any age whatsoever.[95]

b. Physicians and medical researchers engaged in studies that employ various reproductive technologies must ensure that their practices and procedures comply with Catholic teaching. They must never in any way commit, or cooperate illicitly with, acts considered wrong or immoral.

c. Subjects, including those deemed to be near death, must not be subjected to protocols and procedures that will directly hasten their demise or involve other disproportionate risks.

3. The Principle of Respect for the Integrity of Persons

Subjects who participate in medical research deserve the utmost respect and concern. Each person, regardless of social class or medical need, must always be fully and properly respected according to a holistic anthropology; as Pope John Paul II stated, "Health, based on an anthropology that respects the whole person, far from being identified with the mere absence of illness, strives to achieve a fuller harmony and healthy balance on the physical, psychological, spiritual and social level."[96] Individuals who are vulnerable by virtue of their age, education,

---

93. See John Paul II, *Evangelium Vitae*, no. 48: "Life is indelibly marked by *a truth of its own*. By accepting God's gift, man is obliged to *maintain life in this truth* which is essential to it" (emphasis in original). See also no. 89.

94. See ibid., no. 89.

95. See John Paul II, Message to the President of the Catholic Social Weeks of France, November 15, 2001; see also Pope Pius XII, Address to Participants at the Congress of the Italian Catholic Union of Midwives, October 29, 1951, no. 12.

96. Pope John Paul II, Message for the Eighth World Day of the Sick (2000), no. 13.

economic status, medical or psychological condition, or cognitive status must be particularly protected by all physicians and medical researchers.

Guidelines

a. The researcher must not participate in any research paradigm in which the subject is treated as a mere object.[97] The researcher must respect the dignity and nature of the human subject as having the powers of intellect and free will. This fact is the foundation for moral obligations regarding free and informed consent. Generally, both the subject and the researcher must recognize that the subject has moral obligations under the natural law concerning his or her life.[98]

b. The researcher must always be mindful that subjects have a natural law obligation to care for and conserve their health in a manner proportionate to the specific circumstances. At no time should a researcher attempt to compromise this obligation.[99]

c. The subject and not a procedure, process, or product being studied is the most important aspect of every clinical trial.

d. Children and certain other populations have particular vulnerabilities.[100] They may be included in clinical research, for to exclude them is to risk depriving them of the potential benefits they deserve. When they are part of a study, great care must be exercised to protect their well-being and enhance their safety.

e. The potential benefits of any study must weigh against potential risks. When a particular study will not directly benefit a minor or other member of a vulnerable population, the associated risks must be relatively insignificant.

f. The medical researcher and those who assist in medical research must always strive to do good and to avoid causing deliberate harm to subjects in any way.

g. The spirituality and religious beliefs of the subject must be respected by the investigator. It is not permissible to compromise these beliefs unless the investigator will fail in some moral duty of the natural law. For example, in the study of a teratogenic substance, it may be stated that women participants should not become pregnant during the course of the study.[101] The specific method of ensuring that a woman does not become pregnant may be left to the woman, her conscience, and her religious beliefs. However, if she became pregnant and wished to have an abortion, it would not be morally licit for her to have one or for the investigator to recommend her having one.

h. The medical researcher has the moral responsibility to act with a properly formed conscience, and must withdraw from a scientific investigation rather than act against the certain judgment of conscience (see "Guidelines" appendix).[102]

97. See Pope John Paul II, Address to the Pontifical Academy for Life (February 24, 2003), no. 4.

98. See Pius XII, Address to the First International Congress on the Histopathology of the Nervous System, nos. 12–14.

99. See John Paul II, *Evangelium Vitae*, no. 65; and *Catechism of the Catholic Church*, no. 2288.

100. In addition to children, some other populations often considered particularly vulnerable are the mentally ill and cognitively impaired, the dying, the unconscious, pregnant women, and women of child-bearing potential.

101. In listing the permitted methods of avoiding pregnancy, abstinence should always be included and encouraged as the preferred method. Protocols should never require a physician to provide a method of birth control, nor should a subject in a study ever be required to use a method of birth control, contrary to their properly formed conscience in accord with the natural moral law.

102. See *Catechism of the Catholic Church*, nos. 1776–1802; and Joseph Cardinal Ratzinger, "Conscience and Truth," in *Catholic Conscience: Foundation and Formation*, ed. Russell E. Smith (Braintree, Mass.: Pope John Center, 1991), 7–27.

4. The Principles of Generosity and Justice

Physicians and medical researchers must understand that they are instruments through which a loving God cares for His creation. They must always be mindful that their hands are those of Jesus, who cured the sick with compassion, generosity, and understanding. Scientific research should be done for the purpose of serving those who are ill, not solely or primarily for the benefit of the researchers.

Guidelines

a. Research should be conducted according to accepted scientific principles. It must always be deemed necessary and potentially useful. It must never subject an individual to unnecessary or disproportionate risks which overshadow the expected benefit from the research.

b. The researcher must never participate in projects that may involve personal, professional, or financial conflicts of interest. To have a conflict of interest is to treat the human subject as on object of that interest.

c. Studies which may involve immoral cooperation with evil must be avoided. Research that is likely to be the occasion of insurmountable scandal, even though it may not specifically involve immoral cooperation, should also be avoided (see "Guidelines" appendix).

d. Disadvantaged subjects should never be enrolled in clinical trials from which they cannot benefit at least indirectly. They should never compose the research population in a study primarily intended for the benefit of another, more advantaged population.

e. Potential subjects should never be coerced to participate in medical research. Compensation to subjects should never be coercive or excessive.[103] Recruitment methods must not be misleading. Care should be exercised not to use compensation as a tool of exploitation for potential subjects who are unemployed, disenfranchised, or incarcerated or who may lack full capacity to provide consent.

f. A medical researcher should not accept compensation that is disproportionate to the work performed.

g. Medical research must never be undertaken primarily for the purpose of enhancing the influence or reputation of a researcher.

Bibliography

Alessi, Scott. "Debate Continues on Whether Brain Death Signifies End of Life: Ethical and Medical Questions Persist as to Whether Brain Death Truly Marks the End of a Person's Life." *Our Sunday Visitor Newsweekly*, June 12, 2011. http://www.osv.com/tabid/7621/itemid/7993/Debate-continues-on-whether-brain-death-signifies.aspx.

Amariglio, N., A. Hirshberg, B. W. Scheithauer, et al. "Donor-Derived Brain Tumor Following Neural Stem Cell Transplantation in an Ataxia Telangiectasia Patient." *PLoS Medicine* 6 (2009): e1000029.

Andrews, Lori, and Dorothy Nelkin. "Whose Body Is It Anyway? Disputes over Body Tissue in a Biotechnology Age." *Lancet* 351 (1998): 53–57.

Aznar, J., and J. L. Sánchez. "Embryonic Stem Cells: Are Useful in Clinic Treatments?" *Journal of Physiology and Biochemistry* 67 (2011): 141–44.

---

103. Excessive compensation would exceed that which is reasonable and customary to compensate subjects for their time, inconvenience, and other expenditures.

Baeten, J. M., P. M. Nyange, B. A. Richardson, L. Lavreys, B. Chohan, H. L. Martin Jr., K. Mandaliya, J. O. Ndinya-Achola, J. J. Bwayo, and J. K. Kreiss. "Hormonal Contraception and Risk of Sexually Transmitted Disease Acquisition: Results from a Prospective Study." *American Journal of Obstetrics and Gynecology* 185 (2001): 380–85

Beecher, Henry K. "Ethics and Clinical Research." *New England Journal of Medicine* 274 (1966): 1354–60.

Boursiquot, M.-A. "The Real Risks of Oral Contraceptives." *Linacre Quarterly* 78 (2011): 100–104.

Bretzner, F., F. Gilbert, F. Baylis, and R. M. Brownstone. "Target Populations for First-in Human Embryonic Stem Cell Research in Spinal Cord Injury." *Cell Stem Cell* 8 (2011): 468–75.

Carr, L. K., D. Steele, S. Steele, D. Wagner, R. Pruchnic, R. Jankowski, J. Erickson, J. Huard, and M. B. Chancellor. "1-Year Follow-Up of Autologous Muscle-Derived Stem Cell Injection Pilot Study to Treat Stress Urinary Incontinence." *International Urogynecology Journal and Pelvic Floor Dysfunction* 19 (2008): 881–83.

Catholic Medical Association and the National Catholic Bioethics Center. "Catholic Principles and Guidelines for Clinical Research." *National Catholic Bioethics Quarterly* 7, no. 1 (2007): 153–65.

———. *A Catholic Guide to Ethical Clinical Research.* Philadelphia: Catholic Medical Association and National Catholic Bioethics Center, 2008.

Condic, Maureen L. "When Does Human Life Begin? A Scientific Perspective." *Westchester Institute White Paper Series* 1, October 2008. https://www.cedarville.edu/personal/sullivan/bio4410/condic_whitepaper.pdf.

Corbie-Smith, G. "The Continuing Legacy of the Tuskegee Syphilis Study: Considerations for Clinical Investigation." *American Journal of the Medical Sciences* 317 (1999): 5–8.

Diamond, E. F. "The Willowbrook Experiments." *Linacre Quarterly* 40 (1973): 133–37.

Edgar, H., and D. J. Rothman. "New Rules for New Drugs: The Challenge of AIDS to the Regulatory Process." *Milbank Quarterly* 68 S1 (1990): 111–42.

Erdö, F., C. Bührle, J. Blunk, M. Hoehn, Y. Xia, B. Fleischmann, M. Föcking, et al. "Host-Dependent Tumorigenesis of Embryonic Stem Cell Transplantation in Experimental Stroke." *Journal of Cerebral Blood Flow and Metabolism* 23 (2003): 780–85.

French, A. J., C. A. Adams, L. S. Anderson, J. R. Kitchen, M. R. Hughes, and S. H. Wood. "Development of Human Cloned Blastocysts Following Somatic Cell Nuclear Transfer with Adult Fibroblasts." *Stem Cells* 26 (2008): 485–93.

Harris, Gardiner. "Regulators Want Antidepressants to List Warning." *New York Times*, March 23, 2004. http://www.nytimes.com/2004/03/23/health/23DEPR.html?hp.

———. "Diabetes Drug Maker Hid Test Data, Files Indicate." *New York Times*, July 13, 2010. http://www.nytimes.com/2010/07/13/health/policy/13avandia.html.

Hwang, W. S., S. I. Roh, B. C. Lee, S. K. Kang, D. K. Kwon, S. Kim, S. J. Kim, et al. "Patient-Specific Embryonic Stem Cells Derived from Human SCNT Blastocysts." *Science* 308 (2005): 1777–83. Erratum: *Science* 310 (2005): 1769.

Hwang, W. S., Y. J. Ryu, J. H. Park, E. S. Park, E. G. Lee, J. M. Koo, H. Y. Jeon, et al. "Evidence of a Pluripotent Human Embryonic Stem Cell Line Derived from a Cloned Blastocyst." *Science* 303 (2004): 1669–74.

John Paul II, Pope. *Evangelium Vitae, On the Value and Inviolability of Human Life.* Encyclical Letter. March 25, 1995.

———. Message for the Eighth World Day of the Sick. 2000.

———. Address to the Eighteenth International Congress of the Transplantation Society. August 29, 2000. http://w2.vatican.va/content/john-paul-ii/en/speeches/2000/jul-sep/documents/hf_jp-ii_spe_20000829_transplants.html.

———. Message to the President of the Catholic Social Weeks of France. November 15, 2001.

———. Address to the Pontifical Academy for Life. February 24, 2003. http://w2.vatican.va/content/john-paul-ii/en/speeches/2003/february/documents/hf_jp-ii_spe_20030224_pont-acad-life.html.

Kennedy, D. Editorial retraction. *Science* 311 (2006): 335.

Lidegaard, Ø., E. Løkkegaard, A. L. Svendsen, and C. Agger. "Hormonal Contraception and Risk of Venous Thromboembolism: National Follow-Up Study." *British Medical Journal* 339 (2009): b2890.

Lukovic, D., V. M. Manzano, M. Stojkovic, S. S. Bhattacharya, and S. Erceg. "Concise Review: Human Pluripotent Stem Cells in the Treatment of Spinal Cord Injury." *Stem Cells* 30 (2012): 1787–92.

National Commission for the Protection of Human Subjects of Biomedical and Behavioral Research. "The Belmont Report: Ethical Principles and Guidelines for the Protection of Human Subjects of Research." April 18, 1979. http://www.hhs.gov/ohrp/humansubjects/guidance/belmont.html.

Nishihira, H., K. Ohnuma, K. Ikuta, K. Isoyama, A. Kinoshita, Y. Toyoda, M. Ohira, J. Okamura, and F. Nakajima. "Unrelated Umbilical Cord-Blood Stem Cell Transplantation: A Report from Kanagawa Cord Blood Bank, Japan." *International Journal of Hematology* 68 (1998): 193–202.

"The Nuremberg Code." In *Trials of War Criminals before the Nuremberg Military Tribunals under Control Council Law No. 10*. Vol. 2, *The Medical Case; The Milch Case*, 181–82. Washington, D.C.: U.S. Government Printing Office, 1949. Available online at https://www.ushmm.org/information/exhibitions/online-exhibitions/special-focus/doctors-trial/nuremberg-code.

O'Grady, John, and Otto I. Linet. *Early Phase Drug Evaluation in Man*. Boca Raton, Fla.: CRC Press, 1990.

Philpott, S., and R. Baker. "Why the Avandia Scandal Proves Big Pharma Needs Stronger Ethical Standards." *Bioethics* 24 (2010): ii–iii.

Pius XII, Pope. Address to Participants at the Congress of the Italian Catholic Union of Midwives. October 29, 1951.

——. Address to the First International Congress on the Histopathology of the Nervous System. September 14, 1952. http://www.papalencyclicals.net/Pius12/P12PSYCH.HTM.

Pressel, D. M. "Nuremberg and Tuskegee: Lessons for Contemporary American Medicine." *Journal of the National Medical Association* 95 (2003): 1216–25.

Ratzinger, Joseph. "Conscience and Truth." In *Catholic Conscience: Foundation and Formation*, ed. Russell E. Smith, 7–27. Braintree, Mass.: Pope John Center, 1991.

Reubinoff, B. E., M. F. Pera, C. Y. Fong, A. Trounson, and A. Bongso. "Embryonic Stem Cell Lines from Human Blastocysts: Somatic Differentiation In Vitro." *Nature Biotechnology* 18 (2000): 399–404. Erratum: *Nature Biotechnology* 18 (2000): 559.

Rodin, A. E., L. A. Koller, and J. D. Taylor. "Association of Thalidomide (Kevadon) With Congenital Anomalies." *Canadian Medical Association Journal* 86 (1962): 744–46.

Ross, J. S., D. Madigan, K. P. Hill, D. S. Egilman, Y. Wang, and H. M. Krumholz. "Pooled Analysis of Rofecoxib Placebo-Controlled Clinical Trial Data: Lessons for Postmarket Pharmaceutical Safety Surveillance." *Archives of Internal Medicine* 169 (2009): 1976–85.

Rothman, David J. *Strangers at the Bedside: A History of How Law and Bioethics Transformed Medical Decision Making*. New York: Aldine de Gruyter, 2003.

Sangwan, V. S., G. K. Vemuganti, S. Singh, and D. Balasubramanian. "Successful Reconstruction of Damaged Ocular Outer Surface in Humans Using Limbal and Conjuctival Stem Cell Culture Methods." *Bioscience Reports* 23 (2003): 169–74. Erratum: *Bioscience Reports* 124 (2006): 1483.

Schwartz, S. D., J. P. Hubschman, G. Heilwell, V. Franco-Cardenas, C. K. Pan, R. M. Ostrick, E. Mickunas, R. Gay, I. Klimanskaya, and R. Lanza. "Embryonic Stem Cell Trials for Macular Degeneration: A Preliminary Report." *Lancet* 379, no. 9817 (February 25, 2012): 713–20.

Shavers, V. L., C. F. Lynch, and L. F. Burmeister. "Knowledge of the Tuskegee Study and Its Impact on the Willingness to Participate in Medical Research Studies." *Journal of the National Medical Association* 92 (2000): 563–72.

Speirs, A. L. "Thalidomide and Congenital Abnormalities." *Lancet* 1 (1962): 303–5.

Stadtfeld, M., and K. Hochedlinger. "Induced Pluripotency: History, Mechanisms, and Applications." *Genes and Development* 24 (2010): 2239–63.

Takahashi, K, K. Tanabe, M. Ohnuki, M. Narita, T. Ichisaka, K. Tomoda, and S. Yamanaka. "Induction of Pluripotent Stem Cells from Adult Human Fibroblasts by Defined Factors." *Cell* 131 (2007): 861–72.

Trivedi, H. L., V. V. Mishra, A. V. Vanikar, P. R. Modi, V. R. Shah, P. R. Shah, and A. Firoz. "Embryonic Stem Cell Derived and Adult Hematopoietic Stem Cell Transplantation for Tolerance Induction in a Renal Allograft Recipient: A Case Report." *Transplant Proceedings* 38 (2006): 3103–8.

Trivedi, H. L., A. V. Vanikar, U. Thakker, A. Firoze, S. D. Dave, C. N. Patel, J. V. Patel, A. B. Bhargava, and V. Shankar. "Human Adipose Tissue-Derived Mesenchymal Stem Cells Combined with Hematopoietic Stem Cell Transplantation Synthesize Insulin." *Transplant Proceedings* 40 (2008): 1135–39.

Tsubota, K., Y. Satake, M. Kaido, N. Shinozaki, S. Shimmura, H. Bissen-Miyajima, and J. Shimazaki. "Treatment of Severe Ocular-Surface Disorders with Corneal Epithelial Stem-Cell Transplantation." *New England Journal of Medicine* 340 (1999): 1697–703.

United States Conference of Catholic Bishops. *Ethical and Religious Directives for Catholic Health Care Services*. 4th edition. Washington, D.C.: USCCB, 2001.

United States Department of Health and Human Services, Food and Drug Administration, Center for Drug Evaluation and Research (CDER), and Center for Biologics Evaluation and Research (CBER). *Guidance for Industry*, E6, *Good Clinical Practice: Consolidated Guidance*. Rockville, Md.: ICH, 1996. http://www.fda.gov/downloads/Drugs/GuidanceComplianceRegulatoryInformation/Guidances/ucm073122.pdf.

United States House of Representatives, Committee on Energy and Commerce, Subcommittee on Energy Conservation and Power. "American Nuclear Guinea Pigs: Three Decades of Radiation Experiments on U.S. Citizens." October 24, 1986, 99th cong., 2nd sess. http://nsarchive.gwu.edu/radiation/dir/mstreet/commeet/meet1/brief1/br1n.txt.

Urban, David J. "2006 Virginia Commonwealth University Life Sciences Survey." http://lifesciences.vcu.edu/media/life-sciences/docs/ls_survey_2006_report.pdf.

Vinnedge, Debra L. "Aborted Fetal Cell Line Vaccines and the Catholic Family: A Moral and Historical Perspective." Children of God for Life. Updated October 2005. https://cogforlife.org/vaccines-abortions/.

Wadhwa, P. D., H. M. Lazarus, O. N. Koc, J. Jaroscak, D. Woo, C. E. Stevens, P. Rubinstein, and M. J. Laughlin. "Hematopoietic Recovery after Unrelated Umbilical Cord-Blood Allogeneic Transplantation in Adults Treated with In Vivo Stem Cell Factor (R-MetHuSCF) and Filgrastim Administration." *Leukemia Research* 27 (2003): 215–20.

World Medical Association. Declaration of Helsinki, "Ethical Principles for Medical Research Involving Human Subjects." Last amended October 2013. http://www.wma.net/en/30publications/10policies/b3/.

Domenico Francesco Crupi,
Francesco Giuliani, Jere D. Palazzolo,
and Gianluigi Mazzoccoli

---

15. A MODEL OF CATHOLIC CARE— "THE CASA"

The Casa Sollievo della Sofferenza in Italy, founded by St. Pio of Pietrelcina, and its counter-part, Casa San Pio Medical Clinic of Appalachia in Kentucky, provide examples of Catholic health-care centers focused on serving the poor and underserved through medical care, faith, and prayer. Padre Pio was dedicated to providing love, in addition to medical care, in the relief of suffering, and he wanted to create a climate in which patients would experience the love of God and the kindness and compassion of their brothers and sisters given in generous service. His project was realized with the opening of the doors of the Casa in 1956, the construction of which was funded entirely by donations and supported by the prayers of groups throughout the world. Medical professionals working at the Casa perceive it as different from other hospitals, for it has a Christian atmosphere; they seek to relieve suffering through high-quality medical care and also through prayer, love, and moral support of patients, and to exhibit Christian values of charity, humility, respect for life, and sacrifice, with complete dedication and attention to the patient's body and spirit. This chapter offers a concrete example of a model for authentic Catholic care. It is the vision of many in this endeavor that this practice will spread, and additional health-care centers will open in as many places as possible. The U.S. Casa opened its doors in 2011 and continues Padre Pio's mission.—*Editors*

The Casa Sollievo della Sofferenza (Home for the Relief of Suffering), a Catholic health-care delivery system envisioned by St. Pio of Pietrelcina, is "a hospital city technically suitable to the most demanding medical needs," a place in which human knowledge merges with Christian charity.[1] This project, which he referred

---

1. Casa Sollievo della Sofferenza, Editorial Office, *Guide for the Visitor to Padre Pio's Work* (San Giovanni Rotondo, Italy: Casa Sollievo della Sofferenza Editions, 1999), iii.

to as "the Work," consumed his mind and soul for the last decades of his ministry and was the culmination of his own life, which was lived in constant pain from the wounds of Christ in his own hands and feet.

On January 9, 1940, Padre Pio announced his ambitious plans to develop a Home for the Relief of Suffering in the small town of San Giovanni Rotondo in the remote south Italian region of Puglia. The Casa opened its doors on May 5, 1956, as a 300-bed facility, built on the small, sincere, and spontaneous donations and prayers of his followers. He also developed an international network of prayer groups for the support of the Casa and its ministry that currently numbers more than 3,000 groups worldwide and continues to live on and grow today. Padre Pio considered the Casa Sollievo della Sofferenza—his "Work," inspired and blessed by God—to be a haven of relief from suffering for all of God's children in pain in body or soul. It is a model community of Catholic Christian health delivery, and has grown from a regional referral center to one of international renown, thanks to its status as a hospital and research center for the fields of genetic diseases, regenerative medicine, and innovative therapeutics. Today, with more than 1,000 inpatient beds, 2,500 employees, services comparable to most academic research centers of excellence, and more than 50,000 inpatients and 300,000 outpatients each year, the Casa is thriving by God's graces in one of the most remote, most desolate, and poorest areas of Italy, atop Mount Gargano, more than four hours' drive from Rome. In further evidence of growth, the Casa San Pio Medical Clinic of Appalachia, modeled after the original Casa, opened in 2011 to serve the poor and underserved Appalachian region in Kentucky.

The Life of Padre Pio

Padre Pio was born Francesco Forgione on May 25, 1887, to Maria and Grazio Mario Forgione in Pietrelcina, in southern Italy, the fifth of eight children. His father, commonly known as Razio, was a small landowner, and his mother was a woman of great piety. He, too, was devout, even as a child, solemnly consecrating himself to Jesus at age five, and experiencing both celestial visions and attacks by the devil. He entered the Capuchin community at Morcone at age fifteen and received the Franciscan garb of the Order of Friars Minor, taking the name of Fra (Brother) Pio, in honor of St. Pius V, the patron saint of Pietrelcina. At the end of the novitiate year, he took his temporary vows and began his study for the priesthood. His health faltered at this time, and he was obliged to return to his village intermittently for health reasons. His superiors suspected that his health problems were manifestations of a spiritual struggle, but they kept his secret.

Brother Pio was ordained to the priesthood on August 10, 1910, at the Cathedral of Benevento. "I found my heart burning with love for Jesus. How happy was I, how much did I love that day," he later recalled.[2] He returned to Pietrelcina to celebrate

---

2. Padre Pio, *Epistolario* [Letters], ed. Melchiorre da Pobladura and Alessandro da Ripabottoni, vol. 1, p. 47, no. 297. All quotations in this chapter are from this Italian edition; translations are provided by the authors of this chapter. Padre Pio's letters are available in English, edited by Father Gerardo Di Flumeri, OFM

his first Mass; it was there, on September 7, 1910, that he experienced a vision of Jesus and Mary, along with a strong burning sensation in his palms. He had received the wounds of Christ, the stigmata. In confusion, he prayed that he be allowed to suffer like Christ did, but in secret; and his prayer was granted. The wounds disappeared, but the suffering they caused continued. He bore the pain in secret for a year before he told his community's superiors.

The First World War reached Padre Pio in August 1917, when he was inducted into the service and assigned to the 10th Company of the Italian Medical Corps. He served for a time before his ailments returned and he was hospitalized. After a round of sick leaves, interspersed with trips home to Pietrelcina and to various monasteries, he was finally discharged from the army in March 1918 because of double broncho-alveolitis.

In July of that year, responding to Pope Benedict XV's call to all Christians for prayers for the end of the war, Padre Pio offered himself as a victim for that intention. Days later, on August 5, Christ again appeared to him and pierced his side, leaving a physical wound (a transverberation). The following month, his stigmata became visible again, open and bleeding on his hands, feet, and chest.

"What I can tell you about my crucifixion?" he wrote in October 1918.

My God! What a confusion and what humiliation I feel when I try to show somebody what has been done in me.... It all happened in a flash; I felt abandonment with the complete deprivation of everything. What I felt at that moment is indescribable. I thought I would die, and would have died if the Lord hadn't intervened and strengthened my heart, which was about to burst out of my chest! ... I became aware that my hands, feet, and side were pierced and were dripping with blood. You can imagine the torment that I experienced then and that I am almost experiencing every day.... My God, I die of pain, torment, and confusion.[3]

Despite his efforts, Padre Pio could not hide the stigmata this time. Word soon began to spread to the outside world, and crowds of pilgrims began arriving at the monastery to see the miracle and to receive graces from this man who suffered like Jesus. Over the years doctors who examined the wounds were unable to explain their cause, and one physician who tried to "cure" them failed. For the remaining fifty years of his life, they remained intact and continued to bleed.

The fame attracted by Padre Pio's stigmata, along with his spiritual influence, drew detractors as well as believers. Accusations against him poured into the Holy Office (today the Congregation for the Doctrine of Faith), resulting in Vatican-imposed restrictions in 1922. He was obliged to say Mass at varied, unannounced times, and was forbidden to answer letters seeking his spiritual direction. By 1931, doubt about his wounds' supernatural source led the Vatican to completely ban him from celebrating Mass in public and to order his total seclusion in the convent. It was not until early 1933 that Pope Pius XI ordered the ban reversed, saying, "I have not been badly dis-

Cap. (San Giovanni Rotondo, Italy: Padre Pio da Pietrelcina Editions, 1987). For more information on Padre Pio, see also Gherardo Leone, *Padre Pio: A Summary of His Life* (San Giovanni Rotondo, Italy: Casa Sollievo della Sofferenza, 1999).

    3. Padre Pio, *Epistolario*, vol. 1, no. 1093, letter dated October 22, 1918.

posed toward Padre Pio, but I have been badly informed." When Pius XII was elected pope in 1939, he actually began to encourage people to visit Padre Pio.

The crowds returned, seeking a chance to see the saintly priest, to attend Mass, and to have him hear their confessions. He was known as an exceptional confessor, a man with a great ability to provide spiritual guidance and to "read" the inner souls of penitents, who often heard him reminding them of unconfessed sins. If the omission was inadvertent, or dealt with a minor sin, all was well; but if the penitent deliberately held serious sins back, the priest's reproach could be harsh and unyielding. Many times he drove penitents to tears, but there was always a reason, which only that person usually knew.

In 1959, ill health confined Padre Pio to the monastery's second floor, and his spiritual children felt his absence from Mass keenly. He recovered, he said, through the intervention of Our Lady of Fatima, and took up a reduced schedule of Mass and confessions. But around this time, he also became the subject of new attacks on his ministry, this time involving many people close to him. Another investigation by the Vatican led to more restrictions on his spiritual activities. He was essentially isolated from the followers he regarded as his spiritual "children," which was a great mortification for him. His health began to fail, and eventually he was confined to a wheelchair. In September 1968, just a few days after the fiftieth anniversary of his stigmatization, Padre Pio died in his cell, his wounds miraculously healed. Tens of thousands of people flocked to San Giovanni Rotondo for his funeral, and a steady stream of the faithful filed past his body over three days and nights. His grave at the Church of Our Lady of Grace became a site of pilgrimage.

In the years following his death, his reputation for sanctity and miracles grew steadily; and the cause for sainthood got underway. Padre Pio was declared venerable by Pope John Paul II on December 18, 1997, and beatified on May 2, 1999. He was canonized on February 28, 2002. His liturgical feast day is September 23.

Pope John Paul II visited the Home for the Relief of Suffering in 1987, forty years after his initial visit to the site, when construction was still underway. In his address to its staff and patients, he said that the Casa's mission was a true manifestation of Christian love:

The relief of suffering! In this sweet expression is summarized one of the essential perspectives of Christian charity, of brotherly charity that Christ taught us and that must be the distinctive sign of his disciples; that charity whose active practice, especially toward people in need, is fundamental evidence of the credibility of that message of truth, love, and salvation that the Christian must announce to the world. This Work, for which Padre Pio prayed so much, is a wonderful testament to Christian love.[4]

Padre Pio's vision, the pope said, unified medical science with faith and prayer in the service of the sick, acknowledging that suffering is "forever, in a certain mea-

---

4. Pope John Paul II, ai medici e ai malati dell'ospedale "Casa Sollievo della Sofferenza" [To doctors and patients of the Hospital Casa Sollievo della Sofferenza], May 23, 1987, http://www.vatican.va/holy_father/john_paul_ii/speeches/1987/may/documents/hf_jp-ii_spe_19870523_medici-malati_it.html.

sure, a heritage of life on earth." Thus, along with its work to relieve suffering, the Casa's mission must also involve recognition of science's limitations and education on Christian acceptance of suffering. "In this, way," said the pope, "a community founded on Christ's love will be formed: a community full of brotherhood among the ones who cure and the ones who are cured."[5]

Origins of the Casa

Padre Pio knew suffering in all its forms, which is why he dedicated his life to the relief of suffering. It is commonly said that Padre Pio was a very sick child, but in fact this is not true. He had a healthy childhood, and it was not until after he entered the novitiate as a young Capuchin student that he began to suffer from physical deterioration, sickness, lack of appetite, and fever. The symptoms of consumption made themselves known as well, but that ailment was not diagnosed until he did his military service. Even then, for more than two years he alternated between brief periods in service and long convalescences before he was discharged. His illness was so severe that he was forced to return home for long periods, both as a student and as a young priest. Whenever he stayed in the monastery, his ills assailed him with increased intensity, to the extent that his superiors were convinced that he had very little time to live. Because it was thought that he had tuberculosis, the chalice and other vessels with which he celebrated Mass were kept apart for his use alone.

During his ordeals, Padre Pio became profoundly familiar with hospital life, treatment of the sick, and the mentality of doctors; and in his judgment, all were found wanting. Doctors examined their patients without even looking them in the face and pronounced their diagnoses without permitting the patient to speak. His experience in military hospitals was the worst: patients felt abandoned, going for days without being informed about their conditions or their doctor's decisions. Padre Pio likened these hospitals to an exile, a prison sentence. Years later, he recalled, "The doctors dismissed me, giving me only a few weeks to live; and here I am still, thirty years later." He used these words in his ministry to comfort the gravely ill and to give them hope, but his words also implied a condemnation of the system and of ineffectual treatment.

Padre Pio believed that love is the first ingredient in the relief of suffering.

Fifty years of religious life, fifty years mystically bound to the Cross of the Lord, fifty years of devouring flame for the Lord, for his redeemed. What does my soul desire if not to guide all to You, Lord, and to wait patiently for this devouring flame to burn my whole being in the *Cupio Dissolvi*, to be completely in you?[6]

That belief moved this simple, uneducated friar, who had spent his entire life isolated in the monastery of a backward mountain village, to build a large and modern hospital and research center. While equipped with the most advanced facilities for the

---

5. Ibid.
6. Padre Pio, *Epistolario*, vol. 4, no. 922, letter dated January 22, 1953.

scientific response to illness, the hospital had a more transcendent mission: it was designed to express human warmth and understanding of patients' fears and doubts, and to transform the pain, anxiety, and solitude of illness into wellness, hope in God and in one's fellow man, and ultimately joy in life. Padre Pio wanted the Home for the Relief of Suffering to be a first-class hospital, but above all he wished the medicine practiced there to be truly human, and the patients to be treated with warm concern and sincere attention. He knew that people who are ill need more than competent therapeutic care; they need a human and spiritual climate to help them encounter the love of God and the kindness of their brothers and sisters.

A man who, transcending himself, bends over the wounds of his misfortunate brother, raises to the Lord the most beautiful, the most noble prayer, made of sacrifice and love lived. I know that you all are suffering. Take courage! The trust in our Mother is the sure guarantee that she will stretch out her hand to comfort all of us. In every suffering man there is Jesus who suffers! In every poor man there is Jesus who is wretched! In every poor, sick person there is twice Jesus, who is suffering and wretched! Let us always respond lovingly to the needs of our brothers if we want the Lord our God to bless us and bless our families.[7]

Padre Pio's zeal for souls and concern for his suffering brothers and sisters came to life in the Casa. He wished to show that God's "ordinary miracles" take place in and through charity, and the Casa combined compassion and generous service with every available resource of medical science and technology. His vision embraced not only medical staff, but also every person connected with the hospital's construction and operation. Today the hospital still strives to follow this vision.

Padre Pio's desire to relieve suffering dates back to his youth, as evidenced by some of his schoolboy writings. Several of his school compositions describe acts of charity, giving money to the poor; in one of these he even describes the charity shown by nuns and priests in a hospital that seems to foreshadow his own hospital. From the earliest years of his ministry, Padre Pio comforted the sick, suffered with them, and promised to pray for them. Certainly he would have liked to have seen them all cured, and this was the genesis of his dream for the hospital. The first inklings of this project appeared in a 1921 letter Padre Pio wrote to his friend Rev. Peppino Orlando, in which he alludes to asking Orlando for a "sacrifice" which "is for the good of all suffering humanity."[8] We also have the testimony of a young doctor, who as a new graduate frequented San Giovanni Rotondo during this time. One day as the young man stood in the churchyard, Padre Pio looked from the window and, pointing to the mountain, called the young man by name: "Giovanni, do you want to come here?" For many years after, the young doctor asked himself what Padre Pio could have meant. He understood only when the clinic was built.

In the meantime, Padre Pio brought about something more immediate in the village, which suffered from lack of medical facilities. There was at the time nothing worthy of the name "hospital" in the whole of the Gargano region; the nearest hos-

---

7. Pope John Paul II, ai medici e ai malati dell'ospedale "Casa Sollievo della Sofferenza."
8. Padre Pio, *Epistolario*, vol. 4, no. 559, letter dated October 16, 1921.

pital was at Foggia, forty kilometers away. The distance, combined with poor roads and primitive methods of transportation, meant that one went there only in gravest necessity. With the aid of some doctors, Padre Pio transformed an old convent of the Poor Clares into a small but functional hospital. The Hospital of St. Francis, which opened in January 1925, had two wards with about twenty beds all together, along with an operating room. The doctors of the town, including the convent's physician and a local surgeon, donated their time to staff the facility. Though small, the hospital served the needs of the small town for some time, but fell into disuse after a couple of years and finally closed its doors. The structure itself fell victim to a 1938 earthquake, and it seemed that all that remained of Padre Pio's dream was the hospital's dedication plaque, left lying amid the rubble.

But Padre Pio never abandoned his vision. He thought about it continually as his mission became more clear, speaking of it often with the friends who came to visit him during his times of restriction. With some of his more assiduous and dynamic friends, he discussed the project at great length. One evening late in 1939 he brought up the subject with Dr. Mario Sanvico, an agronomist and doctor of commerce from Perugia, and a few others who were visiting at the time. While Padre Pio had spoken to these men about his dream in the past, on this particular evening his words seemed implanted in their minds; and the dream began to take shape. Early the following year, Dr. Sanvico gathered a small group of doctors and others at his humble house near the monastery, to begin laying out plans for a clinic based on Padre Pio's intentions. The group set up a permanent committee, headed by Padre Pio, as founder, and subject to his approval. Other members of this seminal committee were Dr. Sanvico, who served as secretary; Dr. Guglielmo Sanguinetti, technical medical director; and Ida Seitz, director of internal organization. After the meeting, the group traveled to present its results to Padre Pio, who voiced his approval with the words, "This evening my earthly Work has begun. I bless you and all those who will contribute to the Work, which will become bigger and ever more beautiful." While the language may seem flowery, Padre Pio was very conscious of the fact that his vision was now to become a concrete reality, through the help of like-minded, faith-filled people whom he had prepared for this very task.

That evening he spoke to the committee members about the hospital's mission:

"The ills are the children of blame, of the betrayal which man perpetrated against God . . . but God's mercy is great. . . . A single act of man's love for God has so much value in His eyes, that He would think it small to repay him with the gift of the whole creation. . . . Love is only the spark of God in men. . . . the very essence of God embodied in the Holy Spirit. We, miserable creatures that we are, should dedicate to God all the love of which we are capable. . . . Our love, to be worthy of God, should be infinite, but unfortunately only God is infinite. . . . Nonetheless, we must employ all our energies in love, so that the Lord can say to us one day: 'I was thirsty, and you gave me to drink; I was hungry, and you gave me to eat; I was suffering, and you consoled me.'"

After searching in the many pockets of his habit, Padre Pio took out a gold coin he had received that very day from a follower for his works of charity. He presented it to the committee members, saying, "I myself want to make the first offering." Members of the committee and others also contributed their own funds that same evening toward the project.[9]

Thus, on January 9, 1940, in Padre Pio's small Franciscan cell, the Casa Sollievo della Sofferenza was born. Padre Pio himself gave Dr. Sanvico the project's name, Home for the Relief of Suffering. He instructed the committee members to "stay here," and they did so, preparing a base that would allow them to remain close to San Giovanni Rotondo during the building of the Casa.

While the doctors were eager to get construction underway, they were also anxious about undertaking such an ambitious project when Europe was clearly on the brink of another world war. These fears, however, did not stop Padre Pio. The committee set to work, printing a brochure that set out, in several languages, the hospital's aims, accompanied by an image from a painting by Giotto depicting St. Francis giving his coat to a poor man. The brochure described Gargano as a region of pilgrimage where the faithful "seeking direction and peace" had come to find "richness and spiritual light." The Casa, it said, "will thus be a way to show God our gratitude for the graces received in this patch of our country; it will be above all the exchange of the love of the children for the love of the Father."

Dr. Sanguinetti came to San Giovanni Rotondo planning to stay just eight days, but stayed on for forty, assisting Padre Pio's dying father and discussing the project at great length with Padre Pio. When he understood the scope of what was asked of him, he was dismayed, feeling himself unequal to the task. However, he trusted in Padre Pio and took a leap of faith, moving his practice of twenty-seven years to San Giovanni. There, he devoted his days to the project, serving in every role from advisor to driver to newspaper editor. He loved Padre Pio as a brother, and was in turn entrusted with bringing the priest's dream to fruition.

As time went on, all those who moved in the orbit of Padre Pio were informed of the project. A fund for its realization drew donations from people at all levels of society, ranging from small contributions of 30 lire (about $1.50 in 1940, or about $20 today) to large sums from those outside the country, and eventually reaching the level of 1.5 million lire, quite a large sum in those days—nearly $77,000 in 1940, or nearly $1 million today.

As World War II got underway in earnest, it became clear that the project would have to be postponed. To avoid depreciation in the hospital fund, an estate was purchased at Lucera. Dr. Carlo Kisvarday, a pharmacist from Zara who had come to live near Padre Pio and who was serving as the project's bookkeeper, gave his nearby bungalow to be headquarters for the hospital project.

The war in southern Italy was in essence finished by the autumn of 1943, with Allied troops stationed in Gargano. Soldiers of many nationalities came to Padre Pio out of curiosity or devotion. As Italy was gradually liberated, the numbers of ordinary pilgrims also increased; and larger and larger crowds flocked to San Giovanni

---

9. Gherardo Leone, *Padre Pio and His Work*, 3rd ed. (San Giovanni Rotondo, Italy: Casa Sollievo della Sofferenza Editions, 1986), 25.

Rotondo. A sea of broken people began flooding into the monastery, seeking a last ray of hope for bodies, souls, and families crushed by the war. The sick could be counted in the hundreds: victims of tuberculosis, mentally handicapped people, and all sorts of sufferers, seeking healing from Padre Pio. A large sign outside the villa shared by Sanvico and Sanguinetti announced that work on the hospital was imminent. On October 5, 1946, a shareholding company was established with 1 million lire in capital, divided into a thousand shares. Each shareholder signed a document renouncing any profit. While at the bedside of his dying father, Padre Pio gave his blessing to the contract, which soon attracted more signatories.

The hospital site, on the side of the mountain just a few hundred yards from the monastery, was donated by Maria Basilio, who had bought it for 10,000 lire from the mayor of San Giovanni Rotondo, just days after the company's establishment and specifically for the project. Additional acreage was donated by the Serritelli family.

The architectural design was provided by Angelo Lupi, who despite being neither an engineer nor a land surveyor, provided a design that proved most in harmony with the nature of the place. A tall, strongly built man, Lupi typically wore the knickerbockers and big boots of the era, evocative of that generation of men who had endured the harsh reality of war. He and his co-workers on the project certainly had their work cut out for them, as conditions at San Giovanni Rotondo were primitive at best. There was no means of modern communication nor any electrical services. The monastery's beacon was the only light in the night in the small, sparsely inhabited community. Life in the village centered around the monastery's 4 a.m. Mass, celebrated by Padre Pio, for which the villagers rose in the middle of the night.

The first stone was blessed by Padre Pio, with a simple ceremony in the monastery, in the late spring of 1947; and work began under the direction of the same Rev. Peppino Orlando in whom Padre Pio had confided his first ideas about the hospital. Lupi took matters in hand with military discipline, employing able-bodied farm laborers to do the digging. They worked with enthusiasm, often singing a work song they had learned from Rev. Orlando. The structure's foundation required the removal of 75,000 cubic meters of solid rock, which were cut away with dynamite. Despite the doubts of naysayers (such as the doctor at Foggia who said "They're crazy—a hospital on a mountain!") the hospital began to take shape. By the end of 1947, the foundations were laid, and the first walls arose.

The project was financed entirely by donations. No bank loans were available at the time, and even if they had been, Padre Pio would not have pursued them, preferring to rely on divine providence. As it turned out, providence appeared under the name of Barbara Ward, a British journalist for *The Economist* magazine. She had been assigned by her editor to investigate how the European nations were recovering from the war. Her project was financed in part by the United Nations Relief and Rehabilitation Administration (UNRRA). Ward, who was Catholic, had friends in Rome, among them Marquis Bernardo Patrizi, whom she had met in London. Patrizi spoke to Ward of Padre Pio and his work, knowing that she had influential friends in the United States, and encouraged her to visit the hospital site.

The eminent journalist was deeply moved by her visit with Padre Pio and by his efforts to build the hospital. She asked him to pray for the conversion to Catholicism of her Protestant fiancé, Commander Robert Jackson, an Australian who served as delegate-adviser with the United Nations Relief and Rehabilitation Administration.

The United Nations Relief and Rehabilitation Administration's mission was to provide aid for reconstruction in countries damaged by the war, and a hospital was certainly a work of reconstruction. To enlist wider financial support, it was proposed that the hospital be designated as a memorial to an illustrious Italian-American, New York City Mayor Fiorello La Guardia, who had died not long before. This plan, along with funds amounting to 400,000,000 lire ($260,000), an enormous sum at the time, was approved by the U.S. Congress in June 1948. However, as the Italian government had been unaware of the grant, a tangle of red tape ensued; and by the time it was over, the Italian government released just 250 million in lire, paid in installments, and retained the rest. While Padre Pio regarded this government interference as an impropriety, if not outright theft, the funds nonetheless allowed the work to proceed apace.

By September 1949, the hospital was publishing a monthly newsletter to inform donors and other friends of the hospital's progress. This publication soon expanded its subject matter to include the multitude of prayer groups throughout the world, which were established to pray for Padre Pio's intentions and for the hospital's successful completion. The importance of these prayer groups was understood from the beginning as the "other face" of the relief of suffering. Those connected with the hospital recognized that the basis of Christian action must be prayer, and therefore established the Casa as the center for these prayer groups offering their spiritual support.

The work crew, along with Padre Pio and some Italian-American authorities, celebrated the building's first roof covering in early September 1948. The structure was fully roofed in December of 1949, and on June 21, 1950, the sign appeared on the building's facade: *Casa Sollievo della Sofferenza*.

Gradually but perceptibly, the mountain was transformed, as the impressive structure took shape, enhanced by plantings and trees. The construction workers, too, were being transformed from simple farm laborers into skilled workers, who along with their supervisors heeded the siren's call to Mass at the end of the workday every first Friday. By the summer of 1950, the clinic was finished. Barbara Ward visited the site that autumn to see the fruits of the money she had helped procure, and was surprised to discover that the stained glass window of the Madonna in the chapel had been designed to resemble her own face. The resemblance was the idea and work of Angelo Lupi, who, like everyone, considered Ward the hospital's "godmother."

Padre Pio wished to call his projected hospital a "home," to emphasize its mission of offering to its suffering "guests" practical and spiritual assistance, along with medical care. He wanted to avoid the cold impersonality of hospital corridors, the lack of individual bathrooms, and the barracks-like rooms of twenty or more beds. In Padre Pio's Casa, the patients' rooms, each decorated in a different style, were to have four to six beds and adequate personal sanitary services, to make patients feel more at home.

He was adamant that all people involved in the Casa, from the lowliest laborer to the most prestigious medical director, were to be grounded in the concept of human dignity, so that the whole person—body, mind, and spirit—could be treated with respect. Over and over, Padre Pio kept stressing Christ's love. Since Christ gave him the gift of the stigmata as symbols of his Cross and his suffering, Padre Pio had come to regard his wounds as a great privilege that allowed him to suffer with Christ. He wanted all people to share that love and thus to understand that, through suffering, souls are saved. "In this home, the love of God should strengthen the spirit of those who are sick, by means of love for Jesus crucified, which will radiate out from those who assist in healing the infirmities of body and of spirit. Here, patients, doctors, and priests will be reservoirs of love, which will be more abundant inasmuch as it will be shared with others."[10] This vision was not restricted by the building's size limitations; Padre Pio hoped to build a "hospital city." Sanguinetti hoped that it would be the first of many, "the first link in a great chain.... the model for many other innumerable *Casas*, with the same name and above all the same spirit, which must bring love to all of humanity. It is a program that would make us tremble with awe, were it not inspired by God, who is first of all love!"[11]

On July 26, 1954, the hospital opened its emergency ward and outpatient clinic, offering limited services in first aid; routine medical exams; ear, nose, and throat medicine; dentistry; pediatrics; and lab analysis. At this same time, debate was underway on how the hospital should be governed. The Church was unwilling to assume the responsibility, in spite of Padre Pio's wishes. It was finally decided to establish a fifty-member lay council, chosen from among Padre Pio's spiritual "children" and united in a special congregation of the Franciscan Third Order of Santa Maria delle Grazie (Our Lady of Grace). Things were at this point in September 1954 when Dr. Sanguinetti died very suddenly. It was a great shock to Padre Pio, who had depended so much on the doctor's strong character and loyalty. Sanguinetti was replaced by Alberto Galletti, whose management was opposed from the start by Lupi and other directors and was destined to last just a few months. His replacement, Luigi Ghisleri, was an engineer who had no previous connection to the project. He was an industrialist and a manager in the modern sense, with a large range of experience and a network of contacts. Ghisleri immediately found himself in conflict with Lupi, who refused to bend himself to Ghisleri's dictates and who finally asked the administrative council to relieve him of his position. Ghisleri oversaw the clinic's finishing touches, using his influence to obtain the services of internationally renowned physicians. This may not have been what Sanguinetti and the other early founders had in mind initially; they had intended that the medical staff be composed primarily of doctors who were also Padre Pio's spiritual "children." While they may have hoped that the medical staff would be driven by a mission of Christian charity as opposed to a desire for a salary, such a hope was certainly not very viable. In any case, Ghisleri's

10. "Padre Pio to His Children, May 5, 1957, on the First Anniversary of the Inauguration of the Casa Sollievo della Sofferenza," Casa Sollievo della Sofferenza Editions, 2014

11. La Casa Sollievo della Sofferenza, *Bullettin*, no. 7, July 1950.

summons yielded an illustrious medical committee, who chose a staff of doctors from among their own students. Staff preparations lasted for almost a year, with nuns from the Zealous Missionaries of the Sacred Heart of Jesus engaged and trained as nurses.

Seven months later the project lost yet another of its early collaborators, when Dr. Sanvico died at Perugia in April 1955, just a year before seeing Padre Pio's dream become a fully operating reality.

The Home for the Relief of Suffering opened its doors as a 300-bed hospital on May 5, 1956, amid great fanfare. A crowd of fifteen thousand joined many local and Vatican dignitaries and medical luminaries, and Padre Pio celebrated Mass on the site. Cardinal Giacomo Lercaro of Bologna quoted a phrase from the Holy Thursday liturgy:

"Where charity and love are, God is." There is a clear, precise address where God can be found, and we all have so much need of him. And those moments come in life when that need becomes more acute, and our pride, beaten by suffering and humiliation, finally allows us to look for God. Where can we find him? The address is precise: Where charity and love are, God is. Where he passes, where he touches, or better said, where he is allowed to enter, where he is permitted to come, he brings this mark, this unmistakable seal of charity and love. Have you remarked this fact at San Giovanni Rotondo? Yes. Everyone has remarked it; God is here; obviously charity and love are also here.[12]

Padre Pio urged the Casa's benefactors to continue their support for the newly opened hospital.

A new army made by renunciation and love is going to rise for God's glory, and for the solace of sick souls and bodies. Do not take your help away from us; instead, cooperate in this apostolate of relief of human suffering, and God's limitless charity, which is the very light of eternal life, will put together a treasure of light, which Jesus on the cross has left to each one of you. This is a place of prayer and science, where mankind finds itself in crucified Christ as one flock with its shepherd. One step of the route has been taken. Let us not slow our pace; let us promptly answer God's calling for the good cause by complying with our duty: I, our Lord Jesus Christ's useless servant, will keep on praying, and you will keep your great desire for embracing all suffering mankind and presenting it with me to the mercy of the heavenly Father. Your actions will be enlightened grace, with generosity, perseverance in good works, and right intentions.[13]

In conjunction with its opening, the hospital hosted a symposium on cardiac surgery, attended by the world's greatest experts in the field, including believers and non-believers. The participants had a private audience with Pope Pius XII, and at this audience Dr. White, General Dwight Eisenhower's personal physician, told the pope: "Your Holiness, if only every nation could have a Padre Pio!"[14]

In his address to the congress, Pius XII spoke to the physician's role in Christian charity:

---

12. Leone, *Padre Pio and His Work*, 64.
13. Casa Sollievo della Sofferenza, Editorial Office, *Guide for the Visitor to Padre Pio's Work*, iii.
14. Francesco Raimond, "Physician of Body and Soul," *Inside the Vatican* (April 1999): 10–13.

Those who are called professionally to cure and care for souls and bodies soon realize to what degree corporal suffering, in all its aspects, pervades the whole person, reaching the most remote parts of the patient's moral being. It forces the patient to pose again the most fundamental questions concerning our destiny, questions of our attitude regarding God and our fellow men and women, of our individual and collective responsibility, and the sense of our earthly pilgrimage. Medicine that strives to be humane must consider the human being in an integral fashion, body and soul. It is incapable of this by itself, because it has neither the authority nor the mandate which renders it suitable to act in the realms of conscience. It will turn, therefore, to collaborators who can extend its work and bring it to its proper end. The sick person who is placed in ideal conditions, from both a material and a moral point of view, will more easily recognize those who are working for his recovery as auxiliaries of God, concerned with preparing the way for the intervention of grace. Thus will the soul itself be re-stabilized in the fully luminous intelligence of the prerogatives of its supernatural vocation. Only in this condition, truly, will one be able to speak of a genuine relief of suffering.[15]

The hospital's initial departments included general medicine, cardiology, orthopedics, traumatology, pediatrics, urology, obstetrics and gynecology, a surgery unit with two operating theaters, radiology, and physical therapy, along with a transfusion service and research labs. The outpatient ward included surgical, medical, obstetrical-gynecological, pediatric, orthopedic, otological, stomatological, and optical services, with a doctor on duty for first aid. At the foot of the mountain, donated land supported a farm which, to this day, provides the hospital with fresh milk, eggs, poultry, and oil.

The first patient arrived on May 10, but only twenty-five beds were occupied by the end of the month. Perhaps the institution's size and complexity were off-putting to the local people. But then Padre Pio celebrated the feast of Corpus Christi with a procession through the whole clinic, and suddenly the floodgates opened. The Casa Sollievo began filling with patients, and the tide never again stopped. The famous physicians engaged as consultants maintained their contact, offering help and performing procedures at the Casa. Above all there shone the confidence of Padre Pio himself, whose every thought was fixed on this work, and who visited whenever he could to celebrate a baptism, lead a procession, or spend time with the sick. He also regularly attended the theatrical shows that took place several times a year in one of the Casa's rooms for both entertainment and fellowship. In the year following the hospital's opening, Ghisleri gradually began to delegate the hospital's administrative duties to others. At the same time, Padre Pio entrusted Monsignor Giuseppe D'Ercole of the Lateran University with the task of determining a workable legal structure for the hospital's governance. Based on his findings, Padre Pio sent a request to the Holy Father that the hospital's administration be entrusted to the Congregation of the Franciscan Third Order of Our Lady of Grace, in harmony with the donors' wishes. He also requested that upon his death, the Apostolic See accept the Casa's assets and use them to keep the hospital in operation. At the Mass celebrating the hospital's first anniversary, Padre Pio announced that the pope had granted his petition. Moreover, he

15. Leone, *Padre Pio and His Work*, 69–70.

revealed plans for an ambitious extension of the clinic: it would be expanded threefold to include new departments, separate convalescent homes for men and women, and an international study center for the Christian formation of physicians. Padre Pio described the rationale behind this plan:

We must complete this Work so that it becomes a temple of prayer and science, where humankind finds itself in Crucified Jesus as in one flock, under one Shepherd. The Work's children, who gather and pray together in every part of the world according to the spirit of St. Francis and the pope's direction and intentions, must find here their common house for their prayer groups; priests will find here a place for meditation; men, women, and religious will find here houses to improve their spiritual training and their ascent to God, so that God's Love, the ultimate Christian perfection, can live in their faith, detachment, and devotion. Love is the action and voice of the superabundant life that Jesus declared he had come to give to mankind. Let's listen to His invitation: "As my Father has loved me, so I have loved you; remain in my love." Jesus is both our godly teacher and our healing doctor. He is the author of life, who, having died once, now lives triumphant. . . .

If this Work were just solace for bodies, it would just be a model clinic, built through your extraordinarily generous charity. Instead, it is called the living expression of God's love through the expression of charity. The suffering person should live God's love here, wisely accepting his pain in quiet meditation on his destiny toward him . . . who is Light and Love.[16]

A hospital expansion might have seemed a risk, given that the Casa had been open for only a year, but it was in fact a pressing necessity.

Establishing the Casa had been an expensive project, and keeping it functioning required even more funding. Commendatore Angelo Battisti was enlisted to make ends meet, and one of his first measures was to persuade Lupi to resume his previous work with the clinic. At Padre Pio's personal request, Lupi gladly did so. Permission was granted by both the Vatican and the state to restructure the hospital's administration as Padre Pio had proposed, with most of the shares in the name of the Institute for Works of Religion (*Instituto delle Opere di Religione*, or IOR).

On the Casa's second anniversary, Padre Pio pulled a lever in the chapel's sacristy to explode a mine on the mountain, inaugurating the expansion. Work progressed steadily on the new addition, in spite of Padre Pio's extended illness and the upsets of the papal inquiry into his ministry. Lupi worked hard at his duties, but recurring disagreements with others in the administration led him to depart again, this time permanently. In any case, the new construction allowed room for significant expansion of the general medicine department, along with the scientific library and conference hall, and for the establishment of an ear-nose-throat department.

The Casa Today

Casa Sollievo della Sofferenza is today a modern general hospital owned by the Holy See, managed by the Casa Sollievo della Sofferenza Foundation, and operating according to the Italian government health-care system. The hospital, surrounded by

---

16. Casa Sollievo della Sofferenza, Editorial Office, *Guide for the Visitor to Padre Pio's Work*, v–vi.

woods, occupies one hundred thousand square meters and holds nine hundred in-patient beds on nine floors. The outpatient clinic, or *poliambulatorio*, dedicated to Pope John Paul II, is located nearly five hundred meters from the main building and occupies seven floors. The hospital is staffed by twenty-five hundred people, including twenty-two hundred medical professionals who care for the patients directly. The staff includes medical doctors, nurses, technicians, biologists, physicists, chemists, social workers, dietitians, psychologists, and rehabilitation therapists. In addition, ninety researchers work in the hospital's research laboratories.

Padre Pio often exhorted the Casa staff to "bring God to the bed of the ill."[17] This philosophy lives on in the work of the Casa's current chaplains and nuns, some of whom serve as head nurses in the clinical wards and operating rooms. On average, fifty-seven thousand inpatients are admitted to the Casa each year, with ten thousand of these served through a day surgery/day hospital treatment plan. About 17 percent of the patients come from outside the Apulia region. The hospital is also renowned for freely admitting patients from underserved communities and nations, and for its hospitality to the parents of young patients in the onco-hematology unit. It also offers free transportation for patients coming from Bari for radiotherapy.

The Casa is organized in nine clinical departments comprising the following units:

- Cardiological/Vascular Department (cardiology, hemodynamics, cardiological intensive care, vascular surgery, cardiac rehabilitation, interventional radiology),
- Laboratory Department (clinical laboratory, immunology and transfusion, hematological laboratory, thrombosis and hemostasis, medical genetics laboratory, microbiology and virology),
- Emergency Medicine Department,
- Developmental Age Department (medical genetics, obstetrics, neonatology, pediatrics, pediatric onco-hematology),
- Oncohaematology Department (pathological anatomy, hematology, oncology, radiotherapy, oncological nuclear medicine, PET, breast surgery),
- Surgical Sciences Department (abdominal surgery, thoracic surgery, breast surgery, gynecology, urology, orthopedics, intensive care I),
- Medical Sciences Department (internal medicine, dermatology, geriatrics, nephrology, digestive endoscopy, gastroenterology, endocrinology, hepatology, neurology, physical medicine, neuro-rehabilitation),
- Radiological Sciences Department (diagnostic nuclear medicine, radiology, neuroradiology, senology),
- Head and Neck Department (neurosurgery, ophthalmology, dentistry, maxillofacial surgery, otolaryngology, intensive care II).

17. La Casa Sollievo della Sofferenza, Bullettin, issued May 5, 1958, p. 28.

The hospital provides cutting-edge diagnostic and treatment options thanks to its highly qualified professionals and its medical equipment, which includes a surgical robot, linear accelerators, a CT/PET scanner, MRIs (one of them with a 3-Tesla magnetic field), CT scanners, digital angiographers, gamma cameras, and a filmless radiology. The hospital participates in the Integration and Promotion of Italian Hospitals and Health Care Centers Worldwide (IPOCM) project, which promotes the quality improvement of health-care delivery through the supply of teleconsultation and e-learning services to doctors and health personnel in Italian-run health-care centers located in third-world countries.

In October 2009, the hospital management signed a collaboration agreement with the U.S. nonprofit organization Catholic Healthcare International. This agreement is intended to build a network of hospitals in the United States and throughout the world inspired by Padre Pio's vision.

The hospital is committed to the continuing scientific education of all its health-care professionals, as a means of empowering them and improving their service to patients. Each year more than one hundred courses are conducted in the conference room, attended by nearly two thousand people. Many of the hospital's professionals serve as lecturers at Italian universities, and through collaboration with these institutions of higher learning, the hospital hosts academic postgraduate and PhD courses. A special event focused on the relief of suffering is conducted annually to share new treatment and therapy options for acute and chronic pain. The hospital also serves as the general and obstetrical nursing training center for the University of Foggia, and hosts many international students from developing nations, particularly Congo and Benin.

In 1991 the Casa was designated an Italian Research Hospital (IRCCS) for the investigation of genetic and inherited diseases. This brought to fruition yet another dream of Padre Pio's, "to help doctors improve their professional knowledge" through the practice of biomedical science.[18] The research laboratories have conducted studies in a host of pathologies, both rare and common, ranging from diabetes and cancers to Noonan, Joubert, and Mackel syndromes. The institute is directly involved in diagnostic protocols for the screening of common genetic mutations and in gene therapy and transplantation programs. The Casa's nearly ninety researchers have had their findings published in prestigious scientific journals, including the *New England Journal of Medicine, Science, Nature Genetics*, the *American Journal of Human Genetics*, and the *Journal of Neuroscience*. The SCIMAGO World Report 2012 included the hospital in its world list, ranking it ninth in Italy for its scientific output, and first in southern Italy both for total output and high-quality publications. The research activities are mostly funded on a project-by-project basis by the Italian Ministry of Health, entities such as the European Commission, and several public and private funding agencies.

18. Ministerial Decree, July 16, 1991, jointly signed by Italian Minister of Health and by the Minister of the University and Scientific Research.

The outpatient clinic (*Poliambulatorio*) is also home to research laboratories in endocrinology, hemostasis and thrombosis, gastroenterology, medical genetics, gerontology, and oncology. Even more labs in other specialties are located in Rome's Mendel Institute, which was donated to the Casa by Professor Luigi Gedda. Research at the Casa is expected to expand still further in the coming years. While future research will explore regenerative medicine, nanotechnologies, and neural stem-cell treatments for neurodegenerative diseases, the Casa will adhere to Catholic teaching and refrain from the destruction of human embryos to obtain stem cells in its research and therapies.

Thanks to the relevant expertise in this field, the researchers of the hospital obtained funds to build a new research center, the ISBReMIT (Institute for Stem-Cell Biology, Regenerative Medicine and Innovative Therapies), which started its activities in September 2015.

How the Mission of the Casa Is Perceived by Its Professionals

During 2008 a survey was conducted to characterize the extent to which the founding mission of the hospital was perceived by the personnel working in the Casa and the extent to which it influenced the culture of the hospital and the practice of patient care.[19] The study was conducted by Ms. (now Dr.) Nicole Shirilla, who was at the time a student at the University of Pittsburgh. Using a questionnaire, this study found that the respondents were fifty-seven professionals working in the hospital—nineteen physicians, sixteen administrators, twelve nurses, nine researchers, and one chaplain—and the overall average years of work at the hospital was 13.8 years. Of the respondents, 84 percent felt that the mission of the hospital influenced their work; 88 percent believed that the hospital was consistent with its stated mission; 84 percent believed the Casa provided care that was different from other hospitals; and finally, 49 percent considered staff morale to be moderate, while 39 percent considered it to be high or very high

Although the survey involved only a small subset of the hospital staff, it can be considered suggestive of general attitudes, for it confirms the results of a previous analysis on staff climate conducted in the hospital several years before, in 2004. The results suggest the high level at which the mission of the Casa is felt by individuals working in it. This evidence is confirmed by the free-text answers and comments given by respondents to the following questions:

1. What do you think is the mission of this hospital?
2. In your experience, what is the dominant value of this hospital?
3. Why did you choose to work at *Casa Sollievo della Sofferenza*?

Without entering the details of each answer, we present here three summary tables. We classify the answers by core concepts, giving also a glimpse at what the complete answers were.

---

19. Nicole Shirilla, internship thesis (University of Pittsburgh, 2008).

Table 15-1. **View of Hospital Mission**

What do you think is the mission of this hospital?

Core concept	Number of answers	Selection of answers
Addressing explicitly the concept of "suffering"	23	• To accompany in a proper Christian way the patient and his relatives, doing our best to relieve their suffering • To relieve the sufferings of the body with all possible medical tools/devices, and also to help with the spirit of prayer, with the love due to a friend that needs your help • Working having in your mind technical care but mainly moral support to the relief of the sufferings of the patients
Addressing patient-centered care	14	• Giving our best in the field of clinical care and also of the relationship with the person • Humanizing patient care with the support of the best technological standards • Putting the patient at the center of our daily activity
Addressing Padre Pio or the will of the founder	7	• To serve and take care of patients according to the will of our founder, St. Pio, through love and science • To serve the patients in the spirit of the founder, giving a quality level of care from the viewpoint both of humanity and of professionalism
Addressing Christ or Christian way	3	• Taking care of all patients, bringing to their bedside the love of Christ in light of efficiency and efficacy and responsibility in the use of resources • Guiding the patient to live in a Christian way his condition of illness according to the teachings of Jesus crucified
Addressing love or charity	3	• Putting our understanding to the service of charity
Addressing professionalism or excellence	2	• Offering professionalism and competence to solve medical problems

Expanding Padre Pio's "Work" beyond Italy: The Casa USA

In 1950 Dr. Guglielmo Sanguinetti, one of Padre Pio's founding team members and the first technical medical director of the Casa, was quoted in the hospital's monthly magazine as predicting that

The *Casa Sollievo Della Sofferenza* should therefore be the first link in a great chain. It should be the model for many other innumerable *Casas*, with the same name and above all the same spirit, which must bring love to all of humanity. It is a program that would make us tremble with awe, were it not inspired by God, who is above all love![20]

20. La Casa Sollievo della Sofferenza, *Bullettin*, no. 7 , July 1950.

Table 15-2. **View of the Dominant Hospital Value**

In your experience, what is the dominant value of this hospital?

Core concept	Number of answers	Selection of answers
Christian values	8	Charity, Faith, Humility, Respect for life in all its conditions, Sacrifice, Consolation of faith
Commitment toward the patient	7	Complete dedication to the patients Attention to the patient and to humanizing the cure and the care Taking care of the patient in body and spirit
Professionalism	7	Quality of care High medical specialization and competence Efficiency
The founder	4	The extraordinary founder and the spirit that you can find here The presence and benediction of the founder
Relieving suffering	2	To relieve suffering
Spirit of welcome	2	A spirit of welcome

Table 15-3. **Reasons for Choosing to Work at the Casa**

Why did you choose to work at Casa Sollievo della Sofferenza?

Core concept	Number of answers	Selection of answers
Professional environment/opportunities	10	This way I realized my ideal of a profession aware of man as a whole. To have advanced technological medical devices and the possibility to cooperate with high-level professionals. In 70s the hospital appeared to me as a beautiful place and also a starting point to make good health care.
The founder	5	Because the hospital is closest to my point of view regarding the human person and also as a devotion for the saint founder. Because this is the house of God and Padre Pio.
Values of the hospital	3	Because I love patients beyond simple medical care. Because from the first day I put my foot in this place I felt as if I were at home.
Chance	3	It was by chance: I didn't know of the hospital and of Padre Pio before.
Location	2	More than a choice, it was an opportunity to work in my hometown; and I thank God for giving me this opportunity.

Dr. Sanguinetti foresaw a large international network of Casas bringing Padre Pio's spirit, charism and mission to serve the poor and suffering to all corners of the world.

Over fifty years later a small team of health-care leaders in the United States, frustrated by a growing trend toward secularization in the delivery of Catholic health-care services, and inspired by Padre Pio's healing ministry, formed a nonprofit company called Catholic Healthcare International. Sensing a call by Padre Pio, and unwilling to compromise their loyalty and obedience to the Magisterium of the Catholic Church, they adopted Dr. Sanguinetti's prophetic statement as their vision: *to duplicate the Casa Sollievo Della Sofferenza, first in the United States, and then in other countries around the world.* Over the next few years they quietly and methodically laid the groundwork to pursue this ambitious and noble vision.

Dr. Sanguinetti's prediction took a major step toward becoming a reality on October 1, 2009, the feast of St. Thérèse of Lisieux (the Little Flower), when the Casa Sollievo Della Sofferenza entered into a formal collaboration agreement with Catholic Healthcare International to duplicate the Casa in the United States and other countries around the world as a model of faithful Catholic health-care delivery in this secular world. In his homily at the Collaboration Mass, celebrated in Santa Maria Della Grazie Church in San Giovanni Rotondo, Italy, on that day, Cardinal (then Archbishop) Raymond L. Burke, prefect of the Supreme Tribunal of the Apostolic Signatura at the Vatican, made the following comments regarding the importance of this initiative for the Church, the world, and the suffering Jesus being neglected in so many poor souls in our society:

Homes for the Relief of Suffering are so much needed in a culture which more and more views the helpless, the weak, and the sick as a burden for society and even presumes to act against human life, in grave violation of the moral law, for the sake of a more convenient and less burdensome situation. The same culture manifests a godless disregard for the conscience of the health-care worker who is asked to assist in diminishing or taking human life, against the most sacred dictates of his conscience. Understandably, in such a culture, both the suffering and those who care for them lose hope, for they no longer perceive the reality of human suffering as an act of love, united to the Sacrifice of Our Lord, especially through the Sacrament of the Holy Eucharist. How much we need the beacon of sure and enduring hope offered by the Home for the Relief of Suffering![21]

Casa USA: Built on a Foundation of Prayer and Faithfulness to the Church

In the spirit of Padre Pio, the leadership team of Catholic Healthcare International formalized a "Three Pillar Model" as the structure for its campus in the United States, nicknamed the Casa USA. The principal pillars of the Casa USA are (1) the duplication of Padre Pio's hospital, the *Casa Sollievo della Sofferenza*; (2) a regional network of faithful, Catholic physician medical practices; and, (3) a truly faithful, Catholic medical school.

---

21. Raymond Leo Burke, Homily on the Feast Day of St. Thérèse of Lisieux, October 1, 2009.

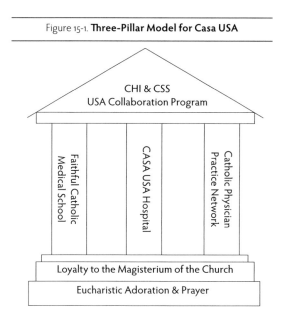

Figure 15-1. **Three-Pillar Model for Casa USA**

As manifestation of the first fruits of the collaboration agreement with Padre Pio's Casa in Italy, the directors of Catholic Healthcare International completed construction and opened the doors of the entirely new, state-of-the-art Casa San Pio Medical Clinic of Appalachia on October 24, 2011. This fully faithful, Catholic, outpatient medical facility is situated in rural Kentucky, in the extremely poor and underserved region of Appalachia. In addition to comprehensive medical care, Casa San Pio provides technical services such as CAT scans, ultrasound, stress testing, X-ray, and laboratory, and a fully electronic medical records system.

As further reflection of their loyalty to the Magisterium of the Church, on July 1, 2013, the directors of Catholic Healthcare International transitioned their personal ownership of Casa San Pio of Appalachia to the Roman Catholic Diocese of Lexington. The clinic is now serving thousands of patients in need of relief of suffering each year as a wholly owned apostolate of the diocese and its bishop.

And Casa San Pio is just the first step: this model of a fully faithful, Catholic medical clinic will be duplicated as an integral component of the campus of the Casa USA in its three-pillar structure. The board of directors of Catholic Healthcare International is currently in the process of finalizing the location for the Casa USA campus. Once the site is identified, the program will first integrate the implementation of a pilgrim shrine as the spiritual and Eucharistic hub for all activities. This shrine will be an authentic replica of the Santa Maria Delle Grazie Church, where Padre Pio celebrated Mass for so many years. This Eucharistic focal hub is intended to manifest the fundamental belief, espoused by Padre Pio, that the success of the Casa would be built upon the foundation of an expansive network of prayer warriors. Long before construction of the Casa in Italy began, he organized a world-wide network of Padre Pio Prayer Groups—currently numbering over three thousand internationally—to storm heaven with prayerful support for the Casa and its mission. He also welcomed his prayer groups to come to San Giovanni Rotondo on pilgrimage to pray with him at the Santa Maria Delle Grazie Church. In similar fashion, the prayer groups and other pilgrims in the United States will travel to the Casa USA shrine to pray for the success of the Casa USA, its health-care professionals, and its most treasured suffering patients, who reflect Jesus in his passion. Perpetual Adoration of the Eucharist will be the keystone of prayer at the shrine, even while the groundwork for the hospital and medical school is being laid, under the planned spiritual direction of a dedicated, cloistered religious group.

The next phase will include the building of the Casa Sollievo della Sofferenza hospital and a Catholic medical school fully faithful to the Magisterium of the Catholic Church. This medical campus will shine as a beacon of light in an increasingly secularized world. It will not only serve the poor and needy in the immediate region and beyond, but will also train physicians to practice as faithful Catholics in all areas of the world, and will serve as a home base for these committed medical professionals to return to be revitalized and strengthened in both spirit and profession.

All of the activities of the Casa USA will be conducted in complete obedience to the local ordinary and to the Magisterium of the Catholic Church, and in compliance with the *Ethical and Religious Directives for Catholic Health Care Services* (ERDs) of the U.S. Conference of Catholic Bishops.[22] This has become an ever-growing issue of concern in the United States as health-care providers and systems continue to forfeit their Catholic identity and distance themselves from full compliance with the teachings of the bishops, creating unfortunate and regrettable scandal for the Church.

The great saint affectionately known as Padre Pio had a humble yet awe-inspiring vision to serve the poor and wretched Jesus in God's suffering and poor children among us. Through his spirit and charism, Padre Pio has planted this burning passion into the hearts and hands of the professionals who serve at the Casa in Italy, and those who visit and observe this very blessed manifestation of charity brought to life. A generation after the death of Padre Pio, the ministry of the Casa Sollievo Della Sofferenza thrives against all odds in its very remote and isolated home atop Mount Gargano, while so many other Catholic health-care apostolates lose their way. And now, while others compromise their mission because of worldly challenges and forfeit their treasured Catholic identities in search of acceptance in society or financial solvency and gain, St. Pio's Casa leads a vibrant initiative toward a renaissance in the delivery of the Catholic health-care services worldwide. As Dr. Sanguinetti expressed so prophetically and eloquently, Padre Pio's "Work" would be "the model for many other innumerable *Casas* . . . which must bring love to all of humanity. It is a program that would make us tremble with awe, were it not inspired by God, who is first of all love!"[23]

---

22. United States Conference of Catholic Bishops, *Ethical and Religious Directives for Catholic Health Care Services*, 5th ed. (Washington, D.C.: USCCB, 2009).

23. La Casa Sollievo della Sofferenza, *Bullettin*, no. 7, July 1950.

The Casa's Future Development

Padre Pio wanted a hospital "technically capable of meeting the most demanding clinical requirements."[24] The Casa has grown over the years and is now undergoing another period of projected growth. Plans are underway to make the hospital more welcoming for pilgrims and prayer groups, as well as for the sick. The projected construction will feature a new reception area, a technological hub with modern equipment, new wards based on today's standards of privacy and comfort, and a new central supply office. To harmonize with the existing structure as well as the natural environment, the buildings will make use of local stone, which absorbs light and changes color depending on the time of day. The sanctuary, located across from the hospital, will emphasize the parallel healing of spirit and body, accented by the ascent of the *Via Crucis* (Stations of the Cross), climbing the mountain, rising toward the sky. The hospital will open onto the city, facing the square, where the path to the Padre Pio Museum begins. A large, bright reception area will welcome visitors and lead to a new meeting center and to a monument dedicated to the Casa's history. Along all the routes dedicated to visitors, spaces for meeting, assembly, and prayer will be provided. On the third floor, the walkways will be dedicated to the circulation of the public, who will find walls lined with portraits of the founder in the art gallery. At the center of the hospital will be the chapel, from which Padre Pio envisioned God's love radiating outward through the entire structure. As he once told the Casa's doctors, "Your mission is to heal the sick. But unless you bring love to the sickbed, I don't believe medicine will be of much use. Take God to the sick. He is more effective than any other treatment."[25]

The north atrium will be the new entrance to the hospital, housing Information and Admittance Services. The new technological hub in the heart of the complex will contain the latest technologies for surgery, ICU, trauma, diagnosis, and laboratory work. The concentration in a single, central block of all the most advanced equipment will allow the hospital to be reorganized on a patient-centric model, with shared resources and technologies and with the capacity to adapt to future developments in medicine. The centrally located research laboratories will facilitate exchanges between physicians and researchers, enabling the rapid transfer of results to their practical applications at the patients' bedside.

The new inpatient rooms will house either two patients or a patient with an assisting relative, closely allied with Padre Pio's vision of the hospital as a "home." Large common areas will provide expansive views of the mountain and the woods outdoors. Padre Pio, when faced with comments that the clinic was too beautiful and luxurious, replied, "Were it possible, I would make the *Casa* of gold, because the sick person is Jesus, and everything we do for the Lord is too little."[26]

Pope Benedict XVI paid the Casa a pastoral visit in June 2009, meeting with

---

24. Casa Sollievo della Sofferenza, Editorial Office, *Guide for the Visitor to Padre Pio's Work*, iii.
25. Antonio Maria Sicari, *Il Secondo Grande Libro dei Ritratti di Santi* (Milano: Jaca Book, 2006), 807.
26. Antonio Maria Sicari, *Il Sesto Libro dei Ritratti di Santi* (Milano: Jaca Book, 2000), 166.

patients, medical and paramedical staff, and administrators. He spoke of Padre Pio's vision of a hospital where "one could experience firsthand that the commitment of science to treating the sick must never be separated from filial trust in God, who is infinitely kind and merciful":

Every time one enters a place of healing, one thinks naturally of the mystery of illness and pain, of the hope of healing and the inestimable value of good health, of which one becomes aware only when it has been lost. In hospitals one sees firsthand the preciousness of our existence, but also its fragility. Following the example of Jesus who travelled throughout Galilee "healing every disease and every infirmity among the people" (Mt 4: 23), the Church, moved by the Holy Spirit from her first days, has considered it one of her duties and privileges to be at the side of those who suffer, cultivating a priority for the ministry of healing.

Illness, which is manifested in so many forms and strikes in different ways, gives rise to disturbing questions: Why do we suffer? Can the experience of pain be considered positive? Who can free us from suffering and death? These are existential questions that more often than not remain humanly unanswerable, since suffering is an enigma that is beyond human reason. Suffering is part of the very mystery of the human person. I emphasized this in the encyclical *Spe Salvi*, noting that: it "stems partly from our finitude, and partly from the mass of sin which has accumulated over the course of history, and continues to grow unabated today." And I added that: "certainly we must do whatever we can to reduce suffering: ... but to banish it from the world altogether is not in our power. This is simply because ... none of us is capable of eliminating the power of evil, ... which ... is a constant source of suffering" (cf. n. 36).

God alone can eliminate the power of evil. Precisely because Jesus Christ came into the world to reveal to us the divine plan of our salvation, faith helps us to penetrate the meaning of all that is human, hence also of suffering. Thus an intimate relationship exists between the Cross of Jesus, the symbol of supreme pain and the price of our true freedom, and our own pain, which is transformed and sublimated when it is lived in the awareness of God's closeness and solidarity.[27]

As everyone is invited to trust in God, abiding in his love and mercy, one cannot deny the power of prayer and the communion it occasions with God and others. "I'm just a friar who prays," Padre Pio once said:

It is prayer, this united strength of all good souls, that moves the world, that renews the consciences, that supports the "Casa," that comforts the suffering, that heals the sick, that sanctifies labor, that elevates health care, that gives moral strength and Christian resignation to human suffering, that spreads the smile and blessing of God on the fainthearted and the weak.[28]

---

27. Pope Benedict XVI, Address to the Sick, the Medical, Paramedical and Administrative Staff of the Health-Care Structure, San Giovanni Rotondo, June 21, 2009, http://www.vatican.va/holy_father/benedict_xvi/speeches/2009/june/documents/hf_ben-xvi_spe_20090621_casa-sollievo_en.html.

28. Casa Sollievo della Sofferenza, Editorial Office, *Guide for the Visitor to Padre Pio's Work*, viii.

O Mary, health of the sick, help, protect, and make blossom my poor Work which is Yours, the Casa Sollievo della Sofferenza, for the glory of God and to the spiritual and material advantage of those who suffer in body and soul.[29]

Bibliography

Benedict XVI, Pope. Address to the Sick, the Medical, Paramedical and Administrative Staff of the Health-Care Structure San Giovanni Rotondo. June 21, 2009. http://www.vatican.va/holy_father/ benedict_xvi/speeches/2009/june/documents/hf_ben-xvi_spe_20090621_casa-sollievo_en.html.

Burke, Raymond Leo. Homily on the Feast Day of St. Thérèse of Lisieux. October 1, 2009.

Casa Sollievo della Sofferenza. *Bullettin*, no. 7 (July 1950).

Casa Sollievo della Sofferenza. Editorial Office. *Guide for the Visitor to Padre Pio's Work*. San Giovanni Rotondo, Italy: Casa Sollievo della Sofferenza Editions, 1999.

John Paul II, Pope. Ai medici e ai malati dell'ospedale "Casa Sollievo della Sofferenza" [To doctors and patients of the Hospital Casa Sollievo della Sofferenza]. May 23, 1987. http://www.vatican.va/ holy_father/john_paul_ii/speeches/1987/may/documents/hf_jp-ii_spe_19870523_medici-malati_ it.html.

Leone, Gherardo. *Padre Pio and His Work*. 3rd edition. San Giovanni Rotondo, Italy: Casa Sollievo della Sofferenza Editions, 1986.

———. *Padre Pio: A Summary of His Life*. San Giovanni Rotondo, Italy: Casa Sollievo della Sofferenza, 1999.

Pio, Padre. *Epistolario* [Letters]. Edited by Melchiorre da Pobladura and Alessandro da Ripabottoni. San Giovanni Rotondo, Italy: Padre Pio da Pietrelcina Editions, 2004.

Raimond, Francesco. "Physician of Body and Soul." *Inside the Vatican* (April 1999): 10–13.

Shirilla, Nicole. Internship thesis. University of Pittsburgh, 2008.

Sicari, Antonio Maria. *Il Sesto Libro dei Ritratti di Santi*. Milan: Jaca Book, 2000.

———. *Il Secondo Grande Libro dei Ritratti di Santi*. Milan: Jaca Book, 2006.

United States Conference of Catholic Bishops. *Ethical and Religious Directives for Catholic Health Care Services*. 5th edition. Washington, D.C.: USCCB, 2009.

29. Padre Pio, January 22, 1953, Ordination Anniversary Card.

CONTRIBUTORS

J. Brian Benestad, PhD, is the D'Amour Chair in the Catholic Intellectual Tradition in the Department of Theology, Assumption College, Worcester, Massachusetts.

Reverend Philip G. Bochanski, MA, MDiv, is the executive director of Courage International in Norwalk, Connecticut. He is also a priest for the Archdiocese of Philadelphia.

Peter J. Colosi, PhD, is an assistant professor of philosophy at Salve Regina University in Newport, Rhode Island.

Domenico Francesco Crupi is the vice president and general manager of Casa Sollievo della Sofferenza Viale Cappuccini in San Giovanni Rotondo, Italy.

Sister Mary Diana Dreger, OP, MD, is an assistant clinical professor of medicine at Vanderbilt University Medical Center. She is also a member of the Dominican Sisters of Saint Cecilia Congregation in Nashville, Tennessee.

E. Wesley Ely, MD, MPH, is a professor of medicine and critical care at Vanderbilt University, the Vanderbilt Center for Health Services Research, and associate director of research for the Tennessee Valley VA Geriatric Research Education Clinical Center in Nashville, Tennessee.

Richard J. Fehring, RN, PhD, FAAN, is a professor emeritus of nursing at the Marquette University College of Nursing, and director of the Marquette University Institute for Natural Family Planning in Milwaukee, Wisconsin.

Ashley K. Fernandes, MD, PhD, is an associate professor of pediatrics and associate director of the Center for Bioethics at The Ohio State University College of Medicine in Columbus, Ohio.

Reverend Patrick Flanagan, CM, PhD, is an associate professor of theology and religious studies at Saint John's University in Jamaica, New York. He is also a member of the Congregation of the Mission (Vincentian Fathers and Brothers).

Francesco Giuliani, MD, is the head of the ICT, Innovation and Research Unit for the Casa Sollievo della Sofferenza Viale Cappuccini in San Giovanni Rotondo, Italy.

Stephen E. Hannan, MD, is a practicing physician in pulmonary and critical care medicine with the Pulmonary, Critical Care, and Sleep Medicine Specialists of SW Florida in Fort Myers, Florida.

Robert A. Mangione, EdD, RPh, is the provost and a professor of pharmacy at Saint John's University in Jamaica, New York.

Dennis M. Manning, MD, is an associate professor of medicine at the Mayo Clinic College of Medicine in Rochester, Minnesota.

Gianluigi Mazzoccoli, MD, is a physician in the Department of Medical Sciences, Division of Internal Medicine and Chronobiology Unit for the Casa Sollievo della Sofferenza Viale Cappuccini in San Giovanni Rotondo, Italy.

Louise A. Mitchell, MA, MTS, is associate editor of *The Linacre Quarterly*, the official journal of the Catholic Medical Association, and an adjunct professor of bioethics.

Medical Student, while a student at the time of initial writing, is now a practicing physician.

Christopher O'Hara, MD, is an assistant professor of pediatrics at the Penn State University College of Medicine, and practices pediatrics at the Penn State Hershey Children's Hospital in Hershey, Pennsylvania.

Jere D. Palazzolo, MHA, is the founder and director of Catholic Healthcare International and Marian Medical Services in Wildwood, Missouri.

Christopher Perro, MD, is a practicing surgeon of otolaryngology in Springfield, Illinois.

James S. Powers, MD, is a professor of medicine at Vanderbilt University, and the associate clinical director of the Tennessee Valley VA Geriatric Research Education and Clinical Center in Nashville, Tennessee.

Kathleen M. Raviele, MD, FACOG, is a practicing gynecologist in Decatur, Georgia.

Peter A. Rosario, MD, is a recently retired physician in the practice of pulmonary and critical care medicine, and volunteer clinical professor of medicine at the Indiana University School of Medicine in Evansville, Indiana.

Leonard P. Rybak, MD, PhD, is a professor of surgery at the Southern Illinois University School of Medicine in Springfield, Illinois.

José A. Santos, MD, is a practicing physician in physical medicine and rehabilitation in San Antonio, Texas.

Wanda Skowronska, PhD, MA, MA, is a psychologist and sessional lecturer at the John Paul II Institute for Marriage and Family in East Melbourne, Victoria, Australia.

John M. Travaline, MD, is a professor of thoracic medicine and surgery at the Lewis Katz School of Medicine at Temple University in Philadelphia, Pennsylvania. He is also a deacon for the Archdiocese of Philadelphia.

William V. Williams, MD, is the president and CEO of BriaCell Therapeutics Corporation; an adjunct professor of medicine at the University of Pennsylvania in Philadelphia, Pennsylvania; and the editor in chief of *The Linacre Quarterly*, the official journal of the Catholic Medical Association. He is also a deacon for the Archdiocese of Philadelphia.

INDEX

abortion, xi, 110, 119; backup to contraception, and cancer, 126; children obtaining, 119, 108n8; complications from, 105, 130–38; counseling after, 367–68, 377; and ectopic pregnancies, 121–24; and emotional distress, 129; grief after, 367–68, 381–84; and human being as product, 65; and the human good, 20–21; and incest, 129; indirect, 122; legalization of, 108; medical, 131–32; and medical practice, 106, 160, 317, 448; and medical research, 456, 458–59, 472; morality of, 122, 129, 146–47; and prenatal diagnosis, 120–21, 129; and rape, 129, 140; reducing rates of, 138; reversing, 132–33; as a right, 108n8; and saving the mother's life, 129; spontaneous, 121; surgical, 131–32; as a violation, 40. *See also* contraception; miscarriage; Plan B

absolute moral norms, 36–37, 40, 44, 61, 66

abstinence, 107, 119, 154, 170, 173, 182, 187, 192–93, 196, 198, 364, 458–59, 472n101; education, 240–41. *See also* chastity

abuse, 249, 382–83, 385–86, 389; emotional, 222; physical, 214, 222, 241; verbal, 216, 241. *See also* research

acne, 106, 108, 111–13, 147, 151, 190, 443

Acts of the Apostles, 17, 72, 78, 408, 420, 426

advance directives, 29, 273, 276–79, 317. *See also* POLST; surrogate

affectivity, 43–44, 46–47

affliction, 5, 7–8, 16, 19, 87, 267

agnosticism, 230

alcohol, 119, 215, 233; abuse of, 135–36, 244–45; impairment due to, 12, 14, 247–48. *See also* substance abuse

Alexander of Hales, 42n32

alienation, 85, 350

allergens, 149

Ambrose, 13, 423–24

American Academy of Pediatrics, 189, 190n76

American Association of Colleges of Pharmacy (AACP), 395

American College of Obstetricians and Gynecologists (ACOG), 105, 118, 120, 124n54, 125n59, 126n63, 139n123, 189, 400, 401n14

American Pharmacists Association, 398

American Psychological Association, 135, 235, 238, 275n45, 385, 466n88

American Society of Reproductive Medicine, 149, 152, 189

amniocentesis, 120

Andresen, Carl, 42

anemia, 114, 116–17, 441

angels, 47, 96n88

anger, 4–5, 13, 15, 26, 212–13, 217–20, 229, 234, 276, 283, 356, 361–62, 380, 385, 387–88

Anointing of the Sick, 9, 70–72, 75–76, 84–87, 90–94, 97–98, 100, 268–69, 308, 310–11, 365

anovulation, 115, 190

anthropology: philosophical, xi–xii, xv, 34, 36, 65–66, 335, 471; theological, 31–34, 37, 40, 47, 56, 65–66, 370, 373, 378

anxiety, 4, 83, 96, 135, 192, 213, 215, 248, 266, 269, 271, 283, 330, 374, 482; as chronic disorder, 292

appetite, desire, 14; rectitude of, 14

appetite: for cigarettes, 244; for food, 5, 271, 481; sexual, 364; suppression, 244

Arinze, Francis, 240

Aristotle, 12–13, 15, 37–39, 41–42, 44, 51n54, 338, 340

artificial insemination: heterologous, 159; homologous, 159

assisted reproductive technology, 105, 121, 157; gamete intrafallopian transfer (GIFT), 158, 159n210; intracytoplasmic sperm injection (ICSI), 158; intrauterine insemination (IUI), 159n210; IVF, 55, 158–59, 337, 380, 384, 404, 452; zygote intrafallopian transfer (ZIFT), 158

atheism, 49, 62n90, 65–66, 209, 230, 246, 309, 367–69

attention deficit disorders, 248–50

Augustine of Hippo, 13–15, 52, 239, 408

Austriaco, N. P. G., 145n145, 333–35, 337n87

autonomy, 4, 13, 19–20, 24–25, 83–84, 210, 228, 273, 278, 295, 342, 399, 433, 439, 445–46, 468. *See also* rights

avarice, 5, 13

axiology, 35–36

baptism, 74, 87–88, 95, 100, 161, 397, 407–8, 426, 489; of Christ, 98

Barrett, Melanie, 196

Barron, Robert, 229–30, 239

basal body temperature, 175, 179, 188, 197–99

Beauchamp, Tom L., 339

beauty, 43–46, 50, 55, 57, 98, 209–10, 215, 230, 421, 431, 482–83, 495, 499; of the body, 235, 217, 227, 235

Belmont Report, 330, 339, 446–49, 462, 466–70

Benedict XVI, Pope: 31–32, 35, 48, 51–52, 55, 57, 62, 87, 89, 202, 237, 321, 334, 351–52, 360n15, 381n45, 390n66, 390n67, 394, 417; *Caritas in Veritate*, 367;

Benedict XVI, Pope (*cont.*)
  Deus Caritas Est, 33n8, 63, 66; *Spe Salvi*, 6, 373, 423n22, 424, 499, 500n27; World Day of the Sick, 87n51, 89n59. *See also* Ratzinger, Joseph
benevolence, 15, 274, 404
Bentham, Jeremy, 36n16
Billings Ovulation Method, 180
bipolar disorder, 135–36, 248
birth, premature. *See* pregnancy
birth control pill, 108, 137, 179–80, 182, 185, 190–91, 230–31. *See also* contraception
births, multiple, 121, 156, 158, 252
blastocyst, 117, 141, 143–44, 146–47, 454, 456
blood, umbilical cord, 453
blood donation, 321, 328, 467n89
blood pressure, 26, 109, 126, 127, 297, 353, 359. *See also* hypertension
Boethius, 42n33, 43, 48–49, 51–52
Bonaventure, 43
bond, family, 59, 284; mother-child, 134–35, 212, 381; parent-child, 226; partner, 59, 134, 242
Bosco, John, 218–19
Boyle, Joseph, 196
brain, traumatic injury, 303, 359–60
brain death, 301–2, 304, 333, 335, 359
breastfeeding, 124, 138, 175, 185–87, 199–201
burden: of caregiving, 269; of communicating with patients, 293; emotional, 299, 385, 389; on health-care system, 272–73, 281; of life, 273, 281; of illness, 80, 86, 262–63, 281, 348, 365, 397, 423; of medical school, 430; of medical practice, 434; of medical research, 439, 447, 465, 469–70; of old age, 265; of a person, 23, 270, 496; of treatment, 21, 24, 271–73, 280–82, 290, 294–300, 304, 307; of utopia, 374
Burke, Greg F., 14, 18, 21n52, 25, 306, 311
Burke, Raymond Leo, 496

cardiopulmonary resuscitation (CPR), 277, 289–92, 294, 297, 304
Cataldo, Peter, 20, 21n50, 130n80, 159n210, 448
catechesis, 76, 92; of medical students, 415, 423, 426–32, 435–37
Catechism of the Catholic Church, 233, 436; abortion, 130–31; amputation, 320; beatitudes, 430; beauty, 430; common good, 28; conscience, 11, 401, 430, 432, 472; discontinuing treatment, 282; duty to parents, 270; dying, 96, 266, 282; faith, 428–30; family, 106–7; forgiveness, 430; goodness, 430; grace, 430; healing, 9, 72, 269; health, 232, 472; Holy Spirit, 430; hope, 431; human dignity, 11, 275; human life, 130 147; human person, 45; image of God, 11, 319–20; knowledge of God, 420, 428; married couples, 106–7; masturbation, 154; moral-ity, 11, 430; mutilation, 320; organ transplants, 334; painkillers, 266; price-gouging, 405; resurrection, 426; sacraments, 70–71, 90–91, 97–100, 269, 310; sexuality, 107, 323, 364; the sick, 63, 72–73, 91–92,
99, 268–69, 310; sin, 11, 98, 430; sterilization, 320; suffering, 8, 98, 266–67, 310; the Trinity, 52–53; truth, 428; virtue, 210, 430–31; vocation, 417
Catholic social teaching, 45, 48, 60, 406
causality, 47, 64, 134, 456n62
CDC. *See* United States Centers for Disease Control
character, 12, 15, 27, 39, 44, 48n49, 224, 228–30, 234, 236, 244, 436, 487
charity, 3, 12–15, 24, 34, 54, 64, 66, 74, 76, 78, 79, 82, 88, 91, 94, 99, 266, 270, 333, 431, 436, 468, 477, 480, 482, 483, 487–88, 490, 494–95, 498. *See also* love
chastity, 78–79, 105, 107, 119, 172–73, 229–31, 233–40, 364–65
Chesterton, G. K., 60
children, preserving innocence of, 216–17, 221, 226, 227, 383
Childress, J. F., 339
chimeras, 65, 332
cholesterol, 112–13
chorionic villus sampling, 120
Clare of Assisi, 261
Clearblue Easy Fertility Monitor, 177, 180, 185, 188. *See also* fertility; monitor
cloning, 65, 450, 454, 460. *See also* somatic cell nuclear transfer
Code of Canon Law, 76, 92, 310–11
cognition, 41, 45, 64, 306, 346–47, 371, 460, 472; dysfunctional, 264, 271, 275–76, 349, 472n100; infant, 213; therapy, 266, 369, 387
Colossians, Letter to the, 16, 19n48, 267
coma, 31, 126, 297, 300–301, 303–5, 311, 359–60, 445. *See also* minimally conscious; persistent vegetative state
comfort, xi, 4, 9, 26, 76, 282, 284, 362, 481–82, 499–500; comforting children, 213–14; dying in, 84, 95, 265–66, 272, 277, 307, 424; in fertility care, 187, 197–98; in grief, 97, 415–16, 425; ministry of 80, 482; in parent-child discussions, 230, 240; in patient-physician discussions, 292, 294, 350. *See also* palliative care
Commendation of the Dying, 92, 95–97
common good, xv, 12, 28–29, 66, 399, 406
communication: biological, 141; of the Christian life, 431; with the elderly, 264; in medical practice, 263, 293, 300, 316–17, 343, 358, 399, 436; in medical research, 470; in NFP, 170, 173, 191–93; parental, 216, 234, 243; of the patient, 277, 290, 292, 295, 340, 349, 358, 378, 388; of the sacraments, 429
communion: of persons, 54, 372; of saints, 29, 99, 431
compassion, 9, 15, 62–63, 81, 83, 85, 94, 99, 101, 139, 209, 217–18, 276, 293–94, 316–17, 320, 351, 374, 386, 395, 397, 416, 433, 473, 477, 482; of Jesus, 8, 70, 72–73
Condic, Maureen L., 131n89, 302n39, 452
Confession, 76, 86–87, 91, 94, 131, 161, 268, 310, 350–51, 356, 365, 384, 397, 480. *See also* forgiveness; reconciliation

confidence: 25, 28, 33, 187, 198, 201, 428, 489; in God, 77, 100

confidentiality, 14, 25, 118, 333, 409, 465. *See also* HIPAA; privacy

conflict, 228, 274, 335, 378, 384, 388, 487; with Catholic teaching, 273, 294, 307, 373, 458; family, 283; between goods, 423; of interest, 442, 448, 460, 465, 473; in office, 160; between principles/ rules, 466, 469; with self-interest, 13–14, 373

Congregation for Catholic Education, 78n21

Congregation for the Clergy, 78, 433n46, 436n54

Congregation for the Doctrine of the Faith: *Dignitas Personae,* 32, 33n9, 34–35, 65n101, 120, 121n39, 146, 147n151, 158, 159n210, 328; *Donum Vitae,* 32–34, 38, 56, 130n85, 153, 158n209, 159n210, 262n1, 322, 328n34, 449; on euthanasia, 253n179, 280n54; on nutrition and hydration, 32n5, 272n38, 307

conscience, 229, 300, 306–7, 421, 432; and anthropology, 45; clauses, 402; and dignity, 11; examining, 349; following, xi, 10, 106, 279n51, 307, 395–96, 400, 410, 422; forming, 281, 307, 400–402, 419, 427, 430–32, 457–58, 462, 472, 500; free, 281, 457–58, 489; rights of, 408, 449, 457, 472, 496

conscientiousness, 25, 309, 335, 444

conscientious objection, 278n51, 396, 403, 409, 441. *See also* rights

consciousness, minimal, 301, 303–4

consent, 14, 27, 371; informed, 29, 133, 316–17, 331, 333–35, 338–40, 342, 402, 441–47, 450–51, 455, 457–66, 470–73; and minors, 118–19; and organ donation, 333–34, 452; and sexual advances, 139, 245

consequentialism, 36

consolation, 6, 76, 80–81, 97, 274, 384, 495

consultation, 14, 194, 273, 292, 307, 319, 403; with family, 455; psychiatric, 274; psychological, 83; with specialist, 126, 279; teleconsultation, 492

contemplation, 56–57, 66, 422

contraception: emergency, 105, 119, 138–47, 400; hormonal, 106–14, 117–18, 140–41, 150, 161, 180, 184, 186–87, 192, 198–200, 202, 404, 448; IUD, 110–11, 117, 181–83, 400; LARC, 111; ring, 111; risks of, 109–11. *See also* Plan B; progestin; sterilization

Council of Trent, 70

courage, xiii, 15, 17, 79, 96–97, 100, 202, 283, 347, 482. *See also* fortitude

covenant, 4, 86, 289, 394, 398–99; marriage as, 363

creation, 6, 11, 38–39, 57, 100, 107, 217, 262, 321, 334, 372–73, 375, 420, 460, 473, 483

Cronin, Daniel. A., 294

Crosby, John F., 45, 46n45, 50n53, 52n58

Cross, of Christ, 8–10, 98–99, 101, 376, 401, 481, 487–88, 499–500

culture, xi, xvi, 18, 33, 209, 219, 224, 228, 235–37, 243–44, 253, 264, 270, 350, 369, 377, 390, 421, 448, 496; of death, 36, 159; of life, 159, 170, 203, 399; of medicine, 246, 433, 493. *See also* social order

deacons, 76, 78, 82, 88, 95, 328

de Lubac, Henri, 49

dementia, 269, 273, 275–76, 306

depression, 23, 26, 109, 111, 134–36, 150, 215, 242, 248, 267, 271, 276, 296, 338, 380, 382; postpartum, 211–12

de Saint-Exupéry, Antoine, 55

detachment, 79, 490

diabetes, 112–13, 177, 156, 297, 300, 332, 341, 346, 441, 445, 492

diet, 22–23, 113, 152, 154, 190, 221–22, 244, 248, 271, 491. *See also* hydration; nutrition; vitamins

disability, xiii, 15, 47–48, 58n78, 74, 81, 125, 129, 139, 262, 311, 317, 343, 346, 348, 356, 365, 376n33, 380, 463, 468, 485

discomfort. *See* comfort; pain

discrimination, xiii, 343, 400

Divine Physician, 161, 269, 416, 418, 429, 431–33, 435, 437

dizziness, 113, 133

DNA, 55–56, 136, 328, 454

DNR, 278, 290, 297

Down syndrome, 120, 129, 459

drug abuse, 135–36, 146, 245–46, 266, 350, 400. *See also* substance abuse

drugs, withdrawn from market, 111, 443, 445, 450. *See also* pharmaceuticals

drunkenness, 13, 244–48

dysmenorrhea, 105, 108, 117–18, 147–48, 150–52

dyspareunia, 147–48, 151–52

economic order, 11, 13, 108n8, 134, 139, 173, 270, 318, 330, 405–7, 409, 472

educators, 13, 250; medical, 425, 427–29, 435–37

egg donation, 55

Emerson, Ralph Waldo, xi

emotional health, 23, 119, 284, 211, 232, 249, 284, 362, 363; problems, 83, 221; stress, 129, 157, 284, 293, 299, 337, 340, 342; suffering, 73, 82, 129, 212, 216, 222, 268, 270, 276, 382, 385–86; support, 120, 212, 243, 282–83

emotions, 15, 44, 96, 192, 211, 217–18, 220, 252, 326, 328, 371, 379–80

end-of-life decisions, 58, 77, 270, 290, 292–93, 295–96, 424. *See also* life

endometriosis, 105, 108, 117–18, 121, 147–54, 157–59, 190–91

endometrium, 115–18, 141–45, 156

Edinburgh Postnatal Depression Scale. *See* depression

envy, 5, 13, 229

Escrivá, Josemaría, 351

Eucharist, 9, 71, 76, 78, 88–89, 95, 310–12, 351, 365, 397, 429, 496–98

eugenics, 22, 108n8

euthanasia, 10, 27, 31, 40, 44, 47, 58–59, 62–64, 253, 277–78, 280, 294–96, 298–99, 316, 332, 384, 404, 448

evangelical counsels, 79. *See also* chastity; obedience; poverty evangelization, 78, 81–82, 160, 350, 407–10, 416, 433; of medical students, 420–26, 435–37

Extreme Unction. *See* Anointing of the Sick

eyesight, 6, 10, 125, 156, 264

Ezekiel, Book of the Prophet, 73, 75

face transplantation, 329–43

faith, profession of, 77, 419, 432

family breakdown, 24, 367–68, 373, 377–82

family planning, 107–8, 142, 160–61; efficacy of NFP, 181–86; natural (NFP), 112, 128, 154, 170–73, 186–203; NFP to achieve pregnancy, 188–89; NFP and marriage, 192–93; philosophy of NFP, 172–73. *See also* rhythm method; Teen STAR

fatigue, 133, 267, 361

Fernandez-Carvajal, Francesco, 348n1, 355, 358

fertility: monitoring, 193–95, 201, 203; preserving, 149, 326. *See also* Clearblue Easy Fertility Monitor; monitor

fetus, 122, 124, 126, 129, 131, 133, 197, 456, 458

fibroid, 114–16, 153

FICA tool, 354–55

follicle stimulating hormone (FSH), 109, 113, 140, 150, 154–56, 174–75, 188

food. *See* nutrition.

forgiveness, 7–8, 71, 90, 92, 217–18, 229, 284, 347, 349, 356, 362–63, 365, 367, 383–89, 415, 430; withholding, 211, 363. *See also* Confession; reconciliation

fortitude, 3, 12–14, 23, 25, 100, 210. *See also* courage

Francis, Pope, 81, 86, 98, 131, 202, 368, 377; *Laudato Si'*, 382; World Day of the Sick, 81n29, 86n40, 86n41, 98n95

Francis of Assisi, 43n39, 60, 261, 484, 490

free choice, 13, 386

free will, 14, 44, 50, 320, 323, 348, 351, 457, 472

generosity, 89, 106–7, 170, 173, 229, 271, 386, 418, 439, 449, 460, 473, 488

Genesis, Book of, 4, 38, 39n24, 53, 107, 219, 399

genetic abnormalities, 120

genetic counseling, 120

gluttony, 4–5, 13, 221, 229, 246, 431

Gomez, José H., 350

Good Samaritan, 3, 18–19, 29, 81–82, 87, 317, 398

Good Shepherd, 70–74, 80, 82, 85, 88, 94–95, 100–101

goodness, 3, 32n5, 33–36, 41, 45, 58, 62n90, 64, 66, 86, 210, 320–21, 372, 388, 401, 419–21, 423, 431–32

grace, 11, 270, 355, 479; in dying, 94, 282, 284, 301; from God, 13–14, 62n90, 72, 82, 271, 348, 356, 373, 376, 389, 419, 423, 430, 478, 484, 488–89; from prayer, xiii; from sacraments, 91, 97–100, 310, 351, 397, 430; in suffering, 94, 320, 365

greed, 229

grief, 4, 7–8, 136, 265, 367–68, 376, 380–84, 415, 423

Guardini, Romano, 48n47

Habermas, Jürgen, 57n75, 65

habit, 12–14, 23, 25, 210, 213, 220, 223–24, 228, 239, 244, 350, 355

habit, eating, 118, 221–22

happiness, 11, 35, 37, 45, 108n8, 210, 219, 228, 239, 268, 325–26, 358, 364, 374, 390, 421, 424, 426, 478

headache, 23, 106, 109, 111

health: obligation to preserve, 4, 24, 290, 472; preserving, 3, 4, 5, 22–24, 28, 232, 281, 290, 371; responsibility for, 23, 27; spiritual, 80, 83, 212, 268, 347–48, 350, 358, 383, 499; virtue of preserving, 24

Health Insurance Portability and Accountability Act (HIPAA), 409

hearing, 6, 10, 125, 264, 375

heart disease, 109–10, 127, 244, 276, 296

hedonism, 36

Hezekiah, 7, 396

Hilgers, Thomas W., 114, 155, 180, 188, 190n80

Hippocratic Oath, 22, 469

Hippocratic tradition, 326, 448, 451, 469

history, spiritual, 268, 294, 309–10

holiness, 4, 98–99, 289, 357, 417, 419

Holy Spirit, 52–54, 72, 79, 90, 96n88, 97–100, 161, 284, 351, 401–2, 407, 430, 483, 500

Holy Trinity, 38, 51–54, 70, 262, 372

honesty, 15, 77, 84, 94, 216, 316, 318, 339, 363, 381, 395, 400, 402, 470–71; dishonesty, 39

hospice, 84–85, 261, 263, 267, 289, 300, 425

hospital administration, 75, 79, 327, 489–90

human chorionic gonadotropin (hCG), 121–22, 124, 141, 156–57, 176

human dignity, 10–11, 13, 27, 40–41, 47, 48, 53, 210, 261–62, 266, 276, 321, 360, 389, 399–400, 404, 428, 487

human papilloma virus (HPV), 231–33

humiliation, 98, 237, 357, 479, 488

humility, 15, 25, 79, 218, 229, 256, 358, 477, 495

hydration, 269, 271–73, 277, 289, 296–97, 300, 306–7, 360; withdrawal of, 272, 300. *See also* diet; nutrition

hypertension, 110, 112, 124, 126–28, 158, 341, 346, 350

hypostasis, 42, 53

hysterectomy, 116, 152, 324

Ignatius Loyola, 23, 24n61

image of Christ 350, 368, 431

imago Dei (image of God), 10–11, 38, 54, 275, 320, 372, 396, 400, 426, 453

implantable cardioverter-defibrillator, 290, 297

imprudence, 20, 26, 431

incarnation, 51, 423

infancy, 15, 87, 124, 128, 133–34, 158, 200, 210–16, 222, 250, 253, 284

infertility, 105–6, 112, 119, 121, 146, 148, 151–59, 170, 172, 176, 178, 182, 185, 188, 190–91, 193–94, 199–200, 321n10, 328

information, withholding, 24, 94, 444, 450, 468

insurance, medical, 14, 26, 319, 405, 409, 431

integrity: of the body, 47, 153, 221, 317, 334; of marriage, 105; of the mind, 221, 465; of the person, 40, 364, 439, 449, 457, 463, 465, 471; of the sexual act, 107, 170–71, 173; of the soul, 47, 221; virtue of, 11, 395, 400, 416, 422, 433, 470

intellect, 27, 43–47, 50, 61, 192, 428, 435, 457, 472

intellectual care, 173, 282–83, 450

intellectual formation, xii, 76, 212, 220, 223, 231, 367, 370n13, 429–30

intelligence, 16, 44, 217, 416, 489

intensive care, 288–93, 295, 308, 311–12, 491, 499

intention, 117, 128, 146, 179, 193, 198, 199, 240, 252, 281, 327, 403–4, 418, 425, 442, 470, 488

in vitro fertilization. *See* assisted reproductive technology

Isaiah, Book of, 4, 7–8, 94, 267

isolation, 73, 83, 85, 99, 265, 284, 306, 338

James, the apostle, 71, 90

jealousy, 4

Jesus: compassion of 8, 70, 72–73; passion of Christ, 8, 71–72, 80, 98–99, 267, 310, 498; resurrection of, 8, 17, 71–72, 89, 94, 98, 100, 372, 426; sacrifice, 3, 10, 100

Job, Book of, 4–7, 16, 374–75

John XXIII, Pope, 28, 130n85, 406

John, Gospel of, 8, 9n6, 54, 72, 88, 94, 100, 397, 422, 424, 430n39, 449

John Paul II, Pope, 32n2, 41, 42n33, 47–52, 56n73, 59, 64, 172n5, 172n6, 202–3, 239, 368, 390, 419n11, 432, 452n40, 472n97, 480, 482, 491; on abortion, 384; on catechesis, 435; on conscience, 422; on conscientious objection, 403; on death, 301–2, 335, 455n59; on euthanasia, 332; *Evangelium Vitae,* 34n11, 57n74, 62n90, 62n92, 195–96, 203n116, 294–95, 321, 332, 333n67, 333n69, 335, 368n6, 384n52, 399, 403, 452n40, 471n93, 472n99; *Fides et Ratio,* 36, 57n76, 301; on forgiveness, 384; on freedom, 320–21, 323; on health, 471; on humanism, 367; on human work, 396; Letter to the Elderly, 261–65, 270, 274; on nutrition and hydration, 306–7; on organ transplantation, 333, 335; to pharmacists, 397n9, 408–9; *Redemptor Hominis,* 57–58; on respect for life, 399; on the sacraments, 429–30; *Salvifici Doloris,* 16–19, 40n27, 63, 74, 82, 85n38, 86, 87, 98, 353, 374–76; on science, 422; theology of the body, 32n2, 38–39, 54, 217, 321; *Veritatis Splendor,* 320, 323, 390, 422; on the vocation of medicine, 416, 426; World Day of the Sick, 74, 75, 77, 80, 81n29, 82, 85, 89, 94, 99–100, 471

joy, 4, 17, 23, 85, 95, 99, 107, 210, 216, 374, 421, 424, 426, 430, 482

Judah, 7

justice, 12–14, 18–19, 20, 22, 27, 37, 39, 41, 94, 123, 210, 343, 385, 389, 399, 405–6, 439, 446–47, 449, 460–66, 468, 469–70, 473; God's, 5, 7

Kantian ethics, 13

Kass, Leon, 10, 15, 22–27, 41n29

Kennedy Institute of Ethics, 4, 19–20

kingdom of God, 8–9, 17, 19, 72, 79, 92, 95, 101, 253, 365, 407, 433, 436

Klaus, Hanna, 241n118

Knaus, Hermann, 178–79

Koterski, Joseph, 42n35

Kowalska, Maria Faustina, 357

Kreeft, Peter, 109n1

labor, early induction of, 105, 124–30

laity, 79–80, 82, 101, 415, 417–18

language: of the body, 107, 321; of creation, 321; decent use of, 160, 236; dehumanizing, 453; development in children, 222–23, 372, 459; of healing, 381; impairment, 275, 293, 303, 349, 357–58; in medical practice, 56, 216, 266, 303, 358, 433; sign, 388

laparoscopy, 157–58

Last Rites. *See* Anointing of the Sick

Lawler, Ronald, 196

Leo the Great, 11

Leo XIII, Pope, 11

Lewis, C. S., 93 94n77, 229, 240

libido, 109

life: end of, 34, 53, 100, 265, 267–68, 271, 277, 282, 289, 290, 298, 300–301, 400, 455; gift of, 23–24, 81, 158, 270, 449, 452, 471; interior, 41, 45, 347, 349, 351, 358; preserving, 5, 21, 45, 54, 290, 295, 306, 421, 437, 451; prolongation of, 5, 22, 74, 272, 277–78, 295, 307, 423–24; sacredness of human, 9, 62n90, 130, 262, 294, 399; spiritual, xvi, 41, 45, 100, 351, 430

life-sustaining therapy, withdrawal of, 289, 291, 294, 298–300

liver, 23, 111, 124, 126, 128, 253, 330, 338, 380, 441, 461

living will, 94, 277. *See also* advance directives

Lombard, Peter, 14

love, 12, 29, 43n39, 50, 53–54, 58–64, 66, 83, 105, 209, 288, 346, 348, 372, 377–78, 401, 415, 439; for the elderly, 261–62, 265, 275; of family, 23, 31–32, 50, 59, 61, 81, 211, 213–14, 216–18, 220–21, 224, 233–34, 249–50, 270, 360, 380; of God, 6–7, 13–14, 47, 60, 84, 365, 368, 399, 417, 478, 483–84; God's love, 54, 71–72, 80, 84, 99, 106, 348, 350–51, 368, 380, 399, 416–17, 420, 428, 436, 477, 481–82, 484, 487–88, 490, 498–500; of neighbor, xii–xiii, 3, 13–14, 18–19, 23, 25, 32–34, 50, 60, 63, 66, 71–72, 74–77, 101, 158, 289, 350, 376, 386, 418, 480, 494, 498; for profession, 28; of self, 23; of spouses, 38–39, 50, 107, 153, 172–73, 193, 214, 227, 230–31, 234–35, 239, 242–43, 328, 452; for the suffering, 266, 268, 274, 283, 310, 360, 368, 424, 477, 495–96, 499

Luke, Gospel of, 8, 18, 54, 72, 76, 85, 89, 317, 394, 397–98

lust, 5, 14, 229, 235, 246

luteal phase, 115, 142–44, 154, 156–57, 190, 200–201

luteinizing hormone (LH), 113–14, 140–45, 146, 150, 154, 156–57, 175–77, 184, 187, 190, 198, 201

MacIntyre, Alasdair, 12

Mark, Gospel of, 8–9, 72, 90, 119, 172, 384, 397

maternal mortality, 128

Matthew, Gospel of, 8–9, 19, 71, 72n4, 73, 75, 172, 210, 235, 347, 350, 356–57, 397, 407, 423, 500

May, William E., 196

McHugh, Paul, 320n5, 325–27

means: disproportionate, 21, 253, 272, 280–82, 290, 295, 300, 304, 306, 317; extraordinary, 21, 277, 280–82, 290, 294–95, 317; ordinary, 21, 277, 280–81, 290, 306, 360; proportionate, 21, 253, 280–81, 290, 304, 306. *See also* burden

medical directive. *See* advance directive; living will

medical school, 13, 20, 33, 66, 106, 202, 415–38, 496–98

medical technology, withdrawal of, 281, 290–91, 297–98, 300–301

medication, withdrawal of, 282

medicine: ends of, 15, 22. *See also* profession; vocation

menopause, 115–16, 137, 148, 175, 184, 186–88, 201

menses, withdrawal period, 109, 113

mental health, xii, 135, 211–12, 248–49, 349

mercy, 217; divine, 77, 80, 86, 136, 357, 365, 384, 389, 483, 488, 500; works of, 72, 105, 217, 415–16

metabolic syndrome, 112

metaphysics, 36

minimally conscious, 301, 303–4. *See also* coma; persistent vegetative state

miracles, 9, 72, 161, 417, 441, 479, 480, 482

miscarriage, 87, 120–21, 123, 133, 137, 148, 456, 458. *See also* abortion

mitochondria, 55–56, 454

modesty, 172, 217, 227, 235–36, 238

MOLST. *See* POLST

monitor, electronic hormonal, 177–78, 184–87, 197–98, 200, 203. *See also* Clearblue Easy Fertility Monitor; fertility

mood disorders, 135, 237

Moraczewski, Albert, 9–10, 15n29, 21, 22n53, 25, 28n75, 130n80, 159n210, 290n2, 301n33, 306n51, 307n56, 404n21

moral certainty, 92–93, 333, 335

moral life, 11, 44, 351

myocardial infarction, 110–11, 297, 333

National Commission for the Protection of Human Subjects of Biomedical and Behavioral Research, 330n47, 339n100, 446, 466n87

National Conference of Catholic Bishops. *See* United States Conference of Catholic Bishops

natural family planning (NFP). *See* family planning

nature: human, 5, 22, 27, 275, 320–21, 323, 327, 370–72, 433, 436; rational, 38, 42–44, 46, 48–49, 50–52, 263, 275

negligence, 5, 14, 437

neighbors, 18, 24, 73, 78, 99, 240, 274, 387, 398, 440–41; love of, 13, 19, 23, 33, 289, 418. *See also* love

neonatology, 119, 125–26, 128–29, 134, 491

Neuhaus, Richard John, 58n80, 61n89

New Testament, 8–9, 17–18, 397

Nuremberg Code, 389, 442, 445–47, 449, 462–63

nursing homes, 74, 79, 87, 90, 93, 261

nutrition, 5, 19, 23, 44–45, 73, 89, 106, 113, 115, 149, 152, 221–22, 228, 244, 271–73, 277, 282, 289, 292, 296, 306–7, 336–37, 360, 365, 388, 406, 429; deficiencies in, 23; spiritual food, 88, 95, 311–12; withdrawal of, 272, 300. *See also* diet; hydration; vitamins

obedience, 78–79, 100; to conscience, 10, 401; disobedience, 61, 218, 408; to Magisterium, 496, 498; social, 22; to truth, 34, 422

occupation, 27, 78–79, 279. *See also* profession

Old Testament, 4–8, 16–17, 267, 394, 396

ontology, 35–36, 41, 321

organs: donation, 277, 318, 321, 328, 334–35, 342, 455; transplantation, 300, 330, 333–34, 337, 455, 467n89. *See also* blood

ovaries, 113–15, 121, 140–41, 147–49, 152, 155, 174, 328; ovarian cysts, 105, 114

ovulation, 108, 113, 117, 150, 198; dysfunctional, 115, 145, 153–57, 179; identification of, 154–55, 173–78, 180, 182–83, 185, 187–88, 190, 194, 199, 201; inducing, 114; irregular patterns, 186, 201; painful, 148; postovulation, 128, 142, 175–76, 179, 182, 187, 194, 199–200; prevention of, 109, 111–12, 139–47, 200, 400; superovulation, 158. *See also* anovulation

pacemaker, 289–90, 297–300. *See also* heart disease

pain, chronic, 152, 263, 341, 346, 356–58, 492

palliative care, 84, 265–67, 280, 300, 326, 362

panic, 136

parenting: authoritative, 218–20; responsible, 106–8, 120, 170–71, 203; selfless, 213

parents, duty to, 270–71

Pascal, Blaise, 55

passion, 11, 13, 15, 230, 233, 322, 498

Passover, 9

pastoral care, xv, 70–102, 317, 350, 356

paternalism, 20, 24, 212, 218

patience, 3, 12, 15, 87, 99, 220, 274, 276, 306, 358

Patient Self-determination Act, 276, 278

Paul VI, Pope: on catechesis, 437; on the Catholic faith, 407; on contraception, 190–91; on dying, 95n85, 96–97; on evangelization, 407, 435, 437; on having children, 172–73, 195; *Humanae Vitae*, xv, 107n4, 107n6, 172n7, 173n8, 173n9, 190n78, 195n95, 196n99, 198n103, 202, 327, 364n19; on marriage, 198, 201; on medical profession, 28–29; on NFP, 173, 196, 202; on procreation, 107; on the sexual act, 364; on sterilization, 327

Paul, Saint, 16, 25, 71, 227, 234, 267, 416, 429, 431

peace, 62, 81, 85, 95, 96n88, 97, 99, 193, 199, 233, 240, 280, 282, 297–98, 326, 384, 386, 400, 484

Pellegrino, Edmund, xi, 12, 13n16, 15, 19, 20n49, 24, 25n64, 26, 28n74, 33–34, 63–64, 66, 299–301, 306

pelvic inflammatory disease, 111, 121, 154, 242

Pentecost, 72

perfection, xii, 11, 13–14, 18, 21, 28, 217, 240, 422, 424, 428, 435, 437, 490

perimenopause. *See* menopause

persistent vegetative state, 31, 47, 272, 301–4, 306–7, 359–60. *See also* coma; minimally conscious

Peter, apostle, 17, 72, 94

pharmacists: John Paul II to, 397n9, 408–9; pharmaceutical care, 393–95, 398; pharmaceutical morality, 398, 400; training, 409

pharmaceuticals, 138, 146–47, 404–5; companies, 14, 250, 405, 445, 448, 451, 456, 458; research, 402, 457

philosophy, xi–xii, xv, 3, 12, 46, 49, 50n53, 61, 65–66, 172, 195, 279n51, 299, 367, 369, 373, 398, 421, 491; Greek, 12, 35, 37–44, 49, 52; relationship with theology, 36, 397; role of, 15, 26; terms, xi, 35, 52. *See also* faith; Kantian ethics; reason; utilitarianism; *and specific philosophical terms*

physician-assisted suicide, xi, 10, 22, 27, 31, 58, 62, 296, 298, 332, 400, 404. *See also* suicide

pituitary gland, 109, 140–41, 174, 186

Pius V, 478

Pius XI, Pope, 202, 394, 479–80

Pius XII, Pope, 93n74, 172n7, 202–3, 280, 290, 333–34, 443, 449n29, 471n95, 472n98, 480, 488–89

Plan B, 138, 140–41, 144, 400. *See also* abortion; contraception

Planned Parenthood, 118, 402

Plato, 13, 25, 39n25

politics, 27, 136, 229, 241, 407, 427; political order, 11, 13, 24, 62n90, 138, 469

POLST, 277, 294–96

polycystic ovary syndrome (PCOS), 105, 108, 112–13, 153, 155–56, 190–91, 200

Pontifical Council for Justice and Peace, 45n44

Pontifical Council for Pastoral Assistance to Health Care Workers, 274n40, 278, 281, 323–24, 368, 416n1, 417nn2–3, 418–19, 421, 422n19, 426n25, 432n44, 433, 434nn48–50, 437

Pontifical Council for the Family, 87, 227

Pope Paul VI Institute, 161

pornography, 216–217, 237–38

positivism, 57, 65

postpartum period, 109, 125, 128, 184–86, 199, 201; depression, 211–12

post-traumatic stress disorder (PTSD), 136, 139, 381

poverty, 10, 15, 78–79, 231, 272, 317, 377, 396, 436, 461, 477–78, 482, 496, 498

pregnancy: and ART, 158; cesarean section, 116, 124–25, 128–29, 158; conception, xvii, 35, 112, 123, 126, 129–31, 139, 140–41, 146–47, 153, 158, 172, 181, 188, 190, 199, 377, 380, 399, 432; and contraception, 142, 150; ectopic, 105, 119, 121–24, 131–32, 157; implantation, 109, 111, 117, 129, 139–41, 143–48, 150, 156–57, 175; increasing rates of, 152, 188–89; inducing labor, 105, 119, 124–29; premature delivery, 124–25, 133–34, 137; and rape, 140; after steriliza-

tion reversal, 157–58; unintended, 181–86, 190, 192, 198–201, 241. *See also* maternal mortality

premarital sex, 230–31, 234, 242–44

premenstrual syndrome, 108, 113

Prentice, David, 56n71

pride, 5, 14, 84, 229, 354, 357–58, 361, 488

priests, 70–71, 74–78, 82–84, 87–88, 90–95, 131, 161, 202, 268–69, 288, 307–8, 310–11, 328, 347–51, 355–56, 358, 363, 383–84, 417, 419, 426, 482, 487, 490

principles: of double effect, 21, 122, 125, 128, 198; of extent, 36

principlism, 19, 349. *See also* autonomy; benevolence; justice

privacy, 92, 131, 331, 333, 337, 396, 433, 464–65, 499. *See also* confidentiality

procreation, 38–39, 53, 105–7, 153, 158–59, 170–72, 190, 197–98, 203, 328, 364, 457

profession, 354; of medicine, xvi, 18, 27–29, 82, 417. *See also* occupation; vocation

profit, 4–5, 13, 404–7, 460, 485

progesterone, 108, 113–15, 121–22, 124, 131–33, 137, 140–47, 151–57, 175, 177, 194

progestin, 108–11, 113, 143, 199–200

progestins, synthetic: drospirenone, 109, 111; levonorgestrel (LNG), 109, 111, 117, 138–45, 147; norethindrone, 109, 151

Project Rachel, 136

proselytization, 289, 310, 350, 407, 436

providence, 6, 485

prudence, 12–15, 172, 210, 304, 312, 458. *See also* wisdom

Psalms, Book of, xi, 7, 43, 57, 70, 86, 96, 384, 388, 399

psyche 5, 23, 26, 227, 316, 324. *See also* soul

psychotherapy, 83, 326, 383, 469

Puchalski, Christina, 309, 354, 363n18

purity, 79, 230, 235

PVS. *See* persistent vegetative state

Rachel's Vineyard, 382

rape, 105, 118–19, 129, 138–40, 145–47, 388

rationing of care, 15

Ratzinger, Joseph, 37, 42, 48n47, 52–54, 57n75, 65, 371n16, 374, 472n102. *See also* Benedict XVI

reconciliation, 350–51, 363, 365, 385, 407. *See also* Confession; forgiveness

redemption, 3, 8, 10, 17, 71, 84–85, 89, 98, 100, 261, 267, 348, 353–54, 373

relationships: doctor and patient, 3–4, 15, 18, 29, 33, 118–19, 130, 153, 161, 209, 264, 268, 278, 289, 292–93, 309–10, 317, 355, 394–95, 398, 400, 432, 442, 463–64, 467, 494; with God, 5, 86, 130, 193, 262, 270, 351, 372, 397, 407, 419–20, 427, 429–30; health-care facility and religious ministers, 82; with others, 45, 51–54, 59–60, 86, 172, 195, 214, 225, 237–40, 242, 246, 270, 274–75, 279, 284, 326, 328, 356, 363, 372, 379, 382, 385; parent and child, 210–13, 216, 223–24, 243–44, 271

relativism, xi, 4, 36–37, 40, 220, 239, 323, 401, 421

reproductive health, 106, 119

research: abuse of subject, 439–42, 444–45, 448, 466; patient withdrawing from, 463, 465; researcher withdrawing from, 472

residency, medical, 106, 433

resurrection, 17, 47, 77, 95, 97, 284, 323, 334, 426

revelation, 49, 86, 373, 375, 402, 427–28

rhythm method, 178–79, 181, 191, 200. *See also* family planning

right and wrong, 25, 35, 65, 220, 234

righteousness, 17

rights, xi, xv, 11, 37, 84, 108n8, 120, 123, 130–31, 147, 153, 236, 267, 276, 283, 307, 319, 322, 357, 386, 399, 403, 406, 408, 444–45, 451, 457, 463, 465; to become parents, 153; to food and water, 271–72; to health care, 23, 241; to information, 318, 439, 445; to life, 41, 62n90, 123, 130, 147, 153, 241, 449, 471; to prepare for death, 283; of self-determination, 342, 399, 439, 445. *See also* autonomy; conscientious objection

Rite for Emergencies, 90, 92

Roman Ritual (*Rituale Romanum*), 70–71, 77, 85–86, 93

Romans, Letter to the, 25, 419, 431

Rybak, E. A., 156n191, 158n205, 316–45

Sabbath, 8

sacraments. *See specific sacraments by name*

sacrifice, 5, 15, 28, 80, 158, 220, 224, 229, 235, 239, 317–18, 376, 403, 406, 416–19, 430, 437, 477, 482, 495

salvation, 7, 9, 11, 17, 19, 73, 77, 87, 99, 136, 350, 396, 402, 436, 480, 500

Saunders, Cicely, 261

Scheler, Max, 44n40, 45, 50n53, 51

Schönborn, Christoph, 49

science, empirical, 55, 241, 440

Scripture, xv, 3, 10, 29, 37, 42, 73, 75, 85, 94, 96, 106, 161, 393, 396–99, 401, 429. *See also* Word of God

Seifert, Josef, 41n29, 42n35

seizures, 109, 221

self-giving, 52, 54, 80, 89, 100–101, 107, 323, 418, 424

Sermon on the Mount, 34

servant, 78, 203, 368, 416

sex education, 216, 227, 234–35, 240, 243

sexual abuse. *See* rape

sexual activity, adolescent, 118–19, 230–44. *See also* Teen STAR

sexual intercourse, withdrawal, 172, 182–83, 196

sexual identity, 118, 320–21, 323, 326–28, 368, 377

sexually transmitted disease, 118–19, 139, 230–32, 241–43, 364

Shakespeare, 26, 229

Shivanandan, Mary, 191n85

sin, 6–9, 11, 71, 86, 90, 92, 94, 96, 211, 219, 240, 270, 347, 353, 365, 373, 384, 430; deadly, 5, 16, 229–30, 239, 480; original, 73, 98

Singer, Peter, 37, 40, 58–62, 66

Sirach, Book of, 4–5, 270, 275, 437

sleep, 7, 23, 197, 213, 303, 359–60, 388, 429

sloth, 5, 14, 229, 431

Smith, Janet E., 131

Smith, Wesley J., 63n94, 64n99

smoking, 23, 136–38, 231, 233, 239, 244, 291; nicotine withdrawal, 364. *See also* substance abuse

social justice, 12

social order, 13, 381, 406, 460. *See also* culture

Socrates, 39–42, 62, 224, 231, 242

solitude, 6, 54, 482

somatic cell nuclear transfer, 454, 460. *See also* cloning

soul, 3, 5, 7, 9, 13, 23, 26, 31–32, 39, 43, 44, 45, 56, 62, 71, 91, 92, 93, 96, 98–101, 211–12, 221, 224, 226, 253, 262, 267, 269, 288, 334, 338, 353–55, 357, 360, 375, 377, 380, 388–89, 430, 449, 478, 480–82, 485, 487–89, 496, 500–501; unity with body, 38, 46–48, 105, 212, 282, 284, 301, 316, 321–23, 327, 368, 371, 421–22, 426. *See also* psyche

Stages of Reproductive Aging Workshop (STRAW), 187–88

sterilization, 20–21, 105–6, 111, 116, 146, 150, 157, 160, 181–82, 190, 192, 197–98, 202, 316–17, 320, 326–27, 404. *See also* tubal ligation; vasectomy

STD. *See* sexually transmitted disease

stroke, 109–11, 244, 304, 325, 346, 360

subjectivism, 36, 386

subjectivity, 39

substance, essence or nature, 42–43, 52–53, 337

substance abuse, 118, 134–35, 244, 246, 266, 336, 364, 382. *See also* alcohol; drug abuse; smoking

Suffering Servant, 7–8, 267, 376

suicide, 134–35, 242, 246, 295, 325, 332, 338. *See also* physician-assisted suicide

Sulmasy, Daniel, 268n21, 299–301, 308–9, 401, 404n21

surgery, transgender, 319–29

surrogate, healthcare, 290, 293–94, 296, 299, 304, 306, 317, 450, 459, 471

Synod of Bishops, 80–81, 419n11

Taking Charge of Your Fertility Charting System, 194

Tamoxifen, 197–98

technology: 65, 234, 399, 422, 449; biotechnology, 32, 55, 58, 281, 289, 364, 457, 482, 499; and lower perception of risks, 231–32; progress, 57, 82, 177, 194–95, 400, 448, 493. *See also* assisted reproductive technology; medical technology

Teen STAR, 241

temperance, 12–14, 23, 210, 233, 364–65

temptation, 11, 57, 65, 83, 96–97, 150, 232, 234, 238, 318, 365, 405, 409

Teresa of Calcutta, 59–60, 62n91, 261, 350, 453

Tertullian, 42

testimony, xvi, 422; expert, 159–60; of faith, 79, 82, 350

theology of the body. *See* John Paul II

therapy: constitutive, 300; life-sustaining, 278, 289, 292–94, 299; occupational, 347, 349; physical, 349, 357, 489; speech, 269, 349; substitutive, 300

Thomas Aquinas, xiii, 11, 13–15, 42–44, 347, 405

Thomasma, David, 12, 13n16, 15, 19–20, 24, 25n64, 26n71, 28n74

thought processes. *See* cognition

thrombosis, 108, 110, 128, 491, 493

transcendence, 43–46, 50, 66, 209, 288, 322, 372, 376, 389, 390, 398, 417, 482

transfiguration, 94

transplantation. *See* face transplantation; organs

Travaline, John, 293n9

tubal ligation, 114, 116, 121, 130, 157

tube feeding, 292, 306, 311–12, 330, 360

twins. *See* births, multiple

TwoDay Method, 185, 194

ultrasound, 112–16, 120–21, 123–24, 131, 133, 142–43, 147, 149, 154, 177–78, 194, 497

United Nations Relief and Rehabilitation Administration, 485–86

United States Centers for Disease Control, 133, 232, 242n122, 247n149, 248, 252n175

United States Conference of Catholic Bishops (USCCB): on abortion, 129; on advance directives, 273, 278, 295; on anencephaly, 129n79; on children, 87; on conscience, 307; on contraception, 150, 171, 190, 197; on cooperation, 403; on dying, 84, 87, 267, 281–83; on early induction of labor, 124; on genetic defects, 120; on healthcare institutions, 81–82, 498; on infants, 87; on human dignity, 275, 400–401; on means of preserving life, 21, 280–81; on NFP, 108, 161, 170–71; on nutrition and hydration, 272, 307; on organ transplantation, 318; on pastoral care, 85, 87; on prolonging life, 272; on priests, 76–77; on rape, 139; on research, 470; on Sacrament of the Sick, 91n67; on sacraments for the disabled, 311n70; on scandal, 403; on sterilization, 150, 197; on suffering, 84, 266–67; surgeons and, 317; on unborn child, 122

USCCB, *Ethical and Religious Directives*, 21, 77, 81–82, 84, 85n37, 87, 91, 108n7, 120, 122, 124, 129, 139, 150, 172–71, 190, 197, 266–67, 272–73, 275n44, 278n51, 280–81, 282n59, 283n61, 283n62, 294–95, 307, 316–18, 403, 470n92, 498

United States Food and Drug Administration, 108, 132, 138, 145, 443–45, 447n24

uselessness: feelings of, 99, 357, 488; of technology, 281

utilitarianism, 36–37, 40, 59–60, 65

vaccinations, 440–41, 456, 457n66, 467n89; HPV, 231–33; morally licit and illicit sources, 250–51; refusal of, 251–53. *See also* human papilloma virus

vasectomy, 22

Vatican Council II, 10, 11n12, 39, 40n26, 54, 56, 62n92, 71, 79, 85, 91n67, 99n98, 107n2, 269n25, 306, 322, 367, 390n65, 401, 420, 423n21, 449n28

venous thromboembolism, 110–11, 116, 325

ventilation, mechanical, 277, 289–92, 296–97, 300, 304, 311

Viaticum, 77, 85–87, 93–96, 311

vices, 4–5, 13–14. *See also specific vices by name*

virtue, 3, 4, 9, 10, 11–16, 22, 27–29, 35, 196, 209, 210, 227, 230, 323, 357, 418, 431; intellectual, 14; moral, 12, 22

virtue ethics, 21, 28

virtues, 3, 12, 14–16, 23, 28, 50, 210, 219, 220, 224, 229, 233, 240, 318, 333, 364, 371, 408, 428, 430–31; cardinal, 12, 14–15, 210, 233; natural, 15; self-control, 193, 214–16, 220, 234, 364; selflessness, 213; theological, 12, 14–15. *See also specific virtues by name*

vitamins, 113–14, 117, 151–52, 271. *See also* diet; nutrition

Vitz, Paul, 368–69, 370n12, 373, 375n27, 390

vocation: of the child, 220; Christian, 79, 89, 397; to consecrated religious life, 79; of the family, 80–81; to life, 158; to love, 66, 158; medical, xii, xv, 18, 82, 269, 348, 416–19, 431–33, 435; of the patient, 377; secular, 79–80, 415; of spouses, 239; supernatural, 11, 489. *See also* occupation; profession

von Balthasar, Hans Urs, 371n16, 376

von Hildebrand, Dietrich, 44n39, 51n54

Weigel, George, 51n54

weight gain, 109, 111–13, 150, 244

WHO. *See* World Health Organization

will, 40, 44, 50, 365, 372, 406, 494; free, 14, 44, 320, 323, 348, 351, 457, 472; of God, 45, 87, 351, 401, 417, 419

wisdom, 4–6, 14, 24, 43, 220, 263, 270, 275, 320, 327, 376, 405–6, 429–30, 434, 436. *See also* prudence

Wisdom, Book of, 96

witness: Catholic, xii, xv, xvii, 209, 261, 288–89, 312, 348, 367–68, 393, 410; to Christ, 72, 82, 94, 101; to concern for the weak, 78; of conscience, 431; of consecrated religious, 79; to faith, 32, 65, 80–81, 98, 360, 401, 416, 435–36, 439; to good of life, 81, 368; of hope, 77; to human dignity, 11, 276, 306; of love, 75, 99, 417, 436; of medical practice, 158, 279, 346, 362, 435; in suffering, 17, 99, 279, 354, 361; to truth, 78, 346, 422, 437; to value of old age, 262. *See also* testimony

Wojtyła, Karol, 39n24, 41, 45, 48–50, 51n54, 63n93, 320n7, 321n9, 328n32

Word of God, 16, 43, 73, 90, 101, 332, 401, 417. *See also* Scripture

World Day of the Sick, 82. *See also* Benedict XVI; Francis; John Paul II.

World Health Organization, 110–11, 141, 154, 180, 183–85, 200n105

World Medical Association, 330n46, 331n48, 442n8, 463n85, 464n86

zygote, 55, 141, 158, 452

Catholic Witness in Health Care: Practicing Medicine in Truth and Love was designed in Garamond, with Hypatia display type, and composed by Kachergis Book Design of Pittsboro, North Carolina. It was printed on 60-pound House Natural Smooth and bound by Sheridan Books of Chelsea, Michigan.